S0-BQM-090

Biological Bases and Clinical Implications of Tumor Radioresistance

Biological Bases and Clinical Implications of Tumor Radioresistance

EDITORS

Gilbert H. Fletcher, M.D.
Professor of Radiotherapy
Division of Radiotherapy
The University of Texas System Cancer Center
M.D. Anderson Hospital and Tumor Institute
Houston, Texas

Carlo Nervi, M.D.
Director
Istituto Medico e di Ricerca Scientifica
Rome, Italy

H. Rodney Withers, M.D., Ph.D.
Professor, Radiation Oncology
Head
Section of Experimental Radiation Oncology
University of California, Los Angeles
Los Angeles, California

ASSOCIATE EDITORS

Giorgio Arcangeli, M.D.
Head, Division of Radiation Therapy
Istituto Medico e di Ricerca Scientifica
Rome, Italy

Francesco Mauro, D.Sc.
Senior Scientist
Laboratorio di Dosimetria e Bofisica
Comitato Nazionale per l'Energia Nucleare
Rome, Italy

Norah duV. Tapley, M.D.
Professor of Radiotherapy
The University of Texas System Cancer Center
M.D. Anderson Hospital and Tumor Institute
Houston, Texas

MASSON Publishing USA, Inc.
New York • Paris • Barcelona • Milan • Mexico City • Rio de Janeiro

Proceedings of the second Rome International Symposium September 21-24, 1980, Rome, Italy

Library of Congress Cataloging in Publication Data
Main entry under title:

Biological bases and clinical implications of tumor radioresistance.

"Proceedings of the 2nd Rome International Symposium, September 21-24, 1980, Rome, Italy—T.p. verso.
Bibliography: p.
Includes index.
1. Cancer–Radiotherapy–Congresses. 2. Radiobiology–Congresses. I. Fletcher, Gilbert Hungerford, 1911- . II. Nervi, Carlo. III. Withers, H. Rodney. IV. Title: Tumor radioresistance.
[DNLM: 1. Neoplasms–Radiotherapy–Congresses. 2. Radiation tolerance–Congresses. W3 RO683D 1980b / QZ 269 R763 1980b]
RC271.R3B56 1983 616.99′40642 82-14819
ISBN 0-89352-179-5

ISBN O-89352-179-5

Library of Congress Catalog Card Number: 82-14819

Printed in the United States of America

FOREWORD

Since the Symposium on "Biological and Clinical Basis of Radiosensitivity" held in Rome in 1971 under the chairmanship of M. Friedman, advances have been made in all the facets of the basic sciences and the clinical knowledge underlying the therapeutic strategies in treatment of human cancers. In addition, a close relationship between the clinical data observed and the basic parameters of radiobiology has been established.

The keynote of the second conference held in 1980 on "Biological Bases and Clinical Implications of Tumor Radioresistance" is the updating of this body of knowledge and its potential implications. The Program Committee, M. M. Elkind, G. H. Fletcher, J. F. Fowler, S. Kramer, C. Nervi, and H. R. Withers, has chosen topics on radioresistance progressing from the cellular level to the level of individual human tumors. The limitations of normal tissue tolerance and attempts to improve the therapeutic ratio by manipulation of the time factor are also covered. Before discussing ways by which results of radiotherapy might be improved by combination with drugs, hypoxic cell sensitizers, or radioprotectors, the present state of that art has been reviewed, giving the results of conventional irradiation and describing some of the ways of maximizing the effectiveness of existing means of treatment including the combination of irradiation and surgery. Finally, the essayists addressed themselves to the problem of clinical trials.

THE EDITORS

CONTRIBUTORS

Gerald E. Adams, Ph.D., D.Sc., Professor of Physics as Applied to Medicine, Institute of Cancer Research, Sutton, Surrey, England

Giorgi Arcangeli, M.D., Head, Division of Radiation Therapy, Istituto Medico e di Ricerca Scientifica, 00191 Rome, Italy

Gerit W. Barendsen, Ph.D., Radiobiological Institute of the Organization for Health Research TNO, 2280 HV Rijswijk, and Laboratory for Radiobiology, University of Amsterdam, 1066 CX Amsterdam, The Netherlands

H. Thomas Barkley, M.D., Associate Radiotherapist and Associate Professor of Radiotherapy, Department of Radiotherapy, The University of Texas System Cancer Center, M.D. Anderson Hospital and Tumor Institute, Houston, Texas 77030

James A. Belli, M.D., Professor of Radiation Therapy, Harvard Medical School, Boston, Massachusetts 02115

Joseph R. Bertino, M.D., American Cancer Society Professor of Medicine and Pharmacology, Departments of Medicine and Pharmacology, Yale University School of Medicine, New Haven, Connecticut 06518

Giovanni Briganti, D.Sc., Director, Laboratorio di Dosimetria Biofiscia, Comitato Nazionale per L'Energia Nucleare, 00060 Rome, Italy

Steven E. Bush, M.D., Chief, Radiation Oncology, Cancer Research and Treatment Center, Principal Investigator of the Pion Project, University of New Mexico, and Assistant Professor of Radiology, University of New Mexico School of Medicine, Albuquerque, New Mexico 87131

John D. Chapman, M.Sc., Ph.D., Director of Radiobiology, Cross Cancer Institute, and Professor of Radiology, University of Alberta, Edmonton, Alberta, Canada T 661Z2

Claire Clarke, Ph.D., Scientific Assistant, Institute of Cancer Research, Sutton, Surrey, England

Kentish B. Dawson, Ph.D., Senior Scientist, Institute of Cancer Research, Sutton, Surrey, England

Juliana Denekamp, B.Sc., Ph.D., D.Sc., Cancer Research Campaign, Gray Laboratory, Mount Vernon Hospital, Northwood, Middlesex HA6 2RN, England

Maurizio D'Incalci, M.D., Research Associate, Instituto di Ricerche Farmacologiche Mario Negri Via Eritrea, 62–20157 Milan, Italy

Stanley Dische, M.D., F.R.C.R., Marie Curie Research Wing for Oncology, Regional Radiotherapy Center, Mount Vernon Hospital, Northwood, Middlesex HA6 2RN, England

J. Dutreix, M.D., Institut Gustave-Roussy, 94805 Villejuif Cedex, France, and Professor, Université Paris-Sud

Mortimer M. Elkind, B.M.E., M.M.E., M.S., Ph.D., Senior Biophysicist, Division of Biological and Medical Research, Argonne National Laboratory, Argonne, Illinois 60439, and Professor, Department of Radiology, The University of Chicago, Chicago, Illinois 60637

Stanley B. Field, B.Sc., Ph.D., Head, Department of Biology, Medical Research Council, Cyclotron Unit, Hammersmith Hospital, London W12 OHS, England

Gilbert H. Fletcher, M.D., Professor of Radiotherapy, Division of Radiotherapy, The University of Texas System Cancer Center, M.D. Anderson Hospital and Tumor Institute, Houston, Texas 77030

Jack F. Fowler, D.Sc., Ph.D., M.Sc., F. Inst. P, Gray Laboratory of the Cancer Research Campaign, Mount Vernon Hospital, Northwood, Middlesex HA6 2RN, England

Allan J. Franko, M.Sc., Ph.D., Research Radiobiologist, Cross Cancer Institute, and Assistant Professor of Radiology, University of Alberta, Edmonton, Alberta, Canada T66 1Z2

W. Göhde, Ph.D., Radiologische Klinik der Universität Münster, Münster, West Germany

Graham Grundy, R.T.T., Data Coordinator, Radiation Oncology Study Center, Philadelphia, Pennsylvania

L.R. Holsti, Department of Radiotherapy and Oncology, University Central Hospital, Helsinki 29, Finland

Shirley Hornsey, D.Sc., F.I. Biol., Medical Research Council, Cyclotron Unit, Hammersmith Hospital, London W12 OHS, England

Neil Howell, Ph.D., Assistant Professor of Radiation Therapy, Harvard Medical School, Boston, Massachusetts 02115

David H. Hussey, M.D., Radiotherapist and Professor of Radiotherapy, Division of Radiotherapy, The University of Texas System Cancer Center, M.D. Anderson Hospital and Tumor Institute, Houston, Texas 77030

Robert F. Kallman, Ph.D., Department of Radiology, Stanford University School of Medicine, Stanford, California 94305

Henry Keys, M.D., Assistant Professor, Department of Radiation Oncology, University of Rochester Cancer Center, Rochester, New York 14642

Morton M. Kligerman, M.D., Professor, Department of Radiation Therapy, University of Pennsylvania School of Medicine, and Staff, Department of Radiation Therapy, Hospital of the University of Pennsylvania, Philadelphia, Pennsylvania

Cameron J. Koch, M.Sc., Ph.D., Research Radiobiologist, Cross Cancer Institute, and Assistant Professor of Radiology, University of Alberta, Edmonton, Alberta, Canada

Makoto Kondo, M.D., Visiting Radiotherapist, The University of New Mexico Cancer Research and Treatment Center, Albuquerque, New Mexico 87131

Simon Kramer, M.D., Professor and Chairman, Department of Radiation Therapy and Nuclear Medicine, Thomas Jefferson University Hospital, Philadelphia, Pennsylvania 19107

John B. Little, M.D., Professor of Radiobiology, Harvard School of Public Health, Boston, Massachusetts 02115

Robert Lustig, M.D., Department of Radiation Therapy, Cooper Medical Center, Camden, New Jersey, and, Assistant Professor, Department of Radiation Therapy and Nuclear Medicine, Thomas Jefferson University Hospital, Philadelphia, Pennsylvania 19107

Moshe H. Maor, M.D., Assistant Radiotherapist and Assistant Professor of Radiotherapy, Division of Radiotherapy, The University of Texas System Cancer Center, M.D. Anderson Hospital and Tumor Institute, Houston, Texas 77030

Francesco Mauro, D.Sc., Senior Scientist, Laboratorio di Dosimetria e Biofiscia, Comitato Nazionale per l'Energia Nucleare, 00060 Rome, Italy

Adam Michalowski, Doc.Dr. Hab.Med., Department of Biology, Medical Research Council, Cyclotron Unit, Hammersmith Hospital, London W12 OHS

David Moylan, M.D., Department of Radiation Therapy and Nuclear Medicine, Thomas Jefferson University Hospital Philadelphia, Pennsylvania 19107

Carlo Nervi, M.D., Director, Instituto Medico e di Ricerca Scientifica, 00191 Rome, Italy

Gustaf Notter, M.D., Department of Radiotherapy, University of Göteborg, Sahlgrenska Hospital, S-413 45 Göteborg, Sweden

F. Otto, Ph.D., Fraunhofer-Institut für Toxikologie und Aerosolforshung, Schmallenberg, West Germany

Jens Overgaard, M.D., The Institute of Cancer Research, Radiumstationen, Nörrebrogade 44 DK-8000 Aarhus C., Denmark

M. Chiara Pardini, D.Sc., Ph.D., Research Associate, Instituto Medico e di Ricerca Scientifico, and Comitato Nazionale per L'Energia Nucleare, Rome, Italy

Lester J. Peters, M.D., Professor and Head, Division of Radiotherapy, The University of Texas System Cancer Center, M.D. Anderson Hospital and Tumor Institute, Houston, Texas 77030

Colin Poulter, M.D., Associate Professor, Department of Radiation Oncology, University of Rochester Cancer Center, Rochester, New York 14642

W.E. Powers, M.D., Professor and Chairman, Department of Radiation Oncology, Wayne State University, Detroit, Michigan

Marcello Quintiliani, M.D., Senior Investigator, Instituto di Tecnologie Biomediche, Consiglio Nazionale de le Ricerche, 00161 Rome, Italy

Philip Rubin, M.D., Professor and Chairman, Department of Radiation Oncology, University of Rochester Cancer Center, Rochester, New York 14642

M. Salmo, Department of Radiotherapy and Oncology, University Central Hospital, Helsinki 29, Finland

E. Schnepper, M.D., Radiologische Klinik der Universität Münster, Münster, West Germany

J. Schumann, Ph.D., Fachklinik Hornheide, Universität Münster, Münster, West Germany

Peter W. Sheldon, Ph.D., Scientific Assistant, Institute of Cancer Research, Sutton, Surrey, England

Alfred R. Smith, Ph.D., Associate Professor, The University of New Mexico Cancer Research and Treatment Center, Albuquerque, New Mexico 87131

Ian J. Stratford, Ph.D., Scientific Assistant, Institute of Cancer Research, Sutton, Surrey, England

Herman D. Suit, M.D., D. Phil., Andres Soriano Director of Cancer Management, Edwin L. Steele Laboratory of Radiation Biology, Department of Radiation Medicine, Massachusetts General Hospital, Harvard Medical School, Boston, Massachusetts 02114

N. duV Tapley, M.D.*, Professor of Radiotherapy, The University of Texas System Cancer Center, M.D. Anderson Hospital and Tumor Institute, Houston, Texas 77030

Howard D. Thames, Jr., Ph.D., Associate Professor, Biomathematics, University of Texas, M.D. Anderson Hospital and Tumor Institute, Houston, Texas 77030

Klaus Rüdiger Trott, Strahlenbiologisches Institut der Universität München and Abteilung für Strahlenbiologie der GSF Neuherberg, West Germany

Maurice Tubiana, M.D., Institut Gustave-Roussy 94800 Villejuif, France

Ingela Turesson, M.D., Department of Radiotherapy, University of Göteborg, Sahlgrenska Hospital, S-413 45 Göteborg, Sweden

A. Wambersie, M.D., Cliniques Universitaires St. Luc, Brussels, and Professor, Université Catholique, Louvain, Belgium

---

*deceased

Ralph R. Weichselbaum, M.D., Associated Professor, Radiation Therapy Department, Harvard Medical School, and Head, Peter Bent Brigham Division, Joint Center, Radiation Therapy Department, Boston, Massachusetts 02115

Stephany Wilson, B.A., Administrator, The University of New Mexico Cancer Research and Treatment Center, Albuquerque, New Mexico 87131

H. Rodney Withers, M.D., Ph.D., Professor, Radiation Oncology, University of California, Los Angeles, California 90024

John M. Yuhas, Ph.D., Professor of Radiation Therapy, Department of Radiation Therapy, University of Pennsylvania, and Children's Cancer Research Center, Children's Hospital of Philadelphia, Pennsylvania 19104

Melvin Zelen, Ph.D., Professor of Statistical Science, Harvard School of Public Health, and Sidney Farber Cancer Institute, Boston, Massachusetts 02115

Contents

CHAPTER 1

Keynote Address: The Problem: Tumor Radioresistance in Clinical Radiotherapy

Lester J. Peters, M.D.[a]
H. Rodney Withers, M.D., Ph.D.[b]
Howard D. Thames, Jr., Ph.D.[c]
Gilbert H. Fletcher, M.D.[a]

Definition

The term "radioresistance" and its converse "radiosensitivity" are simple enough words, but their meanings vary according to the context in which they are used. Historically, tumors were regarded as radiosensitive if they responded rapidly to modest doses of ionizing radiation, while radioresistant tumors showed little or no apparent response even to maximum tolerable doses. Between these two extremes, varying grades of radiosensitivity (more precisely radioresponsiveness) were also recognised. This concept of the terminology, which is still prevalent in the minds of most nonradiotherapists, is well exemplified by Paterson's [15] classification of tumor "species" into the radiosensitive (e.g., lymphomas and seminomas), those of limited radiosensitivity (e.g., the squamous and adenocarcinomas), and the radioresistant (e.g., the sarcomas and melanoma).

[a]Division of Radiotherapy, The University of Texas System Cancer Center, M.D. Anderson Hospital and Tumor Institute, Houston, Texas

[b]Department of Radiation Oncology, University of California, Los Angeles Center for Health Sciences, Los Angeles, Calif.

[c]Department of Biomathematics, The University of Texas System Cancer Center, M.D. Anderson Hospital and Tumor Institute, Houston, Texas

Better understanding of radiation and tumor biology, however, has shown that the rate of response of a neoplasm to irradiation does not necessarily parallel its cellular radiosensitivity. This is because "response" (or volume change following irradiation) depends not only on the number of cells killed, but also on tumor proliferation kinetics, the architecture of the tumor, the mode of cell death, and the efficiency of clearance of dead cells from the tumor mass. Thus, it is not possible to estimate, purely on the basis of volume regression, whether a particular regimen of treatment is more or less effective than another—a fact of considerable importance in the common practice of using "partial response" as an index of therapeutic effectiveness of drugs.

The relationship between the initial volume response of a tumor to a course of fractionated irradiation and its ultimate radiocurability is complex.[7] Clinical data from the M.D. Anderson Hospital suggest that for head and neck tumors, a good initial response carries an improved prognosis, provided the therapist is not lulled into reducing the planned tumor dose. However, there is no doubt that prompt initial regression is not a prerequisite for cure (e.g., in prostatic cancer); in the final analysis the rate of regression of a tumor following irradiation is of much less consequence than whether it is ultimately controlled. Indeed, complete regression may never occur in some "cured" tumors (e.g., chondrosarcomas).

For the purpose of this essay, we suggest the following operational definition of tumor radioresistance: A tumor is clinically radioresistant if it regrows within the irradiated region, regardless of its rate of regression. Since the maximum dose of radiation that can be safely delivered is an inverse function of the treatment volume, it follows that, by this definition, clinical radioresistance is a relative term–the same tumor being relatively more resistant when large treatment volumes are required.

The Problem

The overall magnitude of the radiotherapeutic problem of failure to control local–regional disease is site specific and impossible to quantitate accurately.[19] In general, published clinical results tend to underestimate its absolute frequency because they are usually presented as the crude ratio of recurrences to patients treated, without taking into account deaths from metastatic disease or unrelated causes. Furthermore, reported results from centers of excellence are presumably better than community averages, and there would seem little doubt that a major improvement in radiotherapy results could be achieved simply by more widespread use of refined conventional techniques.

The impact of tumor radioresistance on patient survival depends on the type of cancer in question and the existing level of local–regional disease control. Local control is axiomatically a prerequisite for cure. However, as the efficiency of local treatment increases, the proportion of patients cured for their disease asymptomatically approaches the limit set by the frequency of preexisting metastases. This is true even in sites where uncontrolled local disease is the most common immediate cause of death. For example, of 916 patients with stage 1B-111B carcinoma of the uterine cervix treated at M.D. Anderson Hospital in the years 1964 to 1969, only 46 were documented to have died of pelvic recurrence in the ensuing five years, without concomitant evidence of disseminated disease.[11] The cause of death was not established in 52 other patients, but even if all 52 are assumed to be in this category, the total failure rate in the pelvis only would not exceed 98/916 or 11%. Although it is possible that in some patients metastases were seeded from their recurrences, kinetic considerations make this less plausible than the hypothesis that large and/or biologically aggressive tumors often have the common attributes of radioresistance and an increased likelihood to have metastasized. In such circumstances, the potential for improvement in overall cure rates through better local treatment is quite limited, as exemplified by the preliminary neutron therapy trial results from TAMVEC which showed improved local control, but no survival advantage for patients treated in part with fast neutrons.[16]

Accepting the fact that in certain sites better local disease control *per se* would not dramatically alter cure rates, the quality of life of patients whose primary tumor is successfully treated is undoubtedly improved; and as the efficiency of treatment of disseminated disease increases, local disease control will become more vital in terms of absolute cure. Perhaps of more immediate relevance is that effective methods of reducing tumor radioresistance would permit existing control rates to be achieved at a lower biological cost in terms of the morbidity and complications of treatment, as well as allowing tumors currently considered unsuitable for radiotherapy due to their extent, proximity to, or involvement of vulnerable normal tissues to be successfully treated.

Causes of Clinical Radioresistance

There are many reasons why a tumor may be clinically radioresistant. These will be considered under four headings:

1. Tumor-related factors
2. Host-related factors
3. Technical factors
4. Probabilistic radioresistance

TUMOR-RELATED FACTORS

Number of Clonogenic Cells

The concept of the clonogenic tumor cell derives from experimental assays of cellular reproductive integrity.[6] A clonogenic cell is defined as one which is capable of regenerating the tumor; as such it must either belong to the stem cell compartment or be able to be recruited back into the pool.[12] Since the killing of cells by irradiation is a random phenomenon, tumors with a large number of clonogenic cells will be more difficult to eradicate than those with fewer clonogens of similar sensitivity to irradiation. In practice it is not possible to quantitate the number of clonogens in human tumors, although estimates can be made. For example, in the case of human skin cancers, calculations based on reasonable radiobiological assumptions [Do (for euoxic cells) = 120 to 140, n = 2 to 5], measured values of single dose TCD_{50} of around 1800 rad for tumors of 1 cm^3 volume,[22] and a cell density of $10^6/mm^3$ lead to an estimate of only 1 in 10^3 to 10^4 cells being clonogenic–assuming none to be hypoxic. If this assumption is untrue, the proportion of clonogens would be even lower. Since there is no direct assay for clonogenic cells in human tumors, one cannot predict radioresistance based upon a large number of clonogens. However, the concept involved is exploited in treatment strategies using combinations of surgery and irradiation, or shrinking-field and boost techniques of radiotherapy.[8]

Hypoxia

Hypoxia is the most well-known and clinically quoted cause of tumor radioresistance. All experimental solid tumors contain hypoxic clonogenic cells; and although the proportion varies with tumor type, size, and site of growth, there is overwhelming circumstantial evidence that they exist in most human neoplasms as well.[24] It can be reasonably assumed that when human cancers are controlled by irradiation, the process of reoxygenation during therapy has circumvented the radioresistance of hypoxic cells. What is not established, however, is how frequently treatment failure is ascribable to failure of reoxygenation rather than to one of the many other possible causes. Nonetheless, overcoming tumor-cell hypoxia has been, and continues to be, the rationale upon which most attempts to decrease clinical radioresistance are based.[9]

Tumor Kinetics

Kinetic considerations can account for clinical radioresistance in two ways: (1) rapidly growing tumors may repopulate significantly during a conventional course of treatment, and (2) tumors with slow turnover times may be radioresistant by virtue of poor cellular redistribution in the division cycle between dose fractions.

Clinical support for first cause of radioresistance was provided by Norin *et al.*[14] who achieved far superior control rates in Burkitt's lymphoma when short overall time-treatment fractionation schedules of three times per day were used, rather than with regular daily treatment. Likewise, the results of treatment of inflammatory breast cancer at M.D. Anderson Hospital with accelerated twice-daily fractionation schedules are appreciably better than with the protracted Baclesse technique formerly used.[2] Even tumors that are not rapidly growing may regenerate rapidly following irradiation. Since such a regenerative response cannot at present be predicted, it is a safe policy to avoid excessively protracted or split course regimens.[8]

Clinical evidence of failure of redistribution as a possible cause of tumor recurrence has not been directly adduced. For example,

Dixon *et al.*[5] were unable to correlate pretreatment labelling indices in biopsies with the therapeutic outcome in a series of cancers of the uterine cervix. However, it is hard to dismiss this possible cause of radioresistance since, with fractional doses of 200 rad, aerobic cells synchronised in the most resistant phase of the cell cycle may be more radioresistant than hypoxic cells in the more sensitive phases.[18] Where such a cause of radioresistance is suspected (e.g., in tumors with slow cell turnover), it would be logical to expect a therapeutic gain through the use of high LET radiations.[23] This is supported by clinical data of Breuer.[3]

Intrinsic Radioresistance

By "intrinsic" we mean cellular radioresistance manifested by asynchronous, well-oxygenated populations of tumor cells cultured *in vitro*. Two types of such resistance have been demonstrated—one associated with an apparent increased capacity for "Elkind-type" repair and the other with an increased ability to repair potentially lethal damage. The first type of resistance, manifested by a large shoulder on the radiation cell-survival curve, has been promulgated as a reason for the clinical radioresistance to conventional dose fractions of some human malignant melanomata.[10] This argument has been supported by an analysis of human data showing an increased response rate to irradiation when the incremental fraction size is large ($\geq$600 rad). However, it is important to note that in order for large fractional doses to yield better clinical results than multiple small doses, the initial slope of the survival curve for tumor cells must be shallower, and its shoulder broader, than for the curve for dose-limiting normal tissue cells. When both these conditions exist there can never be a positive therapeutic ratio for treatment by irradiation whatever fractionation scheme is employed; use of large dose fractions or high LET radiations within the reduced total dose limit imposed by late normal tissue tolerance will simply minimize the therapeutic disadvantage.

In contradistinction to the finding of a large shoulder on the survival curve of some melanoma cell lines, Weichselbaum *et al.*[21] reported "conventional" basic survival curve parameters for a range of cultured human tumor cells. Significantly, however, these workers correlated an increased ability to repair potentially lethal damage by plateau phase cultures with clinical radioresistance, and it seems likely that this could be an important cause of treatment failure—also theoretically amenable to high LET radiations.

Reseeding of Irradiated Sites

It is biologically conceivable to sterilize a tumor within the irradiated volume, only to have the area reseeded from a distant tumor focus. Experimentally, it has been well documented that irradiated tissues have a transiently increased ability to support tumor growth; and it is possible that recurrences demarcated by the irradiation portals, which are occasionally seen clinically, could represent this phenomenon.

New Primary Tumor

An apparent cause of clinical radioresistance is the development of a new primary lesion. Second primaries are common in many sites, and it can be impossible clinically to resolve a marginal recurrence from a new tumor.

HOST-RELATED FACTORS

The "Volume Effect"

It has been well understood from the earliest days of radiation therapy that the severity of radiation skin reactions is markedly dependent on the area of the treatment fields. While with megavoltage therapy skin reactions are rarely dose limiting, the frequency of complications in deep-seated tissues and organs is likewise dependent on the volume irradiated, to an extent that is not readily explicable in terms of cellular radiobiology. Thus, when large treatment volumes are required to encompass known or suspected disease, the clinical radioresistance of a tumor increases.

Dose-limiting Normal Tissues

The total biological dose of radiation that can be given to a tumor varies according to the dose-limiting critical organ or tissue in the irradiated volume. Thus, a given tumor may be clinically more radioresistant in one site than in another, depending on the relevant critical normal tissue. This has implications in the treatment of widespread disease, e.g., ovarian carcinoma seeding the peritoneal cavity, where a suboptimal dose must be accepted in part of the treatment volume overlying the kidneys because of local organ sensitivity.

Pathophysiological Factors

Pathophysiological factors may affect tumor radioresistance directly, e.g., by increasing the hypoxic fraction of cells in conditions of anemia[4] or hypoxemia of other causes. In addition, various disease states or old age may prejudice the healing of irradiated normal tissues and so impose a dose limitation which results in apparent tumor radioresistance.

Host Defenses

Attempts to exploit specific or nonspecific immunologically based host defenses in the treatment of human cancer have been almost uniformly unrewarding.[1] Patients rarely manifest evidence of immunological incompetence at the time of their initial treatment; and while some contribution to tumor control by host mechanisms cannot be excluded, it seems unlikely that deficiencies in natural defenses contribute materially to the clinical problem of radioresistance.

TECHNICAL FACTORS

Geographic Miss

By far the most important technical consideration impinging on radioresistance is the necessity to encompass the entire tumor in the treatment volume. Simple calculations show that even a minute geographic miss of say 1 mm^3 in a 5-cm diameter mass limits the surviving fraction of cells to about 1.5×10^5, regardless of the total radiation dose given. It should be emphasized that no matter how sophisticated the beam direction devices used, a geographic miss will guarantee failure, and this possibility is higher when small volume "precision" techniques are used than when shrinking-field methods are employed.

Errors in Dose Delivery

With fractionated treatments extending over many weeks, the possibility of errors in setup is considerable. For example, Kartha *et al.*[13] found by computer monitoring of the parameters of daily treatment that the overall incidence of major accidental errors in field size ($\geq$ 1 cm), gantry angle ($\geq 15^{\circ}$), collimator rotation, ($\geq 10^{\circ}$), or treatment time ($\geq$ 0.5 min) was 3%, and that two-thirds of the patients monitored had at least one major error at some stage during the full course of treatment. Such errors, if not promptly recognized and corrected, could well be the cause of apparent radioresistance.

Machine calibration and dose calculation errors are also disturbingly frequent. Shalek et al.,[17] in a survey of 352 machines at 174 institutions in the United States, found that 77 (22%) had net calibration errors in excess of ± 3% due to errors in one or more of the following categories: chamber correction factor, timer error, field size dependence, source movement mechanism, anomalous source decay, distance indicator, light and radiation beam coincidence, or beam symmetry. Of 768 treatment protocols reviewed, the specified tumor dose was given to within ± 5% in only 88% of the sample, with an extreme range of −56 to +24%. Errors of this magnitude could very easily create the illusion of clinical tumor radioresistance or excessive normal tissue reactions in a given treatment regimen.

PROBABILISTIC RADIORESISTANCE

By definition, tumor cure requires that no clonogenic cells survive to regrow the tumor. Since the killing of tumor cells by irradiation is random, it follows that, for any given tumor, one can define only a probability of control based on the average number of clonogens expected to survive the treatment given, and that no "tumoricidal" dose can be specified. For a completely homogeneous group of tumors exposed to graded doses of irradiation the tumor control probability (TCP) curve is determined by Poisson statistics and is steep over its midrange, increasing from ~10 to ~90% with a dose increment of three times the "effective" D_0 for the tumor cells in question. For daily 200 rad fractionated irradiation of typical well-oxygenated mammalian cells, this dose increment would be expected to be of the order of 1000 to 1500 rad. In practice however, human tumor TCP curves are always flatter than this, and in certain sites no dose response can be defined at all for the overall tumor population (Fig. 1). What this implies is that the populations are heterogeneous with respect to individual tumor characteristics, and that subpopulations of the group of tumors being studied vary in their "radioresistance."

In principle, such differences could result from different causes of radioresistance or from differences in degree of the same cause, particularly clonogen number. The effect in both cases is to flatten the tumor-control probability curve, and to diminish the likelihood of demonstrating an improvement in clinical results with new treatment strategies. For illustrative purposes, we have modelled some hypothetical clinical situations.

First, consider a population of tumors, each of which contains 10^8 clonogenic cells subdivided into four subsets. The first baseline subpopulation which would be clinically "radiosensitive" has a 5% hypoxic fraction which is maintained throughout a fractionated course or irradiation. The tumor cells are moderately radiosensitive and redistribute efficiently so that the surviving fraction in the euoxic compartment after each 200-rad dose fraction is 50%. The tumor-volume doubling time is 70 days with a growth fraction of 20%. The OER at doses of 200 rad is assumed to be 2.5. The second population is rapidly growing, with a growth fraction of 40% and a volume doubling time of 14 days, and is thus more resistant because of repopulation during treatment. Subpopulation three is radioresistant because of inefficient reoxygenation which causes the hypoxic fraction to increase from 5 to 35%, at which level it is subsequently maintained. Finally, the fourth subpopulation is radioresistant because of "intrinsic" cellular radioresistance which results in the net surviving fraction per 200 rad increasing from 50 to 60%. TCP curves pertaining to these four subpopulations are shown in Figure 2 along with overall TCP curve for the whole population, assuming the four subpopulations to be equal in size. (The method of computation of the TCP curves is set out in the appendix.) Figure 2 also depicts the results which would be expected in such a heterogeneous population if treatment were given in conjunction with a radiosensitizer which reduced the OER from 2.5 to 1.5.

The results would not be spectacular, and it is of interest to note the conditions under which such changes would be clinically detectable. Suppose that patients from the heterogeneous group were randomly assigned in equal numbers to two treatment arms—one with and one without the radio-

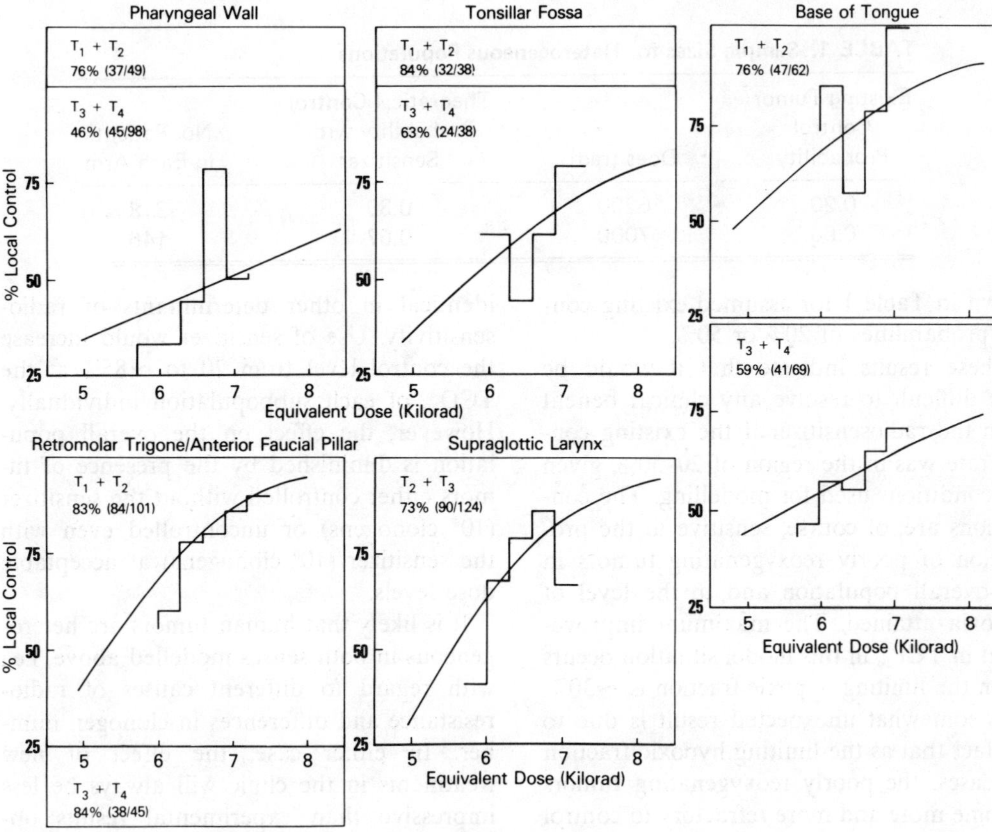

Figure 1. Dose-response relationships for six different populations of human squamous cell carcinomas treated at M.D. Anderson Hospital. Doses were normalised to a '6-week equivalent' dose when different fractionation schemes were used. The curved lines indicate the best fit obtained by computer analysis of the data using Poisson or logistic regression models, while the histograms show the actual proportion of tumors controlled in each 300-rad dose increment. The slopes of the dose-response curves give an indication of the degree of heterogeneity in each tumor population–the shallower the slope, the greater the heterogeneity. The data for T_2 and T_3 tumors of the supraglottic larynx show the steepest dose-response relationship of all the sites analysed, but even for these tumors, the derived "effective D_o" is 2–3 times greater than would be expected for a completely homogeneous tumor population. (Reproduced with permission, *Brit J Cancer*)[20]

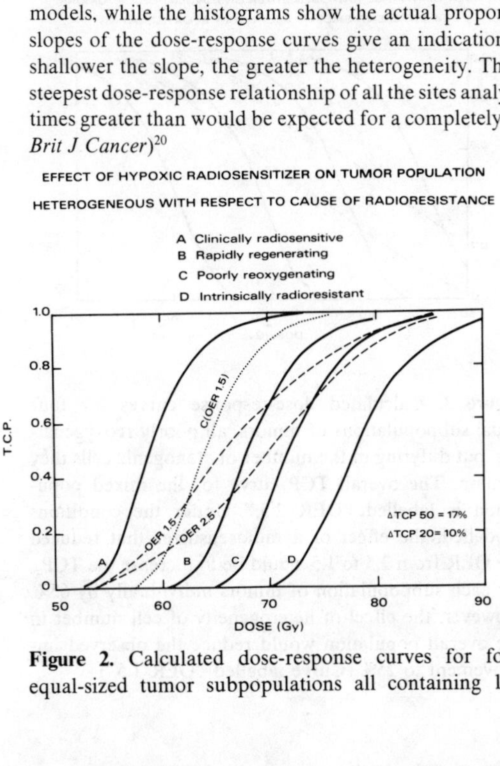

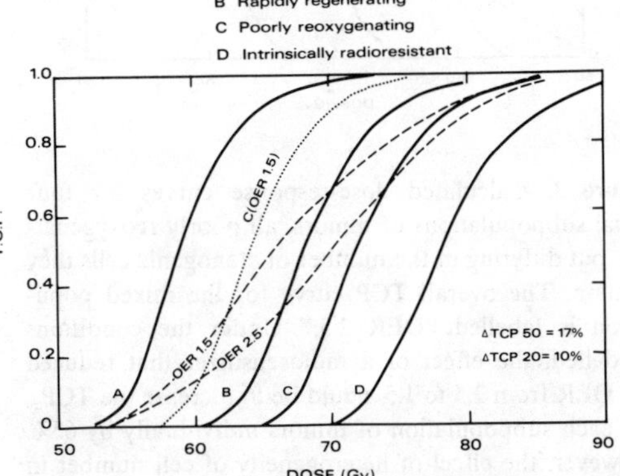

Figure 2. Calculated dose-response curves for four equal-sized tumor subpopulations all containing 10^8 clonogenic cells, but heterogeneous with respect to their cause of "radioresistance." (See text for the parameters used in the calculations.) The dashed line labelled "OER 2.5" is the overall TCP curve for the population as a whole. The use of an hypoxic cell sensitizer would affect only subpopulation C, displacing its TCP curve to the left [curve labelled "C" (OER 1.5)] while the effect on the overall population would be modest, as shown by the dashed line labelled "OER 1.5."

sensitizer–and that each group was treated to the same total dose. How many patients would there have to be admitted to each arm in order that a one-tailed test of difference at the 5% level would be detected with a probability of 0.9? The question is answered by a sample-size calculation as

TABLE 1. Sample Sizes for Heterogeneous Populations

Existing Tumor Control Probability	Does (rad)	Theoretical Control Probability with Sensitizer	No. Patients in Each Arm
0.20	6200	0.30	318
0.50	7000	0.67	146

shown in Table 1 for assumed existing control probabilities of 20% or 50%.

These results indicate that it would be very difficult to resolve any clinical benefit from the radiosensitizer if the existing control rate was in the region of 20–50%, given the conditions used for modelling. The conclusions are, of course, sensitive to the proportion of poorly reoxygenating tumors in the overall population and to the level of hypoxia attained. The maximum improvement in TCP_{20} in this model situation occurs when the limiting hypoxic fraction is ~30%. This somewhat unexpected result is due to the fact that as the limiting hypoxic fraction increases, the poorly reoxygenating tumors become more and more refractory to control even with the sensitizer at doses giving an overall TCP_{20}; and if the hypoxic fraction exceeded ~60%, virtually none of the tumors would be controlled, with or without the sensitizer.

When one considers the effect of increasing the proportion of tumors in the mixed population which reoxygenate poorly (to a limiting 35% hypoxic fraction), the overall improvement in TCP_{20} would gradually increase to 30% if all the resistant tumors (i.e., 75% of the total) were hypoxic, and to 65% if the tumor population were completely homogeneous and hypoxic.

However, even if all the tumors in a population were poorly reoxygenating, the effect of an hypoxic-cell radiosensitizer would be diluted if the tumors varied with respect to their number of clonogenic cells. In Figure 3 we have modelled the effect of a sensitizer on a population consisting of four equal subsets containing 10^6, 10^7, 10^8, and 10^9 clonogens, respectively. All tumors were considered to reoxygenate poorly and to be identical in other determinants of radiosensitivity. Use of sensitizer would increase the control level from 20 to ~85% at the TCD_{20} of each subpopulation individually. However, the effect on the overall population is diminished by the presence of tumors either controlled without the sensitizer (10^6 clonogens) or uncontrolled even with the sensitizer (10^9 clonogens) at acceptable dose levels.

It is likely that human tumors are heterogeneous in both senses modelled above, i.e., with regard to different causes of radioresistance and differences in clonogen number. In either case, the effect of new treatments in the clinic will always be less impressive than experimental results obtained with homogeneous animal tumors.

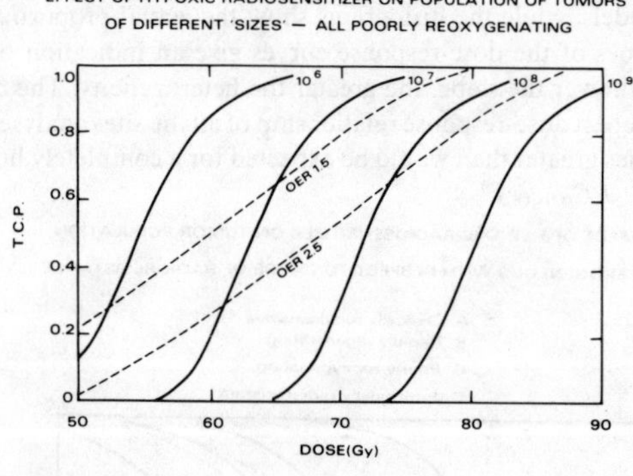

Figure 3. Calculated dose-response curves for four equal subpopulations of tumors, all poorly reoxygenating, but differing in the number of clonogenic cells they contain. The overall TCP curve for the mixed population is labelled "OER 2.5." Under the conditions modelled, the effect of a radiosensitizer that reduced the OER from 2.5 to 1.5 would be to increase the TCP_{20} for each subpopulation of tumors individually by 65%. However, the effect of heterogeneity of cell number in the overall population would reduce the observed improvement to 25% (Curve labelled "OER 1.5").

Conclusion

To overcome clinical radioresistance rationally and consistently we must be able to define the major cause(s) of radioresistance in any given tumor population and adopt appropriate measures, where possible, to counter them. Unfortunately at the present time this cannot be done, and the clinical problem of tumor radioresistance is largely the inability to identify predictively its cause in the individual patient.

Summary

Tumor radioresistance in clinical radiotherapy implies failure to achieve local-regional disease control with radiation doses producing an acceptable degree of morbidity. Such radioresistance may be due to many different causes (biological and technical) which are reviewed in terms of possible remedial actions. Dose-response relationships for human cancers suggest that, in many sites, tumors are heterogeneous with respect to their cure-limiting characteristics. The case is developed that unless the predominant cure-limiting factor can be predicted, little benefit may be seen in trials of new treatment strategies using heterogeneous tumor populations. The fundamental problem of clinical radioresistance is therefore perceived as the inability to identify predictively its cause in the individual patient.

Appendix

The calculations are based on a mathematical model of tumor cell killing by radiation, with concomitant reoxygenation and repopulation of the euoxic moiety. It is assumed that doses are given five times weekly with interfraction intervals of 7/5 days, so that total dose and time are proportional. As a result, the linear decrements in survival that result from fractionated radiation, with slope ln s/d (s = surviving fraction after dose per fraction d), may be scaled to time through the factor (7/5d):

$$\frac{d\, ln\, sf}{d[\text{dose}]} = \frac{ln\, s}{d} = \frac{d\, ln\, sf}{d[(5/7t)d]} = \frac{7}{5d}\quad\frac{d\, ln\, sf}{dt} \qquad 1$$

where sf = surviving fraction at time t.

Let k_x, x, and s_x(k, y, and s_y) denote the initial number, the number at time t, and the surviving fraction after each dose d of euoxic (hypoxic) cells. From (1), the rate of change of x and y due to radiation alone is given by

$$\frac{dx}{dt} = \left(\frac{5}{7}\, ln\, s_x\right) x \quad \text{and} \quad \frac{dy}{dt} = \left(\frac{5}{7}\, ln\, s_y\right) y \qquad 2$$

Exponential repopulation of euoxic clonogens adds a term ax. If hypoxic clonogens are randomly exposed to nutrients and oxygen, reoxygenation will deplete their number exponentially, adding terms ± by so that the resulting differential equation is

$$\frac{dx}{dt} = \left(\frac{5}{7}\, ln\, s_x + a\right) x + by,\ x(0) = k_x;$$

$$\frac{dy}{dt} = \left(\frac{5}{7}\, ln\, s_y - b\right) y;\ y(0) = k_y \qquad 3$$

The solution of (3) is given by

$$x(t) = k_x s_x{}^N e^{at}(1 + b(k_y/k_x)(e^{qt} - 1)/q)$$

$$y(t) = k_y s_y{}^N e^{-bt} \qquad 4$$

where N = number of fractions and

$$q = \frac{5}{7}\, ln\, (s_y/s_x) - a - b \qquad 5$$

When q = 0, (4) reduces to

$$x(t) = k_x s_x{}^N e^{at}\ (1 + b(k_y/k_x)t) \qquad 6$$

The hypoxic fraction H(t) = y(t)/(x(k) + y(t)) is constant if

$$q = b(k_y/k_x) \qquad 7$$

increases with time if

$$q > b(k_y/k_x)$$

and decreases with time if

$$q < b(k_y/k_x)$$

Finally, the probability of tumor cure is the probability of no surviving clonogens per tumor which (assuming random killing) is given by

$$P_{\text{cure}} = \exp[-x(T) - y(T)] \qquad 8$$

where T is the overall treatment time and x(T) and y(T) are computed from equations (4) to (7).

REFERENCES

1. Alexander, P.: Back to the drawing board—The need for more realistic model systems for immunotherapy. *Cancer* **40**:467–470, 1977.
2. Barker, J.L., Montague, E.D., and Peters, L.J.: Clinical experience with irradiation of inflammatory carcinoma of the breast with and without elective chemotherapy. *Cancer* **45**:625–629, 1980.
3. Breuer, K.: In *High LET Radiations in Clinical Radiotherapy*. Supplement to *Eur J Cancer* 1979, pp. 273–276
4. Bush, R.S., Jenkin, R.D.T., Allt, W.E.C., Beale, F.A., Bean, H., Dembo, A.J., and Pringle, J.F.: Definitive evidence of hypoxic cells influencing cure in cancer therapy. *Br J Cancer* **37**:302–306, 1978.
5. Dixon, B., Ward, A.J., and Joslin, C.A.F.: Pretreatment 3H-TdR labelling of cervical biopsies: Histology, staging and tumor response to radiotherapy. *Clin Radiol* **28**:491–497, 1977.
6. Elkind, M.M., and Whitmore, G.F.: *The Radiobiology of Cultured Mammalian Cells* New York: Gordon & Breach, 1967.
7. Fletcher, G.H., and Barkley, H.T.: Prognostic significance of regression rate and clinical status of the tumor at the completion of irradiation. In *Biological Bases and Clinical Implications of Tumor Radioresistance.* New York: Masson, 1983, pp. 129–135.
8. Fletcher, G.H.: Basic clinical parameters. In *Textbook of Radiotherapy*, 3rd ed. G.H. Fletcher, ed. Philadelphia: Lea & Febiger, 1980, pp. 180–218.
9. Fowler, J.F.: New horizons in radiation oncology. *Br J Radiol* **52**:523–536, 1979.
10. Hornsey, S.: The relationship between total dose, number of fractions and fraction size in the response of malignant melanoma in patients. *Br J Radiol* **51**:905–909, 1978.
11. Jampolis, S., Andras, E.J., and Fletcher, G.H.: Analysis of sites and causes of failure of irradiation in invasive squamous cell carcinoma of the intact uterine cervix. *Radiology* **115**:681–685, 1975.
12. Kallman, R.F., Combs, C.A., Franko, A.J., Furlong, B.M., Kelley, S.D., Kemper, H.L., Miller, R.G., Rapachietta, D., Schoenfeld, D., and Takahashi, M.: Evidence for recruitment of noncycling clonogenic tumor cells. In *Radiation Biology in Cancer Research* R. Meyn and H.R. Withers, New York: Raven Press, 1980, pp. 397–414.
13. Kartha, P.K., Chung-Bin, A., Wachtor, T., and Hendrickson, F.R.: Accuracy in patient set-up and its consequence in dosimetry. *Med Phy* **2**:331–332, 1975.
14. Norin, T., and Onyango, J.: Radiotherapy in Burkitt's lymphoma: Conventional or superfractionated regime. *Int J Radiat Oncol Biol Phy* **2**:399–406, 1977.
15. Paterson, R.: *The Treatment of Malignant Disease by Radiotherapy* London: Edward Arnold, 1948.
16. Peters, L.J., Hussey, D.H., Fletcher, G.H., and Wharton, J.T.: Second preliminary report of the M.D. Anderson study of neutron therapy for locally advanced gynaecology tumors. In *High LET Radiations in Clinical Radiotherapy*. Supplement to *Eur J Cancer* 1979, pp. 1–10.
17. Shalek, R.J., Kennedy, P., Stovall, M., Cundiff, J.H., Gagnon, W.F., Grant, W., and Hanson, W.F.: Quality assurance for measurements in therapy, National Bureau Standards, Special Publication 456, pp. 111–118, 1976.
18. Sinclair, W.K.: Dependence of radiosensitivities upon cell age. Brookhaven National Lab. Report, 50203 (C-57), p. 97, 1969.
19. Suit, H.D.: Statement of the problem. Brookhaven National Lab. Report, 50203 (C-57), p. 1, 1969.
20. Thames, H.D., Peters, L.J., Spanos, W., and Fletcher, G.H.: Dose response curves for squamous cell carcinomas of the upper respiratory and digestive tracts. *Br J Cancer* **41**:35–38, 1980.
21. Weichselbaum, R.R., Nove, J., and Little, J.B.: Radiation response of human tumor cells in vitro. In *Radiation Biology in Cancer Research*, R. Meyn and H.R. Withers, eds. New York: Raven Press, 1980, pp. 345–352.
22. Widmann, B.P.: Radiation therapy in cancer of the skin. *Am J Roentgenol* **45**:382–394, 1941.
23. Withers, H.R., and Peters, L.J.: The application of RBE values to clinical trials of high LET radiations. In *High LET Radiations in Clinical Radiotherapy*. Supplement to *Eur J Cancer*, 1979, pp. 257–261.
24. Withers, H.R., and Peters, L.J.: Biological aspects of radiation therapy. In *Textbook of Radiotherapy* 3rd ed., G.H. Fletcher, ed. Philadelphia: Lea and Febiger, 1980, pp. 103–179.

CHAPTER 2

Contribution of the Keynote Discussant

Herman D. Suit, M.D., D.Phil.[a]

In the opinion of this author, the definition of clinical radiation resistance employed by Dr. Peters et al. is not entirely optimal. Rather, it would be more appropriate for the term "clinical radioresistance" to relate to the probability of eradication of tumor of a specific histopathological type and size (or stage) by a specified radiation dose (time, fractionation number, and total dose). Resistance should not be applied to describe a low probability of success. For example, a tumor at one site may not be affected because anatomic site limits dose to a low and ineffective level. Such a tumor is not, in a radiobiologic sense, radiation resistant; it is not amenable to effective therapy. Further, there appear to be real differences in tumors of a given histological type according to anatomic sites in selected situations. For example, a 3-cm diameter squamous cell carcinoma of a buccal mucosa is more readily controlled than a 3-cm diameter squamous cell carcinoma tumor mass that has invaded and destroyed a portion of the mandible. The radiation resistance between the two tumors is different in a radiobiologic sense.

The main point is the assertion that "current treatment failure to achieve local–regional control is not a major stumbling block to cure for most cancers, including those in which uncontrolled disease is the most common immediate cause of death." The implication by the authors is that "cure" is not dependent upon tumor-control probability with reference to the primary tumor. We can accept as fact that cure is not possible in the presence of uncontrolled primary or regional disease. In experimental animal tumor systems, the proportion of long-term survivors increases with tumor control probability. We have examined the incidence of distant metastases in animals who had local control of tumor and the proportion of animals which survived continuously disease free for 200 days. In this stidy 314 mice bearing 8-mm diameter MDH-MCaIV mouse mammary carcinoma growing in the right leg were randomly assigned to receive a single radiation dose of 40–71 Gy. The results are shown in Table 1. Local control frequency increased in an orderly manner with increasing dose of radiation. The proportion of animals that had local control of tumor in the leg but died of metastases in the lung varied between 42 and 28%. The proportion of animals surviving disease free increased from 14 to 55% as radiation dose increased from 60 to 71 Gy. That is, there was a positive correlation between the likelihood of local control of disease and disease-free survival. As local

TABLE 1. Continuously Disease-Free Survival (200 days) after Single-Dose Irradiation of 8mm MCaIV (4)

No. Mice	Dose (Gy)	LC %	DM (w/LC) %	DFS (200 days) %
15	40	0	—	—
15	50	0	—	—
29	60	24	42	14
60	65	55	45	30
110	68	69	28	50
85	71	82	33	55

[a]Andres Soriano Director of Cancer Management, Edwin L. Steele Laboratory of Radiation Biology, Department of Radiation Medicine, Massachusetts General Hospital, Harvard Medical School, Boston, Mass.

TABLE 2. Success of Salvage Surgery for Local Failures of Radiation Therapy

Site	No. Patients	Failures P,N	DM Alone	NED p Salvage Surgery
Tonsillar region (6)	262	132	7	25/42 (61%)
Supraglottis (7)	184	93	12	6/22 (27%)

TABLE 3. Success of Salvage Surgery for Local Failures of Radiation Therapy

Site	Failures/ Patients Treated	Surgical Salvage Attempts	NED (Salvage)	Center	Reference
Bladder (muscular invasive)	240/533	32	25%	M.D.A.H.	3
	27/32	—	2 pts	Royal Marsden	5
	60/85	18	52%	Stanford	2
	258/384	30	48%	Stanford	2
Tonsil	71/140	24	30%	Stanford	8
Base of Tongue	61/104	17	24%	Stanford	8
Uvula and soft palate	15/30	9	44%	Stanford	8
Pharyngeal wall	19/31	2	0/2	Stanford	1
Oral tongue	30/56	5	2/5	Stanford	1
Floor of Mouth	30/58	8	4/8	Stanford	1

control frequency increased, there was a larger pool of animals available for long-term disease-free survival, and we in fact observed this increase in survival.

There are clinical data worthy of comment in this regard. It is instructive to examine the frequency with which local failures of radiation therapy may be salvaged by surgery. If there were no advantage to improved local success of treatment, there would be no salvage of the patients with recurrent disease. Table 2 presents data from two studies by C.C. Wang. There were 262 patients with carcinoma of the tonsillar region and 184 patients with carcinoma of the supraglottic region. Of the patients who had local failure and who were subjected to attempted surgical salvage, the NED rates at >2 years were 25/41 for tonsillar region and 6/22 for the supraglottic region. Table 3 presents several examples from the literature of surgical salvage of radiation therapy failure for patients who had tumors of the bladder, tonsillar region, uvula and soft palate, oral tongue, and floor of mouth.

On review of these various clinical data, I am impressed by two facts: (1) a substantial proportion of the patients who were subjected to a serious attempt at salvage from a local failure have survived disease free for worthwhile periods; and (2) a small proportion of the patients have failed locally and are considered appropriate for subsequent salvage attempts. My reaction is that, had the initial treatment been more successful (fewer local failures), there would be improvement in disease-free survival. Clearly a quantitative estimate of the impact of improved local control cannot be made from this brief review. However, in the opinion of this author, there is no basis for diminished effort at improving the success of local treatments.

REFERENCES

1. Gilbert, E.H., Goffinet, D.R., and Bagshaw, M.A.: Carcinoma of the oral tongue and floor of mouth: Fifteen years' experience with linear accelerator therapy. *Cancer* **35**:1517–1524, 1975.
2. Goffinet, D.R., Schneider, M.J., Glatstein, E.J., Ludwig, H., Ray, G.R., Dunnick, R.R., and Bagshaw, M.A.: Bladder cancer: Results of radiation therapy in 384 patients. *Radiology* **117**:149–153, 1975.

CHAPTER 3

Intrinsic Radiosensitivity of Tumor Cells

Gerrit W. Barendsen, Ph.D.[a]

Despite the large amount of research and numerous discoveries during the past decades concerning cellular responses to ionizing radiations, the basic mechanisms responsible for impairment of clonogenic capacity or cell reproductive death have not yet been fully explained.

It is generally known that x-ray survival curves of bone marrow stem cells, irradiated and assayed *in vitro* or *in vivo,* show a greater sensitivity of these cells as compared with intestinal crypt stem cells or skin stem cells irradiated and assayed *in vivo.* For these different types of stem cells the survival curves mainly represent the sensitivity of noncycling cells; the differences cannot be ascribed to different distributions of cells in the replication cycle, the influence of hypoxia, or to other extracellular conditions. Furthermore, the three cell types are present in the same inbred strain of animals, contain the same amount of DNA, distributed over the same number of chromosomes, with the same genetic information. Consequently, due to lack of better insight, the observed differences in survival curves can only be described as differences in intrinsic radiosensitivity.

In clinical radiotherapy it is well known that lymphomas, leukemias, and seminomas are generally much more sensitive than squamous cell carcinomas of the larynx, adenocarcinomas of the colon, or astrocytomas. Many factors are known that could partially account for these differences in responsiveness, e.g., cell-cycle phase, repopulation rate, oxygenation conditions. However, in view of the knowledge of differences in radiosensitivity among stem cells in normal tissues, it is likely that differences in intrinsic radiosensitivity among tumor cells also play an important role. It is, therefore, important to assess the magnitude of these differences in relation to the influence of other factors, and to stimulate studies of the causes of these differences in intrinsic radiosensitivity among various types of cells.

[a]Radiobiological Institute of the Organisation for Health Research TNO, P.O. Box 5815, Rijswijk, The Netherlands and Laboratory for Radiobiology, University of Amsterdam, The Netherlands.

The Complexity of Damage Induced by Ionizing Radiation in Cells

Lesions produced by ionizing radiations in mammalian cells result from discrete interactions of charged particles with a variety of molecules. Some interactions may produce direct damage in vital molecules; others may yield damage through indirect mechanisms involving radiolytic products of water. Some interactions may produce direct damage in vital molecules; others may yield damage through indirect mechanisms involving radiolytic products of water. Some interactions occur in close proximity to others, e.g., at the end of electron tracks; in other aspects they are distributed approximately at random. Evidently a complex spectrum of damage is produced with respect to the pattern of initial physical energy transfer as well as to primary chemical processes.

Radiation damage manifests itself in a complex spectrum of cellular changes, including chromosome aberrations, mitotic delay, reproductive death, mutations, etc. The sequences of changes between the initiation of various primary processes and their final consequences are not yet clear.

One reason for our failure to obtain a complete description and understanding of the sequences of events that are initiated by energy deposition from ionizing radiations in cells might be that attention has generally been focused on the effects that are observed as cellular damage, rather than on the effects that are not observed, because the cells are capable of repairing lesions and replacing damaged molecules.

In order to illustrate the complexity of these phenomena, it is important to consider a few quantitative aspects of biophysical and biochemical consequences of energy deposition by ionizing radiations in cells and tissues. First, it is of interest to note that for a dose of 1 Gy of low LET radiation delivered to a cell nucleus with a mass of 10^{-10} g, about 100 electrons with an average LET of 1 keV/μm pass through that nucleus and produce a total number of about 20,000 ionizations. If only the DNA in a cell is considered as a vital structure, assuming a mass of 10^{-11} g, the number of electrons associated with a dose of 1 Gy can be calculated at about 20, and the number of ionizations is equal to about 2000. The average energy transfer involved in the production of an ion pair, which is of the order of 10 eV, is adequate to break most types of chemical bonds. Consequently many types of damage can be induced in a variety of molecules in cells, and such a diversity has indeed been observed. For instance, damage to DNA includes single-strand breaks, double-strand breaks, base damage, DNA-DNA and DNA-protein crosslinks. In addition, various types of damage can be induced in other biological macromolecules, in membranes, etc.

It is evident, however, that the many and diverse chemical changes induced in mammalian cells by a dose of 1 Gy do not all result in lesions that are lethal to the cell. A dose of 1 Gy of x-rays will cause reproductive death in only 10 to 50% of the cells, depending on the type of cell investigated. It follows that, in the majority of cells irradiated with a dose of 1 Gy, all chemically altered molecules are repaired or rendered ineffective with respect to impairment of the reproductive integrity. For cells that have lost the capacity for unlimited proliferation after a moderate dose of 1 Gy of low LET radiation, it must also be concluded that, except for one or a few lesions, most of the damaged molecules are repaired, restored in their function, or replaced by normal cellular metabolism. For single-strand breaks in DNA it has been demonstrated that complete repair occurs, while for double-strand DNA breaks 90% repair has been observed for low LET radiation.[3]

To visualize the variety of changes induced by a dose of radiation, a schematic representation is given in Figure 1. This figure shows a hypothetical frequency spectrum of changes of different severity with respect to their influence on cell reproductive capacity. This degree of severity may be associated with the type of molecule that is affected (e.g., DNA, protein or membrane), with the type of chemical changes in the molecule (e.g., a single-strand break or a double-strand break in a DNA molecule), and with the spatial association of damaged molecules (e.g., depending on the ionization density). Many lesions must be assumed to be of little consequence to a cell–e.g., dam-

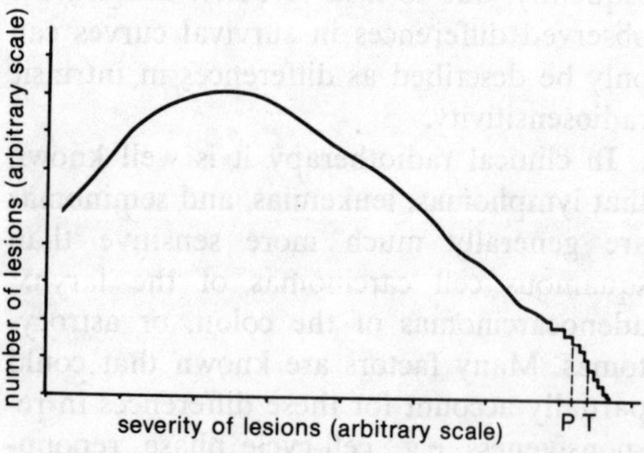

Figure 1. Hypothetical spectrum of lesions in cells irradiated with 2 Gy of x-rays (T indicates threshold beyond which lesions cause cell reproductive death, and P indicates threshold for lesions which are only lethal in specific conditions, e.g., if repair is diminished). Spectrum is assumed to represent all lesions in 100 cells combined.

age to a protein that can be replaced by normal synthesis pathways. Other lesions might be repairable, and no further consequences are observed. Various types of lesions might cause some damage to the reproductive capacity but might not be severe enough to definitely impair the production of an unlimited number of descendents–e.g., the result is small colony formation *in vitro*. This phenomenon is possibly related to a reduced growth rate of recurrent tumors after very high doses. Finally, various types of severe lesions are produced (e.g., yielding dicentric chromosomes), which lead to loss of cellular clonogenic capacity. It is evident, however, that only a very small fraction of all the molecular changes induced by a dose of ionizing radiation are actually effective in causing cell reproductive death, while the great majority of damaged molecules is repaired or rendered harmless. This applies, for instance, to single-strand as well as double-strand breaks of DNA.

The conclusion of these considerations is that mammalian cells have a very large capacity to repair lesions or to render them ineffective. It is also understandable in this perspective of a wide spectrum of lesions that a considerable number of lesions are induced which are close to a threshold of severity beyond which cells cannot cope with the damage. This is indicated in Figure 1 by the range between P and T on the scale of severity. This implies that relatively small changes in the capacity for repair can cause major changes in the fraction of cells inactivated. If, for example, 98% of all changes are repaired or rendered ineffective in optimal conditions, and if a slight reduction in repair capacity is caused by a change in cellular conditions, yielding only 96% of all changes to be repaired, then the effectiveness of this dose of radiation in causing cell inactivation has increased from 2 to 4%–i.e., a difference in effectiveness by a factor of 2 will be observed. It is also expected that among different types of cells, even among those derived from the same animal with equivalent chromosomal structure and information, considerable variations in radiosensitivity may be observed due to relatively small differences in the capacity to repair or replace damaged molecules or structures. It is not surprising, therefore, that the comparison of different types of cells in similar conditions shows differences in radiosensitivity of similar magnitude as observed for a given cell type irradiated and cultured in different conditions–e.g., with respect to oxygenation conditons, culture conditions allowing repair of sublethal or potentially lethal damage, or stage in the intermitotic cycle. In the next sections we will discuss evidence that such differences indeed occur among cells from different tumors.

Differences in Cell-Survival Curves among Cells from Experimental Tumors

In Figure 2 cell-survival curves are shown for a number of cell lines in culture which have been derived from different types of tumors in rats and mice.[3] It is evident that significant differences are observed between the x-ray survival curves and somewhat smaller differences between survival curves for the same cell types irradiated with 15-MeV neutrons. These curves can be analyzed in a variety of ways and can be described by various equations.

A most significant characteristic is that all curves start with an initial negative slope at low doses. This implies that any model that is used to derive cell-survival-curve equations must incorporate an exponential term: e^{-a_1D}. Thus,

$$S/S_o = e^{-a_1D}$$

At doses in excess of 2 Gy of x-rays a significant increase in slope is commonly obtained for survival curves of many types of cells, but not for all types.

This increase in slope can be described by a formula with a quadratic term in the exponent:

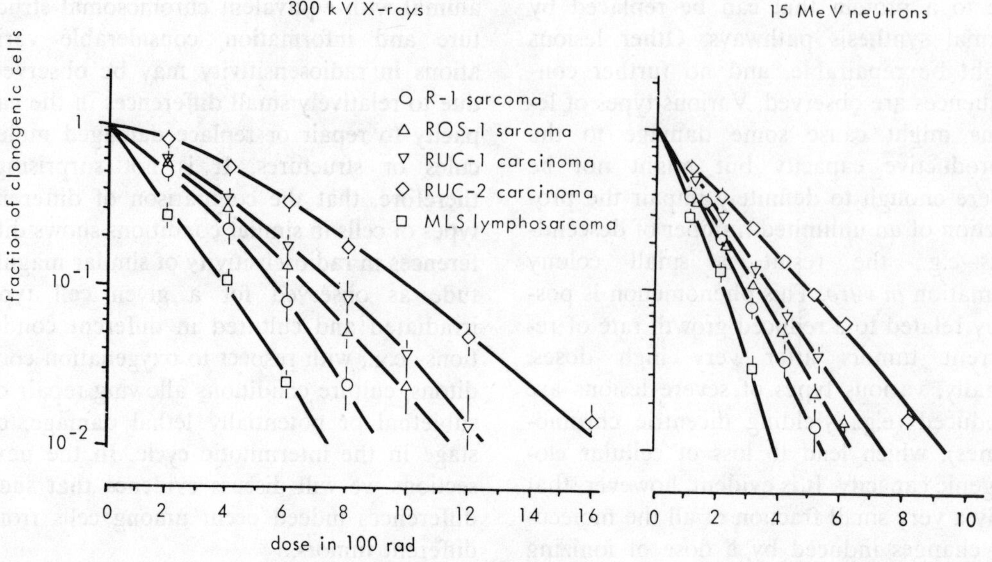

Figure 2. Survival curves of cells in culture derived from different types of animal tumors obtained with *(a)* 300 kV x-rays and *(b)* 15 MeV neutrons.

$$S/S_o = e^{-a_1 D - a_2 D^2}$$

However, this formula frequently is only adequate as a fit to data on fractions of surviving cells between 1 and 0.1. If one also attempts to fit data on lower fractions of surviving cells between 10^{-1} and 10^{-3}, equation (2) frequently yields values of a_1 that are too small or values of a_2 that are too large. The region of fractions of surviving cells below 10^{-1} can generally be better represented by a multitarget model yielding:

$$S/S_o = e^{-a_1 D}[1-(1-e^{-bD})^N]$$

For radiations of high LET the simple exponential term $e^{-a_1 D}$ dominates more strongly, and a_2 or b are relatively of lesser significance.

It is important to note that these formulas can be used without assuming a specific mechanism of action. In Table 1 a number of parameters are presented derived from the x-ray survival curves of Figure 2 and a few other cell lines. They show very significant differences especially for the initial slopes represented by D_o or a_1, but also for the final slopes, extrapolation numbers and D_o/D_o' values, as well as the values of a_2.

In order to investigate the differences in intrinsic radiosensitivity between various cell lines for fractionated irradiations, doses of 1 Gy were given at 2-hour intervals. A few results are presented in Figure 3. It is also evident that significant differences directly related to differences in a_1 or D_o (initial) are obtained with fractionated treatments.

It is worthwhile to mention that a few of the cell lines mentioned in Table 1 have also been irradiated in plateau phase cultures. For R-1 cells and RUC-2 cells very little difference was observed in comparison with corresponding cells in exponentially growing cultures.

Significance of Differences in Intrinsic Radiation Sensitivity of Different Cells for Responses of Tumors to Radiotherapy

The cell lines for which cell-survival

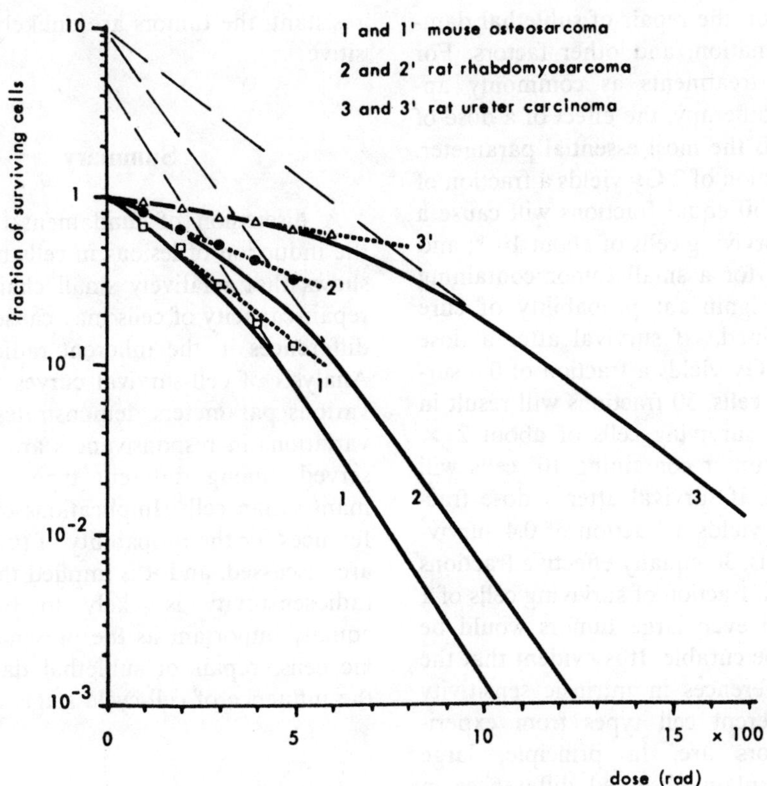

Figure 3. X-ray survival curves of different cell lines. Curves 1, 2, and 3 are single doses of 300 kV x-rays; curves 1′, 2′, and 3′ represent 100 rad of 300 kV x-rays per fraction given at 2-hour intervals.

TABLE 1. Parameters of X-Ray Survival Curves of Cells in Culture Derived from Different Experimental Tumors

Type of Tumor	a_1 ($\times 10^1$) (Gy^{-1})	a_2 ($\times 10^2$) (Gy^{-2})	a_1/a_2 (Gy)	D_o (initial slope	N (extrapolation number)	D_o' (slope at high doses)	D_o/D_o'
R-1	1.8	3.7	4.0	5.5	10	1.3	4.2
RUC-1	1.2	2.3	5.0	8.5	20	1.5	5.7
RUC-2	0.8	1.0	8.0	12.0	20	2.2	5.5
ROS-1	1.8	3.6	5.0	5.5	4.0	1.6	3.3
RMS-1	2.2	5.4	4.1	4.5	10	1.1	4.1
MLS-1	3.6	2.5	14.5	2.8	5.0	1.2	2.3

curves are presented in Figure 2 can all be inoculated in animals and yield tumors with a variety of growth characteristics.[4] It is evident that the tumors grown from resistant cell lines are expected to be less responsive to x-ray treatments than tumors grown from sensitive cell lines. However, with respect to growth delay induced by single doses of x-rays, many other factors (e.g., the fraction of hypoxic cells, the rate of repopulation by surviving cells, and others) play a part.[1]

The response to fractionated treatments

will depend on the repair of sublethal damage, reoxygenation, and other factors. For fractionated treatments as commonly applied in radiotherapy, the effect of a dose of about 2 Gy is the most essential parameter. If a dose fraction of 2 Gy yields a fraction of 0.5 survival, 30 equal fractions will cause a fraction of surviving cells of about 10^{-9}; and consequently for a small tumor containing 10^8 cells, a significant probability of cure may be attained.[2] If survival after a dose fraction of 2 Gy yields a fraction of 0.6 surviving tumor cells, 30 fractions will result in a fraction of surviving cells of about 2×10^{-7}, and a tumor containing 10^8 cells will not be cured. If survival after a dose fraction of 2 Gy yields a fraction of 0.4 surviving tumor cells, 30 equally effective fractions will result in a fraction of surviving cells of 1×10^{-12}, and even large tumors would be expected to be curable. It is evident that the observed differences in intrinsic sensitivity between different cell types from experimental tumors are, in principle, large enough to explain observed differences in responses among different types of tumors. More research on the causes of these differences in intrinsic sensitivity is required because it might provide important insight into differences in radioresistance of tumors in men.

The data and ideas presented and discussed in this contribution should not be interpreted as suggesting that other causes of radioresistance (e.g., repair of subeffective and sublethal damage, the presence of hypoxia, and repopulation during protracted treatments) are not important. If a tumor consists of cells that are intrinsically sensitive with respect to impairment of the clonogenic capacity, the dose required for local control may well be higher than expected from the cellular response, due to the factors mentioned. On the other hand, if a tumor consists of cells that are intrinsically radioresistant, the tumors are unlikely to be sensitive.

Summary

A discussion of fundamental aspects of the induction of lesions in cells by radiation shows that relatively small changes in the repair capacity of cells may cause important differences in the inherent radiosensitivity. Analysis of cell-survival curves in terms of various parameters demonstrates that wide variations in responsiveness are indeed observed among different types of cultured mammalian cells. Implications of these differences for the probability of tumor control are discussed, and it is implied that intrinsic radiosensitivity is likely to be at least equally important as the presence of hypoxic cells, repair of sublethal damage, and the influence of cell-cycle stage.

REFERENCES

1. Barendsen, G.W.: Variations in radiation responses among experimental tumors. In *Radiation Biology in Cancer Research.* R.E. Meyn and H.R. Withers, eds. New York: Raven Press, 1980, pp. 333–343.
2. Barendsen, G.W., and Broerse, J.J.: Experimental radiotherapy of a rat rhabdomyosarcoma with 15 MeV neutrons and 300 kV x-rays. I. Effects of single exposures. *Eur J Cancer* **5**:373–391, 1969.
3. Barendsen, G.W., and Broerse, J.J.: Differences in radiosensitivity of cells from various types of experimental tumors in relation to the RBE of 15 MeV neutrons. *Int J Radiat Oncol Biol Phys* **3**:211–214, 1977.
4. Barendsen, G.W., Janse, H.C., Deys, B.F., and Hollander, C.F.: Comparison of growth characteristics of experimental tumors and derived cell cultures. *Cell Tissue Kinet* **10**:1–7, 1977.
5. Cole, A., Meyn, R.E., Chen, R., Corry, P.M., and Hittelman, W.: Mechanisms of cell injury. In *Radiation Biology in Cancer Research.* R.E. Meyn and H.R. Withers, eds. New York: Raven Press, 1980, pp. 33–58, 333–343.

CHAPTER 4

The Role of Potentially Lethal Damage Repair in Human Tumor Radiocurability

Ralph R. Weichselbaum, M.D.[a]
John B. Little, M.D.[b]

Radiocurability of a human tumor may depend on many of the following parameters: (1) total dose, fraction schedule, dose distribution, and dose rate; (2) tumor size; (3) characteristics of tumor cells (to include inherent cellular radiosensitivity, cell-cycle distribution of cycling cells, and the presence of noncycling but clonogenically viable cells; (4) repair of sublethal and potentially lethal damage; (5) hypoxia; and (6) immunologic and hormonal influences of the host.

Our discussion will center on the repair of potentially lethal radiation damage, and the application of density-inhibited, plateau or stationary phase human cell cultures to experimental tumor radiotherapy. We will first discuss briefly our experience in the investigation of the intrinsic radiosensitivity of human tumor cell populations *in vitro*. Table 1 shows radiosensitivity of exponentially growing human tumor cells *in vitro*. Except for one human melanoma line, we have found no human tumor lines to be unusually radioresistant, and under no experimental conditions have we observed a large extrapolation number ($\bar{n}$). On the other hand, some human leukemia and lymphoma cell lines examined in our laboratory are radiosensitive relative to these solid tumors.[9]

TABLE 1. Radiosensitivity of Exponetially Growing Human Tumor Cell Lines *IN VITRO.*

Cell Line	Tumor Type	D_o	$\bar{n}$
TX-4	Osteosarcoma	145	1.8
SAOS	Osteosarcoma	135	2.2
TX-7	Medulloblastoma	135	1.5
TX-14	Medulloblastoma	131	1.6
TX-13	Glioblastoma	143	1.4
MCF-7	Breast carcinoma	134	1.3
LAN-1	Neuroblastoma	149	1.2
MEL-H	Melanoma	150	2.5
PAS	Hypernephroma	131	1.2
C-32	Melanoma	220	1.6
176	Lymphoma	69	5.3

The above data suggest that, aside from lymphoma and an occasional melanoma, differences in intrinsic radiosensitivity of human tumor cells as measured in exponentially growing cultures is not a major factor in determining the differences in therapeutic response. Other laboratories have reported a seminoma to be sensitive as well as an occasional resistant tumor line; but in general the results have been in agreement with ours.[5,10,11]

We have also examined the enhancement in survival that occurs when a radiation dose is split with an interval of several hours between fractions. This enhancement has been interpreted as resulting from the repair of sublethal damage induced by the first dose in cells that survive the initial exposure. This has been postulated to be a major factor in human tumor radiocurability. Split-dose recovery experiments *in vitro* are

[a]Associated Professor, Radiation Therapy Department, Harvard Medical School, Head, Peter Bent Brigham Division, Joint Center, Radiation Therapy Department, Boston, Mass.

[b]Professor of Radiobiology, Harvard School of Public Health, Boston, Mass.

usually performed on exponentially growing cells. Since the extrapolation number on our human tumor cells was relatively small compared to some animal lines, we thought that the *in vitro* shoulder might underestimate the split-dose recovery response. However, experiments performed on several human tumor lines showed that the extrapolation numbers accurately reflected the amount of split-dose recovery measured in these cells.[8]

The low-dose region of the survival curve is important to the clinical radiotherapist since clinical doses are usually considered to be near the shoulder of the radiation survival curve. No systematic differences have been demonstrated in human tumors regarding the repair of (1) sublethal damage or (2) intrinsic radiosensitivity, with the exception of the above-mentioned tumors. (*Note*: Lymphoma and seminoma cells, like their benign counterparts, may die an intermitotic death.) We therefore expanded our study to stationary phase cells to explain a cellular component of radiocurability.

Potentially Lethal Damage Repair

Enhancement of survival after delay of subculture of cells irradiated in a density-inhibited state is referred to as the repair of potentially lethal damage (PLDR) and is analogous to liquid holding recovery in bacteria. Little[2,4] proposed plateau phase cultures *in vitro* as models of *in vivo* tumors and pointed out that in these cultures human tumors are in an anatomic and physiologic state which approaches more closely their *in vivo* counterparts.

PLDR has been demonstrated in animal tumors and established cell lines, and we wished to examine whether PLDR reflected a molecular repair process in human cells. Table 2 shows x-ray and UV PLDR recovery in normal diploid fibroblasts; fibroblasts from patients with ataxia telangiectasia, an autosomal recessive disease characterized by oculocutaneous telangiectasia and unusual sensitivity to X-irradiation, and a defect in the repair of gamma radiation in fibroblasts from these patients; and fibroblasts from patients with xeroderma pigmentosum (XP), an autosomal recessive disease associated with a sensitivity to the effects of UV light *in vivo* and *in vitro*. This sensitivity is due to a defect in the excision repair pathway.

As can be seen, XP fibroblasts did not perform UV PLDR and AT fibroblasts performed minimal x-ray PLDR compared to normal controls. Patients from the XP vari-

TABLE 2. Radiation Sensitivity and Repair of Potentially Lethal Damage in Human Diploid Fibroblast Strains

Clinical Classification	D_o (X-Ray)	Enhancement after X-Ray	Survival D_o (Ultraviolet Light)	Survival Enhancement after Light
Normal skin fibroblasts	149 ± 7	4.13 ± 0.02	31 ± 6	4.33 ± 0.34
Skin fibroblasts from ataxia telangiectasia	46 ± 3	1.78 ± 0.13	29 ± 3	3.10 ± 0.55
Skin fibroblasts from xeroderma pigmentosum (XP) (group A)	160 ± 17	4.63 ± 1.04	6 ± 1	0.96 ± 0.15
XP skin fibroblasts (group C)	—	—	8 ± 1	0.91 ± 0.21
XP skin fibroblasts (variant)	—	—	20 ± 1	2.30 ± 0.40

ant proficient in excision repair were also proficient in UV PLDR, leading us to the conclusion that potentially lethal damage repair reflects a molecular repair phenomenon like the excision repair pathway for the UV system, and a molecular but as yet undetermined process for gamma repair. Thus, we felt that the examination of human cells in a density-inhibited system approximated the physiologic state of at least some component of human tumors–i.e., nondividing or slowly dividing cells–and that this cellular recovery phenomenon reflects the activity of, and thus the capacity for, a molecular repair process. Furthermore, the "one-dose" experiments more closely approximate repair seen in clinical fractionation schemes than classical "two-dose" experiments where doses are separated by only 4 to 6 hours.[7]

Experiments were performed with cells in a density-inhibited state. Under these circumstances most cells are in the G_1 phase of the cell cycle. Once the cells in the culture dish became confluent, the nutrient medium was changed daily for three days to assure density inhibition. It is important to point out that this differs from nutritional depletion or drug inhibition of cell proliferation. Under these conditions, cells may not be uniformly arrested in G_1. In addition, such factors do not approach the physiologic state. Cells were irradiated and subcultured at low densities at various times from 0 to 24 hours after treatment to assay for colony formation. Only those colonies containing 50 or more cells were scored as survivors.

Results

Our results may be divided into (1) radiocurable tumors and (2) nonradiocurable tumors.

The radiocurable tumors, including two breast lines (MCF-7 and MDA) and a neuroblastoma line, did relatively small amounts of PLDR (Fig. 1). The other tumor lines were derived from tumors which are relatively incurable by radiotherapy (glioblastoma, hypernephroma, osteosarcoma, etc.). These cell lines did significantly more PLDR than the radiocurable tumors (Fig. 2). However, a subset of nonradiocurable tumors including melanoma and osteosarcoma did significantly more PLDR than the other lines examined. These two

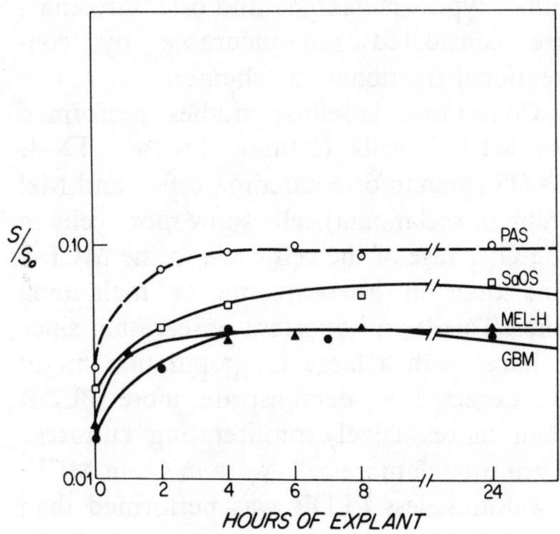

Figure 1. PLDR following X-irradiation in human tumor cell lines: PAS, a hypernephroma (O); SaOS, an osteosarcoma (□); MEL-H, a melanoma (▲); and GBM, a glioblastoma (●).

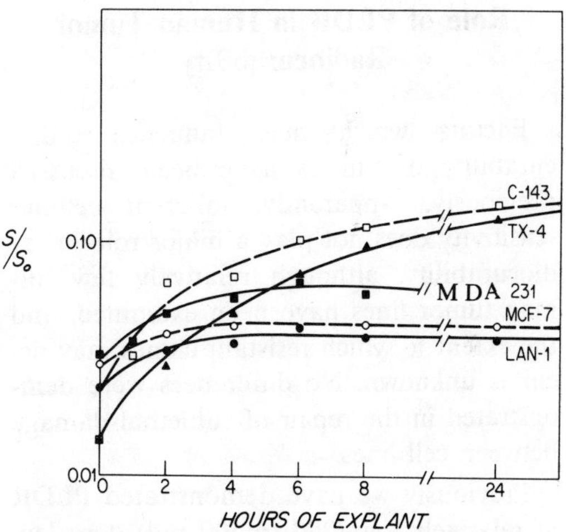

Figure 2. PLDR following X-irradiation in human tumor cell lines: C-143, a melanoma (□); TX-4, an osteosarcoma (▲); MDA-231, a carcinoma of the breast (■); MCF-7, a carcinoma of the breast (O); and LAN-1, a neuroblastoma (●).

tumor types–melanoma and osteosarcoma–are considered radioincurable by conventional fractionation schemes.

Continuous labelling studies performed on MCF-7 cells (human breast), TX-4, SAOS (human osteosarcoma cells), and Mel (human melanoma) cells show more cells in the G_1 phase of the cell cycle in the MCF-7 line than in osteosarcoma or melanoma lines. This is an important observation since cultures with a large G_1 population might be expected to demonstrate more PLDR than more actively proliferating cultures.[3] Even though more cells were in G_1 in MCF-7 cultures, less PLDR was performed than in melanoma or osteosarcoma, and we therefore postulate that PLDR recovery is a repair phenomenon characteristic of cell phenotype.

Role of PLDR in Human Tumor Radiocurability

Factors which may influence radiocurability of tumors have been discussed previously. Apparently, inherent cellular sensitivity does not play a major role in radiocurability, although relatively few human tumor lines have been examined, and the extent to which resistant clones may occur is unknown. No differences were demonstrated in the repair of sublethal damage between cell lines.

Previously we have demonstrated PLDR at relatively low (200 to 500 rad) dose levels.[6] One might envision that even a three-to four-fold recovery over a 30 fraction treatment scheme might render a tumor quite incurable. If some human tumors have PLDR characteristics of TX-4 or the melanoma line C-143, this would render a tumor quite incurable. It should be pointed out that there is a heterogeneity of radiocurability within all cell types (melanoma, osteosarcoma, breast).

Some of the radiocurable tumors have the same PLDR characteristics as normal human diploid fibroblasts. It must be recalled that the normal tissue/tumor ratio generally consists of volume effects–i.e., a small volume of many normal tissues can be irradiated to high doses and large volumes can only receive small doses (hopefully, the entire tumor is irradiated); therefore, the most important characteristic is the cellular repair capacity of the tumor and not necessarily a comparison of tumor to normal tissue ratio.

It is impossible to determine what relationship cloned *in vitro* tumor cell lines have to the PLDR capacity of the parent tumors *in situ*. However, other characteristics of these lines are similar to the tumors from which they were derived–i.e., melanoma makes melanin, breast carcinoma has hormone receptors and produces alpha-lact-albumin, etc. It is not unreasonable to assume that the repair characteristics are similar, especially since radiosensitive patients with ataxia telangiectasia have demonstrated radiosensitivity *in vitro* and XP patients sensitive to UV light have similar responses *in vitro* with demonstrated molecular repair defects. Therefore, the radiobiologic parameters of cells *in vitro* may be similar to those observed *in vivo*.

The extent to which PLDR accounts for radiocurability is likely to vary from tumor to tumor since *in vitro* there appears to be variability within cell phenotypes. Also, the extent to which *in vivo* tumors contain cells analogous to density-inhibited cells *in vitro* will bear direct relevance to PLDR in human tumor radiocurability. It would appear that even a small amount of PLDR in a significant population of cells would render a tumor quite incurable, especially over a protracted fractionation scheme. Fowler has commented that PLDR should not be discounted in any treatment scheme.[1]

Conventional survival curve theory may be overemphasized in human tumor radiobiology since relatively few cell lines derived from solid tumors are either sensitive or resistant, and mathematical models for survival curves may have been constructed for biological event without sufficient data. Furthermore, the repair of sublethal damage, i.e., conventional two-dose repair, may not bear the biologic relevance once thought.

Radiocurability is undoubtedly a highly complex function, although for many common tumors (head and neck, cervix) tumor size is the most important determinant of radiocurability. Whether this decrease in radiocurability is strictly due to greater numbers of cells or due to an increase in the hypoxic function or cells which resemble *in vitro* plateau phase cells or both has yet to be determined.

Summary

Radiation survival-curve parameters on exponentially growing human tumor cells examined in our laboratory are relatively homogeneous: D_o = 131 to 150; n = 1.2 - 2.2 with the exception of a single melanoma line (D_o = 220) and a lymphoma line (D_o = 69). The repair of potentially lethal damage repair (PLDR) has been studied in nine human tumor cell lines. Tumors considered clinically radiocurable perform less PLDR than tumors not generally considered radiocurable, although heterogeneity of PLDR exists within tumor cell phenotypes. The possible role of PLDR in human tumor radiotherapy is discussed.

ACKNOWLEDGMENTS

This work was supported by Grants CA-21848 and CA-11751 from the National Cancer Institute.

We thank Ms. Annie Schmit for expert technical assistance.

REFERENCES

1. Fowler, J.F.: Symposium summary. In *Radiation Biology in Cancer Research* R.E. Meyn and H.R. Withers, eds. New York: Raven Press, 1980, pp. 645–654.
2. Little, J.B.: Repair of sublethal and potentially lethal radiation damage in plateau phase cultures of human cells. *Nature* **224**:804–806, 1969.
3. Little, J.B., and Hahn, G.M.: Life cycle dependence of radiation repair of potentially lethal damage. *Int J Radiat Biol* **23**:401–7, 1973.
4. Little, J.B., Hahn, G.M., Frindel, E., and Tubiana, M.: Repair of potentially lethal damage *in vitro* and *in vivo*. *Radiology* **106**:689–694, 1973.
5. Smith, I.E., Courtenary, D., Mills, J., and Peckham, M.S.: *In vitro* radiation response of cells from four human tumors propagated in immune suppression mice. *Radiat Res* **38**:390–392, 1978.
6. Weichselbaum, R.R., Little, J.B., and Nove, J.: Response of human osteosarcoma *in vitro* to X-irradiation: Evidence for unusual cellular repair activity. *Int J Radiat Biol* **31**:295–299, 1977.
7. Weichselbaum, R.R., Nove, J., and Little, J.B.: Deficient repair of potentially lethal damage in ataxia telangiectasia and xeroderma pigmentosum fibroblasts. *Nature* **291**:261–262, 1978.
8. Weichselbaum, R.R., Nove, J., and Little, J.B.: Radiation response of human tumor cells *in vitro*. In *Radiation Biology in Cancer Research* R.E. Meyn and H.R. Withers, eds. New York: Raven Press, 1980, pp. 345–351.
9. Weichselbaum, R.R.: Manuscript in progress.
10. Weininger, J., Guichard, M., Joly, A.M., Malaise, E.P., and Lachet, B.: Radiosensitivity and growth parameters *in vitro* of three human melanoma strains. *Int J Radiat Biol* **34**:285–290, 1978.
11. Wells, J., Berry, R.J., and Laing, A.H.: Reproductive survival of explanted human tumor cells after exposure to nitrogen mustard or X-irradiation; differences in response with subsequent subculture *in vitro*. *Radiat Res* **69**:76–78, 1977.

CHAPTER 5

The Relationship of Cell-Cycle Phase Progression Delay to Cell Inactivation after X-Ray and Neutron Irradiation

W. Göhde, Ph. D.[a]
J. Schumann, Ph.D.[b]
F. Otto, Ph.D.[c]
E. Schnepper, M.D.[d]

The irradiation of proliferating cells leads to changes in the composition of the cells concerning their position in the cell division cycle.[2,5,8] The ability of this cytobiological response to influence the clinical response to therapeutic irradiation has been noted.[7,12] The idea to employ such cell-cycle phenomena in radiotherapeutic schedules is still controversial[14,15] since the fundamental work of Bergonié and Tribondeau.[1] Due to new cytobiological techniques, we have been able to improve our knowledge about tumor cell biology under *in vitro* and *in vivo* conditions.[5,10] This might lead to a better understanding of the extent that cell-cycle parameters influence *in vivo* response to irradiation.

It is obvious that considerations about influencing cell-cycle parameters must be related to cells that are kinetically influenced but still clonogenic. The second important precondition is that cells in the different phases of the cell-division cycle have a different radiosensitivity. Both parameters are investigated under *in vitro* conditions: data for human tumors under *in vivo* conditions are nearly nonexistent, representing a remarkable gap in our knowledge about tumor cell radiobiology.

The radiosensitivity of the different cell-cycle phases is shown in Figure 1, taken from a paper of Sinclair.[11] This example shows for hamster (lung) fibroblasts *in vitro* a difference between S-phase cells and G_1- and G_2-phase cells in the response to irradiation. Under ideal experimental conditions the ratio of the surviving fractions can amount to a factor of 40. The curves in Figure 1 demonstrate that for this cell type the different dose-response curves are almost parallel. Thus, it is likely that different cells have different abilities to repair sublethal damage. From the radiotherapy point of view the difference in radiosensitivity is more pronounced in the small dose range. In contrast to this parallel shape of the different dose-response curves, other cell lines can show different D_0 values for the different cell-cycle stages.[13]

The relationship of irradiation-induced cell-cycle phase progression delay to cell inactivation is more difficult to investigate under *in vivo* conditions; there are no relevant data available at the moment.

[a]Radiologische Klinik der Universität Münster, W. Germany.

[b]Fachklinik Hornheide, Universität Münster, W. Germany.

[c]Fraunhofer-Institut für Toxikologie und Aerosolforschung, Schmallenberg, W. Germany.

[d]Radiologische Klinik der Universität Münster, W. Germany.

The comparison of the effects of x-rays and neutrons on proliferating cells shows, *in vitro* and *in vivo*, drastic changes in the composition of the cells concerning their position in the cell cycle.[2,8] The quality of these changes, as in G_2 arrest and S-phase delay, are principally the same for both noxae;[2,8] the shape of the survival curves, on the other hand, is different. We have used an *in vitro* system to demonstrate to what extent cell-cycle phenomena are combined with cell inactivation. Tumor treatment schedules with radio- or chemotherapy which consider cell-cycle phenomena have to be based on data for the clonogenicity of such cells which show cell-cycle phase progression delay after a previous step of treatment.

Materials and Methods

L-929 cells were grown logarithmically in TC-199 medium containing 10% newborn calf serum. The cells were irradiated with 250 kV x-rays (0.5 mm Cu-filter, 2 Gy per minute) or with neutrons from the accelerator of the Abteilung für biophysikalische Strahlenforschung der Gesellschaft für Strahlen- und Umweltforschung in Frankfurt. The neutron energy was 1.5 to 15 MeV. The dosimetry was performed according to Kühn.[6] The cell survival was studied with the colony-forming test. In addition, irradiated cells were harvested at different times after exposure. The composition of the cell samples concerning the different cell-cycle phases was analyzed by measuring the single-cell DNA content in at least 30,000 cells in each sample. These measurements were performed with a pulse cytophotometer (FCM) developed by these authors.[2,5]

A special problem concerns the dose-response curves for the kinetic effect of cells. The main difficulty is that logarithmically growing populations of cells *in vitro*, as well as in tumors, contain different target cells which can react with different types of kinetic changes and which can show those

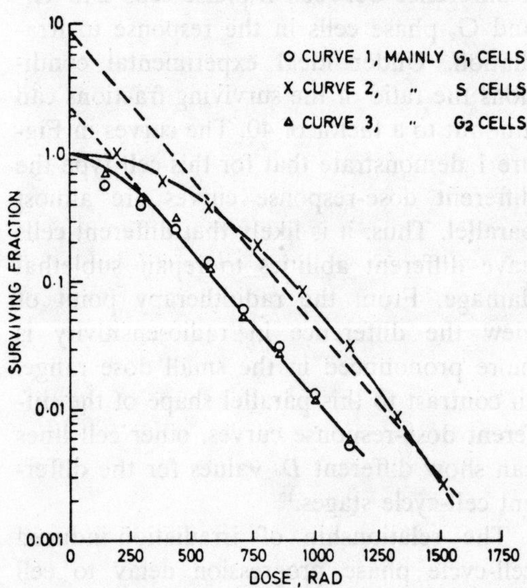

Figure 1. Survival curves of Chinese hamster (lung) fibroblasts irradiated in air during the three phases of the cell cycle.[11]

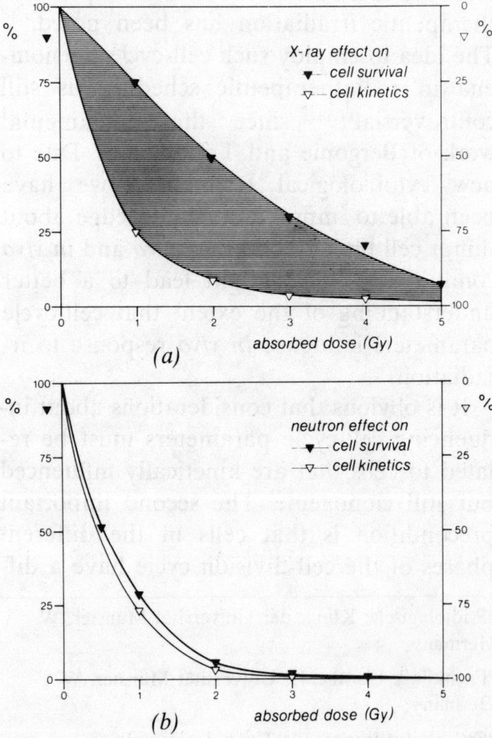

Figure 2. Dose-response curves in a lin-lin-plot for (*a*) x-rays and (*b*) fast neutrons. The open triangles represent cell kinetics; the closed triangles represent the cell inactivation.

changes at different times after exposure. The dose-response curves for the kinetic effects, shown in Figure 2, are based on the following consideration: the L-929 cells have a overall cell cycle time of 16 hours which also can be seen in Figure 3. The S-phase and (G_2 + M)-phase transition time is about 10 hours. If a logarithmically growing cell population is analyzed 10 hours after exposure, each treated S-, G_2-, and M-phase cell has had the chance to divide into two daughter cells. At the same time all treated G_1-phase cells move forward in the cell-division cycle and reach the S phase. Previous investigations[2,8] and Figure 3 show that x-rays and neutrons do not induce a G_1-phase delay at doses used in these investigations. Thus, 10 hours after exposure all detected G_1-phase cells have divided after irradiation. The dose-response curves for the kinetic effects of cells shown in this paper represent the percentages of treated S- and (G_2 + M)-phase cells which have divided within 10 hours after exposure. These figures contain about 70% of the treated cell population. The other 30% of cells were G_1-phase cells at the time of treatment. They show their kinetic effects at later times—at times when those effects interfere with fluctuations of cell-cycle phase frequencies from other groups of cells. This difficulty in counting the kinetic effects for the whole cell population can be overcome using centrifugal elutriation which we have applied to analyze the adriamycin effect on cell kinetics and cell inactivation.[4]

In addition to the presented kinetic and inactivation experiments, time-lapse photography was performed to follow the cell-division and cell-cycle times of irradiated individual L-929 cells.

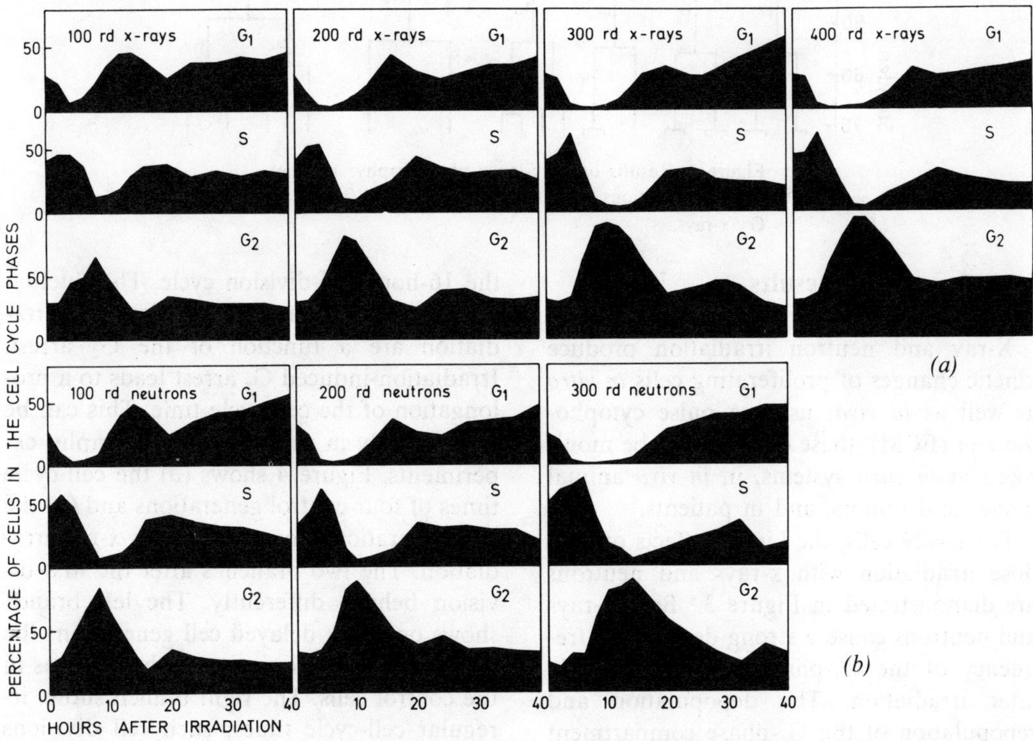

Figure 3. The effect of (*a*) x-ray and (*b*) neutron irradiation on the frequency of L-929 cells in the various cell-cycle phases. The cell-cycle distributions were measured with the pulse cytophotometer every 2 hours after treatment.[2]

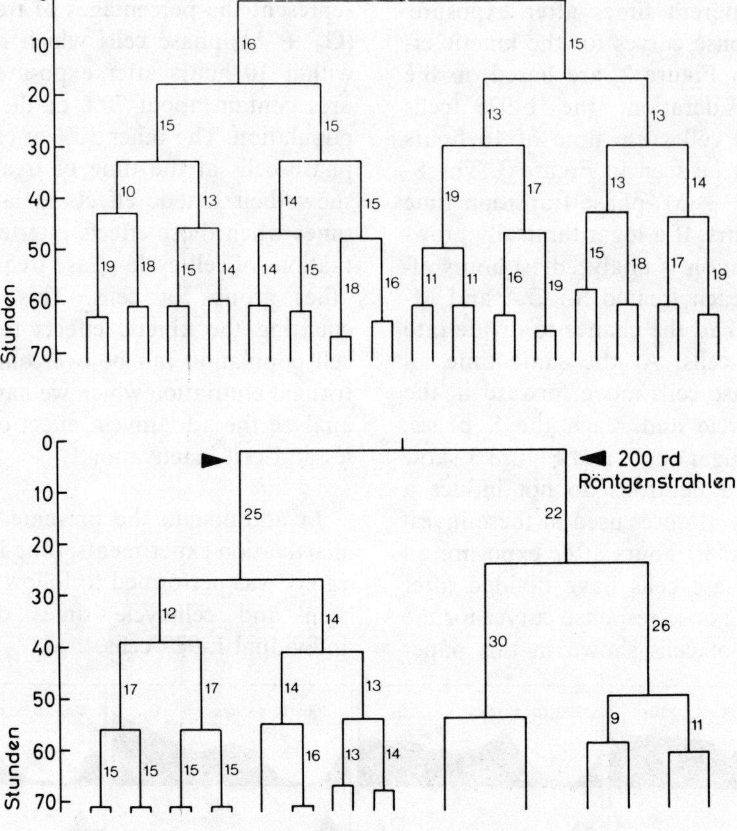

Figure 4. Results of time-lapse photography: number of cell generations *(a)* without treatment and *(b)* after 2 Gy x-rays.

Results

X-ray and neutron irradiation produce kinetic changes of proliferating cells *in vitro* as well as *in vivo*; using a pulse cytophotometer (FCM), these changes can be monitored in *in vitro* systems, in *in vivo* animal tissues and tumors, and in patients.[5]

For L-929 cells, the kinetic effects of low-dose irradiation with x-rays and neutrons are demonstrated in Figure 3.[8] Both x-rays and neutrons cause a strong decrease in frequency of the G_1-phase cells immediately after irradiation. The depopulation and repopulation of the G_1-phase compartment shows, in both cases, almost identical patterns. This pattern reflects the irradiation-induced G_2 arrest with a maximum frequency of G_2-phase cells after 10 to 12 hours into the 16-hour cell-division cycle. The fluctuations of the S-phase frequencies after irradiation are a function of the G_2 arrest. Irradiation-induced G_2 arrest leads to a prolongation of the cell-cycle time. This can be seen directly in time-lapse photography experiments. Figure 4 shows (*a*) the cell-cycle times of four control generations and (*b*) the cell generation times after 2 Gy x-ray irradiation. The two branches after the first division behave differently. The left branch shows only one delayed cell generation; the following cell-cycle times are the same as in the control cells. The right branch shows irregular cell-cycle times; such cell divisions produce preferentially cells which have lost their clonogenicity.[9]

The aim of this investigation was to analyze the quantitative relationship of cell

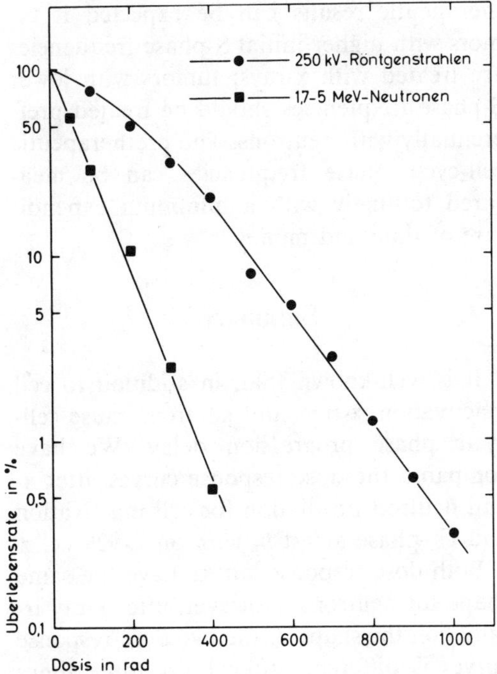

Figure 5. Survival curves of L-929 cells treated with x-rays and with fast neutrons.

inactivation and induction of cell-cycle phase progression delay. The x-ray- and neutron-induced cell inactivation is shown in Figure 5. The dose-response curves have extrapolation numbers of 1 for neutrons and 3,5 for x-rays. The RBE at 1% survival is 2,3.

To describe the kinetic effect quantitatively we have used the G_1-phase cell frequency 10 hours after irradiation. At this time all treated S-phase and (G_2 + M)-phase cells have had the chance to divide. The dose-response curves for the kinetic effect shown in Figure 2 contain the percentages of all treated S-phase and (G_2 + M)-phase cells which have divided within 10 hours after treatment. In Figure 2 the cell-survival curves are also shown in a lin-lin-plot.

The survival curves and kinetic effect curves for x-ray-treated L-929 cells are different. Thus, in the case of x-rays, more cells show kinetic effects than are inactivated. The absolute difference between these two curves has a maximum at about 1 Gy; only 25% of the cells are killed, whereas 75% of the treated S- and (G_2 + M)-phase cells show cell-cycle phase progression delay. Because the treated G_1-phase cells are not counted in this figure, a minor correction of the amount of the kinetic effect might be necessary. The treated G_1-phase cells show their G_2 arrest at a different time after treatment. The effect overlaps with other cycle phase fluctuations. Models have to be developed to describe the kinetic effects quantitatively for the whole cell population.

The neutron data shown in Figure 2 (*b*) demonstrate that there is no difference in the cell inactivation and induction of cell-cycle phase progression delay. About the same frequency of cells which are delayed (as defined before) are also inactivated. It is likely to assume for neutron irradiation that cells showing cell-cycle phase progression delay have lossed their clonogenicity.

X-ray- and neutron-induced kinetic effects show about the same dose-response curves. Both curves fit nicely the neutron survival curve. Thus, in a lin-log-plot, the kinetic-effect curves do not have a shoulder in both cases.

Discussion

The analysis of x-ray-induced cell-cycle phase progression delay and cell inactivation shows no close correlation of these two effects to each other for L-929 cells. At low x-ray doses, far more cells show a delay in the cell-cycle phase progression than are inactivated. For the quantitative analysis the presented dose-response curves do not contain the 30% cells in the G_1 phase at the time of treatment. Further experiments, e.g., using centrifugal elutriation of the different cell-cycle phases and separate experiments with sorted cells, will also allow us to take into account the G_1-phase cells.[4] But it can be assumed that the shape of the dose-response curves for the kinetic effect will not be very different from the above data.

For neutron irradiation we found similar dose-response curves for both the cell inactivation and kinetic effect. The data show that cell kinetic considerations in fractionation schedules are valid for x-rays, but they will not have any influence if neutrons are used. Neutron irradiation causes the same kinetic effects as x-ray irradiation. But in the case of x-rays many of the arrested cells temporarily in the G_2 phase keep their ability to form colonies.

The size of the group of x-ray-irradiated synchronized cells is dose dependent; the duration of the cell-cycle block is also dose dependent. Fractionation schedules which consider cell kinetic parameters should use relatively low x-ray doses given with time intervals in the range of the duration of the S phase. This ensures that cells which are temporarily blocked in the x-ray-sensitive phase of the cell cycle–the G_2 and M phase–are still viable after the first dose fraction and can be inactivated more effectively with the next treatment. This can reduce the dose for the same degree of inactivation. This model will be more effective in tumors because of their higher S-phase frequencies in comparison to the related normal tissue.[10] The relatively low single doses increase the therapeutic range, and more dose fractions can reach more proliferating cells–even such cells which are triggered from the nonproliferating into the proliferating compartment.

For this model one has to take into account the maximal difference of x-ray sensitivity of the various cell-cycle stages. The difference in the sensitivity is more pronounced in the first part of the dose-response curve, in the region of the shoulder. This difference can reach an isoeffective dose difference of a factor of two as seen in Figure 3. This higher dose-reduction factor in the beginning of the dose-response curves is a further argument for using more frequent small x-ray doses in therapeutic regimen. Based on these considerations, better therapeutic results can be expected if tumors with higher initial S-phase frequencies are treated with x-rays; tumors with lower S-phase frequencies should be treated preferentially with neutrons. The pretherapeutic cell-cycle phase frequencies can be measured routinely with a minimum expenditure of time and money.[10]

Summary

It is well-known that, in addition to cell inactivation, x-rays and neutrons cause cell-cycle phase progression delay. We have compared the dose-response curves after x- and neutron irradiation for cell inactivation and G_2-phase arrest *in vitro* on L-929 cells.

Both dose-response curves have the same shape for neutrons. However, after x-ray irradiation the shape of the two dose-response curves is different; after 1 Gy three times more cells are arrested temporarily in the G_2 phase of the cell-division cycle than are inactivated. The x-ray-induced kinetic effect leads to cell synchronization for the majority of cells.

The therapeutically usable range between the kinetic effect and cell inactivation could be utilized in treatment schedules if relatively low-dose fractions are used with time intervals in the range of the S-phase and $(G_2 + M)$-phase duration. The data suggest that dose fractionation of neutron irradiation, considering cell-cycle phenomena, will not be successful. Tumors with a relatively high initial frequency of S-phase cells should be treated with x-rays; tumors with lower S-phase frequencies should be administered for neutron treatment preferentially.

ACKNOWLEDGMENTS

This work was supported by the Arbeitsmeinschaft für Krebsbekämpfung im Lande Nordrhein-Westfalen, Düsseldorf, W. Germany.

REFERENCES

1. Bergonié, J., and Tribondeau, L. (translation by G. H. Fletcher): Interpretation of some results of radiotherapy and an attempt at determining a logical technique of treatment. *Radiat Res* **11**:587, 1959. (Originally published in 1906.)
2. Göhde, W.: Automation of cytofluorometry by use of the Impulsemicrophotometer. In *Fluorescence Techniques in Cell Biology* Berlin: Springer-Verlag, 1973, p. 79.
3. Göhde, W.: Zellzyklusanalysen mit dem Impulscytophotometer: Der Einflub chemischer und physikalischer Noxen auf die Proliferationskinetik von Tumorzellen. Thesis, Medical Faculty, University of Münster, 1973.
4. Göhde, W., Meistrich, M., Meyn, R., et al.: Cell-Cycle Phase-Dependence of Drug-Induced Cycle Progression Delay. *J Histochem Cytochem* **27**:470, 1979.
5. Göhde, W., Schumann, J., Büchner, T., Otto, F., and Barlogie, B.: Pulse cytophotometry: Application in tumor cell biology and clinical oncology. In *Flow Cytometry and Sorting* New York: Wiley, 1979, p. 599.
6. Kühn, H.: Aspects in practical neutron dosimetry with ionizing chambers. *Biophysik* **10**:229, 1973.
7. Madoc-Jones, H., and Mauro, F.: Age responses to x-ray, vinca alkaloids, and hydroxyurea of murine lymphoma cells synchronized in vivo. *J Nat Cancer Inst* **45**:1131, 1970.
8. Otto, F., and Göhde, W.: Effects of fast neutrons and x-ray irradiation on cell kinetics. In *Pulse-Cytophotometry II* Ghent: European Press, 1976, p. 244.
9. Sasaki, H., and Yoshinaga, H.: Study of proliferation kinetics of irradiated mammalian cells incorporating time-lapse photography. In *Fraction Size in Radiobiology and Radiotherapy* Munich: Urban and Schwarzenberg, 1974, p. 38.
10. Schumann, J., Göhde, W., and Straub, C.: Cytogenetic and cytokinetic characterisation of malignant melanoma (in press).
11. Sinclair, W. K.: Radiation effects on mammalian cell populations in vitro. In *Radiation Research* Amsterdam: North-Holland Publishing Company, 1966, p. 607.
12. Sinclair, W. K., and Morton, R. A.: X-ray sensitivity during the cell generation cycle of cultures of Chinese hamster cells. *Radiat Res* **29**:450, 1966.
13. Terasima, T., and Tolmach, L. J.: Variation in several responses of HeLa cells to x-irradiation during the division cycle. *Biophys J* **3**:11, 1963.
14. Trott, K. R.: Einige strahlenbiologische Aspekte der "Synchronisationstherapie" in der Tumorbehandlung. *Strahlentherapie* **42**:568, 1971.
15. Whitmore, G. F., Gulyas, S., and Botond, J.: Radiation sensitivity throughout the cell cycle and its relationship to recovery. In *XVII Animal Symposium on Fundamental Cancer Research, M. D. Anderson Hospital and Tumor Institute* Baltimore: Williams and Wilkins, 1965, p. 423.

CHAPTER 6

Antineoplastic Drugs and Radiation: Comparison of the Phenomena Determining the Effectiveness of Fractionated Treatments

Francesco Mauro, D.Sc.[a]
Giovanni Briganti, D.Sc.[b]
Carlo Nervi, M.D.[c]

The differential lethal effects of fractionated treatments depend upon a succession of partially overlapping cellular phenomena. In the case of ionizing radiation, an updated list of these phenomena would include the following:

1. Radiosensitivity—"intrinsic" cellular
2. Response according to the initial shape of the survival curve
3. Oxygen effect and reoxygenation
4. Repair from sublethal damage
5. Repair from potentially lethal damage
6. Age response and reassortment through the cell cycle
7. Recruitment of quiescent cells into cycle
8. Repopulation.

In recent years the radiation response has been reanalyzed according to these postirradiation events, with the hypothesis being that the effectiveness of radiotherapy would lie not in any greater intrinsic sensitivity of tumor cells to radiation, but in the schedule and modality of radiation delivery. Therefore, at least some of the R's of radiotherapy have been adequately reinvestigated.[17,36] This has been especially true for phenomena related to the proliferative state of normal and tumor tissue and, in a more general way, to the increasingly evident proliferative heterogeneity of human solid tumors.

The relative weight of each phenomenon in determining the end response to fractionated doses is still open to further research and debate, especially with regard to reoxygenation, reassortment, and recruitment. The fact remains that such an approach has furnished a useful framework to discuss biological rationales for new radiotherapy schemes and eventual manipulation of postirradiation events.

By analogy, the same general approach could be used to discuss the effectiveness of fractionated administrations of cytotoxic drugs. Of course, some important considerations should be taken into account: the first deals with pharmacodynamics; and the second concerns the fact that cytotoxic agents can be considered only approximately as "radiomimetic" and therefore not depending, in their action, upon the same categories of cellular phenomena (oxygen effect and reoxygenation being possible examples). Nevertheless, the description of the

[a]Senior Investigator, Laboratorio di Dosimetria e Biofisica, Comitato Nazionale per l'Energia Nucleare, Rome, Italy.
[b]Director, Laboratorio di Dosimetria e Biofisica, Comitato Nazionale per L'Energia Nucleare, Rome, Italy.
[c]Director, Istituto Medico e di Ricerca Scientifica, Rome, Italy.

TABLE 1. The R's of Chemotherapy

Drug-sensitivity, "intrinsic" cellular	Yes, according to mechanisms
Shape of the survival curve	?
Oxygen effect and reoxygenation	Possibly irrelevant
Repair from sublethal damage	?
Repair from potentially lethal damage	Yes, somewhat important[a]
Age-response and reassortment	Yes, very important[b]
Recruitment	Possibly important
Repopulation	Yes

[a] Ray et al., 1975; Barranco et al., 1975
[b] Madoc-Jones and Mauro, 1974; Hill, 1978

cell-cycle age-responses to cytotoxic agents has supplied the initial rationale for a less empirical administration of antineoplastic drugs—a fact lending favor to the validity of a cellular approach to the problem of establishing optimal drug administration schedules.

The state of the art with regard to the R's of chemotherapy is summarized in Table 1. In the present work an attempt is therefore made to collect the data about, and to discuss some of the neglected R's of, chemotherapy, using the same comparative approach for the phenomena determining the effectiveness of fractionated treatments for both radiation and antineoplastic drugs.

The Shape of Drug Survival Curves

Sigmoid survival curves, characterized by a shoulder region preceding the exponential part of the curve (which appears linear on a semilog plot), are typical of mammalian cells exposed to radiation *in vitro* and *in vivo*. The shoulder is generally associated with the requirement for accumulation of sublethal damage and the ability of the cell to repair it. Conversely, actual absence of such a shoulder in the curve—a fact seldom reported, perhaps related to anoxia—is associated with the lack of ability to accumulate sublethal damage. It is not clear at this time whether this association consistently applies to radiation survival curves only. However, a variety of recent observations has evidenced, in the region of low doses of radiation, an initial "nonzero" negative slope of the survival curve.[9] Sigmoid survival curves are also given by cells exposed to some cytotoxic drugs, especially alkylating agents,[7,23] including the instance of a shoulderless, simple exponential survival curve.[27] However, in the majority of cases tested, cytotoxic drugs—and especially antimetabolites and antibiotics—elicit survival curves described as biphasic,[3] hyperbolic,[6] or even exponential with a "negative" shoulder.[32] In some instances the curve exhibits an initial shoulder or threshold region, followed by a tract that, because of the uncertainties in the experimental points, can fit more than one plotting schema.

As far as cytotoxic drugs are concerned, an interpretation of the survival curve shape in terms of a detailed theoretical model is not yet at hand. In comparison to X-irradiation, chemical agents present the additional difficulty of yielding survival variations as a function of both exposure time (at a fixed, initial drug concentration) and drug concentration (during a fixed exposure time or for "continuous" exposures). *In vitro* as well as *in vivo* drug concentration may or may not remain constant—in terms of biologically active drugs—as a function of the time after administration. The situation approaches that of a radiation delivered at a relatively low, continuously decreasing dose rate. Finally, while the use of the integral-dose concept of "C × T" (at least in fractionation experiments) is a correct indica-

TABLE 2. Classification of Antineoplastic Drugs

Agent	Shape of the Survival Curve[a] Log	Plateau	Reference
Nitrogen mustard	A		Sakamoto and Elkind, 1969
Ethylmethanesulfonate	A	B	Hahn, 1969
McCCNU	B	A	Barranco, 1977
Rubidazone	A		Drewinko et al., 1979
Cis-platinum (II)	A		"
VP-16-213	A		"
3,3 Dimethlyltriazeno-o-benzoic acid	A		"
Cyclophosphamide	B		Dewys and Knight, 1969
Sulfur mustard	B		Mauro and Elkind, 1968
Methylmethanesulfonate	B	A	Hahn, 1969
CCNU	B		Drewinko et al., 1969
BCNU	B		"
L-Phenylalanine mustard	B		"
Yoshi 864	B		"
Cyclohexanecarboxylic acid, 4-(3-(2-chloroethyl)-3-nitrosoureido), *cis*	B		"
X-Rays	B	A/B	
Bleomycin	C	C	Mauro et al., 1974
Adriamycin	C[b]	C[b]	
Actinomycin D	C[b]	C[b]	
Camptothecin sodium	C		Drewinko et al., 1979
m-(di-(2-chloroethyl)-amino)-L-phenylalanine	C		"
Metronidazole	C[b]	B[b]	
Misonidazole	C[b]	B[b]	
ICRF 159	C		
Hydroxyurea	D		Drewinko et al., 1979
Methotrexate	D		"
O2, 2'-Cyclocytidine	D		"
Prednisolone	D		"

[a] Operational classification of survival curve shape (see Fig. 1): type A = simple exponential; type B = sigmoid; type C = biphasic ($1D_o$ higher than $2D_o$), hyperbolic, or with a "negative" shoulder preceding an exponential tract; type D = exponential with a final plateau

[b] Data from the authors' laboratory

tion,[1,35] it is not often easy and clear-cut. Recently, the opportunity of classifying antineoplastic drugs according to their survival curve shape—without theoretical implications as far as mechanisms are concerned but at least in operational terms only—has been advocated.[8,21] A classification of antineoplastic drugs according to their survival curve shape (essentially *in vitro* observations) is summarized in Figure 1 and Table 2.

Fractionation Effects of Antineoplastic Drugs

We have attempted to correlate the following kind of data from the literature and/or our unpublished laboratory work: (1) the shapes of the survival curves of various antineoplastic agents; (2) the presence or absence of an initial shoulder (including the "negative" shoulder); and (3) variation

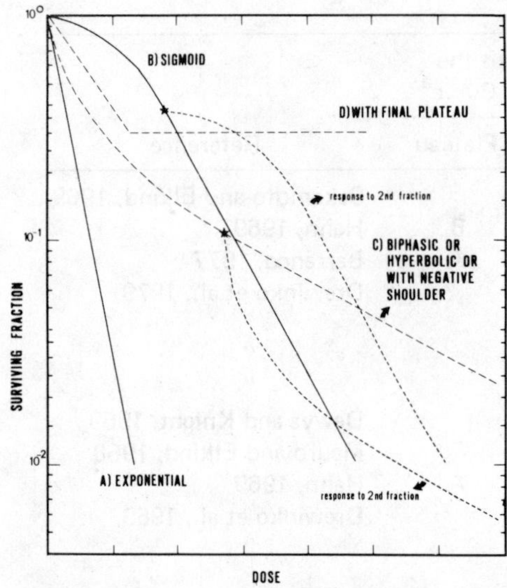

Figure 1. Operational Classification of Survival-Curve Shapes: type A = simple exponential; type B = sigmoid (initial shoulder followed by an exponential tract); type C = biphasic, hyperbolic, or with a "negative" shoulder preceding an exponential tract (see text); type D = exponential followed by a final plateau. In the case of the type-B curve, an example of response to a second dose fraction in a two-dose experiment is also reported. A response to a second dose fraction is also illustrated for a type-C ("negative" shoulder) curve. In the latter instance, the phenomenon is operationally contrary to the repair of sublethal damage, and can be described as "potentiation" by fractionation.

in survival observed after two-dose experiments.

Whenever possible, the information was taken from tests on either log- or plateau-phase cultures, and eventually from *in vivo* systems.

The data are reported in Table 3 (*in vitro*) and Table 4 (*in vivo*, hemopoietic stem cell system). They appear to indicate that a functional classification of cytotoxic agents according to the characteristics of the initial part of the survival curve (present, absent, or "negative" shoulder, independent from the actual overall shape of the curve) can be correlated, at least in operational terms, to the cellular response after two-dose (or multifraction) exposures. In particular, the possibility has to be taken into consideration that at least some cytotoxic agents, eliciting a survival curve with an initial upward concavity, induce a type of cellular damage that can be enhanced by fractionation ("potentiation" by fractionation). As originally proposed for bleomycin,[31,32] this could be due to a rapid, reversible induction of cellular resistance by the agent. Our own tests appear to exclude only the hypothesis of the involvement of differential sensitivity through the cycle.

Recruitment

Recruitment is definitively an attractive phenomenon and, hypothetically, may well explain some clinical observations on kinetic changes after cell-number reduction by antineoplastic therapy[19] or in recurrence vs. primary cell population. However, useful data are very scanty and refer to a handful of agents administered to malignant systems: (1) araC,[13] (2) bleomycin,[24] and (3) cyclophosphamide.[20] Even in the case of radiation, the relative importance and actual presence of recruitment in experimental tumor systems is still under discussion.[14,16] Therefore, some specific information, along the lines presented below, is badly needed to describe this elusive phenomenon, especially from the point of view of chemotherapeutic application.

1. Agent-specificity of recruitment: Are all cytotoxic agents also recruiting agents? Can other agents, such as chalones or hormones, be used as recruiting agents? (at this juncture screening has been reported only for the hemopoietic system.[34])
2. Dose-dependence of recruitment
3. Age-response characteristics of the reentry into cycle[5,22]
4. Methods of distinguishing recruitment from induced phenotypic resistance followed by outgrowth.

TABLE 3. Survival-Curve Shape and Fractionation Effect[a,b,c]

	Log	Plateau	Log	Plateau	Log	Plateau	*In Vivo Tests*
Alkylating Agents, Type A	A	A	0	0	0	0	
Alkylating Agents, Type B	B	B	+	+	+	+	
X-Rays	B	A/B	+	+/0	+	0	*
Bleomycin[d]	C	C	–	–	–	–	*
Adriamycin[d,e]	C	C	–	–	–	–	*
Metronidazole[d]	C	B	–	+	–	+	
Misonidazole[d,f]	C	B	–	+	–	+	

[a]Shoulder: + present; 0 no shoulder; – absent

[b]Fractionation effect: + increase in survival; 0 no variation; – decrease in survival

[c]Two-dose *in vitro* experiments have been performed either in full medium at 37°C or in buffer and/or room temperature so as to discriminate variations in survival due to cell-cycle age-response.

[d]Data from authors' laboratory

[e]The fractionation effect observed for adriamycin is dose dependent.

[f]Data from authors' laboratory; see also Stratford, 1978.

TABLE 4. Data on Hemopoietic Stem Cell System

	% Cells S Phrase	D_{37}(mg/kg)	*n*	Treatment Schedule (mg/kg)	Survival Ratio
Bleomycin					
CFU_s	4–8	630 ± 40	0.84	400 + 8 hr (control)	1.0[a]
				200 + 4 hr + 200 + 4 hr	1.2[a]
CFU_s-ENDX-stim.	50	960 ± 55	0.13	640 + 8 hr (control)	1.0[b]
				320 + 4 hr + 320 + 4 hr	0.57[b]
CFU_c	51	960 + 70	0.66	400 + 8 hr (control)	1.0[b]
				200 + 4 hr + 200 + 4 hr	0.44[b]
Adriamycin					
CFU_s	5–10	25 ± 5	1.2	28 + 8 hr (control)	1.0[a]
				14 + 4 hr + 14 + 8 hr	0.8[a]
CFU_c	51	20 ± 1	0.82	28 + 48 hr (control)	1.0[b]
				14 + 24 hr + 14 + 24 hr	0.3[b]

[a]T-test not significant

[b]T-test significant ($P < 0.01$)

[c]Exposure time chosen according to time-survival curve

Elements for Discussion

The aim of the present paper was to propose some working hypotheses on antineoplastic drug lethal effects so that the problem of fractionation effectiveness of chemical agents could be approached in "radiobiological" terms. The data presented appear to indicate that the effectiveness of drug fractionated treatments can be ascribed, as in the instance of radiation, to a series of partially overlapping cellular phenomena—some of which are typical of chemical agents only (limited "radiomimicry"). The phenomena relevant to fractionation effectiveness can be summarized as follows:

1. Shape of the survival curve
   a. Type B would imply that drug concentrations that are too low may

yield clinically irrelevant killing effects.[8]

b. Type C would imply that drug concentrations that are too high may not yield a clinically appreciable increase in killing effects; of course, differences should be allowed for various mechanisms responsible for this particular survival curve shape: (1) actual stage-specificity of the lethal effect; (2) heterogeneity of cell population with regard to drug sensitivity, independent from the cell position in the cycle; or (3) rapid, reversible induction of cellular resistance.

2. Drug persistence within the cell (adriamycin and anthracycline antibiotics being typical examples)
3. Repair from sublethal damage, when active
4. "Potentiation" by fractionation, at least for some antineoplastic drugs exhibiting a type-C survival curve. In these instances, multiple pulsed administrations of relatively low drug doses could be clinically more advantageous than the usual administrations repeated at relatively long intervals (e.g., the traditional 1-week interval); of course, such an approach would be valid only if, after a certain time, the biologically active agent becomes unavailable on the tumor site.
5. Repair from potentially lethal damage, when active (preferentially on nonproliferating cells?)
6. Age-response and reassortment (the main conditioning factor being the fraction of proliferating cells) according to:
   a. Differential killing through the cycle
   b. Differential proliferative block(s) in the cycle
   c. Resumption of cell progression along the cycle
7. Differential response of proliferating vs. nonproliferating cells
8. Differential response of euoxic vs. hypoxic or anoxic cells, if indeed existing in the case of (some) chemical agents[12,26,28]
9. Recruitment (?) in tumor vs. normal tissues and parasynchronous fluctuations taking place in the so-called "prereplicative"[5] and/or other "transition" phases
10. Repopulation
11. Induced phenotypic resistance (see Chapter 38). The occurrence of such a phenomenon would point to an important difference between radiation and drugs; in fact, in the case of radiation, while small decreases in inherent radiation response may be induced during the course of treatment (or resistant cells may be selected as treatment progresses), there is essentially no evidence that significant radiation resistance (or sensitization) develops during treatment; at least one reason for this is that radiation penetrates; however, with conventional chemotherapy spread over weeks or months, the induction and outgrowth of resistent clone of cells may become a likelihood after drug treatments,[10] due to a variety of reasons (physiological, transport, and/or genetic changes).

An example of how this complex of phenomena can qualitatively affect the results of a fractionated treatment with a single agent is shown in the schema of Table 5 for bleomycin. Unfortunately, the rank order of importance of the various phenomena is still open to discussion.

It must be clear, however, that to recognize the relevance of these phenomena in determining the response to a drug fractionated treatment should not mean an underestimation of other phenomena of a more specifically pharmacological nature, such as the kinetics of drug availability on the site,[29] the metabolic change of an agent into an active or inactive derivative, etc. Apart from the pharmacological problems, a "radiobiological" approach underlines the importance of further problems:

TABLE 5. Bleomycin: Effect of Several Phenomena on Overall Survival

<table>
<tr><th></th><th>High Fraction Proliferating Cells</th><th>Low-Fraction Proliferating Cells</th></tr>
<tr><td>Shape of Survival Curve (Type C)</td><td colspan="2">↑</td></tr>
<tr><td>Repair from Sublethal Damage</td><td colspan="2">–</td></tr>
<tr><td>"Potentiation" by Fractionation</td><td colspan="2">↓</td></tr>
<tr><td>Repair from Potentially Lethal Damage</td><td>↑</td><td>↑↑</td></tr>
<tr><td>Age-Response and Reassortment</td><td>↓</td><td>–</td></tr>
<tr><td>Proliferating vs. Nonproliferating Response</td><td>↓</td><td>–</td></tr>
<tr><td>Euoxic vs. Hypoxic or Anoxic Response</td><td colspan="2">?</td></tr>
<tr><td>Recruitment</td><td>–</td><td>↑</td></tr>
<tr><td>Parasynchronous Fluctuations after Recruitment</td><td>–</td><td>↓</td></tr>
<tr><td>Reoxygenation (after Radiation, prior to Drug)</td><td colspan="2">?</td></tr>
<tr><td>Repopulation</td><td colspan="2">↑</td></tr>
</table>

1. The question of the "time-of-assay" in experimental design and, as a matter of fact, of the "time-of-subsequent-administration" in clinical schemes: The delicacy of the timing is self-evident, as rightly emphasized by Twentyman[33] with regard to repair from potentially lethal damage *in situ*, standard suggestions being not yet available.
2. With regard to combined treatments, enhanced cell killing could be dependent not only upon the molecular characteristics of intracellular damage interaction per se,[10] but on the overlapping and preemption of the various mechanisms affecting the response to fractionation.
3. Synergistic effects should not be described only in empirical terms; the high number of mechanisms interfering with the cellular response to an agent administered subsequently to another agent may well lead to the emergency of a high number of "false" superadditive results.

The general feeling is that, with respect to biologically oriented radiation therapy, there is still a long way to go for a less empirically based chemotherapy.

This is even more true if we consider the amount of information available on radiobiological phenomena that, after all, refer only to one agent among a plethora of agents.

A Note of Caution

From 1972 to 1980 drug-survival curves and age-responses have been continuously rechecked at C.N.S. Casaccia's Laboratory—the data being kept as unpublished or personally quoted results. The data have been generally obtained on V79, CHO, and/or HeLa cell lines. Many of the traditional (and some of the new) antineoplastic drugs have been tested and retested. The following critical conclusions can be drawn with regards to drug response:

1. Drug effectiveness is line dependent and can even change in the same line according to its age in terms of transplant number (checks have been made with frozen down samples).
2. Drug effectiveness is medium, serum, temperature, and proliferation dependent.
3. Age-response often depends on the synchronization method and sometimes is dose dependent; some line-dependent differences are possible.
4. Survival-curve shape(s) can vary according to (1) and (2) above.

In spite of these limitations, some general conclusions remain valid or can be reintroduced, mainly:

1. Various shapes of survival curves are

possible and can be associated with (empirical) groups of drugs.
2. Often, the survival-curve shape is *not* exponential or sigmoid, even if so reported in the literature; it is necessary to recognize that, in the past, curves were expected to be linear on the semilog plot and, accordingly, a "preferential" fitting was used.
3. Almost all drugs exhibit some kind of age-response.
4. The age-response of the majority of drugs can be described as stage-preferential-specificity, *not* as actual stage-specificity.
5. The qualitative aspects of the various age-responses can often be associated with (empirical) groups of drugs.

In vitro systems can only be considered as models for studying antineoplastic drugs, with scarse similarity to *in vivo* systems. Furthermore, agent-effectiveness seems to present gross variations in traditional vs. newly developed clonogenic test systems (see Chapter 46). It is likely that many of the same limitations apply to *in vivo* experimental systems, especially if murine or rodent in origin. A strict (quantitative and qualitative) similarity between experimental and clinical response can neither be suggested nor implied.

Acknowledgments

Critical comments and suggestions by Drs. M.M. Elkind and B. Drewinko have been essential in preparing the manuscript and are greatly appreciated. The collaboration of Drs. G. Levi, A. Sacchi, and G. Zupi in some of the reported experiments is dutifully acknowledged.

Summary

In the last ten years the criteria for effective radiotherapy regimens have been rediscussed by analyzing the dependence of radiation response upon the radiobiological phenomena affecting the results of fractionated treatments. In the original definition of H.R. Withers, these phenomena have been referred to as the four R's of radiotherapy, and today we suspect that their number may be higher than that. By analogy, and in spite of the fact that chemical cytotoxic agents are seldom radiomimetic in the strict sense of the word, a similar general analysis could be used to discuss the effectiveness of fractionated administrations of antineoplastic drugs. However, information is only available for the cell-cycle age-dependence of lethal and kinetic effects and the repair from potentially lethal damage induced by these agents. In the present work, an attempt is made to discuss some of the neglected R's of chemotherapy, with the aim of establishing (not exclusively empirical) criteria for drug scheduling and of clarifying some of the observations on interaction between agents. In particular, with regard to antineoplastic drugs, published and unpublished information is available not only for the well-known phenomenon of reassortment, but also for the shape of the survival curve, recovery (or potentiation) between dose fraction, and recruitment. Some advantages (and pitfalls) can be evidenced when applying this kind of radiobiological approach to chemotherapy.

REFERENCES

1. Barranco, S.C.: *In vitro* responses of mammalian cells to drug-induced potentially lethal and sublethal damage. *Cancer Treat Rep* **60**:1799–1810, 1976.
2. Barranco, S.C.: Cell kill and recovery in exponentially growing and stationary phase cells. In *Growth Kinetics and Biochemical Regulation of Normal and Malignant Cells* B., Drewinko and R.M., Humphrey, eds. Baltimore: Williams & Wilkins, 1977, pp. 689–703.
3. Barranco, S.C., Gerner, E.W., Burk, K.H., and Humphrey, R.M.: Survival and cell kinetic effects of Adriamycin on mammalian cells. *Cancer Res* **33**:11–16, 1973.

4. Barranco, S.C., Novak, J.K., and Humphrey, R.M.: Studies on recovery from chemically induced damage in mammalian cells. *Cancer Res* **35**:1194–1204, 1975.
5. Baserga, R.: *Multiplication and Division in Mammalian Cells* New York: M. Dekker, 1976.
6. Berenbaum, M.C.: Dose-response curves for agents that impair cell reproductive integrity: A fundamental difference between dose-response curves for antimetabolites and those for radiation and alkylating agents. *Antibiot Chemother* **15**:426–433, 1969.
7. DeWys, W.C., and Knight, N.: Kinetics of cyclophosphamide damage: Sublethal damage repair and cell-cycle-related sensitivity. *J Natl Cancer Inst* **42**:155–163, 1969.
8. Drewinko, B., Roper, P.R., and Balrogie, B.: Patterns of cell survival following treatment with antitumor agents *in vitro. Eur J Cancer* **15**:93–99, 1979.
9. Elkind, M.M.: The initial part of the survival curve: Implications for low-dose, low-dose-rate radiation response. *Radiat Res* **71**:9–23, 1977.
10. Elkind, M.M.: Fundamental questions in the combined use of radiation and chemicals in the treatment of cancer. *Int J Radiat Oncol Biol Phys* **5**:1711–1720, 1979.
11. Hahn, G.M.: Radiochemotherapy of cell cultures containing cycling and non-cycling cells. *Front Radiat Ther Oncol* **4**:17–23, 1969.
12. Harris, J.W., and Shrieve, D.C.: Effects of Adriamycin and X-rays on euoxic and hypoxic EMT-6 cells *in vitro. Int J Radiat Oncol Biol Phys* **5**:1245–1248, 1978.
13. Hartmann, N.R., Dombernowsky, P., and Bichel, P.: Resting cells L1210 and JB1 ascites tumors with special emphasis on recycling. *Cancer Treat Rep* **60**:1861–1870, 1976.
14. Hermens, A.F., and Barendsen, G.W.: Effects of ionizing radiation on the growth kinetics of tumors. In *Growth Kinetics and Biomedical Regulation of Normal and Malignant Cells* B. Drewinko and R.M. Humphrey, eds. Baltimore: Williams & Wilkins, 1977, pp. 531–545.
15. Hill, B.T.: Cancer chemotherapy: The relevance of certain concepts of the cell cycle kinetics. *Biochim Biophys Acta* **516**:389–417, 1978.
16. Kallman, R.F.: Text of discussion after the paper presented by A.F. Hermens. In *Growth Kinetics and Biochemical Regulation of Normal and Malignant Cells* B. Drewinko, and R.M. Humphrey, eds. Baltimore: Williams & Wilkins, 1977, pp. 545–546.
17. Kallman, R.F.: Facts and models applied to tumor radiotherapy. *Int J Radiat Oncol Biol Phys* **5**:1103–1109, 1979.
18. Madoc-Jones, H., and Mauro, F.: Site of action of cytotoxic agents in the cell life cycle. In *Handbook of Experimental Pharmacology* Vol. 38/1, A. Sartorelli, and D. Johns, eds. Berlin: Springer-Verlag, 1974, pp. 205–219.
19. Mauer, A.M., Murphy, S.B., and Hayes, F.A.: Evidence for recruitment and synchronization in leukemia and solid tumors. *Cancer Treat Rep* **60**:1841–1843, 1976.
20. Mauer, A.M., Murphy, S.B., Hayes, F.A., and Dahl, G.V.: Scheduling and recruitment in malignant cell populations. In *Growth Kinetics and Biochemical Regulation of Normal and Malignant Cells* B. Drewinko, and R.M. Humphrey, eds. Baltimore: Williams & Wilkins, 1977, pp. 855–864.
21. Mauro, F.: Effetti del frazionamento della dose di radiazioni o farmaci antineoplastici su colture di cellule in fase logaritmica o di plateau di crescita. In *Radiobiologia dei Tumor* C. Biagini, and M. DiPaola, eds. Rome: E.M.S.I., 1978, pp. 168–173.
22. Mauro, F., Briganti, G., and Zupi, G.: A rationale for the search of the missing agent in cancer combination therapy. In *International Symposium on Radiobiological Research Needed for the Improvement of Radiotherapy* M. Beck, ed. Vienna: I.A.E.A., 1977.
23. Mauro, F., and Elkind, M.M.: Comparison of repair of sublethal damage in cultured Chinese hamster cells exposed to sulfur mustard and X-rays. *Cancer Res* **28**:1156–1161, 1968.
24. Mauro, F., Falpo, B., Briganti, G., Elli, R., and Zupi, G.: Effects of antineoplastic drugs on plateau-phase cultures of mammalian cells. 2. Bleomycin and hydroxyurea. *J Natl Cancer Inst* **52**:715–722, 1974.
25. Ray, G.R., Hahn, G.M., Bagshaw, M.A., and Kurkjian, S.: Cell survival and repair of plateau-phase cultures after chemotherapy. *Cancer Treat Rep* **57**:473–475, 1975.
26. Roizin-Towle, L., and Hall, E.J.: The effect of bleomycin on aerated and hypoxic cells *in vitro*, in combination with irradiation. *Int J Radiat Oncol Biol Phys* **5**:1491–1494, 1979.
27. Sakamoto, K., and Elkind, M.M.: X-ray and nitrogen mustard independent action in Chinese hamster cells. *Biophys J* **9**:1115–1161, 1969.
28. Shrieve, D.C., and Harris, J.W.: Effects of bleomycin and irradiation on euoxic and hypoxic cells. *Int J Radiat Oncol Biol Phys* **5**:1495–1498, 1979.
29. Siemann, D.W., and Sutherland, R.M.: A comparison of the pharmacokinetics of multiple and single dose administration of adriamycin. *Int J Radiat Oncol Biol Phys* **5**:1271–1274, 1979.
30. Stratford, I.J.: Split dose cytotoxic experiments with misonidazole. *Br J Cancer* **38**:130–136, 1978.
31. Takabe, Y., Katsumata, T., and Watanabe, M.: Lethal effect of bleomycin on cultured mouse L cells: Comparison between fractionated and continuous treatment. *Gann* **63**:645–646, 1972.
32. Terasima, T., Takabe, Y., Katsumata, T., Watanabe, M., and Umezawa, H.: Effect of bleomycin on mammalian cells. *J Nat Cancer Inst* **49**:1093–1100, 1972.

33. Twentyman, P.R.: Timing of assays: An important consideration in the determination of clonogenic cell survival both *in vitro* and *in vivo*. *Int J Radiat Oncol Biol Phys* **5**:1213–1220, 1979.
34. van Putten, L.M.: Recruitment, une arme à double tranchant dans la chimiothérapie du cancer. *Bull Cancer* **60**:131–142, 1973.
35. Wheeler, K.T., Levin, V.A., and Deen, F.D.: The concept of drug dose for *in vitro* studies with chemotherapeutic agents. *Radiat Res* **76**:441–458, 1978.
36. Withers, H.R.: The 4 R's of radiotherapy. *Adv Radiat Biol* **5**:241–271, 1975.

CHAPTER 7

Contribution of the Discussion Initiators

Ralph R. Weichselbaum, M.D.[a]
Mortimer M. Elkind, B.M.E., M.M.E., M.S., Ph.D.[b]

L.J. Peters carefully defined clinical terms necessary to stress the problem of local failure in clinical radiation oncology. He separates technical from biological factors and presented meaningful definitions for the terms "radioresistance" and "radiosensitive." He divides the biologic parameters as follows:

1. Tumor-related factors such as hypoxia, cell kinetics, and intrinsic sensitivity (including repair competence)
2. Host factors, such as dose-limiting normal tissue effects, as they relate to tumor volume and to host defense mechanisms
3. Probabilistic radioresistance–that is, heterogeneous tumor populations that have some probability of developing resistance during therapy for any of the reasons noted above.

Peters suggests that each tumor may require an individual therapeutic strategy for optimal treatment based on the foregoing considerations, and he emphasized the complexity of the dose-response function for individual tumors.

[a]Associated Professor, Radiation Therapy Department, Harvard Medical School, Head, Peter Bent Brigham Division, Joint Center, Radiation Therapy Department, Boston, Mass.

[b]Senior Biophysicist, Division of Biological and Medical Research, Argonne National Laboratory, Argonne, Ill., Professor, Department of Radiology, The University of Chicago, Chicago, Ill.

H.D. Suit stressed that one never obtains a cure without local control and pointed to animal data suggesting that local recurrence should be viewed as distinct from the development of distant metastases.

G.W. Barendsen described a range of radiobiologic parameters of animal tumors of different histiologic types. These include the R-1 sarcoma, the ROS-1 sarcoma, the RUC-2 carcinomas, and the MLS lymphosarcoma. Barendsen stresses that a dose fraction of 200 rad, which may yield only small differences in single-dose surviving fractions, can result in large changes in net surviving fractions after multiple fractions. He further emphasizes that the initial slope is an important radiobiologic parameter.

R.R. Weichselbaum reviewed the multivariate complexity of human tumor radiocurability. He describes radiation survival-curve parameters (n, D_o) for cells derived from a variety of human tumors of varying radiocurability. Most of the cell lines in exponential growth gave relatively homogeneous survival-curve parameters (n = 1.2–2.2, D_o = 131–150 rad). However, a human lymphoma line showed an unusual radiosensitivity *in vitro* (D_o = 69 rad), and a human melanoma line displayed on unusual radioresistance (D_o = 220 rad).

The repair of potentially lethal x-ray damage was described in nine human tumor cell lines by Weichselbaum. A melanoma line and an osteosarcoma cell line affected significantly more (10-fold recovery) repair of potentially lethal damage than lines from three tumors considered to be radiocurable (two breast cancer lines and one neuroblastoma line). Six tumor lines from tumors not considered radiocurable were intermediate in their ability to repair potentially lethal damage (three- to five-fold recovery).

W. Göhde employed L-929 cells to investigate the relationship of irradiation-induced cell-cycle phase-progression delay and cell inactiovation. He concluded that progression delay through the cell cycle and cell inactivation show no close correlation, and at low x-ray doses more cells show delay than inactivation. A multifractionation low-dose scheme, as suggested by Göhde, might employ small single x-ray doses given within time intervals of the duration of the S phase to take advantage of radiation-induced parasynchronization and specific cell-cycle sensitivities to x-rays. Göhde also suggested that flow cytometry could be used to measure the relationship of proliferating to noncycling cells within individual tumors.

F. Mauro suggested that efficacy of radiation treatment schemes is not related to greater intrinsic radiosensitivities of tumor cells but to the schedule and modality according to which the radiation is applied. He also stressed that factors such as repair, recruitment, repopulation, reassortment, and reoxygenation may assume new importance. He drew an analogy between the fractionated administration of radiation and cytotoxic drugs, and emphasized certain pharmacodynamic and cellular differences. Mauro attempted to design scientific rationales for the employment of certain chemotherapeutic regimens based upon: (1) the shape of drug survival curves (this includes repair of damage and cellular drug sensitivity as reflected by curve shape); (2) fractionation effects of antineoplastic drugs; and (3) cell recruitment.

Mauro reviewed the shapes of four basic drug survival curves–simple exponential, sigmoid, biphasic, and exponential with a final plateau. He suggested the equation of biologic and pharmacologic concentration × time (C × T) information to initiate time/dose (concentration) relationships for combination drug regimens.

The final discussion of the session centered on whether assays of clones resistant to chemotherapy and/or radiation therapy are possible, and whether flow cytometry could provide an adequate assay of the kinetic determinants of the cells in individual human tumors. The apparent differences between the repair of sublethal damage *in vivo* and *in vitro* were discussed as well as the ultimate importance of local control in the therapeutic regimen. For most human tumors of different histological subtypes tumor size was felt to be the major determinant of radiocurability. The emergence of resistant clones to drugs or to ionizing radiation, as well as the repair of potentially lethal damage in large vs. small tumors, was also discussed.

CHAPTER 8

Keynote Address: Hypoxic Cells in Reoxygenation: Role of Radiation Resistance

Herman D. Suit, M.D., D.Phil.[a]

The problem to be discussed is whether viable and hypoxic cells exist in human tumors and represent a cause for an important proportion of the failures of conventional (low LET) radiation therapy (1.5–3 Gy per fraction) to achieve permanent local control of the treated lesion. There has been a high and sustained interest in biologic and radiobiologic studies of hypoxia in tumor tissue since 1953 when Gray et al.[12] called attention to the radiation sensitizing power of oxygen and the possibility that hypoxic cells were present in human tumors but not to an important extent in most normal tissue. At that time, Scott[24] showed that the response of Ehrlich ascites tumor transplants in legs of mice to single radiation doses was increased by allowing the animal to respire oxygen at increased pressure during the irradiation. The enhancement of response was greater for tumor than for skin. Thomlinson and Gray[37] subsequently demonstrated that necrotic regions were observed in human bronchogenic carcinomas at distances from capillaries which corresponded to the calculated diffusion length of oxygen. They posited that adjacent to the necrotic region there would be viable and hypoxic cells which could be a cause of recurrence of tumor following treatment.

[b]Director of Cancer Management, Massachusetts General Hospital. Harvard Medical School, Boston, Mass.

Since then, there has been extensive documentation of the fact that oxygen is a potent sensitizer of lethal response of mammalian cells to low LET radiation.[13] Much evidence has accumulated for the presence of hypoxic cells and their importance to the radiation response of murine tumors, and to a lesser extent of human tumors. This evidence includes polarographic estimates of tissue pO_2,[5,18] reduced levels of oxyhemoglobin in the erythrocytes in tumor capillaries,[42] radiobiologic estimates of the proportion of tumor cells which are hypoxic,[19] modification of response of tumor to radiation by hyperbaric oxygen,[26,41] and chemical hypoxic cell sensitizers (such as misonidazole[1,8]) and the use of high LET radiations.[9]

Determination in quantitative terms of the role of hypoxic cells in the response of human tumor tissue to fractionated irradiation is not feasible because of the complexity of parameters of radiation response. These parameters are listed in Table 1. In examining the results of a particular treatment, it is essential to allow for the fact that observed local control frequency is derived from the treatment of a population of spontaneous tumors, each with a unique profile of values for the listed parameters. Due to the number of important parameters (and to the fact that many of them are interdependent, e.g., reoxygenation, repair, and proliferation), I will consider for this review

TABLE 1. Parameters of Response of Tissue to Fractioned Irradiation

1. Number of viable cells
2. Distribution of values for the parameters of cellular radiation sensitivity.
   a. *Do, n* (parameters of the multitarget, single-hit model)
   b. Age-response function
   c. Age-density distribution
   d. Distribution of pO_2 (OER, reoxygenation)
3. Kinetics and magnitude of repair of radiation damage
   a. Sublethal damage
   b. Potentially lethal damage
   c. "Slow repair"
4. Proliferation kinetics of the surviving cells
   a. Growth fraction
   b. Cell-loss factor
   c. Distribution of cell-cycle times
5. Magnitude and character of the host reaction against tumor

only studies of the efficacy of hyperbaric oxygen, tourniquet hypoxic, or the chemical sensitizer of hypoxic cells to modify the response of tumor tissue *in vivo.* Any observed enhancement of tumor response due to the use of these modalities can be accepted as proof that hypoxic cells are important factors. The absence of an improvement does not mean that hypoxic cells were not significant factors. Cytotoxicity of oxygen is considered to be negligible, and the induced cytotoxicity by tourniquet-produced hypoxia or by the chemical sensitizer is judged to be of minor importance. Reference will not be made to investigations of experimental or clinical radiation therapy using high LET radiation beams because repair kinetics and age-response functions are LET dependent. Hence, superior results might be due to factors other than a low OER and as such cannot unequivocally be ascribed to overcoming, in part, the hypoxic cells.

Hyperbaric Oxygen and Chemical Sensitizers of Hypoxic Cells in Murine Tumor Systems

There is now extensive evidence that in unperturbed murine tumors there are viable and hypoxic cells. In a review of this subject by Kallman,[19] the proportions of hypoxic cells in 12 tumor systems were listed as in the range of 1 to 50%. Kallman,[20] in his discussion of this paper, expands on this from a more recent view of the subject.

A wide variety of murine tumors (adenocarcinoma, sarcoma, and squamous cell carcinoma) have been investigated to assess the efficacy of respiration of oxygen at one to four atmospheres of pressure absolute to increase the efficacy of single- or multidose radiation. Table 2 is a listing of results of several studies. In all instances where fractionated irradiation was used in combination with $O_2$3ATA (respiration of oxygen at three atmospheres of pressure absolute), a positive enhancement ratio was observed. In an intensive investigation of fractionated irradiation combined with $O_2$3ATA using 8-mm isotransplants of MDAH-MCa IV, enhancement ratios (TCD50 aIR/$O_2$3ATA) were found to be in the range of 1.6 to 2.0 for radiation given in 2 to 10 fractions over total time periods of 3 to 18 days.[26] Of special interest is the enhancement ratio at low doses per fraction, namely ≃ 2 to 3 Gy. The only data known to the author dealing with this point are also from an experiment using the MCa IV (8-mm isotransplants). Radiation was administered in 24 equal doses with three fractions per day (intertreatment interval of 4 hours) and an overall treatment

TABLE 2. Laboratory Studies of the Effect of Respiration of Oxygen at 1 to 4 ATA on the Response of Murine Tumors to Irradiation

Tumor System	O_2 Pressure (ATA)	Dose Fraction Number	Positive ER[a]	Reference
C3H	1	6	No	DuSault (1963)
Spontaneous MCa (autochthonous)	3	6	Yes	DuSault (1963)
C3H MCa	1	2	Yes	Inch (1970)
DBAG tumor	3	1	No	Goldfeder (1960)
DBAH tumor	3	1	No	Goldfeder (1960)
R1B5 sarcoma	1 to 4	1	Yes	Thomlinson (1967)
Ehrlich tumor	3 to 4	1 to 3	Yes	van den Brenk (1967)
C3H MCa	3	2[b]	Yes	Howes (1969)
C3H MDAH MCa IV	1	10	Yes	Suit (1972)
	3	1 to 24	Yes	Suit (1977)
C3H FSaI	3	1,10	Yes	Suit (1967)
C3H MDAH SCC	3	1	No	Suit (1967)
		10	Yes	Suit (1967)
DBA-MCa	3	1	No	Suit (1967)
		10	Yes	Suit (1967)
C3H SCCVII	3	5,10	Yes	(unpub.)

[a] ER is enhancement ratio.
[b] Only the second dose was given under $O_2$3ATA conditions.

time of 8 days. The enhancement ratio using local control of tumor was 1.3 (TCD50 air/$O_2$3ATA), and this obtained for dose per fraction of ≃ 4 Gy. Figure 1 shows the plot of median recurrence times as a function of dose per fraction for radiation administered under $O_2$3ATA or air of control conditions. At 2.25 to 5 Gy per fraction, enhancement ratios in terms of recurrence time were ≃ 1.4.[32] These results document that at ≃ 2 to 3 Gy per fraction, $O_2$3ATA modifies the response to radiation, at least for this one tumor system.

There has also been extensive evaluation of the chemical sensitizers metronidazole and misonidazole to increase the response of murine tumors to local irradiation. Stone and Withers[25] were among the first to report a clearly positive enhancement ratio (for metronidazole). Fowler and Denekamp[8] summarized much of the data in the literature relating to enhancement ratios for misonidazole injection when given 1, 2, 3, 5, 10, or 20 equal dose fractions. There was a ten-

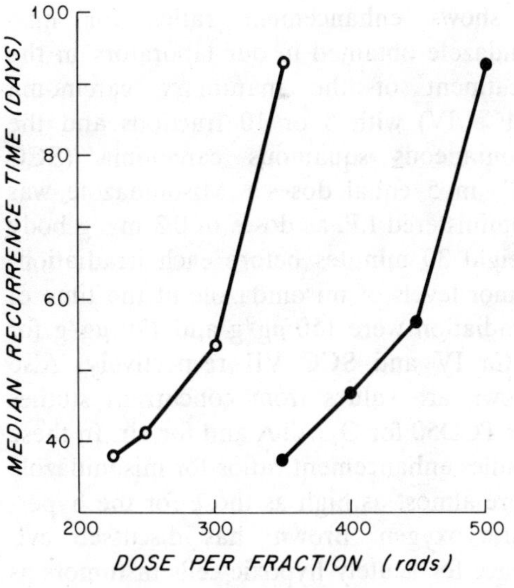

Figure 1. Efficacy of respiration of O_2 at 30 psi in modifying recurrence times of mammary carcinoma. Radiation was given in 24 equal doses, three fractions a day, with 4 hours between treatments given in any one day. Open circles = O_2 30 psi; full circles = air.

TABLE 3. ER for $O_2$3ATA and Misonidazole in the Fractionated Radiation Treatment of MCa IV and SCC VII

Tumor/ Treatment	TCD50 Values (Gy)			ER	
	Air	Misonidazole[a]	$O_2$3ATA[b]	Misonidazole	$O_2$3ATA
MCa IV					
6 mm/ ν=5; t_i=1d	75.8 (67.3 . . . 85.4)[c]	47.8 (35.8 . . . 63.8)	38.6 (30.4 . . . 48.9)	1.58	1.96
8 mm/ ν=5; t_i=1d	97.6 (84.7 . . . 112)	63.1 (49.8 . . . 80.1)	62.4 (50.4 . . . 77.1)	1.55	1.56
8 mm/ ν=10; t_i=1d	108.6 (96.1 . . . 122.8)	64.6 (54.8 . . . 76.2)	60.7 (55.5 . . . 66.5)	1.68	1.79
SCCVII					
6 mm/ ν=5; t_i=1d	134.8 (127.7 . . . 142.2)	95.2 (89.2 . . . 101.6)	85.4 (69.4 . . . 105.3)	1.42	1.58

[a] Misonidazole (0.3 mg/g BW) was administered I.P. at 30 minutes before irradiation.
[b] Mice were anesthetized by an I.P. injection of 0.05 mg/g BW of sodium pentobarbital.
[c] 95% confidence intervals.

dency for the observed enhancement ratio to decrease with fractionation number–i.e., enhancement ratios for single doses were often in the range of 1.7 to 2.1, but for treatment in 5 or 10 equal doses enhancement ratios were in the range of 1.0 to 1.7. Table 3 shows enhancement ratios for misonidazole obtained in our laboratory in the treatment of the mammary carcinoma (MCa IV) with 5 or 10 fractions and the spontaneous squamous carcinoma (SCC VII) in 5 equal doses.[29] Misonidazole was administered I.P. as doses of 0.3 mg/g body weight 30 minutes before each irradiation; tumor levels of misonidazole at the time of irradiation were 150 μg/g and 170 μg/g for MCa IV and SCC VII respectively. Also shown are values from concurrent studies for TCD50 for $O_2$3ATA and for air. In these studies enhancement ratios for misonidazole were almost as high as those for the hyperbaric oxygen. Brown[2] has discussed evidence for acutely hypoxic cells in tumors as being the critical tumor cells in tumor response. He suggested that they might be produced by temporary closing of capillaries. If so, chemicals such as misonidazole, which are metabolized slowly, would be expected to have a greater access to these foci of hypoxic cells than would molecular oxygen. He predicted that such chemical sensitizers would accordingly be more effective as sensitizers of hypoxic cells than would oxygen. In the MCa IV and SCC VII tumor system, $O_2$3ATA achieves enhancement ratios at least as high as does 0.3 mg/g BW of misonidazole; this result indicates that, at least in this tumor system, oxygen has access to the "critical" hypoxic cells.

Clinical Studies

The least ambiguous evidence as to the role of hypoxic cells in the success of clinical radiation therapy are results from radiation therapy administered while patients respire oxygen at high pressure or to patients under conditions of tourniquet-produced hypoxia. There are in fact substantial data from prospective randomized clinical trials for patients who were irradiated either under air conditions or while respiring oxygen at 3 atmospheres absolute (unanesthetized). These have been reviewed previously and will be considered here only briefly.[34] Table 4 shows the results of the Cardiff Second Trial

TABLE 4. Hyperbaric Oxygen and Radiation Therapy in Treatment of Head and Neck Cancer[a]

	HPO[b]	AIR[c]
Patients	51	52
Local Control of Primary Lesion (2 Years)	65%	47% ($0.1 > p > 0.05$)
Survival (2 Years)	71%	50% ($p < 0.02$)

[a] Data from Cardiff Second Trial (See Henk et al., 1977).
[b] Dose = 10 fractions of 4 Gy given over 22 days.

TABLE 5. Local Control and Survival at 4 Years in Patients with Stage III Carcinoma of the Uterine Cervix Treated by Radiation and Hyperbaric Oxygen[a]

		Local Control			Survivors		
Center	No. Patients	$O_2$3ATA	Air	p Value	$O_2$3ATA	Air	p Value
Glasgow	127	87%	60%	0.01	50%	37%	0.1
Mt. Vernon	56	76%	46%	0.04	39%	28%	0.66

[a] Watson et al., 1978

of hyperbaric oxygen in the treatment of squamous cell carcinoma of the head and neck region.[15] The treatment protocols were $O_2$3ATA, 4 Gy × 10 in ≃ 22 days; air or control, 2 Gy × 30 in 6 weeks. There was an increase in local control rate ($0.1 > p > 0.05$), and a significant increase in the survival ($p < 0.02$). There was no evidence of an increased normal tissue reaction in the oxygen series. This improvement in results is substantiated by their first trial in which both the air and the $O_2$3ATA arm were administered in 10 doses of ≃ 4 Gy.[14] There have been several studies of $O_2$3ATA and radiation therapy in the treatment of carcinoma of the uterine cervix. The Medical Research Council Trial (UK) was based on separate trials at Portsmouth, Oxford, Glasgow, and Mount Vernon.[44] Different fractionation schedules and total dose were used in each of these trials. Survival and local control frequencies were higher in the hyperbaric oxygen patients than in the air or control patients in each trial. Table 5 presents the local control survival results from the Glasgow and Mount Vernon trials; these are referred to specifically because relatively conventional fractionation schedules were employed. As shown, local control rates were significantly higher in the $O_2$3ATA patients. Survival, however, was not significantly greater in either study alone; if the data for the two studies were pooled, they would show a significant difference in favor of the $O_2$3ATA patients.[34] A small advantage for the $O_2$3ATA patients was found in the trial sponsored by the Radiation Therapy Oncology Group with respect to disease-free survival.[23] No advantage for hyperbaric oxygen was reported in the trials of hyperbaric oxygen and radiation therapy in treatment of carcinoma of the uterine cervix by Fletcher et al.,[7] Glasburn et al.,[10] or Ward et al.[43]

One center has performed two trials of hyperbaric oxygen and radiation therapy in the treatment of carcinoma of the bronchus and reported positive results in each (see Table 6). There was no improvement of results of radiation therapy of carcinoma of the urinary bladder by hyperbaric oxygen in one large trial;[3] in two limited studies there was an advantage (not significant) for hyperbaric oxygen treating carcinoma of the bladder.[22,39]

In summary there is evidence from prospective clinical trials that radiation administered to patients respiring O_2 at 3ATA is

TABLE 6. Hyperbaric Oxygen and Radiation Therapy in Treatment of Squamous Cell Carcinoma of Bronchus[a]

Survival at 2 Years				
Dose	ν[b]	Patients	HPO	AIR
6000 rad	40	51	14.8%	8.3%
3600 rad	6	123	24.6%	12.4%

[a]Data from St. Mary's General Hospital (Portsmouth) Trial (see Cade and McEwan, 1978).
[b]ν = number of fractions.

more effective than radiation alone in the treatment of patients with carcinomas of the head and neck region and of the bronchus. The evidence is mixed for carcinoma of the uterine cervix, and no apparent benefit is seen for carcinoma of the bladder. In contrast to the data from clinical investigations, studies based upon laboratory animal tumors have regularly demonstrated a substantial enhancement ratio for $O_2$3ATA combined with fractionated irradiation. One obvious technical difference between the treatment of patients and of mice is that the former have been conscious and the latter anesthetized. In a limited series of experiments in our laboratory using the mammary carcinoma (MCa IV) and squamous cell carcinoma (SCC VII), $O_2$3ATA has been more effective with radiation when the host mice have been anesthetized (sodium pentobarbital at 0.05 mg/g BW I.P.); for a preliminary report, see Suit et al.[30] Provided these data can be confirmed with other tumor systems and fractionation schedules, the potential value of anesthesia in clinical application of hyperbaric oxygen could be considered.

Radiation Therapy Under Tourniquet Hypoxic Conditions For Sarcomas of Bone and Soft Tissue

Local control of osteosarcoma following 140 Gy administered under conditions of tourniquet-induced hypoxia (14 fractions in 43 days) was achieved in only one of four patients, i.e., there were three local regrowths.[27] Local control was obtained in each of three patients followed for more than 12 months after 160 Gy (16 fractions in 50 days); however, the late fibrosis was unacceptably severe. Survival in these patients whose tumors were treated to 140 or 160 Gy was short because of development of distant metastasis; accordingly, long-term assessments of local control by this approach has not been made. The technique was discontinued by those authors because of the observed frequency of local failure and the severity of late changes in the 160-Gy group. In a clinical trial of tourniquet-induced hypoxia and radiation therapy for sarcoma of soft tissue there was no evident advantage for the tourniquet hypoxic patient; good results were obtained in the control and the study arm.[33] In that series, treatment was administered postsurgery (to a small residual cell number); this was in contrast to the use of the tourniquet technique in the treatment of osteosarcoma where the radiation was the sole modality and was therefore used in the treatment of a large mass of sarcoma tissue. Clinical studies by van den Brenk[40] also failed to yield evidence of a clear gain by the use of the tourniquet technique. In summary the available evidence does not indicate a therapeutic gain by administering radiation with tourniquet-technique conditions.

Clinical Testing of Chemical Sensitizers of Hypoxic Cells

The data from two clinical trials of the chemical sensitizer of the hypoxic cells indicate a modest gain. Urtasun et al.[38] employed metronidazole in combination with radiation therapy in the treatment of high-grade gliomas and reported significant prolongation of median survival time. Survival in the control group was, however, not as high as that obtained in most centers using a conventional approach. At this meeting, Kogelnik and Karcher[21] reported significant prolongation in median survival time for patients with supratentorial astrocytomas of grades III and IV treated by misonidazole and radiation. Although the observed survival time for the misonidazole and radiation group is superior to that expected for radiation alone, it is comparable to that being obtained by the combination of chemotherapy (CCNU) and radiation. Dr. Kogelnik indicated to me that his group is evaluating protocols for combining misonidazole with chemotherapy and radiation. These limited data indicate that there is a modification of response of human tumor tissue to radiation by combining radiation with these chemical sensitizers, and as such are indicative of the presence and clinical importance of hypoxic cells in the high-grade glial tumors. Obviously there is too little research, based on only one type of tumor, and too short an observation period to warrant general conclusions about the value of the hypoxic cell sensitizers.

Summary

Results from experiments on murine tumors performed by a variety of investigators have demonstrated that (1) there are hypoxic and viable cells present and (2) respiration of oxygen at increased pressure or administration of chemical sensitizer of hypoxic cells (i.e., metronidazole or misonidazole) in combination with fractionated irradiation achieved significant reduction in the TCD50 values. In review of the studies of human tumors, emphasis was placed on examination for evidence that the maneuvers which overcome, to an important extent, the impact of hypoxic cells in murine tumors succeed when applied clinically. This is true because at present we cannot directly determine the role of hypoxic cells in the failures of conventional radiation therapy. Data from clinical trials are not entirely consistent but do indicate that for some human tumors local results are improved by combining radiation with hyperbaric oxygen or chemical sensitizers. These tumors include carcinomas of the head and neck, bronchus and high-grade gliomas. The results for hyperbaric oxygen and radiation in the treatment of carcinoma of the uterine cervix are mixed and must be classed as only suggestive. For carcinomas of the urinary bladder (hyperbaric oxygen and radiation) and for osteosarcoma (radiation under tourniquet conditions) the available results are equivocal.

ACKNOWLEDGMENTS

This work supported in part by DHEW Grant #CA13311.

REFERENCES

1. Adams, G.E., Fowler, J.F., and Wardman, P., eds.: *Hypoxic Cell Sensitizers in Radiobiology and Radiotherapy. Br J Cancer* **39**. London: H.K. Lewis, 1978.
2. Brown, J.M.: Evidence for acutely hypoxic cells in mouse tumors, and a possible mechanism of reoxygenation. *Br J Radiol* **52**:650–656, 1979.
3. Cade, I.S., and McEwen, J.B.: Clinical trials of radiotherapy in hyperbaric oxygen at Portsmouth (1964–1976). *Clin Radiol* **29**:333–338, 1978.
4. Cade, I.S., McEwen, J.B., Dische, S., Saunders, M.I., Watson, E.R., Halnan, K.E., Wiernik, G., Perrins, D.J.D., Sutherland, I.H.: Hyperbaric oxygen in radiation therapy: A medical research coun-

cil trial of carcinoma of the bladder. *Br J Radiol* **51**:876–878, 1978.

5. Cater, D.B.: Effect of breathing high pressure O_2 upon tissue O_2 tension in rat and mouse tumors. *Acta Radiol* **1**:233–253, 1963.
6. DuSault, L.A.: The effect of oxygen on the response of spontaneous tumors in mice to radiotherapy. *Br J Radiol* **36**:749–754, 1963.
7. Fletcher, G.H., Lindberg, R.D., Caderao, J.B., Wharton, J.T.: Hyperbaric oxygen as a radiotherapeutic adjuvant in advanced cancer of the uterine cervix. *Cancer* **39**:617–623, 1977.
8. Fowler, J.F., and Denekamp, J.: A review of hypoxic cell radiosensitization in experimental tumors. *Pharmacol Ther* **7**:413–444, 1979.
9. Fowler, J.F., Sheldon, P.W., and Denekamp, J.: Optimum fractionation of the C3H mouse mammary carcinoma using x-rays, the hypoxic cell radiosensitizer Ro-07-0582, or fast neutrons. *Int J Radiat Oncol Biol Phys* **1**:579–592, 1976.
10. Glassburn, J.R., Brady, L.W., and Plenk, H.P.: Hyperbaric oxygen in radiation therapy. *Cancer* **39**:751–765, 1977.
11. Goldfeder, A., and Clarke, G.E.: The response of neoplasms to X-radiation in vivo at increased oxygen tension. *Radiat Res* **13**:751–767, 1960.
12. Gray, L.H., Conger, A.D., Ebert, M., Hornsey, S. and Scott, O.C.A.: The concentration of oxygen dissolved in tissues at the time of irradiation as a factor in radiotherapy. *Br J Radiol* **26**:638–648, 1953.
13. Hall, E.J., ed. *Radiobiology for the Radiologist* Hagerstown, Maryland: Harper & Row, 1978, pp. 79–92.
14. Henk, J.M., Kinkler, P.B., and Smith, C.W.: Radiotherapy and hyperbaric oxygen in head and neck cancer. *Lancet* 101–103, 1977.
15. Henk, J.M., and Smith, C.W.: Radiotherapy and hyperbaric oxygen in head and neck cancer. *Lancet* 104–105, 1977.
16. Howes, A.E.: An estimation of changes in the proportions and absolute numbers of hypoxic cells after irradiation of transplanted C3H mouse mammary tumors. *Br J Radiol* **42**:441–447, 1969.
17. Inch, W.R., McCredie, J.A., and Sutherland, R.M.: Effect of duration of breathing 95% oxygen plus 5% carbon dioxide before X-irradiation on cure of C3H mammary tumor. *Cancer* **25**:926–931, 1970.
18. Jamieson, D., and van den Brenk, H.A.S.: Oxygen tension in human malignant disease under hyperbaric conditions. *Br J Cancer* **19**:139–150, 1965.
19. Kallman, R.F.: The phenomenon of reoxygenation and its implications for fractionated radiotherapy. *Radiology* **105**:135–142, 1972.
20. Kallman, R.F.: Discussion of hypoxia and reoxygenation in radiation resistance of solid tumors. In *Biological Bases and Clinical Implications of Tumor Radioresistance* G.H. Fletcher and C. Nervi, eds. New York: Masson, 1983, pp. 55–60
21. Kogelnik, H.D., and Karcher, K.H.: High dose irradiation and misonidazole in the treatment of glioblastoma multiforme: Preliminary report. Unpublished data.
22. Plenk, H.P.: Hyperbaric oxygen radiation therapy: Time-dose schedules and present status. In *Fraction Size in Radiobiology and Radiotherapy* T. Sugahara, L. Revesz, and O.C.A. Scott, eds. Baltimore: Williams & Wilkins, 1974.
23. Radiation Therapy Oncology Group Progress Report, 1976–1978.
24. Scott, O.C.A.: The response of tumors and normal tissues of the mouse to X-radiation delivered to animals breathing oxygen. *Br J Radiol* **26**:643–645, 1953.
25. Stone, H.B., and Withers, H.R.: Metronidazole: Effect on radiosensitivity of tumor and normal tissues in mice. *J Natl Cancer Inst* **55**:1189, 1975.
26. Suit, H.D., Howes, A.E., and Hunter, N.: Dependence of response of a C3H mammary carcinoma to fractionated irradiation on fractionation number and intertreatment interval. *Radiat Res* **72**:440–454, 1977.
27. Suit, H.D., and Lindberg, R.: Radiation therapy administered under conditions of tourniquet-induced local tissue hypoxia. *Am J Roentgenol* **102**:27–37, 1968.
28. Suit, H.D., Lindberg, R., Suchato, C., and Oxenne, A.: Radiation dose fractionation and high pressure oxygen in radiotherapy of the DBA mouse mammary carcinoma. *Am J Roentgenol Radiol Ther Nucl Med* **99**:895–899, 1967.
29. Suit, H.D., Maimonis, P., Michaels, H.B., and Sedlacek, R.: Comparison of hyperbaric oxygen and misonidazole in fractionated irradiation of murine tumors. *Radiat Res.* In press.
30. Suit, H.D., Maimonis, P., Rich, T.A., and Sedlacek, R.S.: Anesthesia and efficacy of hyperbaric oxygen in radiation therapy. *Br J Radiol* **52**:244, 1979.
31. Suit, H.D., Marshall, N., and Woerner, D.: Oxygen, oxygen plus carbon dioxide and radiation therapy of a mouse mammary carcinoma. *Cancer* **30**:1154–1158, 1972.
32. Suit, H.D., and Orsi, L.: The efficacy of hyperbaric oxygen in modifying the response of tissue to irradiation in doses of 200–400 rad per fraction. 6th L.H. Gray Memorial Conference Proceedings. London: Institute of Physics, 1975, pp. 208–287.
33. Suit, H.D., and Russell, W.O.: Soft part tumors. *Cancer* **39**:830–836, 1977.
34. Suit, H.D., and Scott, O.C.A.: Hyperbaric oxygen and irradiation—Review of laboratory experimental and clinical data. In *Progress in Radio-Oncolology.* K.H. Karcher, H.D. Kogelnik, and H.J. Meyer, eds. Stuttgart-New York: Georg Thieme Verlag, 1980, pp. 150–161.
35. Suit, H.D., and Suchato, C.: Hyperbaric oxygen

and radiotherapy of a fibrosarcoma and of a squamous cell carcinoma of C3H mice. *Radiology* **89**:720–726, 1967.

36. Thomlinson, R.H., and Craddock, E.A.: Response of experimental tumor to x-rays. *Br J Cancer* **21**:108–123, 1967.
37. Thomlinson, R.H., and Gray, L.H.: The histological structure of some human lung cancers and the possible implications for radiotherapy. *Br J Cancer* **9**:539–549, 1955.
38. Urtasun, R.C., Band, P.R., Chapman, J.D., Wilson, A.F., Marynowski, G. and Starreveld, E.: Metronidazole as a radiosensitizer. *N Engl J Med* **295**:901, 1976.
39. van den Brenk, H.A.S.: Hyperbaric oxygen in radiation therapy: An investigation of dose-effect relationships in tumor response and tissue damage. *Am J Roentgenol* **102**:8–26, 1968.
40. van den Brenk, H.A.S.: The oxygen effect in radiation therapy. *Curr Top Radiat Res* **5**:197, 1969.
41. van den Brenk, H.A.S., Elliott, K., and Hutchings, J.: Effect of single and fractionated doses of x-rays on radiocurability of solid Ehrlich tumor and tissue reactions in vivo for different oxygen tensions. *Br J Cancer* **16**:518–534, 1962.
42. Vaupel, P., Manz, R., Muller-Kliesler, W., and Grunewald, W.A.: Intracapillary HbO_2 saturation in malignant tumors during normoxia and hyperoxia. *Microvasc Res* **17**:818–891, 1979.
43. Ward, A.J., Dixon, B., and Stubbs, B.: A clinical appraisal of hyperbaric oxygen in cervix cancer. *Br J Radiol* **51**:150–151, 1978.
44. Watson, E.R., Halnan, K.E., Dische, S., Saunders, M.I., Cade, I.S., McEwen, J.B., Wiernik, G., Perrins, D.J.D., Sutherland, I.: Hyperbaric oxygen and radiotherapy: A Medical Research Council trial in carcinoma of the cervix. *Br J Radiol* **51**:879–887, 1978.

CHAPTER 9

Contribution of the Keynote Discussant: Hypoxia and Reoxygenation in the Radioresistance of Solid Tumors

Robert F. Kallman, Ph.D.[a]

In order to examine the importance of reoxygenation, it is necessary first to consider a number of fundamental questions. Some of these we can answer and some we cannot. Some are qualitative and some are quantitative. Among these important questions are the following:

1. Acknowledging that solid tumors contain hypoxic cells, how good is the quantitative evidence that significant numbers of cells are hypoxic? The word *significant* must be considered from both the statistical and biological standpoints.
2. Is the number of hypoxic cells related to tumor type? Tumor size? Degree of malignancy? Location? State of the host? To other variables?
3. Is the hypoxic fraction an invariant property of a given tumor? Or does it depend upon the variables listed above, or upon others?
4. When cells are demonstrably hypoxic, is this hypoxia a chronic condition or an acute one? Or, to what extent is acute hypoxia present, and how much of a problem does it constitute? If we grant that tumor cells experience acute hypoxia, how long does this condition last? And therefore, of what concern is it to radiotherapy?

When considering these and related questions we make a number of assumptions. The assumption that cellular hypoxia is indeed of primary importance rests upon an abundance of solid and convincing evidence. It is probably best demonstrated by the multiphasic survival curve that is obtained when solid tumors are irradiated *in vivo* and cell survival is assayed by a variety of methods. A morphological context for data such as this was established originally by Thomlinson and Gray[10] and elaborated on by many subsequent workers. Certain quantitative characteristics of this "classical" kind of corded morphology are perhaps best found in the paper by Tannock.[9] Thus, one can envision corded tumors with central capillaries and others with peripheral capillaries; and in either case the diffusion of oxygen from these capillaries establishes a gradient in local oxygen concentration.

All tumors are not corded, however. Indeed, much of the quantitative laboratory work that provides relevant information about hypoxic fractions and reoxygenation was done with noncorded tumors. As an example, in the EMT6 tumor it may be seen that the tumor cells are disposed in sheets or bundles. In the RIF-1 tumor we again fail to see a distinct corded morphology. Nonetheless, these and many other tumors that have been subjected to rigorous experimentation have proven to have significant numbers of severely hypoxic cells. This neither violates important laws nor gives cause for alarm.

[a]Department of Radiology, Stanford University School of Medicine, Stanford, Calif.

Clearly, tumor cells are fed by capillaries, whatever the histopathologic arrangement of cells might be, and, just as clearly, it is conceptually reasonable to suppose that there can be cells just beyond the range of effective oxygen diffusion from blood capillaries.

About 8 years ago we first reviewed the state of knowledge about proportions of hypoxic cells, and there were relatively few quantitative studies which could be cited at that time.[6] Very recently, Moulder and Rockwell[8] have undertaken to review critically the evidence for hypoxic fractions in a variety of tumors and by a variety of methods, and I should like to dwell at length on their excellent and comprehensive analyses. Basically, they have reanalyzed all available data and have done so using common mathematical techniques. Hypoxic fractions have been estimated by either of three methods: (1) comparison of survival curves for tumor cells irradiated *in situ* in air-breathing and nitrogen-asphyxiated animals; (2) analysis of TCD_{50} of normal tumors and tumors whose blood flow has been interrupted by clamping; and (3) analysis of the growth curves of normal and clamped tumors after they have been irradiated. As Moulder and Rockwell[8] have pointed out, all of these methods share a number of basic assumptions—namely, that both aerobic and hypoxic cells survive according to single-hit (single- or multitarget) kinetics, that oxygen is dose modifying, that naturally occurring hypoxic cells have the same radiation response as cells made hypoxic artificially, and that adequate hypoxia may be induced by asphyxiation of the host animal or by clamping off the blood flow in a living animal.

The paired survival curve method demands that the viability (i.e., survival) of cells be determined in an environment different from the tumor in which they resided when irradiated. Before one can compare a pair of survival curves, three important conditions must be satisfied: (1) there must be at least three points on each curve (2) doses used in generating the all-hypoxic (i.e., nitrogen-asphyxiated) curve must overlap with those used to generate the air-breathing curve; and (3) both curves must be linear and parallel, although linearity cannot of course extend back to zero dose. Moulder and Rockwell have identified 16 tumors which have provided data reported in at least that many publications, data that satisfied the conditions I have just enumerated. I shall not name all these tumors or authors who have reported them, for the paper to be published by Moulder and Rockwell will give all of this documentation in considerable detail. In the summary compiled by these authors, the paired survival-curve method has yielded a wide range of hypoxic fractions, allowing for only a few generalizations to be made. There seems little relationship between the size of the hypoxic fraction and tumor type: sarcomas and carcinomas do not differ in any systematic way. Hypoxic fractions vary downwards from almost 100% to less than 0.1%, but the majority seem to lie between about 5 and 40%. The hypoxic fraction may depend upon the site in which the tumor is grown, as intramuscular tumors seem to have fewer hypoxic cells than intradermal tumors of the same type. When rigorous criteria are used for analysis of TCD_{50} data, one sees, it seems to me, even greater heterogeneity of hypoxic fractions, and regrowth assays give highly variable hypoxic fractions.

Several important generalizations were drawn by Moulder and Rockwell. All of the techniques used for hypoxic-fraction determination have limitations and potential artifacts associated with them. When different techniques were used with the same tumor, different results were obtained—although occasionally the results may have looked similar. There was no obvious pattern in the differences generated by the use of different methods (i.e., one method did not always give higher or lower fractions than another). There was no obvious dependence on tumor size as long as the tumors were macroscopic; the data suggest that the hypoxic fraction is smaller in microscopic-sized tumors. And there was no obvious dependence of hypoxic fraction on tumor growth or histology. Of the 27 tumor systems surveyed, 23 had hypoxic fractions compatible with the range 2–37%, 10 may have had less than 1%, and 5 may have had less than 0.1%.

I have dwelled at some length on the question of hypoxic fractions simply because these are the data one must have in order to describe the process of reoxygenation, for after all, reoxygenation is defined as a change in hypoxic fraction from high to low. I think it is also important to recognize the limitations associated with different methods of determining the hypoxic fraction for the obvious reason that one would like to extend these studies to tumors growing in the human host. Of the three main methods, only one–namely, regrowth–is applicable to humans; and this method seems to suffer from serious deficiencies.

Despite this fact, some notable attempts have been made to use tumor growth/regrowth data to derive estimates of the hypoxic fraction. Recently, Denekamp et al.[3] have estimated the hypoxic fractions of 14 mouse tumors from regrowth data. They used three different methods and obtained a provocative set of data. One of these methods necessitates measuring growth delays in the presence and absence of hypoxic-cell radiosensitizers, but this also necessitates making a number of basic assumptions about survival-curve parameters. It must be recognized that there are two major sources of uncertainty in this approach–uncertainties associated with the manner in which tumor-regrowth curves are obtained[1] and, of course, the uncertainties inherent in the assumptions about survival-curve parameters. Uncertainties apply to the other two methods of calculating hypoxic fractions from regrowth data; nonetheless, these three methods have yielded a reasonably consistent set of hypoxic fraction estimates, and the authors admittedly offer these with reservations or strong qualifications. Some of the 14 tumors were reported to have very few hypoxic cells by all three methods (e.g., SA S), while another (SA FA), had a high hypoxic fraction by all three methods. However, still others showed great variability (e.g., CA RH, which had a small hypoxic fraction, approximately 2%, by one method and 15–25% by the others). Using this same approach, Denekamp et al.[2] made several estimates of the hypoxic fraction in multiple subcutaneous metastases of a squamous carcinoma of the cervix in a patient. The authors present a wide choice of hypoxic fractions which vary according to assumptions about tumor cell D_0 and extrapolation number; and assuming these to be 380 rad and 10, respectively, they report a best estimate of 12–20% hypoxic cells in this tumor. This exercise in calculations and assumptions should be regarded as a noble experiment, but one that is fraught with almost insuperable difficulties if it is to be applied in a practical way. In other words, survival-curve parameters are simply not known in advance for any tumor which might be found in a patient, nor is it possible to deduce these from simple observations. Making incorrect assumptions can lead to erroneous conclusions, and this could jeopardize the life of the patient if one treatment plan were chosen over another in the case of such erroneous pretherapeutic data and calculations.

What, then, do we know about the rate or kinetics of reoxygenation? Even if we assume that any of these estimates of the hypoxic fraction are accurate, do they tell us anything about how this important parameter changes during the course of radiotherapy? Despite the paucity of hard data, one can make rather sophisticated models and plans, and these are exemplified in the elegant review by Fowler and Denekamp.[5] Quite simply, they consider the effectiveness of sensitizers in tumors (capable of poor, moderate, or good reoxygenation) as a function of the hypoxic fraction (low to high) that is characteristic of the unirradiated tumor. Despite the fact that, with anything less than good reoxygenation, the hypoxic

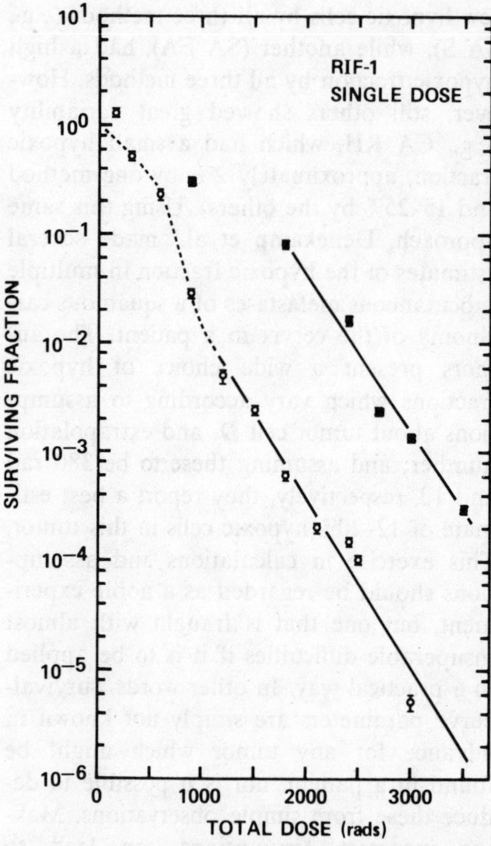

Figure 1. Survival curves of RIF-1 tumor cells irradiated *in vivo*. Surviving fractions were determined by counting colonies that grew *in vitro* from single tumor cells. Circles = tumors irradiated in living air-breathing mice; squares = tumors irradiated in nitrogen-asphyxiated mice.

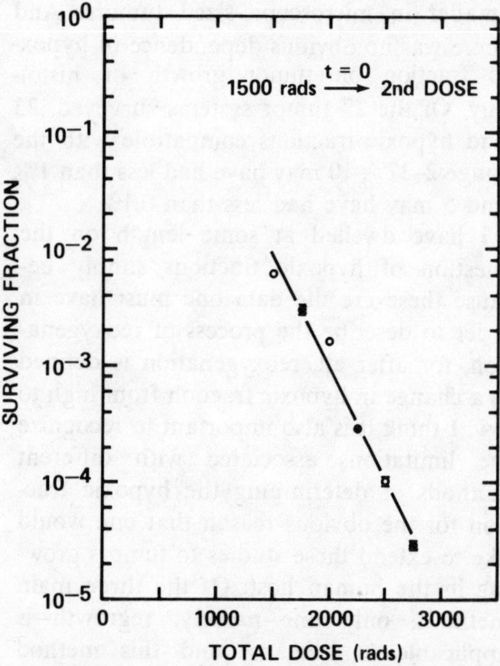

Figure 2. RIF-1 tumor cell surviving fraction as a function of radiation dose, for tumors irradiated with 1500 rad (air-breathing) plus a second irradiation of the same tumors in air-breathing (circles) or nitrogen-asphyxiated (squares) mice. The second dose was administered 5 minutes after the first.

fraction should increase progressively during the course of fractionated radiotherapy, they conclude that radiosensitizers are best used at the beginning of treatment. The reason is simple: We do not know *a priori* when and how any tumor will reoxygenate.

Our knowledge of reoxygenation kinetics has not really advanced much since 1974 when I reviewed this subject.[7] Then, most tumors appeared to reoxygenate rapidly, and one, an osteosarcoma,[11] did not begin reoxygenation for at least 3 or 4 days. We have recently examined the reoxygenation kinetics of another tumor, RIF-1, which exhibits a rather interesting and perhaps significant behavior.[4] This tumor has a very small hypoxic fraction, 0.8%, which necessitates using a somewhat higher conditioning dose–namely, 1500 rad. A lower dose simply does not deplete the tumor of well-oxygenated cells sufficiently to allow the study of reoxygenation kinetics. The single-dose survival curve of the tumor is shown in Figure 1, along with the survival curve of cells irradiated in nitrogen-asphyxiated animals; it is from the vertical distance between these parallel curves that we calculate the hypoxic fraction to be 0.8%. When we give graded test doses immediately after 1500 rad, we get the survival data shown in Figure 2 which leads us to conclude that the cells that survived 1500 rad were essentially all from the hypoxic compartment. One hour later (see Fig. 3) the curves have moved apart, yielding a hypoxic fraction of 50%. The data that we have obtained to date are given in Table 1. It is obvious that there is very rapid reoxygenation during the

TABLE 1. Hypoxic Fraction of the RIF-1 Tumor at Different Times after a Conditioning Dose of 1500 Rad

Time (Hours)	1500 Rad RIF-1
0	106
1	50
6	45
14	67
24	48
48	46
(without conditioning irradiation)	0.8

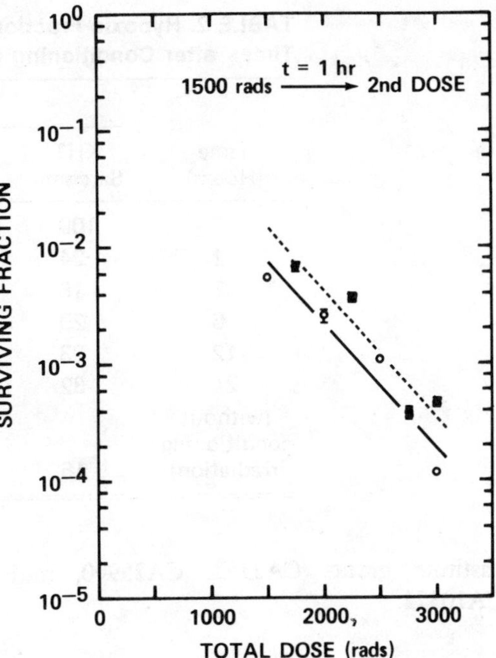

Figure 3. RIF-1 tumor cell surviving fraction as a function of radiation dose, for tumors irradiated with 1500 rad (air-breathing) plus a second irradiation of the same tumors in air-breathing (circles) or nitrogen-asphyxiated (squares) mice. The second dose was administered 1 hour after the first.

first hour and that nothing much happens beyond that for at least the next 2 days.

Of course, we do not know how typical these kinetics are, whether they depend upon the very low hypoxic fraction prior to irradiation or whether there is any correlation with the hypoxic fraction in any untreated tumor. This prompts us to look back at our old data (see Table 2). Until these recent RIF-1 experiments, we had concluded that reoxygenation which follows a single dose of 1000 rad was complete within 12 to 24 hours. These data show that there indeed was extensive reoxygenation after about 12 to 24 hours in every case, but in no case did the hypoxic fraction return to its pre-irradiated level. At the time we published these data, we did not think of these differences as significant–comparing pre-irradiated with postirradiated hypoxic fractions. (These numbers have rather wide confidence limits, so that it is impossible to state with certainty that numbers like 16 and 23%, for example, are different.) However, it is rather striking that we rarely obtained postirradiated hypoxic fractions that were as low as those found in unirradiated tumors. These data, and especially our most recent findings for the RIF-1 tumor, lead us to suggest that perhaps reoxygenation may not be as efficient as we thought as a means of restoring an irradiated tumor to its inherent radiosensitivity. We are fully aware of the many qualifications built into the inferences that we might draw from such experiments, and not the least of these stems from the fact that we used a single conditioning dose that is much larger than doses commonly used in clinical radiotherapy. We do know very little about the efficiency of reoxygenation in tumors which are accumulating their radiation doses progressively over the course of time–by daily or near-daily fractionated schedules. While we intend to examine reoxygenation kinetics under these circumstances, until we do, data such as these suggest that even good reoxygenation does not eliminate the need for effective adjuvants, notable hypoxic-cell radiosensitizers.

ACKNOWLEDGMENTS

Original research covered in this paper was supported by USPHS National Cancer

TABLE 2. Hypoxic Fractions of 3 Mouse Tumors at Different Times after Conditioning Doses of 1000 or 2000 Rad.

	1000 Rad			2000 Rad
Time (Hours)	KHT Sarcoma	KHJJ Carcinoma	EMT6 Sarcoma	EMT6 Sacroma
0	100	67	61	86
1	24	34	44	79
3	18	32	29	81
6	29	21	35	79
12	23	31	24	87
24	32	34	46	29
(without conditioning irradiation)	16	19	35	

Institute grants CA3353, CA25990, and CA10372.

REFERENCES

1. Begg, A.C.: Analysis of growth delay data: Potential pitfalls. *Br J Cancer* **41**:93–97, 1980.
2. Denekamp, J., Fowler, J.F., and Dische, S.: The proportion of hypoxic cells in a human tumor. *Int J Radiat Oncol Biol Phys* **2**:1227–1228, 1977.
3. Denekamp, J., Hirst, D.G., Stewart, F.A., and Terry, N.H.A.: Is tumor radiosensitization by misonidazole a general phenomenon? *Br J Cancer* **41**:1–9, 1980.
4. Dorie, M.J., and Kallman, R.F.: Reoxygenation of the RIF-1 tumor. *Radiat Res* **83**:376–377, 1980.
5. Fowler, J.F., and Denekamp, J.: A review of hypoxic cell radiosensitization in experimental tumors. *Pharmacol Ther* **7**:413–444, 1979.
6. Kallman, R.F.: The phenomenon of reoxygenation and its implications for fractionated radiotherapy. *Radiology* **105**:135–142, 1972.
7. Kallman, R.F.: The oxygen effect and reoxygenation. In *Proceedings of the 11th International Cancer Congress* (Florence, Italy, 1974). Excerpta Medica International Congress Series No. 353, 5:136–140, 1974.
8. Moulder, J.E., and Rockwell, S.C.: Survey of published data on the hypoxic fractions of solid rodent tumors. *Radiat Res* **83**:376, 1980.
9. Tannock, I.F.: Oxygen diffusion and the distribution of cellular radiosensitivity in tumors. *Br J Radiol* **45**:515–554, 1972.
10. Thomlinson, R.H., and Gray, L.H.: The histological structure of some human lung cancers and the possible implications for radiotherapy. *Br J Cancer* **9**:539–549, 1955.
11. Van Putten, L.M.: Oxygenation and cell kinetics after irradiation in a transplantable osteosarcoma. In *Effects of Radiation on Cellular Proliferation* Vienna: IAEA, 1968, pp. 493–505.

CHAPTER 10

The Fraction of Hypoxic Clonogenic Cells in Tumor Populations

J.D. Chapman, B.Sc., M.Sc., Ph.D.[a]
A.J. Franko, B.Sc., M.Sc., Ph.D.[b]
C.J. Koch, B.Sc., M.Sc., Ph.D.[c]

It has been suggested that the oxygen concentration in tumor cells might be critical for the successful treatment of human cancers by ionizing radiation.[21] In fact, some clinical evidence (briefly reviewed in the following section) indicates that hypoxia (or low oxygen tension) is a controlling factor in the radiocurability of some cancers. Experimentalists have demonstrated that hypoxia occurs in most animal tumors, and several techniques which measure the presence of clonogenic hypoxic cells in animal tumors have been developed. Although a wealth of information has been produced about the fraction of hypoxic cells in animal tumors, the reoxygenation of tumor cells after radiotherapy, and physical and chemical techniques which circumvent hypoxic cell radioresistance, the practice of clinical radiotherapy has not, to date, been significantly improved through this information. Most techniques for measuring the presence of hypoxic cells in tumors are either highly invasive or destructive, and consequently are difficult to export to the clinic.

[a]Director of Radiobiology, Cross Cancer Institute, Professor of Radiology, University of Alberta Medical School, Edmonton, Alberta, Canada.
[b]Radiobiology Program, Cross Cancer Institute, Assistant Professor of Radiology, University of Alberta Medical School, Edmonton, Alberta, Canada.
[c]Radiobiology Program, Cross Cancer Institute, Assistant Professor of Radiology, University of Alberta Medical School, Edmonton, Alberta, Canada.

Oncologists would benefit from knowledge of the extent and distribution of hypoxic cells throughout individual tumors. Such information could be useful in the design of treatment strategy–for example, in deciding whether or not to employ hypoxic-cell radiosensitizers and/or high-LET radiations. Ideally, one would like to obtain the distribution of hypoxic cells throughout each tumor at a microscopic level (or at least at a resolution of ± 1 mm) using a noninvasive technique. Unfortunately current technology cannot achieve these goals.

Two recently developed techniques could alter this situation. The measurement of intracellular ^{31}P in ATP molecules (a signal which is strongly dependent upon intracellular pH) by nuclear magnetic resonance imaging techniques is currently being researched and developed to measure hypoxia in human tumors. As well, the new class of drug, known as hypoxic-cell radiosensitizers, shows promise for identifying hypoxic, clonogenic cells in tumors by virtue of the fact that these drugs become covalently bound to cellular macromolecules by a metabolic process unique to hypoxic cells. Evidence is presented which suggests that radioactively labelled hypoxic sensitizers could become a useful tool in tumor biology and possibly, with the use of nuclear medicine techniques, a clinical assay for hypoxic cells in human cancers.

Clinical Evidence for Hypoxic Cells in Tumors

The work of Thomlinson and Gray[59] emphasized that the histological structure of some human cancers suggested the presence of hypoxic cells and, potentially, an inherent resistance to treatment with ionizing radiations. The early discussions of the clinical evidence for hypoxic cells in human cancer have been reviewed.[30,47,57,62]

Recent evidence for hypoxic cells in human tumors has come from clinical studies with new therapies directed against radioresistant hypoxic cells. Van den Brenk[61] and Henk and Smith[23] have reported on clinical trials which compared tumor response for patients breathing air or hyperbaric oxygen at the time of radiation treatment. The dose fractionation scheme was similar for both patient groups, and the improved local control obtained with hyperbaric oxygen therapy was evidence for hypoxic cells in these tumors.

Urtasun et al.[60] showed that when the hypoxic-cell radiosensitizer metronidazole was given to patients prior to radiation treatment for glioblastoma multiforme, a significant increase in survival time was observed compared to patients treated with the same course of radiation therapy without the sensitizer. This result was indirect evidence for hypoxic, clonogenic cells (in advanced human brain tumors) which could control, at least in part, the response to treatment. Several randomized phase III studies with the hypoxic-cell radiosensitizers metronidazole and misonidazole are currently in progress in several countries to evaluate any beneficial role these drugs might have in the radiotherapy of various human cancers.

Another recent evidence for hypoxic cells in human tumors is the role of anemia and pretherapy transfusion on the cure rate of carcinoma of the cervix.[10] Patients with Stage IIb and III disease and hemoglobin levels during treatment of 12 g% or less had a significantly higher pelvic recurrence rate and also a lower cure rate than patients whose hemoglobin levels were 12 g% or greater. Correction of the anemic state by pretherapy transfusions reduced the rate of pelvic recurrence and increased the cure rate to levels comparable to patients with normal hemoglobin levels. This study indicates that tumors in anemic patients are probably more hypoxic and more radioresistant than tumors in patients with normal blood parameters. Consequently, the state of anemia should be corrected by transfusion in most patients who are to be treated with radiation.

Techniques for Determining Hypoxia in Animal Tumors

TUMOR HISTOLOGY AND OXYGEN PHARMACOLOGY

The number of hypoxic cells in a tumor is determined by several factors, including (1) the relative rates of proliferation of capillary endothelial cells and tumor cells, (2) the oxygen content of the blood and rate of blood flow, (3) the rate of oxygen consumption by normal and tumor tissues, (4) the rate of oxygen diffusion through tissues, and (5) the rate of cell death which results from hypoxia. Thomlinson and Gray[59] have discussed these factors as they possibly relate to the histology of some human lung cancers. Tannock[53-56] studied the effects of pO_2 on cell-proliferation kinetics in two transplanted mouse tumor systems. His work demonstrated that the microarchitecture of the animal tumors was almost identical to that of some human tumors examined by R. H. Thomlinson. Furthermore, he showed that the proliferating zone of tumor cells occurred within a 100 ± 30 μm radius around mouse blood vessels, a distance which closely corresponded to theoretically computed oxygen diffusion distances. Labelling index, proliferating zone radius, and tumor growth rate were all lowered if animals were made to breathe air which contained only 10% oxygen. These studies provided conclusive evidence that oxygen concentration was an important factor in tumor-growth kinetics and that histology was a useful tool for studying such effects. Proliferating cells in tumor sections were identified by the autoradiography of incorporated ^{3}H-thymidine. Unfortunately, no label specific for hypoxic-viable cells was available at the time of these studies; consequently, these cells were not specifically identified in these tumor sections. Although these studies provide valuable information for tumor biologists and cell kineticists, the diagnosis or treatment of human cancer has not directly benefited from this work.

DIRECT MEASUREMENT OF LOW pO_2 WITH OXYGEN ELECTRODES

The polarography of oxygen involves the reduction of oxygen at a noble metal surface (cathode) with a driving voltage established via a reference anode (e.g., Ag/AgCl). For intratumor or even intracellular oxygen measurements the cathode is usually fabricated as an open-ended, glass-covered gold or platinum microelectrode with the anode reference separated physically from the cathode (usually at the skin surface). The physical separation partially defeats the purpose of the reference electrode as large potential changes can exist between the cathode and anode and result in artifactual changes in cathode current. In addition, the oxygen reduction occurs in discrete steps so that chemicals which interact with superoxide or hydrogen peroxide can alter the apparent oxygen concentration. Interfering chemicals can also increase or decrease the polarographic current, and "poisoning" of the cathode surface by proteins can occur. The measurement of oxygen concentrations by electrodes implanted into animal tissues is not, consequently, totally independent from biomolecular influences.

Cater et al.[11,12] have measured low oxygen concentrations in human tumors by means of oxygen electrodes. Such measurements with electrodes directly confirmed the prediction that hypoxic regions would occur in rapidly proliferating tissues which could outgrow their vasculature. The electrodes used in this early work were relatively large and measured an oxygen concentration which was an average of over several thousands of cells in the tumor. Microelectrodes have been developed but numerous measurements are required over the whole volume of the tumor in order to map the hypoxic zones. Of course, the great limitation of this technique is that it is highly invasive, and the implantation of the electrode can introduce oxygen and yield false measurements.

Attempts have been made to solve some of the technical problems associated with the polarography of oxygen. Some microelectrodes have been fabricated with self-contained anode references[5,6] in a manner similar to the development by Clark et al.[17] of larger membrane-covered electrodes. However, it seems that the smaller the electrodes are constructed the greater are the uncertainties in absolute oxygen measurements. In fact, quantitative measurements with these new microelectrodes of oxygen in the range of radiobiological hypoxia (0.1–2.0 micromolar) have not been convincing. Another approach to the problem of physical separation of anode and cathode has been to make a microelectrode containing two electrically isolated cathodes–one for the actual reduction and the other to monitor the anode-cathode voltage.[1] This advance has been made possible by the manufacture of suitable dual-channelled, glass capillary tubing.

The invasiveness of most techniques for measuring oxygen concentrations in tissue has been eliminated at the expense of detailed knowledge of oxygen concentrations at large depth from the skin surface. One method involves measuring the surface oxygen tensions at several points simultaneously.[32] With a sufficiently large number of electrodes it is possible to make estimates of the subsurface distribution of oxygen concentrations. Another application of surface measurements yields data on the average subsurface oxygen concentration in the capillary bed and the oxygen diffusion constant of the intervening tissue.[33] Although these methods of oxygen concentration measurement represent significant methodological advances, it is still not possible to monitor tumor and normal tissue oxygen concentrations on a routine basis and with the detail that would be useful to oncologists.

MEASUREMENTS OF TUMOR-CELL RADIORESISTANCE

The first radiobiological measurements of hypoxic-cell fractions in animal tumors were performed almost 20 years ago,[25,42] and this technique has been reviewed by Kallman[31] and most recently by Moulder and Rockwell.[41] Three different variations of this technique are in current use. All involve the comparison of estimates of numbers of cells surviving after irradiation of tumors in unperturbed animals and of tumors whose cells have been made hypoxic by local occlusion of blood flow or asphyxiation of the host. At doses which kill all the oxygenated cells in unperturbed tumors, the increase in cell survival observed in those tumors made artificially hypoxic is equated with the fraction of previously oxygenated cells. This equality depends on several assumptions which might not be valid in all cases, including equal inherent radioresistance for chronically and artificially hypoxic cells[27] and equal degrees of hypoxia for the chronically and artificially hypoxic cells.[9]

The technique with potentially the greatest accuracy uses cellular survival curves from tumors irradiated under the two conditions. If the curves are parallel, the hypoxic-cell fraction can be obtained directly from the separation of the curves. The technique requires the disaggregation of tumors to single cells; so it is assumed that this yields representative samples of the viable hypoxic and oxygenated cells.[43] Cell survival can be measured by colony formation *in vitro*[46] and in lungs[28] or by scoring tumor formation from progressively diluted inocula of the cell suspension (end-point dilution).[25,42]

The other two techniques use the radiation response of tumors left *in situ* to estimate the number of surviving cells in normal and artificially hypoxic tumors. This eliminates the problems inherent in the disaggregation of tumors, but involves additional assumptions. The radioresistance of hypoxic cells *in situ* must be estimated, either from actual survival curves (which is often impossible), or by choosing a reasonable value.[63] The procedure of clamping to produce artificial hypoxia must not affect the survival of cells by affecting blood flow after the release of the clamp or by permitting the accumulation of toxic agents in the tumor. This can be tested by measuring the effect of clamping on the growth of unperturbed tumors.

Both regrowth delay and tumor cure can be used to estimate the hypoxic fraction *in situ*. With tumor cure, the difference between the doses required to cure 50% of normal and artificially hypoxic tumors is used to estimate the difference in the surviving fractions which is ascribed to the normally well-oxygenated fraction of cells.[51] With regrowth delay, a similar procedure is used, based on the difference in dose required to produce a given regrowth delay.[58] In this case, a further assumption made is that any effects of irradiation of the host tissues on regrowth delay are equal for unperturbed and artificially hypoxic tissues. This assumption may not be true if direct damage to normally oxygenated tissue such as blood vessels can be protected by artificial hypoxia. It is also assumed that the surviving cells regrow at the same rate, which seems unlikely to be true immediately after irradiation.[4,24] These techniques provide an estimate of the "effective" hypoxic fraction in terms of the influence of hypoxic cells on the radiocurability of the tumor. The actual proportion of living hypoxic cells might be quite different if some of the hypoxic cells in unperturbed tumors are doomed because of their growth conditions,[3,26] or if their capacity for repair of potentially lethal damage is different from that of artificially hypoxic cells which become oxygenated as soon as blood flow is restored.[22,34,39] These potential problems are not present in the survival-curve technique.

These techniques have been applied to over two dozen different tumor systems (reviewed recently by Moulder and Rockwell).[41] A few tumors have very few hypoxic cells (less than 1%), while a few contain 50% or more hypoxic cells. There are estimates of hypoxic fractions for three tumors by the survival-curve technique and one by the *in situ* technique. In all cases the values are different by factors ranging from 2 to 50. The *in situ* technique gave the largest value for one of the three tumors[39] and the smallest for the others,[36,37,40,45,58] so no consistent pattern can be predicted at this time. The disagreements must be due to the failure of some of the assumptions, but to decide which technique gives the "correct" value appears to be difficult,[8,38] unless all techniques are applied simultaneously and additional work is performed to test some of the assumptions.

The determination of hypoxic fraction by various measurements of tumor-cell radioresistance is the most widely employed technique used in tumor biology today. Nevertheless, this technique is totally destructive and cannot be applied to clinical oncology.

IMPROVED TUMOR RESPONSE AFTER HYPERBARIC OXYGEN THERAPY

The studies of Gray et al.[21,59] prompted the investigation of elevated oxygen levels at the time of radiation treatment on tumor radioresponse. Experiments performed with four different animal tumors[49] indicated an increase in tumor radiosensitivity if irradiations were performed under conditions of high pressure oxygen. The radiosensitizing effect of hyperbaric oxygen was diminished as the radiation dose was fractionated,[50] suggesting that reoxygenation of hypoxic cells in animal tumors occurred over the time of the fractionated treatment. These basic studies are evidence for hypoxic, clonogenic cells in solid tumors, and the technique of high pressure oxygen radiotherapy has been exported successfully to some clinics only with extreme persistence.[23,61] In fact, this technique of circumventing hypoxic-cell radioresistance has not, as yet, had a major impact on the practice of clinical radiotherapy.

INFLUENCE OF ANEMIA AND PRETHERAPY TRANSFUSION ON TUMOR RADIORESPONSE

Hill et al.[28] have demonstrated that hemoglobin level can influence the radiation response of an animal tumor. This result is evidence for hypoxic cells in animal tumors, and retrospective clinical investigations (reviewed above) show that anemia can influence the clinical response to radiotherapy. Pretherapy transfusion for anemia should be considered an essential procedure for all cancer patients who have a chance for radiocure.

INCREASED TUMOR RESPONSE WITH HYPOXIC-CELL RADIOSENSITIZERS

The identification of drugs which could selectively radiosensitize hypoxic mammalian cells[2] made possible the demonstrations that some sensitizers could greatly improve the radiosensitivity of several animal tumors.[7,44,48] Hypoxic-cell radiosensitizers have become an extremely useful tool in animal tumor biology and have provided a wealth of information about the existence of clonogenic, hypoxic cells (and their reoxygenation) in several tumor models. The sensitizing effect of these drugs is usually smaller with fractionated courses of radiation.[18,20] This result has been interpreted as evidence for reoxygenation.

As previously discussed, metronidazole and misonidazole are currently being studied in several randomized clinical cancer trials in several countries, but a few more years are required to determine if hypoxic sensitizers can improve the radiocurability of some human cancers.

FLUORESCENCE OF SPECIFIC CELLULAR MOLECULES

Another technique for identifying and studying hypoxic cells involves the measurement of oxygen-dependent intracellular chemical change. Changes in spectral absorption, fluorescent emission, and electron spin resonance signals have been investigated. A quantitative description of the distribution of oxygen concentrations near the surface has been made by observing the tissue reflectance,[16] and estimates of the average redox state of several thousand cells at a depth of up to 850 μm has recently been achieved using a solid-state, light-pipe spectrophotometer.[29] Although similar techniques have been utilized to monitor oxygen concentrations in tumors where the geometry can be adapted to absorption or emission techniques, the tumors must often be perfused to eliminate red-cell absorption. Thus, the technical complexities of this approach for the evaluation of hypoxia in tumors have not been overcome, and these techniques are not available to clinicians today.

Novel Methods for Measuring Hypoxia in Tumors

NMR DETECTION OF HYPOXIA

Specific concentrations of chemicals and biochemicals can be detected in living tissues by nuclear magnetic resonance spectroscopy (NMR). Computerized reconstructions of NMR signals obtained in several directions across whole animals have resulted in images of specific organs and body functions.[19] Cellular ATP levels which vary systematically with intracellular pH are being investigated with NMR measurements of ^{31}P to determine if tumor hypoxia and possibly necrosis can be detected (C.R. Shonk, personal communication). Preliminary results indicate that the signal-to-noise ratio between hypoxic and oxygenated cells in tumors is very low, and technical developments may be required before NMR can be applied routinely for the detection of hypoxia in cancers. The advantage of this technique is that a measure of the extent of tumor hypoxia might be obtained by a relatively harmless, noninvasive procedure.

COVALENT BINDING OF RADIOACTIVELY LABELLED SENSITIZERS TO HYPOXIC CELLS

Hypoxic-cell radiosensitizers were shown to become selectively bound to the macromolecules of hypoxic cells by metabolism-induced[35] and radiation-induced[15] reactions. Radiation-induced binding was used to identify hypoxic cells in multicellular spheroids,[52] although the total radiation dose and dose-rate employed in this study complicates the interpretation of the result. Recently, the criteria for exploitation of the "sensitizer-binding phenomenon" as a tool for tumor biology and as a possible nuclear medicine procedure have been defined.[13,14]

Experiments have been performed which measured the kinetics of radiation-induced and metabolism-induced binding of ^{14}C-misonidazole to hypoxic-cell macromolecules. Briefly, radiation-induced binding of the sensitizer to hypoxic cells is relatively independent of the concentration of sensitizer (over the range 1–500 μm) and is linear with dose up to several kilorad. Metabolism-induced binding of sensitizer to hypoxic cells is strongly dependent upon sensitizer concentration and is linear with time up to at least 4 hours. These studies showed that the amount of ^{14}C-misonidazole bound to cells after 2 hours of hypoxic metabolism was equivalent to the amount bound by several kilorad of radiation. Consequently, our most recent efforts have involved studies into the metabolism-induced process of sensitizer binding, exclusively.

Multicellular spheroids of Chinese hamster V79 cells (~0.6 mm diameter) were incubated for 3 hours at 37°C in the presence of 50 μM ^{14}C-misonidazole (specific activity 144 mCi/mg, generously supplied by Hoffman LaRoche, Nutley, N.J.). Spheroids were removed from the labelled medium by sedimentation, washed with unlabelled media, fixed, embedded, and sectioned according to standard procecures. Sections mounted on microscopic slides were dipped in liquid emulsion (Kodak NTB3) and exposed for 10, 17, and 30 days. Figure 1 shows a section of either a small spheroid or the edge section of a large spheroid. The autoradiographic procedure has produced very few grains in the emulsion overlaying the cells indicating that very little ^{14}C-misonidazole was bound and retained in this section. In contrast, Figure 2 shows an autoradiograph of a larger spheroid with evidence of pyknotic cells and necrosis in the center. An abundance of ^{14}C-misonidazole was bound and retained in cells several layers deep in the spheroids, surrounding the pyknotic and necrotic region. Examination of several serial sections from this spheroid preparation indicates that the pattern of retained radioactivity is consistent from section to section and could indicate the presence of metabolizing hypoxic cells in the spheroids.

EMT-6 tumors were grown at different sites in BALB/c mice from inocula of different numbers of cells. When the largest tumor had grown to ~0.5 cm diameter, the animal was injected with ^{14}C-misonidazole to achieve a maximum plasma concentration of ~50 μM. Additional radioactive drug was administered at 1 and 2 hours to

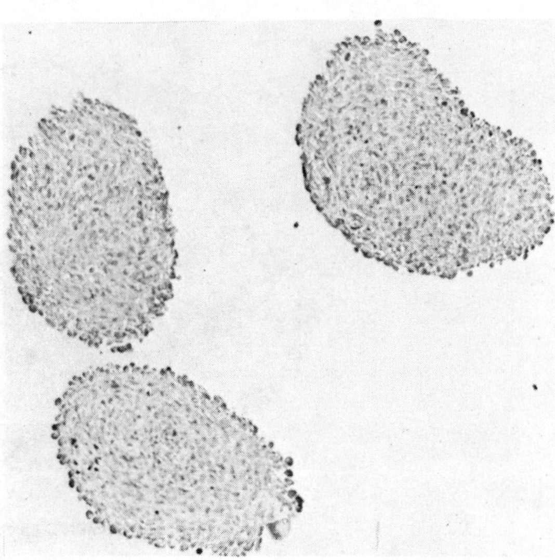

Figure 1. An autoradiograph of Chinese hamster V79 spheroids exposed to ^{14}C-misonidazole for 3 hours.

simulate an exposure of the hypoxic tumor cells to a constant concentration of ~50 μM ^{14}C-misonidazole. At 3 hours after the initial drug injection the animal was sacrificed, and the tumors were excised and fixed in buffered formalin. The tumors were washed with buffered formalin to dilute and remove the unbound ^{14}C-misonidazole, then fixed, embedded, sectioned, and mounted on microscopic slides for autoradiography as described above for spheroids.

Figures 3, 4, 5, and 6 show autoradiographs (exposed for 17 days) of four different EMT-6 tumors of various size. The smallest tumor (approximately 1.5 × 0.5 mm) has histological features of a simple subcutaneous spheroid. There is no evidence that the injected tumor cells had intercepted any existing vasculature, and this small tumor has a relatively large region of central necrosis. The rim of bound ^{14}C-misonidazole is several cell layers below the surface of the tumor and might indicate the location of metabolizing hypoxic cells. The medium-sized tumors (3 to 4 mm diameter) shown in Figures 4 and 5 have strikingly different patterns of bound sensitizer which can possibly be related to the tumor vasculature. Examination of over 50 serial sections of the tumor shown in Figure 4 shows that the rim

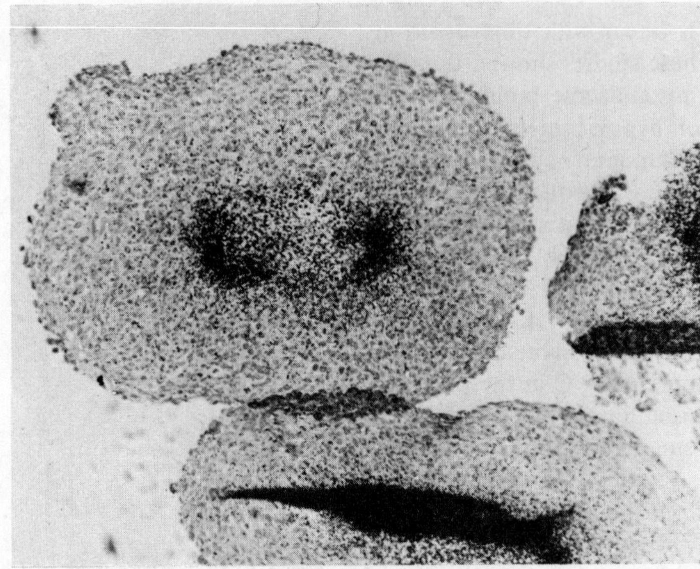

Figure 2. An autoradiograph of Chinese hamster V79 spheroids exposed to ^{14}C-misonidazole for 3 hours.

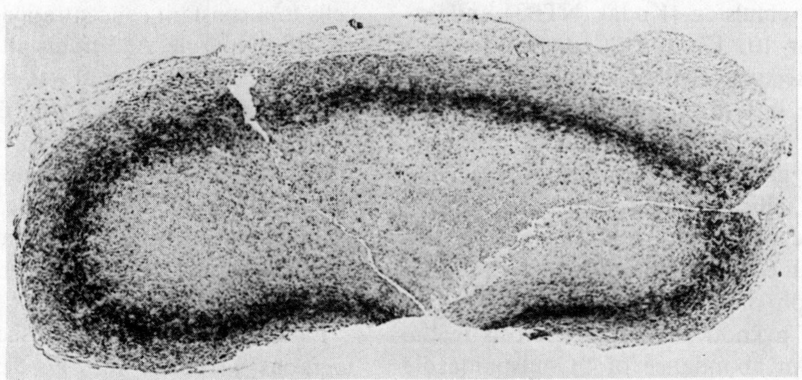

Figure 3. An autoradiograph of an EMT6 tumor (1.5 × 0.5 mm) in a BALB/c mouse exposed to ^{14}C-misonidazole for 3 hours.

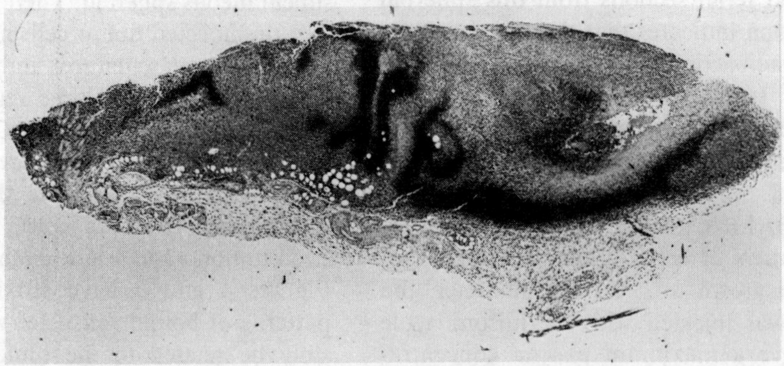

Figure 4. An autoradiograph of an EMT6 tumor (4.0 × 1.5 mm) in a BALB/c mouse exposed to ^{14}C-misonidazole for 3 hours.

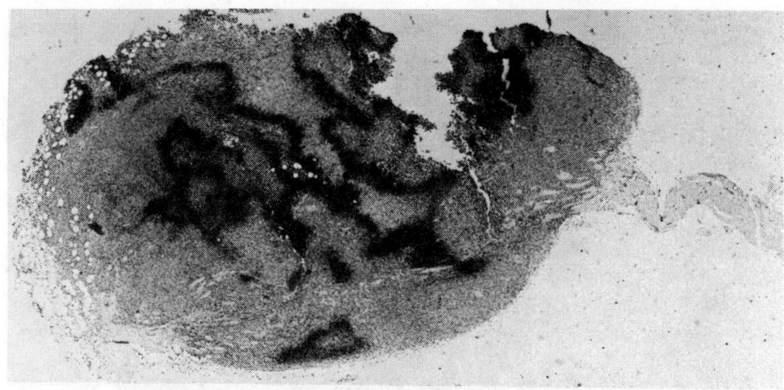

Figure 5. An autoradiograph of an EMT6 tumor (4.0 × 2.5 mm) in a BALB/c mouse exposed to ^{14}C-misonidazole for 3 hours.

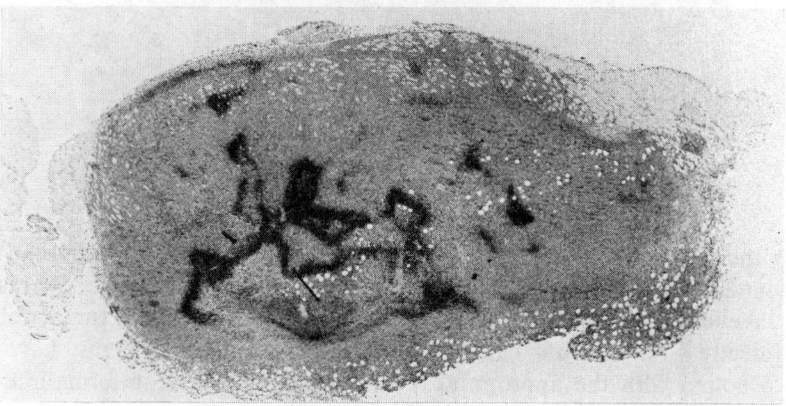

Figure 6. An autoradiograph of an EMT6 tumor (5.0 × 3.0 mm) in a BALB/c mouse exposed to ^{14}C-misonidazole for 3 hours.

of bound sensitizer around the blood vessel near the center of the tumor moves with the position of that vessel in the section. Three-dimensional reconstructions of zones within the tumor which bind sensitizer are technically feasible. The pattern of bound sensitizer in the largest tumor (~ 5 mm diameter, Figure 6) again shows an extremely complex pattern which correlates with tumor necrosis and vasculature. Sensitizer-binding near the surface of the tumor is evident, possibly indicating a site of future surface necrosis. Figure 7 shows a high-power photomicrograph of the edge of the smallest tumor shown in Figure 3. It is clear that the amount of sensitizer bound to cells at a depth of 10 to 15 cells is at least 10 times higher than the amount bound over the necrotic region, and over 20 times higher than that bound to cells near the tumor surface. If this bound sensitizer is truly a marker for the viable hypoxic cells in tumors, then the signal-to-noise ratio of 10 or more might be adequate for exploitation by nuclear medicine techniques.

These preliminary studies on metabolism-induced binding of radioactively labelled sensitizers to hypoxic cells are encouraging in that a specific marker for viable hypoxic cells in tumors may have been identified. Such a marker could be exploited in the study of tumor-cell biology and tumor-cell kinetics. If we can show that it is from such labelled cells that tumor regrowth occurs (after treatments which eliminate the oxygenated and proliferating tumor-cell com-

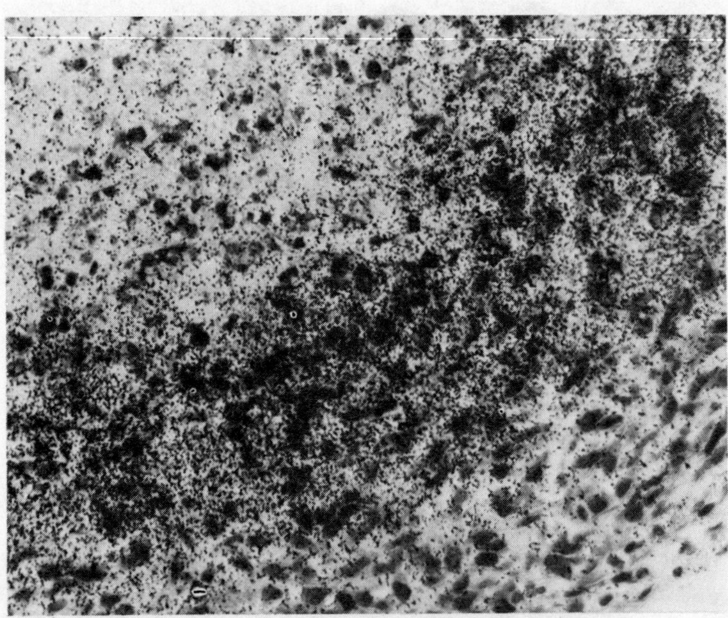

Figure 7. A higher power photomicrograph of the edge of the EMT6 tumor shown in Figure 3.

partments), then a specific marker for tumor cells resistant to treatment may have been found. By labelling the appropriate hypoxic sensitizer (ideally with a serum half-life in man of < 6 hours) with the appropriate γ-emitting radionuclide (e.g., ^{77}Br, whose half-life is ~ 57 hours), a nuclear medicine assay for hypoxia in human tumors might be developed. Patients could be injected with radioactively labelled sensitizer on a given day and scanned one or two days later for bound and retained activity in tumor. Total retained activity could indicate the extent of tumor hypoxia, distribution of activity within tumors could possibly map the intratumor hypoxic regions, and micrometastases of a dimension comparable to the tumor shown in Figure 3 might be detectable.

This new technique is being researched as a tool for tumor biology and as a clinical procedure in nuclear medicine at the Cross Cancer Institute, Edmonton because of its possible utilization as a prognostic aid in tumor-treatment design and outcome.

Summary

The studies on hypoxic cells controlling the radiocurability of human cancer have been briefly reviewed. Several techniques developed to study tumor-cell hypoxia in animal model systems have provided a wealth of basic information, but few of these techniques have had any impact on the clinical practice of radiotherapy. The preliminary evidence that hypoxic-cell sensitizers become covalently bound to hypoxic metabolizing cells in tumors may indicate that a marker for "treatment-resistant" tumor cells has been found. If this marker can be successfully labelled with a γ-emitting radionuclide, a nuclear medicine assay for hypoxic cells in human tumors could become a clinical reality. Such a procedure would be useful in the diagnosis and treatment-planning of cancer.

ACKNOWLEDGMENTS

The new research reported in this chapter was performed with the skillful technical assistance of Bert Meeker, Ron Moore, and Janet Sharplin. The assistance of Shirley Dawson and Karl Liesner in preparing the manuscript is appreciated. Research was supported from the Alberta Heritage Savings and Trust Fund (Applied Cancer Research) and the National Cancer Institute of Canada.

REFERENCES

1. Acker, H., Sylvester, D., Dugan, E., and Durst, G.: The bitumen PO_2 electrode—a new method to manufacture PO_2 needle electrodes. In *Oxygen Transport to Tissue* vol. III, I.A. Silver, M.E. Recinska, and H.I. Bicher, New York: Plenum Press, 1978, pp. 3–8.
2. Adams, G.E.: Chemical radiosensitization of hypoxic cells. *Br Med Bull* **29**:48–53, 1973.
3. Barendsen, G.W., and Broerse, J.J.: Experimental radiotherapy of a rat rhabdomyosarcoma with 15 MeV neutrons and 300 kv x-rays. I. Effects of single exposures. *Eur J Cancer* **5**:373–391, 1969.
4. Barendsen, G.W., Roelse, H., Hermens, A.F., Madhuizen, H.T., van Peperyul, H.A., and Rutgers, D.H., Clonogenic capacity of proliferating and nonproliferating cells of a transplantable rat rhabdomyosarcoma in relation to its radiosensitivity. *J Natl Cancer Inst* **51**:1521–1526, 1973.
5. Beebe, C.H., Liston, M.D., and McKinley, E.W.: U.S. Patent 3,098,813, Electrode, 1963.
6. Bicher, H.I., and Knisely, M.H.: Brain tissue reoxygenation time demonstrated with a new ultramicro oxygen electrode. *J Appl Physiol* **28**:387–390, 1970.
7. Brown, J.M.: Selective radiosensitization of the hypoxic cells of mouse tumors with the nitroimidazole metronidazole and RO-07-0582. *Radiat Res* **64**:633–647, 1975.
8. Brown, J.M., and Howes, A.E.: Comparison of tumor growth delay with cell survival. *Br J Radiol* **47**:509–510, 1974.
9. Brown, J.M., Twentyman, P.R., and Zamvil, S.S.: The response of the RIF-1 tumor to x-irradiation (cell survival regrowth delay and tumor control), chemotherapeutic agents and activated macrophages. *J Natl Cancer Inst* **64**:605–611, 1980.
10. Bush, R.S., Jenkin, R.D.T., Allt, W.E.C., Beale, F.A., Bean, H., Demko, A.J., and Pringle, J.F.: Definitive evidence for hypoxic cells influencing cure in cancer therapy. *Br J Cancer* **37**: Suppl. III, 302–306, 1978.
11. Cater, D.B.: Oxygen tension in neoplastic tissues. *Tumori* **50**:435–444, 1964.
12. Cater, D.B., and Silver, I.A.: Quantitative measurements of oxygen tension in normal tissues and in the tumors of patients before and after radiotherapy. *Acta Radiol* **53**:233–256, 1960.
13. Chapman, J.D.: Hypoxic sensitizers—implications for radiation therapy, *N Engl J Med* **301**:1429–1432, 1979.
14. Chapman, J.D., Raleigh, J.A., Pedersen, J.E., Ngan, J., Shum, F.Y., Meeker, B.E., and Urtasun, R.C.: Potentially three distinct roles for hypoxic cell sensitizers in the clinic. In *Radiation Research,* S. Okada, M. Imamura, T. Terashima, and H. Yamaguchi, eds. Tokyo: Japanese Association for Radiation Research, 1979, pp. 885–892.
15. Chapman, J.D., Reuvers, A.P., Borsa, J., Petkau, A., and McCalla, D.R.: Nitrofurans as radiosensitizers of hypoxic mammalian cells. *Cancer Res* **32**:2616–2624, 1972.
16. Cheung, P.W., Takatani, S., and Ernst, E.A.: Multiple wavelength reflectance oximetry in peripheral tissues. In *Oxygen Transport to Tissue,* vol. III. I.A. Silver, M.E. Recinska, and H.I. Bicher, New York: Plenum Press, 1978, pp. 69–75.
17. Clark, L.C., Wolf, R., Granger, D., and Taylor, Z.: Continuous recording of blood oxygen tensions by polarography. *J Appl Physiol* **6**:189–193, 1953.
18. Denekamp, J., and Harris, S.R.: The response of a transplantable tumor to fractionated irradiation I. X-rays and the hypoxic cell radiosensitizer RO-07-0582. *Radiat Res* **66**:66–75, 1976.
19. Dwek, R.A., Campbell, I.O., Richards, R.E., and Williams, R.J.P., eds: *NMR in Biology.* London: Academic Press, 1977.
20. Fowler, J.F., Adams, G.E., and Denekamp, J.: Radiosensitizers of hypoxic cells in solid tumors. *Cancer Treat Rev* **3**:227–256, 1976.
21. Gray, L.H., Conger, A.D., Ebert, M., Hornsey, S., and Scott, O.C.A.: Concentration of oxygen dissolved in tissues at time of irradiation as a factor in radiotherapy. *Br J Radiol* **26**:638–648, 1953.
22. Hahn, G.M., Rockwell, S., Kallman, R.F., Gordon, L.F., and Frindel, E.: Repair of potentially lethal damage *in vivo* in solid tumor cells after x-irradiation. *Cancer Res* **34**:351–354, 1974.
23. Henk, J.M., and Smith, C.W.: Radiotherapy and hyperbaric oxygen in head and neck cancer: Interim report of second clinical trial. *Lancet* **2**:104–105, 1977.
24. Hermens, A.F., and Barendsen, G.W.: The proliferative status and clonogenic capacity of tumor cells in a transplantable rhabdomyosarcoma of the rat before and after irradiation with 800 rad of x-rays. *Cell Tissue Kinet* **11**:83–100, 1978.
25. Hewitt, H.B., and Wilson, C.W.: Survival curves for tumor cells irradiated *in vivo. Ann NY Acad Sci* **95**:818–827, 1961.
26. Hill, R.P.: Radiation-induced changes in the *in vivo* growth rate of KHT sarcoma cells: Implications for the comparison of growth delay and cell survival. *Radiat Res* **83**:99–108, 1980.
27. Hill, R.P., and Bush, R.S.: A new method of determining the fraction of hypoxic cells in a transplantable murine sarcoma. *Radiat Res* **79**:141–153, 1977.
28. Hill, R.P., Bush, R.S., and Yeung, P.: The effect of anemia on the fraction of hypoxic cells in an experimental tumor. *Br J Radiol* **44**:299–304, 1971.
29. Ji, S., Chance, B., Nishiki, K., Smith, T., and Rich, T.: Micro-light guides: A new method for measuring tissue fluorescence and reflectance. *Am J Physiol* **236**:144–156, 1979.

30. Kallman, R.F.: Repopulation and reoxygenation as factors contributing to the effectiveness of fractionated radiotherapy. *Front Radiat Ther Oncol* **3**:96–108, 1968.
31. Kallman, R.F., The phenomenon of reoxygenation and its implications for radiotherapy. *Radiology* **105**:135–142, 1972.
32. Kessler, M., and Gruenwald, W.: Possibilities of measuring oxygen pressure fields in tissue by multiwire platinum electrodes: *Prog Res Res* **3**:147–152, 1968.
33. Kimmich, H.P., Spaan, J.G., and Kreuzer, F.: Directly heated transcutaneous oxygen sensor, In *Oxygen Transport to Tissue*, vol. III. I.A. Silver, M.E. Recinska, and H.I. Bicher, New York: Plenum Press, 1978, pp. 25–30.
34. Little, J.B., Hahn, G.M., Frindel, E., Tubiana, M.: Repair of potentially lethal radiation damage *in vitro* and *in vivo*. *Radiology* **106**:689–694, 1973.
35. McCalla, D.R., Reuvers, A., and Kaiser, C.: Mode of action of nitrofurazone. *J Bacteriol* **104**:1126–1134, 1970.
36. McNally, N.J.: A low oxygen-enhancement ratio for tumor-cell survival as compared with that for tumor-growth delay. *Int J Radiat Biol* **22**:407–410, 1972.
37. McNally, N.J.: A comparison of the effects of radiation on tumor growth delay and cell survival. The effect of oxygen. *Br J Radiol* **46**:450–455, 1973.
38. McNally, N.J.: Tumor growth delay and cell survival "in situ." *Br J Radiol* **47**:510–511, 1974.
39. McNally, N.J., and Sheldon, P.W.: The effect of radiation on tumor growth delay, cell survival and cure of the animal using a single tumor system. *Br J Radiol* **50**:321–328, 1977.
40. Martin, D.F., Moulder, J.E., and Fisher, J.J.: Tumor response endpoints in the BA 1112 rat sarcoma. *Br J Cancer* **41**: Suppl. IV, 271–274, 1980.
41. Moulder, J.E., and Rockwell, S.C.: Survey of published data on the hypoxic fractions of solid rodent tumors (abstract). *Radiat Res* **83**:376, 1980.
42. Powers, W.E., and Tolmach, L.J.: A multicomponent x-ray survival curve for mouse lymphosarcoma cells irradiated *in vivo*. *Nature* **197**:710–711, 1963.
43. Rasey, J.S., and Nelson, N.J.: Response of an *in vivo–in vitro* tumor to x-rays and cytotoxic drugs: Effect of tumor disaggregation method on cell survival. *Br J Cancer* **41**: Suppl. IV, 217–221, 1980.
44. Rauth, A.M., and Kaufman, K.: *In vivo* testing of hypoxic radiosensitizers using the KHT murine tumor assayed by the lung-colony technique. *Br J Radiol* **48**:209–220, 1975.
45. Reinhold, H.S.: Quantitative evolution of the radiosensitivity of cells of a transplantable rhabdomyosarcoma in the rat. *Eur J Cancer* **2**:33–42, 1966.
46. Rockwell, S., and Kallman, R.F.: Cellular radiosensitivity and tumor radiation response in the EMT-6 tumor cell system. *Radiat Res* **53**:281–294, 1973.
47. Rubin, P., and Casarett, C.W.: *Clinical Radiation Pathology* vols. 1 and 2. Philadelphia: W.B. Saunders, 1968.
48. Stone, H.B., and Withers, H.R.: Metronidazole: Effect on radiosensitivity of tumor and normal tissue in mice. *J Natl Cancer Inst* **55**:1189–1194, 1975.
49. Suit, H.D.: Hyperbaric oxygen in radiotherapy of four mouse tumors. In *Proceedings International Conference Radiation Biology and Cancer,* T. Sugahara, ed. Radiation Society of Japan, 1967, pp. 39–43.
50. Suit, H., Lindberg, R., Suchato, C., and Ozenne, A.: Radiation dose fractionation and high pressure oxygen in radiotherapy of the DBA mouse mammary carcinoma. *Am J Roentgenol Rad Ther Nucl Med* **99**:895–899, 1967.
51. Suit, H.D., and Maeda, M.: Hyperbaric oxygen and radiobiology of a C3H mouse mammary carcinoma. *J Natl Cancer Inst* **39**:639–652, 1967.
52. Sutherland, R.M., and Durand, R.E.: Hypoxic cells in an *in vitro* tumor model *Int J Radiat Biol* **23**:235–246, 1973.
53. Tannock, I.F.: A study of the relationship between vascularity, oxygen tension, and cell proliferation characteristics in experimental tumors. Ph.D. Thesis, University of London, 1968.
54. Tannock, I.F.: The relation between cell proliferation and the vascular system in a transplanted mouse mammary tumor. *Br J Cancer* **22**:258–273, 1968.
55. Tannock, I.F.: A comparison of cell proliferation parameters in solid and ascites Ehrlich tumors. *Cancer Res* **29**:1527–1534, 1969.
56. Tannock, I.F.: Effects of pO_2 on cell proliferation kinetics. In *Time and Dose Relationships in Radiation Biology as Applied to Radiotherapy.* Brookhaven National Laboratory, Upton, N.Y., 1970, pp. 215–224.
57. Thomlinson, R.H.: Changes of oxygenation in tumors in relation to irradiation. *Front Radiat Ther Oncol* **3**:109–121, 1968.
58. Thomlinson, R.H., and Craddock, E.A.: The gross response of an experimental tumor to single doses of x-rays. *Br J Cancer* **21**:108–123, 1967.
59. Thomlinson, R.H., and Gray, L.H.: The histological structure of some human lung cancers and the possible implications for radiotherapy. *Br J Cancer* **9**:539–549, 1955.
60. Urtasun, R.C., Band, P., Chapman, J.D., Feldstein, M.L., Mielke, B., and Fryer, C.: Radiation and high-dose metronidazole in supratentorial glioblastomas. *N Engl J Med* **294**:1364–1367, 1976.
61. van den Brenk, H.A.: Hyperbaric oxygen in radiation therapy. An investigation of dose-effect relationships. *Am J Roentgenol* **102**:8–26, 1968.

62. van Putten, L.M.: Tumor reoxygenation during fractionated radiotherapy: Studies with a transplantable mouse osteosarcoma. *Eur J Cancer* **4**:173–182, 1968.

63. Wheldon, T.E.: Can dose-survival parameters be deduced from *in situ* assays? *Br J Cancer* **41**: Suppl. LV, 79–87, 1980.

CHAPTER 11

Nitroimidazoles as Hypoxic-Cell Radiation Sensitizers and Cytotoxic Agents

Gerald E. Adams, Ph.D., D.Sc.[a]
Claire Clarke, Ph.D.[b]
Kent B. Dawson, Ph.D.[c]
Peter W. Sheldon, Ph.D.[d]
Ian J. Stratford, Ph.D.[e]

The possibility that the relative radiation resistance of hypoxic tumor cells may be a major limiting factor in the local control of some human tumors treated with fractionated radiotherapy has been recognized for over a quarter of a century. Although clinical evidence of the hypoxic cell problem is still rather sparse, there is now little doubt that, in many experimental rodent tumors, hypoxia is certainly the largest single factor influencing tumor response to radiation, even with multifraction radiation. Hypoxic cells, which are present in most rodent solid tumors and probably most human solid tumors as well, arise as a result of tumor-cell proliferation essentially outstripping the development of the vascular supply of the tumor. They occur in and around areas of tumour necrosis where oxygen access is poor. Cells may also become temporarily hypoxic by normal variations in capillary blood flow.

[a]Professor of Physics as Applied to Medicine, Institute of Cancer Research, Sutton, Surrey, England
[b]Scientific Assistant, Institute of Cancer Research, Sutton, Surrey, England
[c]Senior Scientist, Institute of Cancer Research, Sutton, Surrey, England
[d]Scientific Assistant, Institute of Cancer Research, Sutton, Surrey, England
[e]Scientific Assistant, Institute of Cancer Research, Sutton, Surrey, England

Hypoxic cells are dangerous because of their relative radiation resistance. These cells are in a resting state and most will eventually die of nutrient deprivation. Subsequent to, or during radiation treatment, however, tumor regression can occur, and cells which were previously hypoxic can become reoxygenated, enter cycle, and provide a focus for regrowth of the tumor.

Evidence that hypoxia can influence response in clinical radiotherapy has been provided by various studies,[5] including some employing radiation treatment in hyperbaric oxygen.[9,19] Other methods aimed at overcoming hypoxia include the use of unconventional fractionation regimes aimed at optimizing reoxygenation processes during treatment, radiotherapy with high-energy neutrons, and radiation-sensitizing drugs. Chemical agents which increase the radiation sensitivity of hypoxic tumor cells without increasing radiation damage to well-oxygenated normal tissue would be an inexpensive method of overcoming hypoxic-cell radiation resistance. If free of complications, they could be used routinely in radiotherapy without the need for investment in specialized hardware.

There are now many compounds of diverse chemical structure that are known to function as hypoxic-cell sensitizers *in vitro.*

The most promising group currently available—certainly the most well-studied group—includes the nitroimidazoles. In particular, the 2-nitroimidazole misonidazole has been shown to act as a potent hypoxic-cell sensitizer in many different types of experimental tumor systems and is currently in widespread clinical trial as a sensitizer in radiotherapy.

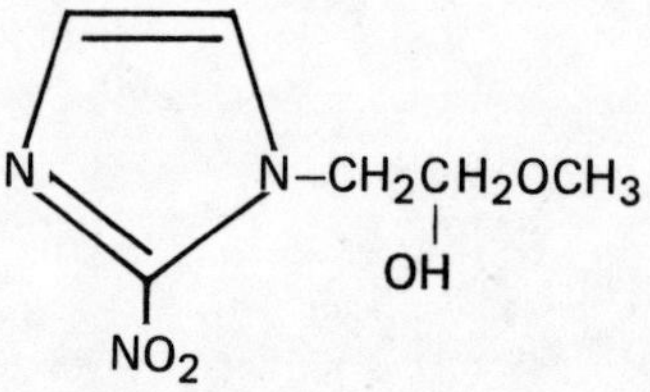

N $N-CH_2CH_2OCH_3$
OH
NO_2

Misonidazole

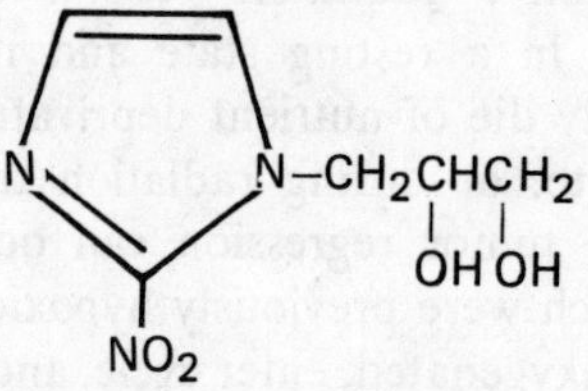

N $N-CH_2CHCH_2$
OH OH
NO_2

Desmethyl Misonidazole
(Ro 05-9963)

Many laboratory studies have established that these compounds mainly act as oxygen-mimetics in that the mechanism of sensitization occurs via fast radiation-induced, free-radical reactions. At least in part, these reactions increase the radiation damage to intracellular DNA which in turn leads to a greater efficiency of cell-killing. Sensitization occurs *only* in hypoxic cells, and this is the major rationale behind their application in radiotherapy since potentiation of normal tissue radiation damage should not be a problem. Thus far, results of ongoing clinical studies are reassuring in this respect.

The generality of sensitization by misonidazole observed in many diverse experimental tumor model systems demonstrates that hypoxic-cell radiation resistance is a common feature of most solid tumors. In some cases, however, reoxygenation occurring during fractionated treatment can greatly reduce the total number of hypoxic cells, and this is reflected in the smaller sensitization sometimes observed under these conditions. It is also likely that reoxygenation may reduce the extent of hypoxia in the clinical situation. It is most unlikely, however, that reoxygenation alone can eliminate entirely the hypoxia problem.

Clinical Limitations of Misonidazole

It is now clear that the neurotoxic properties of misonidazole will prevent the drug from being used at dosages sufficient to give maximum sensitization irrespective of the treatment regime chosen. Currently, most drug regimes limit total dosage to a maximum of 12 g/m^2. The individual dose per fraction will obviously depend on the number of fractions given. Therefore, the greater the number of fractions, the lower the drug-dose per fraction and the attainable enhancement ratio. In conventional treatment—e.g., those employing 30 radiation fractions with misonidazole administered before each treatment—the dose of drug per fraction is 0.4 g/m^2. This leads to tumor levels of about 20–25 $\mu g/g$ which would predict maximum enhancement ratios of no greater than about 1.3. Not surprisingly, some of the current trials employ treatment regimes where the drug is given in a smaller number of fractions, thereby permitting larger individual amounts to be administered. In 10 fraction treatments, for example, tumor levels of about 50–60 $\mu g/g$ may be attained which should lead to higher enhancement ratios. In some situations however, reoxygenation will decrease the hypoxic fraction, and the enhancement ratios will be reduced.

It has been shown that phenytoin influences the pharmacokinetics of misonidazole.[18,20,21] Patients receiving phenytoin show a marked reduction in the half-life of misonidazole, although peak levels are unchanged. Since neurotoxicity in man is probably a function of the total tissue exposure to misonidazole, reduction of half-life without reduction of peak tumor levels could increase therapeutic ratios.

An obvious requirement for the development of improved radiosensitizers is an understanding of the factors influencing their neurotoxic properties. It is necessary to have available a suitable animal model which would enable reliable quantitative comparisons to be made of the neurotoxic potentials of different compounds. Several biochemical methods have been developed for detecting chemically induced peripheral neuropathies.[8] These methods involve the measurement of the enzymes β-glucuronidase and β-galactosidase in nervous tissue. This can be done either by measurement of activities in homogenized preparations of whole nerves[10] or by an *in situ* cytochemical technique.[6] It is known that the activities of both these enzymes greatly increase during the second phase of Wallerian degeneration, i.e., during the period of proliferation of Schwann cells and macrophages. Since the majority of chemically induced neuropathies appear to be of the Wallerian type, there are grounds for believing that an increase in the activity of these enzymes in animals treated with nitroimidazoles indicates the development of peripheral neuropathy.

Desmethyl Misonidazole (Ro 05-9963)

The compound desmethyl misonidazole (9963), in which the terminal methoxy group in the side chain is replaced by hydroxyl, is the major metabolite of misonidazole. Numerous studies both *in vitro* and *in vivo* have shown that this compound is also a potent sensitizer. Some new data using a tumor-cure end point are shown in Figure 1.

The experimental details of the technique have been published by Sheldon and Hill.[12] Briefly, fragments of the anaplastic MT tumor were implanted subcutaneously over the sacral regions of the backs of female WHT/Ht mice. The mice were selected for treatment when the tumors had attained a mean diameter of 5–6 mm. Either misonidazole or 9963 was injected I.P. at 0.3 mg/g (in 0.5 ml saline/25 g mouse) 60 and 45 minutes respectively before local irradiation of the tumor. These intervals are known to be optimal.[13] The unanesthetised mice were restrained in lead boxes and their tumors locally irradiated with 240 kV x-rays (HVL 1.3 mm Cu; 3.9 Gy/min). Tumor response was assayed at 80 days and tumor control plotted as a function of radiation dose. The dose required for 50% control (TCD_{50}) was computed using the logit method of maximum likelihood.[16]

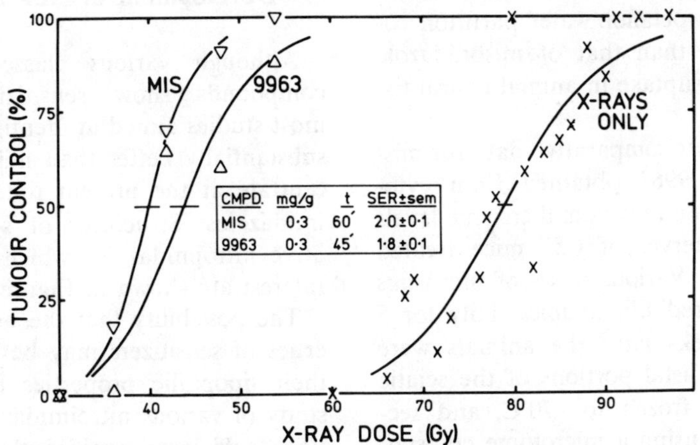

Figure 1. Response of the MT tumor to single doses of x-rays; effect of misonidazole and Ro 05-9963 given 60 and 45 minutes respectively before irradiation.

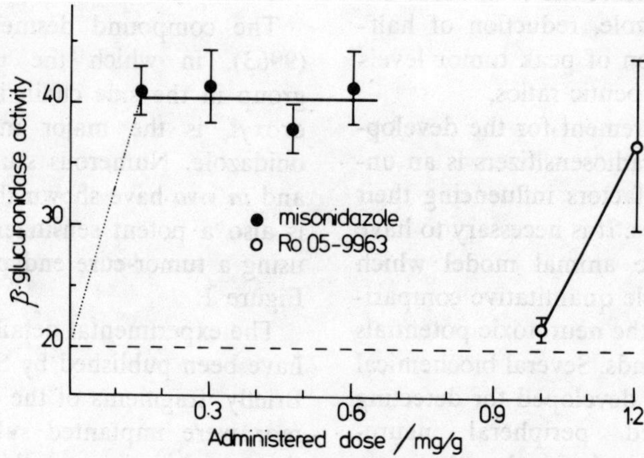

Figure 2. Elevation of enzyme activity in peripheral nerve of WH mice treated with five daily doses of misonidazole and Ro 05-9963. Enzyme activity assayed 4 weeks after dosing.

The TCD_{50} for mice treated with x-rays alone is 78.9 ± 0.7 Gy (see Fig. 1). A single dose of 0.3 mg/g of 9963 or misonidazole reduces the TCD_{50} values to 43.9 ± 1.6 Gy and 40.0 ± 1.2 Gy which correspond to enhancement ratios of 1.80 ± 0.07 and 1.97 ± 0.06 respectively. Misonidazole is marginally more effective than 9963 in this system.

NEUROTOXIC PROPERTIES OF 9963

There is evidence that some nitroimidazoles with octanol/water partition coefficients lower than that of misonidazole show decreased uptake in animal neural tissue.[4]

Figure 2 shows comparative data for misonidazole and 9963 obtained from cytochemical studies on lysozomal enzyme levels in peripheral nerves of C57 mice treated with each drug. Various doses of the drugs were administered I.P. to mice daily for 5 days. Four weeks later the animals were killed and the distal portions of the sciatic nerves excised, frozen to −70°C, and sectioned (10 μm) using a microtome cryostat. Activity of β-glucuronidase was assayed by the *in situ* technique referred to above. It can be seen in Figure 2 that misonidazole doses as low as 0.15 mg/g daily caused a doubling in enzyme activity, whereas with 9963 daily doses of 1.2 mg/g were required. These results suggest that 9963 is less neurotoxic than misonidazole, although whether or not this will be reflected clinically remains to be seen. However, clinical studies with this drug are now under way, and preliminary data are presented by Dische in Chapter 40.

Development of New Sensitizers

Although various classes of chemical compounds show sensitizing properties, most studies aimed at identifying sensitizers substantially better than misonidazole concentrate at the present time on the nitroimidazoles. Structures of some representative nitroimidazoles which are of current interest are shown in Figure 3.

The possibility that the neurotoxic properties of sensitizers may be associated with their lipophilic properties has led to the study of various nitroimidazoles with partition coefficients significantly less than that of misonidazole. The compound SR 2508 (Stanford Research Institute)[3] shows a sensitizing efficiency *in vivo* comparable to that

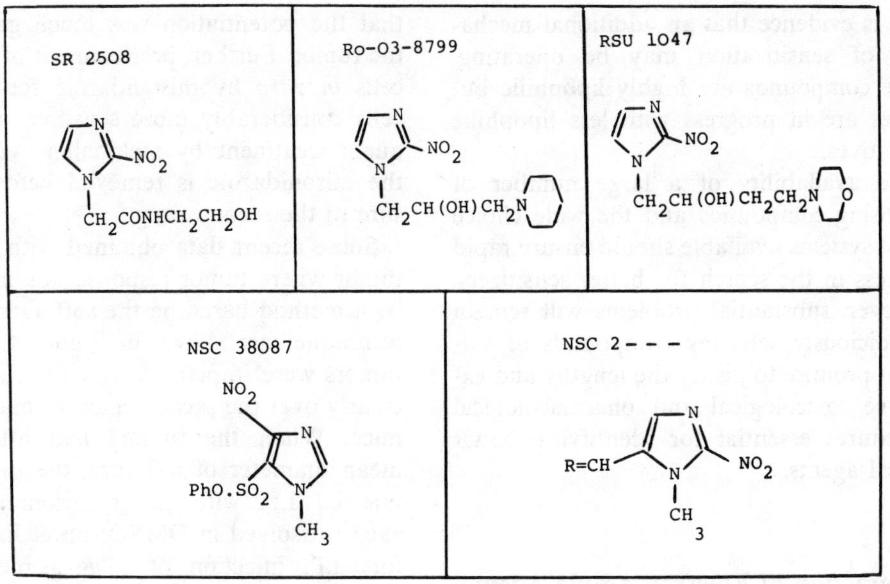

SR 2508	Ro-03-8799	RSU 1047
$CH_2CONHCH_2CH_2OH$ (2-nitroimidazole, NO_2)	$CH_2CH(OH)CH_2N$ (piperidine) (2-nitroimidazole, NO_2)	$CH_2CH(OH)CH_2CH_2N$ (morpholine, O) (2-nitroimidazole, NO_2)
NSC 38087: NO_2, PhO.SO_2, N–CH_3	NSC 2- - - : R=CH, NO_2, N–CH_3	

Figure 3. Structures of some nitroimidazoles of current interest.

of misonidazole, but has a substantially higher LD_{50} value (i.e., less toxic). Its low lipophilicity (P = 0.046) is reflected in the relatively low uptake in brain tissue in the mouse.

The Roche compound 8799 and the Sutton compound RSU 1047 are related. The former is a member of a series of promising β-hydroxy propanolamine derivatives,[14] shows good sensitizing properties *in vivo* and *in vitro*, and is superior to misonidazole in its hypoxic/cytotoxic properties. The compound RSU 1047 is a derivative from a series of nitroimidazoles where the influence of side chain length is being investigated.[1] Its efficiency is comparable to misonidazole, but in the lysozomal enzyme assay it appears to be less neurotoxic. Its partition coefficient (0.2) is intermediate between misonidazole and 9963.

It is now well established that the major factor influencing sensitization efficiency *in vitro* is the redox properties of hypoxic-cell sensitizers of this type. Electron-affinity correlations have been helpful, particularly in identifying promising compounds in the nitroimidazole series. An example of a general group where sensitizing efficiency is substantially greater than that of misonidazole is the 5-substituted 2-nitroimidazole structure shown in Figure 3. Interest in this group stems from an earlier observation of very high activity in the Lepetit compound L8711, a 5-aldehydo-2-nitroimidazole.[2] This is in line with its high one-electron reduction potential. However, the compound is fairly toxic in aerobic mammalian cell cultures. A series of related compounds with the R=CH group substituted in position 5 has been synthesized in our laboratory (Gibson, unpublished research). Several of these show sensitizing efficiencies an order of magnitude or more greater than that of misonidazole. Some compounds are particularly promising because of their low lipophilicities, and further studies are in progress.

An atypical series of nitroimidazoles is represented by the NCI compound 38087. It has been shown that 4-nitroimidazoles substituted in position 5 with various sulphonamide or sulphonate groups show sensitizing efficiencies up to two orders of magnitude greater than that of misonidazole,[1] although their electron affinities are similar. The reasons for this are still not clear, although there is evidence that an additional mechanism of sensitization may be operating. These compounds are highly lipophilic but studies are in progress with less lipophilic derivatives.

The availability of a large number of promising compounds and the wide choice of test systems available should ensure rapid progress in the search for better sensitizers. However, substantial problems will remain in judiciously selecting compounds of sufficient promise to justify the lengthy and expensive toxicological and pharmacological procedures essential for identifying better clinical agents.

Interaction of Electron-Affinic Agents with Cytotoxic Drugs

It is now well established, following original observations by Sutherland,[17] that nitro-containing, electron-affinic sensitizers are generally much more cytotoxic to hypoxic cells than are oxic cells. This prompted the speculation[17] that drugs of this type could have potential value in combination chemotherapy if hypoxic cells were resistant or inaccessible to some of the cytotoxic drugs used in cancer chemotherapy. Indeed, there is now substantial evidence that hypoxia can induce chemoresistance in some cases. However, additional evidence now accumulating strongly suggests direct interaction between electron-affinic compounds and other cytotoxic agents, particularly alkylating drugs.

Results from several laboratories have shown potentiation of tumor response to melphalan, cyclophosphamide, and other alkylating agents when misonidazole is also administered to the tumor-bearing mice. In studies of Rose et al.,[11] for example, misonidazole (1 mg/g) given immediately before melphalan increased the response of Lewis lung tumors to the melphalan with a dose-modification factor of two. Although some enhancement was also observed in normal tissue response, it was concluded that the potentiation was much greater in the tumor. Further, pretreatment of hypoxic cells *in vitro* by misonidazole renders the cells considerably more sensitive to subsequent treatment by melphalan even when the misonidazole is removed before exposure to the second drug.[15]

Some recent data obtained with the MT tumor where tumor response was measured by a method based on the soft agar cloning technique[7] are shown in Figure 4. Briefly, tumors were implanted as a brei intramuscularly over the sacral region of male WHT mice. When the tumors had attained a mean diameter of 6–7 mm, the mice were injected I.P. with either misonidazole or 9963 (dissolved in DMSO) immediately before I.P. injection of 5 μg/g melphalan. Eighteen hours later, the tumors were excised, cellular suspensions prepared, and the cells plated onto soft agar for incubation. Plating efficiency was 90%, and cell survival was expressed as CFU/g.

Melphalan (5 μg/g) with DMSO reduced cell survival to 3.6×10^{-2} (see Fig. 4), but no significant toxicity was observed with either misonidazole or 9963 dissolved in DMSO or with DMSO alone. However, when either misonidazole or 9963 was administered with melphalan, tumor-cell survival was greatly reduced. At 1 mg/g misonidazole the dose-modification factor was about 2, and even at 10% of this dose a

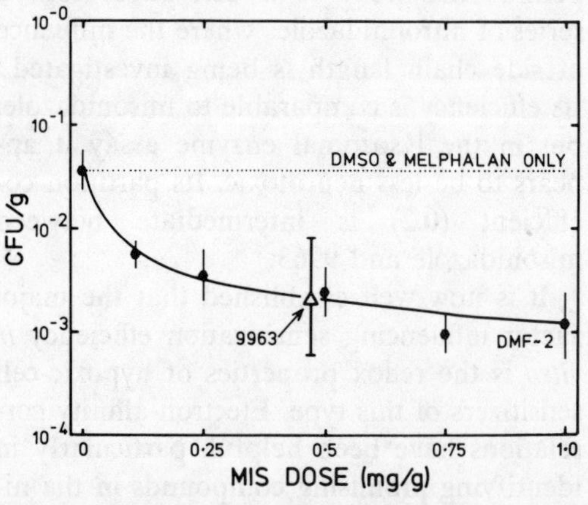

Figure 4. Potentiation by misonidazole of the cytotoxic effect of melphalan in MT tumors in WH mice.

DMF of 1.5 is still evident, suggesting that potentiation might be achievable with misonidazole used at doses within the clinical range.

It is far too early to say whether this type of drug interaction will have any therapeutic value in oncology. Certainly much further work is required, particularly with normal tissue systems. Nevertheless, recent laboratory evidence that the effect can be found with a variety of experimental tumors, electron-affinic agents, and alkylating drugs is certainly encouraging.

ACKNOWLEDGEMENTS

We wish to thank Dr. C.E. Smithen of Roche Products Ltd. for supply of misonidazole and Ro 05-9963, and Miss E. Batten and Miss D. Scottow for excellent technical assistance.

REFERENCES

1. Adams, G.E., Ahmed, I., Fielden, E.M., O'Neill, P., and Stratford, I.J.: The development of some nitroimidazoles as hypoxic cell sensitizers. *Cancer Clin Trials* **3**:37–42, 1980.
2. Adams, G.E., Flockhart, I.R., Smithen, C.E., Stratford, I.J., Wardman, P., and Watts, M.E.: Electron-affinic sensitization VII: A correlation between structures, one-electron reduction potentials and efficiencies of nitroimidazoles as hypoxic cell radiosensitizers. *Radiat Res* **67**:9–20, 1976.
3. Brown, J.M., and Lee, W.W.: Pharmaco-kinetic considerations in radiation sensitizer development. In *Radiation Sensitizers: Their Use in the Clinical Management of Cancer.* Brady, ed. New York: Masson, 1980, pp. 2–13.
4. Brown, J.M., and Workman, P.: Partition coefficients as a guide to the development of sensitizers which are less toxic than misonidazole. *Radiat Res* **82**:171–190, 1980.
5. Bush, R.S., Jenkins, R.D.T., Allt, W.E.C., Beale, F.A., Bean, H., Dembo, A.J., and Pringle, J.F.: Definitive evidence for hypoxic cells influencing cure in cancer therapy. *Br J Cancer* **37**: Suppl. III, 302–306, 1978.
6. Clarke, C., Dawson, K.B., Sheldon, P.W., Chaplin, D.J., and Stratford, I.J.: A quantitative cytochemical method for assessing the neurotoxicity of the radiosensitizer misonidazole. In *Radiation Sensitizers: Their Use in the Clinical Management of Cancer.* Brady, ed. New York: Masson, pp. 245–249, 1980.
7. Courtenay, V.D.: A soft agar assay for Lewis lung tumor and B16 melanoma taken directly from the mouse. *Br J Cancer* **34**:39–45, 1976.
8. Dewar, A.J., and Moffett, B.J.: Biochemical methods for detection of neurotoxicity. A short review in *Pharmacological Methods in Toxicology,* G. Zbinden, and F. Gross, eds. Oxford: Pergamon Press, 1979.
9. Henk, J.M., and Smith, C.W.: Radiotherapy and hyperbaric oxygen in head and neck cancer. *Lancet* 104–105, 1977.
10. Rose, G.P., Dewar, A.J., and Stratford, I.J.: A biochemical method for assessing the neurotoxic effects of hypoxic cell radiosensitizers: Experience with misonidazole in the rat. *Br J Cancer* **42**: 890–899, 1980.
11. Rose, C.M., Millar, J.L., Peacock, J.H., Phelps, T.A., and Stephens, T.C.: Differential enhancement of melphalan cytotoxicity in tumor and normal tissue by misonidazole. In *Radiation Sensitizers: Their Use in Clinical Management of Cancer.* Brady, ed. New York: Masson, 1980, pp. 250–257.
12. Sheldon, P.W., and Hill, S.A.: Hypoxic cell radiosensitizers and tumor control by x-ray of a transplanted tumor in mice. *Br J Cancer* **35**:795–808, 1977.
13. Sheldon, P.W., and Hill, S.A.: Further investigations of the effects of the hypoxic cell radiosensitizer, Ro 07-0582 on local control of a mouse tumor. *Br J Cancer* **36**:198–205, 1977.
14. Smithen, C.E., Clarke, E.D., Dale, J.A., Jacobs, R.S., Wardman, P., Watts, M.E., and Woodcock, M.: Novel (nitro-1-imidazolyl) alkanolamines as potential radiosensitizers with improved therapeutic properties. In *Radiation Sensitizers: Their Use in Clinical Management of Cancer* Brady, ed. New York: Massson, 1980, pp. 22–32.
15. Stratford, I.J., Adams, G.E., Horsman, M.R., Kandaiya, S., Rajaratnam, S., Smith, E., and Williamson, C.: The interaction of misonidazole with radiation, chemotherapeutic agents or heat: A preliminary report. In *Radiation Sensitizers: Their Use in Clinical Management of Cancer* Brady, ed. New York: Massson, 1980, pp. 276–281.
liminary report. *Cancer Clin Trials* (in press).
16. Suit, H.D., Shalek, R.J., and Wette, R.: Radiation response of C3H mouse mammary carcinoma evaluated in terms of cellular radiation sensitivity. In *Cellular Radiation Biology.* Baltimore: Williams & Wilkins, 1965, pp. 514–530.
17. Sutherland, R.M.: Selective chemotherapy of non-cycling cells in an *in vitro* tumor model. *Cancer Res* **34**:3501–3503, 1974.
18. Wasserman, T.H., Phillips, T.L., Van Raalte, G., Urtasun, R., Partington, J., Kozoit, D., Schwade,

J.G., Gangji, D., and Strong, J.M.: The neurotoxicity of misonidazole: Potential modifying rôle of phenytoin and dexamethasone. *Br J Radiol* **53**: 172–173, 1980.

19. Watson, E.R., Halnan, K.E., Dische, S., Saunders, M.I., Cade, I.S., McEwen, J.B., Wiernik, G., Perrins, D.J.D., and Sutherland, I.: Hyperbaric oxygen and radiotherapy. A Medical Research Council Trial in Carcinoma of the Cervix. *Br J Radiol* **51**:879–887, 1978.
20. Workman, P.: Effects of pre-treatment with phenobarbitone and phenytoin on the pharmacokinetics and toxicity of misonidazole in mice. *Br J Cancer* **40**:335–353, 1979.
21. Workman, P., Bleehen, N.M., and Wiltshire, C.R.: Phenytoin shortens the half-life of the radiosensitizer misonidazole in man. *Br J Cancer* **2**:302–304, 1980.

CHAPTER 12

Radiosensitizers Other Than Nitroimidazoles

Marcello Quintiliani, M.D.[a]

Radiosensitizers other than nitroimidazoles include a large number of compounds, widely different in structure and biological activity.

On the whole, radiosensitizers can be classified, according to an advisory group convened by IAEA in 1975, as follows:[11]

1. Radiosensitizers specific for hypoxic cells
   a. Electron-affinic agents
   b. Membrane-specific agents
2. Analogues of DNA precursors
   a. Incorporated into DNA
   b. Not incorporated into DNA
3. Radiation-activated cytotoxic compounds
4. Factors which modify cellular regulatory processes
   a. Inhibitors of repair
   b. DNA-binding and intercalating compounds
   c. Inhibitors of natural radioprotection
   d. Hyperthermia

While the classification neither excludes the existence of other types of drugs nor implies that the groups are mutually exclusive, we shall refer to it for the purpose of the present discussion. This will deal with a limited number of nonnitroimidazole compounds belonging to one or another of the classes reported above. The reasons for this approach can be summarized as follows:

1. Apart from nitroimidazoles, no single compound, or class of compounds, has been identified during the last few years as a real breakthrough in the applications of radiosensitizers to radiotherapy.
2. Some of the compounds recently investigated, however, seem to be worthy of further investigation, while others, already extensively studied, offer the opportunity of discussing the requisites for the use of sensitizers in radiotherapy on the basis of practical experience.

This author has tried to center his discussion on true radiosensitizers alone, avoiding as far as possible examples of enhanced drug–radiation interactions (as the applications of chemotherapeutic drugs and radiation are discussed elsewhere in this volume). In addition, the choice of compounds strictly reflects the personal views of the author.

Chlorpromazine

Among the sensitizers specific for hypoxic cells, some attention can be devoted to chlorpromazine (CPZ), one of the so-called membrane-specific agents. Compounds in this class include anesthetics, analgesics, and tranquilizers, and have been investigated mainly by Singh and his associates at BARC in Bombay.

CPZ is probably the most interesting of this class of compounds. According to She-

[a]Senior Investigator, Istituto di Tecnologie Biomediche, Consiglio Nazionale delle Richerche, Rome, Italy

noy et al.,[14] CPZ markedly increased the lethal effect of radiation on anoxic *E. coli* B/r cells as well as that on Yoshida ascites sarcoma cells and thymocytes from rat, as revealed by the erythrosin-exclusion test. Moreover, the drug displayed a definite cytotoxicity vs. anoxic bacterial cells[14] and two experimental tumors in mice.[7,17] Such toxicity markedly increased under acutely hypoxic conditions in one of the two experimental tumors. With regard to interactions with radiation, CPZ showed a synergistic effect on fibrosarcoma and a sensitization effect on mouse sarcoma 180 A.[7,17] As far as the mechanism involved is concerned, evidence has been produced showing that the sensitizing effect requires OH radicals and is likely to be due to long-lived radical cations formed on reaction of CPZ with the same OHs.[15,21] In any case, the drug has a quite distinct chemical behavior from electron-affinic compounds, being rather an electron donor.

Quite independently from these studies, it has been reported by other investigators that CPZ is an active radiosensitizing agent against some experimental malanotic tumors.[23] This activity seems to be related to the melanotropic nature of CPZ and to its selective localization in melanine-rich tissues. Two hypotheses have been proposed to explain the radiosensitizing activity of CPZ toward melanomas. The first holds that melanotic cells are radioresistant because of the stable free radical nature of melanine which enables it to capture damaging radiation-induced free radicals preventing them from reacting with critical targets in cells. Sensitization occurs because CPZ forms a charge-transfer complex with melanine, masking its free radical nature and thus eliminating its scavenging ability. The second hypothesis attributes instead the sensitization to the *in situ* formation of CPZ transients which then attack melanotic cells due to the preferential localization of CPZ in such cells.[4]

Analogues of DNA Precursors Incorporated into DNA

The best known of this class of compounds are derivatives of thymine by substitution of the methyl group in 5 position with Cl, Br, or I. Among the derivatives, the nucleoside bromo-deoxy-uridine (BUdR) is the most extensively studied because it is the least toxic. The halogen-uracil derivatives can be incorporated by competition into the DNA of dividing cells in place of thymine, particularly in the presence of a suitable antimetabolite inhibiting the endogenous synthesis of thymidine; this makes the cells more sensitive to lethal effects of radiation[18]. Sensitization is only due to the halogenated base incorporated in DNA and proportional to the extent of thymine substitution (which is evidence in favor of the critical role of DNA in cell-killing by radiation). Evidence has been produced that cells incorporating 5-BU exhibit increased radiosensitivity and decreased capacity of recovery from sublethal damage.[6] It has been shown that substituted DNA is more susceptible to radiation damage[9] and that, in some cases, the presence of 5-BU interferes with the DNA-repair systems which operate in irradiated cells.[10] The molecular mechanism of biological sensitization is not yet fully understood however. During the 1960s attempts were made in the United States and Japan to apply 5-BUdR sensitization in cancer radiotherapy. Because of its rapid degradation in the liver, BUdR was given intraarterially before each exposure to x-rays and tumors to be treated were restricted to advanced cases of oral cavity and orofaringeal cancer[1] and to brain tumors.[8] Reports on the American trial concluded that, while striking responses were observed in some of the tumors thus treated, prohibitively intense mucous membrane reactions developed consistently enough to suggest that the normal mucosal epithelium of the mouth and pharinx, after intensive irradiation, turns over at a rate close to, and possibly exceeding, that of squamous cell carcinomas arising in these sites—making it unlikely that the analogs would be incorporated differentially into the tumor cells to a clinically useful degree. Brain tumors have been evaluated somewhat more optimistically in spite of side effects such as depilation, radiodermatitis on the catheterized side of the forehead, and onychomadesis of fingernails. 5-BUdR, however, has not been used in conjunction with radiotherapy during the last few years, at least to the author's knowledge.

Iodine-Containing Radiosensitizers

Compounds in this class of sensitizers, which include a wide variety of inorganic and organic chemicals containing iodine in their molecule, have been called "radiation-activated cytotoxic compounds" because their sensitizing activity is due to the transient species formed by their reaction with radiation-induced primary water radicals.[12] These transients are very likely iodine or iodine-containing radicals; they are probably able to attack critical biological structures more effectively and selectively than water radicals alone—resulting in sensitization. As an example of this mechanism, the radiolysis of the simplest iodine sensitizer, I^-, can be mentioned. The process goes as follows:

$$I^- + OH \rightarrow I^\bullet + OH^-$$

$$I^\bullet + I^- \rightarrow I_2^-$$

$$I_2^- + I_2^- \rightarrow I^- + I_3^-$$

As a result, OH radicals are replaced by the radicals $I^\bullet$ and I_2^- which are responsible for the radiosensitization.[12] The third reaction shows how I_2^- decays to form two stable species if not reacting with any substrate.

Iodine-containing compounds are probably the most versatile radiosensitizers with regard to their ability to enhance the response to radiation of a variety of biological systems and end points (ranging from enzyme inactivation to 30 days lethality in mammals).[12]

In view of possible practical application of iodine-containing sensitizers, some interest was originated by the recent demonstration that iodinated contrast media used in radiology also belong to this class. These compounds, generally derivatives of triiodobenzoic acid, are very well known with regard to their pharmacology and toxicology; they can be administered, mainly intravenously, in large amounts without undesiderable side effects.

The experimental data for contrast media available at this time indicate their radiosensitizing activity with respect to survival of bacterial and mammalian cells and to growth inhibition of mouse fibrosarcoma. Experiments on mammalian cells in culture, using V 79 cells and iothalamic acid, have shown that the sensitizing effect is dose modifying and near to a maximum of 100 mM ITA with an enhancement ratio of about 2 (whether cells are anoxic or fully oxigenated).[19] The indifference of the sensitizing activity to the presence or the absence of oxygen is a general feature of iodine-containing sensitizers. In some conditions, however, particularly with bacteria, the sensitizing activity is much larger in oxic than in anoxic cells.[20] The experiments on mouse fibrosarcoma[14] were also carried out using ITA, injected directly into the tumor mass in the amount of 200 mg prior to radiation. This was given either as a single or double dose; tumor-bearing animals were submitted to a second exposure when the tumor mass reached the minimum size after the first irradiation. These experiments tested, in addition to ITA, a membrane-specific drug such as procaine-HCl. Both ITA and procaine, in combination with x-rays, induced reduction in tumor size greater than that induced by radiation alone. The cure-rate increased from 19% in animals only irradiated to 52% in animals treated with ITA. These rather preliminary observations have not thus far been followed up by further reports.

Conclusion

The data reported above fully justify the statement made in the introduction that none of the nonnitroimidazole radiosensitizers discovered during the last few years seem to bear the promise of major improvements in radiation therapy. The so-called membrane-specific drugs, and in particular chlorpromazine, are probably worthy of further investigation. Perhaps the most interesting feature of CPZ is the interaction of the drug with melanine and the possibility that it can be used in the treatment of melanotic tumors. Recent investigations have shown that 7-hydroxy chlorpromazine, a major metabolite of the drug, has a greater melanine affinity than CPZ and is a better sensitizer for a melanotic experimental tumor than CPZ.[4] This observation has stimulated efforts to modify the CPZ structure in order to arrive at a molecular pattern providing optimum sensitization and a minimum of negative side effects. CPZ is in fact not deprived of adverse effects, including skin photosensitivity, melanine deposition, retinal damage, and ocular opacity.

The data relative to 5-BUdR have been reported, in spite of the fact that 5-BUdR is not likely to be the object of future applications in combinations with radiotherapy, because clinical experience accumulated so far contains important information relevant to the use of radiosensitizers. The fundamental point is that no therapeutic advantage can be expected unless an induced alteration of response acts differentially. This principle is one of the main reasons why it is very difficult to envisage any possible future applications for iodine-containing sensitizers, particularly for iodinated contrast media. The experimental evidence thus far available does not indicate that they could sensitize tumor cells preferentially with respect to normal cells.

One could speculate on the possible means of artificially inducing selectivity; the simplest of those means is probably that of administration by selective catheterism which has been already applied to radiological contrast media for diagnostic purposes.[22] At this moment, however, a further question arises: Is there any point in trying to sensitize euoxic tumor cells? According to some clinicians the main problem in the local control of primary tumors is that posed by hypoxic cells. If so, there is no future for sensitizers not specific for such cells. Admittedly a lot more research would be required before one could ascertain whether iodinated contrast media could be amenable to therapeutic exploitation in the treatment of well-oxigenated tumor cells. However, before undertaking such research an answer to the question posed above would be required.

Summary

Among the large variety of nonnitroimidazole-sensitizing agents, no single compound or class of compounds, has been identified during the last few years as a real breakthrough in the application of radiosensitizers to radiotherapy. In the author's opinion, however, a limited number of compounds are worthy of consideration, namely:

1. *Chlorpromazine* (CPZ)–some evidence indicates that CPZ can specifically increase the radiosensitivity of melanotic cells; it is, in fact, active in sensitizing to radiation some experimental melanomas; the possibility of using some convenient CPZ derivative in the treatment of human melanotic tumors is being explored.
2. *5-Bromodeoxy-uridine*–this nucleoside, which contains a bromine-substituted uracil and is incorporated, in place of

thymine, into DNA of dividing cells, has already been used as a radiosensitizer in human cancer therapy. However, clinical applications have been practically halted because sensitization occurred experimentally both in tumors and healthy tissues, showing that no therapeutic advantage can be expected unless an induced enhancement of the radiation response acts differentially.

3. *Iodinated contrast media* (ICM)–like other iodine-containing compounds, the radiosensitizing activity of ICM is due to the iodine-containing transient species formed by irradiation at expense of the original compound. The available data do not indicate that ICM can be applied in human radiotherapy.

ACKNOWLEDGEMENTS

Thanks are due to Mr. A. Mancini for assistance in preparing the manuscript.

REFERENCES

1. Bagshaw, M.A., Doggett, R.L.S., Smith, K.C., Kaplan, H.S., and Nelsen, T.S.: Intraarterial 5-bromodeoxyuridine and x-ray therapy. *AJR* **99**:886–894, 1967.
2. Cooper, M., and Mishima, Y.: The radio-response of malignant melanomas pretreated with chlorpromazine. In *Biology of Normal and Abnormal Melanocytes* T. Kawamura, T.B. Fitzpatrick, M. Seiji, eds. Baltimore: Univ. Park Press, 1971, pp. 141–147.
3. Cooper, M., and Mishima, Y.: Increased *in vitro* radiosensitivity of malignant melanoma induced by *in vivo* administration of chlorpromazine. *Br J Dermatol* **86**:491–493, 1972.
4. Damsker, J.I., Maklis, R., Brady, L.W., and Nodiff, E.A.: Radiosensitization of malignant melanoma. I. The effect of 7-hydroxychlorpromazine on the *in vivo* radiation response of Fortne's melanoma. *Int J Radiat Oncol Biol Phys* **4**:821–824, 1978.
5. Djordjevic, D., and Szybalski, W.: Genetics of human cell lines. III. Incorporation of 5-bromo and 5-iododeoxyuridine into the DNA of human cells and its effect on radiation sensitivity. *J Exp Med* **112**:509–531, 1960.
6. Elkind, M.M.: DNA damage and mammalian cell killing. In *Symposium on DNA Repair Mechanisms* Keystone, Colorado, 1978, pp. 447–480.
7. George, K.C., Srinivasan, V.T., and Singh, B.B.: Cytotoxic effect of chlorpromazine and its interaction with radiation on a mouse fibrosarcoma. *Int J Radiat Biol* **38**:661–665, 1980.
8. Hoshino, T., Nagai, M., Soto, F., Sano, K., and Watari, T.: Bromouridine as a radiosensitizing agent of malignant brain tumors. In *Radiation Protection and Sensitization* H.L. Moroson, and M. Quintiliani, eds. London: Taylor and Francis, 1970, pp. 492–497.
9. Kaplan, H.S.: DNA-strand scission and loss of viability after X-irradiation of normal and sensitized bacterial cells. *Proc Nat Acad Sci USA* **55**:1442–1446, 1966.
10. Lett, J.T., Coldwell, I., and Little, J.G.: Repair of X-ray damage to the DNA in *Micrococcus Radiodurans*: The effect of 5-bromodeoxyuridine. *J Mol Biol* **48**:395–408, 1970.
11. *Modification of Radiosensitivity of Biological Systems* Vienna: IAEA, 1976, pp. 207–209.
12. Quintiliani, M.: Molecular mechanisms of radiosensitization by iodine-containing compounds. In *Advances in Chemical Radiosensitization* Vienna: IAEA, 1974, pp. 87–103.
13. Shenoy, M.A., George, K.C., and Singh, B.B.: Studies on chlorpromazine. A hypoxic cell sensitizer and a potent cytotoxic drug. BARC/I-555, Bombay, India, 1979.
14. Shenoy, M.A., George, K.C., Singh, A.B., and Gopal-Ayengar, A.R.: Modification of radiation effects in single-cell systems by membrane-binding agents. *Int J Radiat Biol* **28**:519–526, 1975.
15. Shenoy, M.A., and Gopalakrishna, K.: Biochemical aspects of radiation sensitization of *E. coli* B/r by chlorpromazine. *Int J Radiat Biol* **33**:587–593, 1978.
16. Shenoy, M.A., and Singh, B.B.: Hypoxic cytotoxicity of chlorpromazine and the modification of radiation response in *E. coli* B/r. *Int J Radiat Biol* **34**:595–600, 1978.
17. Shenoy, M.A., and Singh, B.B.: Cytotoxic and radiosensitizing of chlorpromazine hydrochloride in sarcoma 180 A. *Indian J Exp Biol* **18**:791–795, 1980.
18. Szybalski, W.: Radiosensitizing effect of the halogenated thymidine analogs. In R.F. Kallman, ed., Research in Radiotherapy. Approaches to Chemical Sensitization, Washington, D.C.: Nat'l Acad. Sci., Nat'l Research Council, 1961, pp. 162–80.
19. Simone, G., Pini, L., Tamba, M., et al.: and Quintiliani, M.: Radiosensitization by iothalamic acid in single cell systems (abstract). *Radiat Environ Biophys* **17**:331, 1980.
20. Simone, G., and Quintiliani, M.: Iodinated radiological contrast media as radiosensitizers. *Int J Ra-*

diat Biol **31**:1–10, 1977.

21. Wilson, R.L.: (Personal communication).
22. Wirtanen, G.W.: Percutaneous transbrachial artery infusion catheter techniques. *Am J Roentgenol Rad Ther Nucl Med* **117**:696–700, 1973.

CHAPTER 13

Contribution of the Discussion Initiator: Quantitative Aspects of Tumor Radioresistance Related to the Presence of Hypoxic Cells

Gerrit W. Barendsen, Ph.D.[a]

It is now generally accepted that many solid tumors contain fractions of hypoxic cells which are important with respect to the radioresistance of these tumors to treatments with single doses of photons. Experimental and clinical evidence on the fractions of hypoxic cells is taken up in Chapter 10. Chapter 11 deals with the properties of various hypoxic-cell sensitizers as well as developments of new sensitizers.

With respect to the influence of hypoxic cells on responses of tumors to fractionated radiation treatments, the phenomenon of reoxygenation after individual dose fractions as observed in many tumors is of crucial importance. The extent of reoxygenation and the rate at which it proceeds are likely to depend on several factors. At least three mechanisms can be envisaged in this respect.

The first, as studied by Thomlinson and Gray, holds that, at specific distances from blood vessels, tumor cells are deprived of oxygen due to the limitation of oxygen diffusion and inadequate vascularisation. As a consequence, cells at distances larger than 100–150 μm from blood vessels are expected to be chronically hypoxic. Reoxygenation after a dose of radiation would result from killing of oxygenated cells, shrinkage of tumors and subsequent improvement of oxygen supply to previously hypoxic cells. This mechanism would be consistent with a rather slow reoxygenation process, occurring within several days.

In recent years attention has been drawn to the possibility that insufficient oxygen supply to tumor cells might be caused by a second mechanism–abrupt changes in blood flow in capillaries. This would result in temporary transient hypoxia of cells in many areas in tumors, not all of them associated with necrotic zones. Such intermittent hypoxia might be consistent with a rapid reoxygenation occurring within minutes or hours. With this type of cellular oxygen deprivation in tumors, fractionated treatments with low LET radiation would be expected to be effective, and the influence of hypoxic-cell radiosensitizers would be much smaller as compared to single large doses. While a gain factor of 2.0 or larger might be expected for nonreoxygenating or slowly reoxygenating tumors, this factor might decrease to values between 1.1 and 1.3 for fast reoxygenating tumors.

A third mechanism which might cause tumor cells to become hypoxic would be an increased metabolism during specific parts of the cell cycle. If oxygen supply is less than optimal in many areas of tumors, then

[a]Radiobiological Institute of the Organisation for Health Research TNO, P.O. Box 5815, Rijswijk, The Netherlands

Laboratory for Radiobiology, University of Amsterdam, Plesmanlaan 121, Amsterdam, The Netherlands

a temporarily increased consumption in individual cells might reduce the oxygen concentration in the cell nucleus sufficiently to cause an increase in radioresistance. With this mechanism it is expected that reoxygenation occurs relatively fast, i.e., within a few hours. Consequently, the effectiveness of fractionated radiotherapy would be influenced to a smaller extent by such intermittent hypoxia as compared with slow reoxygenation in tumors.

It is important to note, however, that even a modest gain factor of 1.1 to 1.3 might be very significant if local control probability increases rapidly with the radiation dose (as suggested for cancer types with relatively little heterogeneity). Furthermore, a specific advantage of hypoxic-cell sensitizers might be the possibility to use somewhat larger doses per fraction than are commonly employed in clinical radiotherapy. In this respect the question whether large doses per fraction could be beneficial should be considered.

With respect to sensitizers which are not specifically acting on hypoxic cells, M. Quintiliani correctly points out in Chapter 12 that the main problem is to obtain a sensitizer that discriminates between cells in tumors and cells in normal tissues. Recent literature suggests that the simultaneous administration of radiation and chemotherapeutic agents–some of which are also radiosensitizers–has not been very successful in this discrimination, and more advantage is expected from the sequential administration of radiation and chemotherapy. In several experimental tumors sensitization has been observed by factors of 1.1 to 1.5, but similar factors have been observed for normal tissue responses. Thus, a definite advantage is difficult to predict.

CHAPTER 14

Prediction and Quantification of Tumor Response

Juliana Denekamp, B.Sc., Ph.D., D.S.c.[a]

The prediction of tumor response can be considered in two categories: the general prediction for a group of patients and the specific prediction of the prognosis for an individual patient. Many factors are known to be of general prognostic value; these are listed in any controlled clinical trial so that the patients will be allocated to the two treatments that are being compared, without a bias to one or the other. Among the factors considered to be important are the tumor histology, grade and stage, size and site, and host factors, such as age, sex, and general condition (e.g., hemoglobin level). These factors have been shown to influence the response to treatment within a group of patients when all are treated with a similar protocol, and therefore they need to be allocated equally to each arm of a trial.

Shrinkage and Prognosis

The question of early prediction of the prognosis for an individual patient is a much more difficult problem. Clinicians instinctively feel that rapid regression is a good prognostic sign, but this does not appear to be true for all tumors. Table 1 summarizes some of the experimental and clinical data relating to shrinkage. In animal studies using large single doses of radiation, it has been clearly shown that there is no correlation between shrinkage within the first week and the local control or recurrence of individual tumors.[27,29] This is not surprising since a 12-mm diameter tumor shrinking dramatically to 1.2 mm diameter will only represent the loss of three decades of cells (i.e., down to 0.1% of the original volume), whereas the difference between a cured or a recurrent tumor will represent cell-killing of seven to nine decades of cells (i.e., survival of 10^{-7} or 10^{-9} cells; see Fig. 1). Shrinkage after single doses gives more

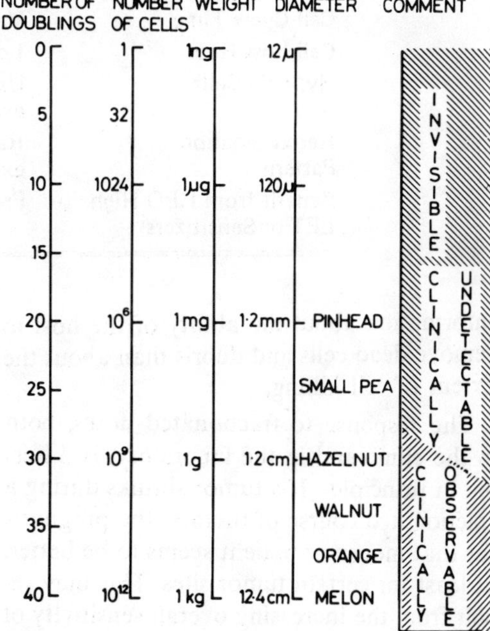

Figure 1. Diagram illustrates that most of the life history of a tumor occurs while it is clinically undetectable. If every tumor cell is clonogenic, 10^9 cells must be eradicated in a 1g tumor to achieve local tumor control. Shrinking from 1g to 1 mg (or from 1.2 cm diameter to 1.2 mm) only represents the loss of three decades of cells (from Denekamp[10]).

[a]Gray Laboratory of the Cancer Research Campaign, Mount Vernon Hospital, Northwood, Middlesex

TABLE 1. Shrinkage as a Predictor of Local Control After Radiotherapy

No	Thomlinson, 1960	Single dose	Rats
No	Suit et al., 1965	Single dose	Mice
Yes	Denekamp, 1977	Fractionated	Mice
No	Suit et al., 1965	Fractionated	Human head and neck
Yes	Dische et al., 1980	Fractionated	Human cervix
Yes	Marcial et al., 1970	Fractionated	Human cervix
Yes	Grossman et al., 1973	Fractionated	Human cervix
Yes	Breur (private communication)	Fractionated	Human cervix
Yes/No	Friedman, 1939; 1955; 1967	Fractionated	Human various sites
Yes	Sobel et al., 1976 (at 2 to 3 months)	Fractionated	Human head and neck
Yes	Dawes, 1980	Fractionated	Head and neck
No	Quivey et al., 1980	Fractionated	Pancreas

TABLE 2. Shrinkage and Cell-Proliferation Kinetics: Effect on the Radiation Response of Rodent Tumors

	Sarcomas	Carcinomas
Shrinkage after irradiation with a large single dose	after Delayed	ir Immediate
Growth Rate	Usually Fast	Usually slow
Median Volume Doubling Time	Mice = 3 days Man = 41 days	Mice = 6 days Man = 75 days
Cell-Cycle Time	Varies with T_D	Varies little
Cell-Loss Rate	Low or none	Very high
Hypoxic Cells	Usually 10–20% *except* in slow SA	Usually 10–20% even in slow CA
Reoxygenation Pattern	Rapid but not extensive	Rapid and extensive
Benefit from HBO High LET or Sensitizers	Probably great	Possibly not much

information about the ability of the host to remove dead cells and debris than about the extent of cell killing.

The response to fractionated doses, both in the clinic and in the laboratory, is different in principle.[7] If a tumor shrinks during a fractionated course of therapy the prognosis for that mouse or patient seems to be better, at least for certain tumor sites. This may result from the increasing overall sensitivity of shrinking tumors due to reoxygenation of hypoxic cells (or recruitment of noncycling cells) as the intercapillary distances shrink and the nutrient supply improves.[10] Thus, the shrinking tumor may become more sensitive to subsequent doses of radiation, and this may lead to an improved prognosis rather than shrinkage being an indicator of the extent of cell kill.[7]

The rate of shrinkage of tumors is related to the histology in a rather general way, although considerable variations may be seen within one histological type. In animals, sarcomas shrink least rapidly, carcinomas shrink within days, and lymphosarcomas may appear to "melt" or disappear overnight. These different shrinkage patterns probably relate to the cell kinetics of the tumor, and particularly to the cell-loss factor in the unirradiated tumor. Table 2 and Figure 2 summarize some of the characteristics of experimental sarcomas and carcinomas. The high natural cell-loss factor in carcinomas may lead to rapid shrinkage after a

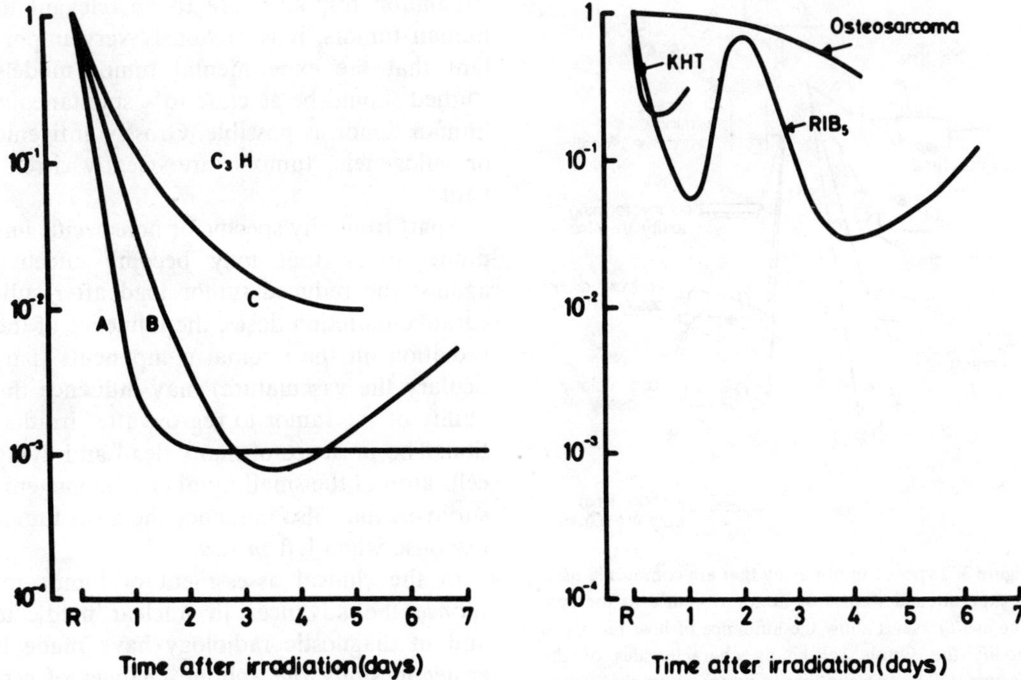

Figure 2. Reoxygenation kinetics of six experimental tumors. The proportion of hypoxic cells, normalized to 100% immediately after a large dose of irradiation, is shown as a function of time. All three C3H carcinomas, which shrink rapidly, show extensive reoxygenation to below the original preirradiation level. The three sarcomas, which shrink more slowly, show more variable and less extensive reoxygenation (from Denekamp[7]).

large radiation dose, which in turn can lead to extensive reoxygenation. Of the six tumors in which reoxygenation kinetics have been measured (Fig. 2), the three carcinomas show rapid and extensive reoxygenation, whereas the three sarcomas show less extensive reoxygenation.[7,10] Although the shrinkage patterns of different histological types of tumors are important, there are also differences within one tumor type, as was illustrated with fractionated irradiation of the C3H mouse mammary carcinoma.[7] Even though a highly significant correlation could be demonstrated between shrinkage and cure, it would not have been adequate to predict the outcome for any individual animal, as was noted by Suit and Walker.[28]

Other factors that have been used clinically as early prognostic indicators include histological assessment of the percentage of viable cells, the proportion of differentiated cells, the cell density, or the change in the uptake of tritiated thymidine partway through therapy.[1,15,31] All of these parameters are believed by some workers to have some prognostic value, but they may give a significant proportion of false negatives and hence cannot be used in a "fail-safe" way to radically alter the mode of treatment for those patients with a poor prognosis. Until the false-positive or false-negative rates are very low, e.g., 5–10%, it will not be possible to use any of these factors to select a group of patients whose prognosis on conventional therapy is poor, and who can therefore be submitted ethically to a more radical and potentially hazardous alternative form of treatment.[4,28] Nevertheless, some of these factors may be useful as early indicators of a trend when two sides of a clinical trial are being compared.

Quantitation of Tumor Response

In order to assess the efficacy of any treat-

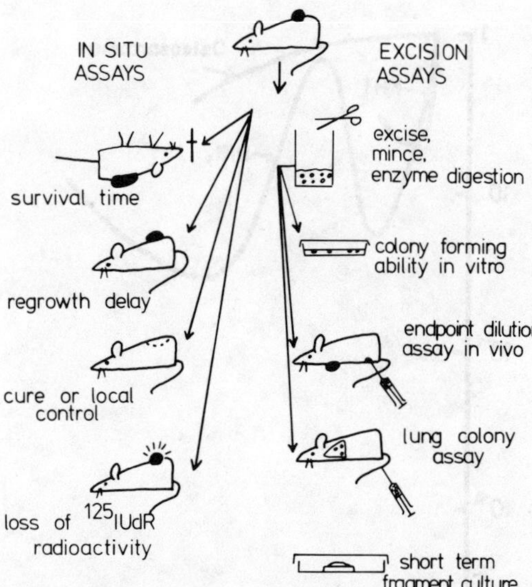

Figure 3. Types of tumor assay that are commonly used in experimental studies of tumor response to therapy. The *in situ* assays allow the influence of host factors to modify the simple cell-killing characteristics of the treatment. The excision assays, which allow the surviving fraction to be determined with precision, may include artifacts because the cells are removed from their milieu after treatment (from Denekamp[8]).

ment or to compare one treatment with another, it is necessary to quantify the response of the tumor. Figure 3 summarizes the many techniques that are available for this in the laboratory. These can be divided broadly into two groups: those involving assessment of the tumor *in situ* in the treated host; and those that require that the tumor be excised, disaggregated into a single-cell suspension, and the clonogenic ability of the cells assayed *in vitro* or in other recipient mice.

In Situ Assays

The *in situ* assays (e.g., growth delay or local control of transplantable tumors) can obviously be applied most readily in the clinic; these have the advantage of measuring the response of the tumor together with any modification by postirradiation changes in the milieu or by any host factors. If the host factors in mice that influence postirradiation responses are to be relevant to human tumors, it is obviously very important that the experimental tumor models studied should be as close to a spontaneous human tumor as possible. Grossly antigenic or allogeneic tumors are clearly irrelevant.[8,9,17,23]

Apart from any specific or nonspecific immune attack that may become effective against the reduced tumor load after subcurative radiation doses, the influence of the radiation on the stromal components (particulary the vasculature) may influence the ability of the tumor to regrow after irradiation. The presence of many dead and dying cells around the small number of clonogenic survivors may also influence the gross tumor response when left *in situ*.

In the clinical assessment of tumor response the advances in nuclear medicine and in diagnostic radiology have made it easier to study the volume changes of certain tumors. Most of the techniques, however, have a resolution of 1–2 mm in a linear dimension which will not allow the detection of a tumor mass containing one million potentially clonogenic cells (see Fig. 1). Thus, their usefulness in determining whether a tumor has been totally eradicated must be questioned. Tumor-specific marker proteins may be more useful for detecting low tumor cell numbers, but there is not yet good evidence for a constant proportionality between the blood levels of the marker and the clinically detectable tumor load.[20] Furthermore, the number of tumors producing an identifiable ectopic marker is still very limited.[3]

Excision Assays

The excision assays have the advantage of giving precise estimates of the surviving fraction of clonogenic cells. If the assay is performed *in vitro*, or as lung colonies after intravenous injection, they also have the advantage of speed. There are several reasons

TABLE 3. Comparison of *In Situ* and Cloning Assays[a]

Parameter	Results Agree	Results Differ	Reference
Surviving fraction to predict tumor cure	Rhabdomyosa		Reinhold and DeBree, 1968
	Rhabdomyosa R1		Barendensen and Broerse, 1969
		MT	McNally and Sheldon, 1977
		EMT 6	Rasey et al., 1977
		EMT 6	Rockwell and Kallman, 1973
Hypoxic fraction		KHT	Field and Kallman (unpub.)
		RIB5C	McNally, 1975
		SA F	McNally, 1973
		MT	McNally and Sheldon, 1977
Oxygen-Enhancement ratio		RIB5	McNally, 1972
		RIB5C	McNally, 1973
Misonidazole SER	SA F		McNally, 1975
	WHFIB		McNally (unpub.)
		MT	McNally and Sheldon, 1977
Neutron RBE		RIB5C	McNally, 1975
		Rhabdomyosa R1	Barendsen and Broerse, 1969
		EMT 6	Rasey et al., 1977
Repair capacity		WHFIB	McNally et al., 1979

[a]For references see Denekamp[8]

why such an accurate estimate of surviving fraction may be unrepresentative of the effect that would have been observed if the tumors had been left *in situ*. The post-irradiation conditions are changed when the tumors are excised; this can influence repair of potentially lethal damage, survival and/or reoxygenation of hypoxic cells, and recruitment of nondividing cells. The yield of cells obtained with disaggregation techniques seldom exceeds 1–10% of the original tumor population, and there is still some doubt about whether this is always a representative sample.[21] Even within this small sample the plating efficiency of apparently viable cells may be as low as 10–20%. These factors and the relative merits of the different techniques have been discussed in detail in the proceedings of the 9th L.H. Gray Conference.[9]

Excision techniques are not readily applicable to all animal tumors and cannot yet be applied to human tumors. The tumor cells from rodent tumors often have been "trained" to grow *in vitro* and *in vivo*,[22] and the details of the disaggregation procedures have to be worked out for each tumor. Thus, although excision techniques are attractive as accurate quantitative assays, they are not easily applicable in the clinic, nor are they necessarily relevant. The quantitative assessments of repair capacity, RBE, sensitization by misonidazole, etc. are often not identical when measured for the same tumor using both *in situ* and excision assays (see Table 3).

Another technique that can be used to assess the intrinsic radiosensitivity of human tumor cells involves xenografts—i.e., human tumor cells grown in immune-suppressed or naturally immune-deficient athymic mice (see Fig. 4). Many tumors have now been grown and passaged in such mice; they appear to retain their cytogenic and biochemical characteristics and histological appearance. However they do not retain the original growth rate, as they would not grow to a measurable size within the limited life span of the nude mouse (about 1 year). These tumors are effectively chimeras because the vasculature and supporting stromal elements are supplied by the mouse; up to 35%

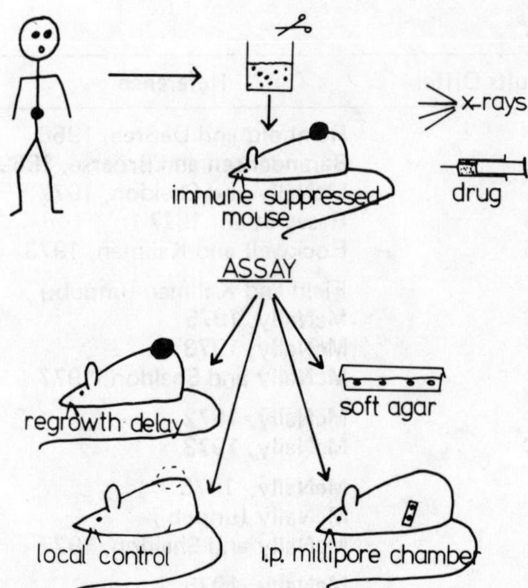

Figure 4. Methods of assaying established xenografts of human tumor cells growing in immune-deprived mice. After treating the xenografted tumor *in situ*, assessments of the tumor response *in situ* or by excision assays may be used (from Denekamp[8]).

of the tumor can consist of mouse cells.[33] When xenografted tumors have been established they can be assayed *in situ* or by an excision technique in the same way as for other rodent tumors (see Fig. 4). The excision techniques are becoming more popular because they avoid the potential problems of returning immunocompetence in immune-deprived mice and of natural killer cells in nude mice.[26] These NK cells occur in larger numbers in nude mice than in other mice, presumably to compensate for the lack of T-cell-mediated immunity.

While xenografts allow intrinsic cellular sensitivities to be compared for different types of tumor, the factors that depend upon growth rate or the vascular supply (e.g., hypoxic fraction, growth fraction, distribution around the cell cycle, and drug access) are likely to be poorly reproduced in the xenograft model. For chemotherapy, where the biochemical characteristics of the individual tumor cells may dominate the response to certain drugs, the xenograft may be useful, but its advantage over short-term cell cultures is not clear. Its usefulness for experimental radiotherapy appears to be no better than that of a range of animal tumors, and possibly less useful because of the small numbers available.

Clinical Trials: The Use of Two Dose Levels

For the comparison of new and old forms of therapy it is usual in controlled clinical trials for a single dose level to be chosen for the new form of therapy, and for this to be compared with the response to the standard dose of conventional treatment. In order to compare the two-treatment modalities, both tumor response and the normal tissue complications need to be carefully documented in both arms of the trial. If the clinicians setting up the trial have chosen very wisely on the basis of whatever pretrial information was available, they may achieve a higher local control rate with exactly the same complication rate as they are accustomed to find in conventional radiotherapy. With an input of several hundred patients and a follow-up period of 5 years (total time = 10 years) they may then be able to prove that the new treatment is better than the old.

If the initial "guestimate" of a dose level is poor (because of a lack of appropriate data at the time the trial is set up), the result of 10 years work may be inconclusive. The higher local tumor control may be accompanied by more morbidity, or a lower level of tumor control may be achieved accompanied by a reduction in normal tissue complications. Such a frustrating result has been obtained in several carefully designed clinical trials.[5,16] It could be avoided if two closely spaced dose levels were used in the new treatment (e.g., the best "guestimate" ±3 to 5%) and compared to the standard dose in the conventional arm.[14] If the upper dose level were grossly overdosing the normal tissues, this would be detected quite

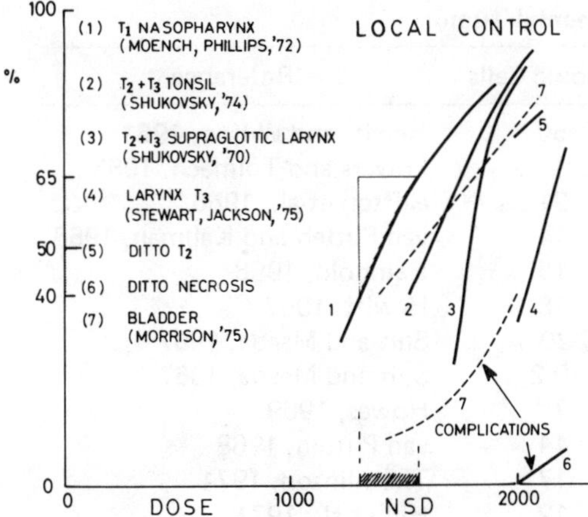

Figure 5. Percent of local control in human tumors as a function of radiation dose, normalized to nominal standard doses by means of the Ellis NSD formula. The steepness of the dose-response curves varies from one site to another. The steepest dose-response curve is that of Schukovsky,[25] and the flattest is that of Morrison.[19] (Data compiled by J.F. Fowler via personal communication with author.)

soon from early skin or mucosal reactions, although these do not always reflect the late complications that will occur. While a three-arm trial of this kind will clearly require even more patients to be assessed, it will ultimately yield far more information, both about the trial itself and about the steepness of the dose-response curves for human tumors and normal tissues. After 80 years of radiotherapy there is still a sad paucity of data concerning the slope of such dose-response curves (see Fig. 5). While the data of Schukovsky[25] is often quoted, in which a 10% increase in nominal standard dose gave an increase in local control rate of 50%, other curves are much less steep. This is particularly true of the data of Morrison[19]—the only example where a variation in dose level was deliberately planned while keeping other important factors (e.g., tumor size) constant.

Therapeutic Gain: How Little is Useful?

For the planning of radiobiological research that might make significant contributions to improving clinical radiotherapy, it is of vital importance to know how much increase in effective dose is needed to obtain a significant increase in local tumor control or in patient survival. Many of the applied areas of radiobiology relate to the question of hypoxic radioresistance. It now seems quite clear that hypoxic cells exist before treatment in most animal tumors (see Table 4) and also in the human tumors that have been studied in the nitroimidazole trials.[2,30,32]

If hypoxic radioresistance (equal to a dose-modifying factor of 2.5–3.0) is the cause of clinical radioresistance to fractionated radiotherapy, then hyperbaric oxygen, fast neutrons, and the electron-affinic radiosensitizers all hold a promise of improvements. With misonidazole, although the dose that can be administered clinically is limited by neurotoxicity, serum levels can be achieved in six fractions that would be expected to give a Sensitizer Enhancement Ratio (SER) for hypoxic cells in excess of 1.7. This is illustrated in the upper part of Figure 6 where the SER values for a totally hypoxic cell population are indicated. At low radiation doses, however, the survival curve for a mixed population of oxic and hypoxic cells is dominated by the more sensitive subpopulation, i.e., the oxic cells. Thus, the observed enhancement ratio (SER′) for a small single dose to a mixed population will be much lower than that expected for a fully hypoxic population. If repeated small doses are given, the oxic population will rapidly be depleted and the hypoxic cells will come to dominate the response, *unless* reoxygenation occurs between successive doses. Therefore, the measured SER′ value will depend critically on the pattern of reoxygenation rather than on the presence of hypoxic cells at the start of a course of therapy.

The relative advantage of a few large fractions or of many small fractions of x-rays and misonidazole have recently been

TABLE 4. Proportion of Hypoxic Cells in Experimental Tumors

Tumor Identification		% Hypoxic Cells	Reference
CBA sarcoma F		>50	Hewitt and Wilson, 1961
Gardner lymphosarcoma		1	Powers and Tolmach, 1963
Adenocarcinoma MTG-B		21	Clifton et al., 1966
C3H sarcoma KHT		14	van Putten and Kallman, 1968
Rhabdomysarcoma BA1112		15	Reinhold, 1966
Squamous carcinoma D		18	Hewitt, 1967
C3H mammary	(250 mm^3)	>20	Suit and Maeda, 1967
Carcinoma	(0.6 mm^3)	0.2	Suit and Maeda, 1967
C3H mammary carcinoma		7	Howes, 1969
Osteosarcoma C22LR		14	van Putten, 1968
Fibrosarcoma RIB5		17	Thomlinson, 1971
Fibrosarcoma KHT		12	Hill et al., 1971
Carcinoma KHJJ		19	Kallman, 1974
Sarcoma EMT 6		35	Kallman, 1974
C3H mammary	(females)	1	Fowler et al., 1975
Carcinoma	(males)	17	Fowler et al., 1975
CBA Sarcoma F	(*in situ*)	<10	McNally, 1975
	(excised)	50	McNally, 1975
Squamous	(intradermal)	<1	Peters, 1976
Carcinoma G	(subcutaneous)	>46	Peters, 1976
WHT anaplastic 'MT'	(*in situ*)	>80	McNally and Sheldon, 1977
	(excised)	5	McNally and Sheldon, 1977
Carcinoma DC		10–30%	Denekamp et al., 1980
Carcinoma RH		2–25%	Denekamp et al., 1980
CBA carcinoma NT		7–18%	Denekamp et al., 1980
Sarcoma S		<0.01%	Denekamp et al., 1980
Sarcoma S (fast variants)		1–30%	Denekamp et al., 1980
Sarcoma FA		30–70%	Denekamp et al., 1980
Sarcoma BS 2b		5–25%	Denekamp et al., 1980

[a]These values have been derived from the published SER data using the method described by Denekamp et al.[11]

considered by using a computer simulation of the response of a mixed population with various assumed cell-survival parameters and patterns of reoxygenation.[13] This analysis enabled the influence of each parameter on the likely clinical outcome to be assessed. With misonidazole, in spite of the lower drug dose that can be given with many small fractions, it appeared that for most simulations 30 fractions with sensitizer would be the best treatment, although the gain might be very small. This is illustrated for one set of parameters in Figure 7. The conclusion depends critically on the reoxygenation pattern and on the repair capacity of the cells, for neither of which is any information available in human tumors.

If an ideal radiosensitizer were available (i.e., one which sensitized to the full sensitivity of oxic cells and which was completely non toxic), the total dose of sensitizer would not be limited, and hence the maximum SER could be expected with all fractionation schemes. The observed SER′ would still depend upon the pattern of reoxygenation, however. This is illustrated in Table 5 for a tumor population with a very low repair capacity (n = 2). In this case the full SER (2.7) would be achieved with many small fractions if there were no reoxygenation. If even moderate reoxygenation occurs, however, (e.g., of 20% of the hypoxic cells each day), the SER′ is reduced to 1.6 to 1.9.[12] If the reoxygenation processes are

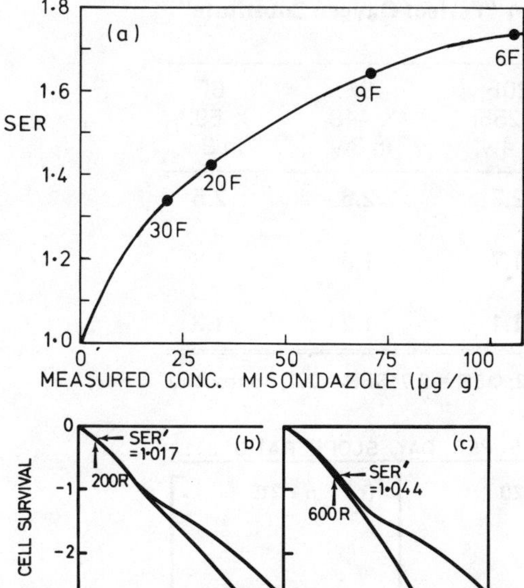

Figure 6. Sensitizer Enhancement Ratio (SER) as a function of misonidazole concentration for a purely hypoxic population. (*a*) The SER achievable with the clinical serum levels obtained with 6, 9, 20, or 30 fractions are indicated. Panels (*b*) and (*c*) show how these SER′ values are reduced at low radiation doses if the population consists of 90% well-oxygenated and only 10% hypoxic cells (from Denekamp et al.[13]).
SER = x-ray dose without drug/x-ray dose with drug to achieve the same cell kill for a hypoxic population.
SER′ = observed ratio of x-ray doses for a mixed population of oxic and hypoxic cells.

sufficiently effective to return the hypoxic fraction to its initial 10% before each fraction, then the SER′ values are reduced much further, to 1.1 - 1.3.

Table 5 illustrates two parameters about which we need information before we can predict the likely usefulness of techniques aimed at overcoming the radioresistance of hypoxic cells. The extent of reoxygenation during a course of radiotherapy is clearly of great importance in determining the gain that can be expected. Direct visualization of hypoxic, clonogenic cells, and hence estimates of hypoxic fractions, are at present impossible to obtain. A considerable quantity of radiobiological data is needed to deduce this parameter indirectly for animal tumors, and there are some questions about the validity of assuming that clamping makes tumor cells uniformly radioresistant.[24] The technique described in Chapter 10 offers the promise of directly identifying viable hypoxic cells; this might enable us to determine whether hypoxic cells persist in human tumors throughout a course of radiotherapy. In the meantime, however, the extent of shrinkage during the treatment may be our best indication of effective reoxygenation due to reduced intercapillary distances.

The other parameter of importance illustrated in Table 5 is the steepness of the dose-response curves which is directly related to the size of the SER′ that could be useful. If the human tumor dose-response curves are as steep as that obtained by Schukovsky[25] (see Fig. 5), then an SER′ of 1.1 would be of considerable clinical value. If they are as shallow as those obtained by Morrison[19] or by Moench and Phillips[18] than an SER′ of 1.1 would be of little value and an SER′ of 1.3 to 1.5 might be needed to give a significant clinical gain. This illustrates how important clinical dose-response data are. These can only be obtained by careful quantitation of the local tumor response *in situ*. They would be obtained faster and more reliably by the deliberate inclusion of more than one dose level for tumors that are identical in all respects (e.g., grade, site, and size). It is to be hoped that such dose-response data will become available from some of the careful clinical trials that are currently in progress.

Summary

This paper briefly reviews the methods of assessing tumor response in the clinic and in experimental animal tumors. The predictive value of histological parameters and of gross tumor shrinkage are discussed. Macroscopic measurements of tumor shrinkage appear to have predictive value even though they are a poor indication of the survival of small foci of tumor cells which can lead to local

TABLE 5. Gain (SER') Expected from "Perfect Oxygen Substitute": SER - OER[a]

Assumed Reoxygenation Pattern	30F × 192r in 6w.	20F × 255r in 4w.	9F × 440r in 3w.	6F × 599r in 3w.
None	2.7	2.7	2.6	2.5
Moderate (20% per day)	1.6	1.7	1.9	1.8
Effective (Back to 10%)	1.1	1.1	1.2	1.3

[a] Assumptions: D_o = 135r; D_s/D_o = 3; n = 2; OER = 2.7; SER = 2.7; no toxicity

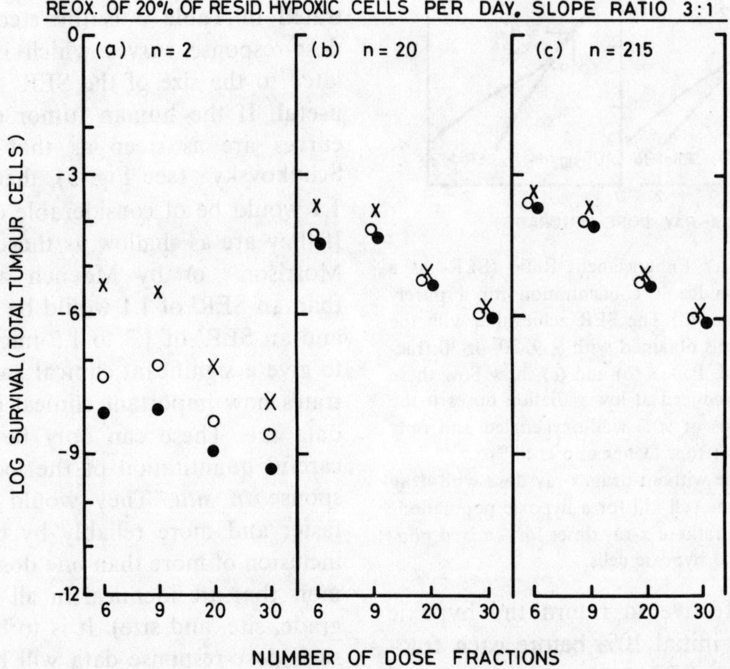

Figure 7. Calculated values for the surviving fraction of tumor cells that should be achieved with four of the proposed clinical regimes. Although the maximum advantage of the sensitizer (cf. circles and crosses) is seen with a few large doses, the maximum cell kill is seen with many small doses of radiation and drugs (from Denekamp et al.[13]).

recurrence. Their usefulness probably relates to the indication of underlying alterations in blood flow and nutrient supply.

The importance of the reoxygenation pattern in determining tumor response is stressed. This will influence the response to conventional radiotherapy and will determine the benefit that will be obtained from misonidazole, fast neutrons, or hyperbaric oxygen. Methods of measuring the hypoxic fraction part way through a course of therapy would be of great predictive value.

The importance of dose-response curves for human tumors and for normal tissue morbidity are stressed. The use of three-arm clinical trials (with two dose levels in the new treatment group) would lead to the acquisition of such data. This approach would minimize the risk that the clinical trials would be inconclusive. It would also indicate how much tumor radiosensitization or normal tissue protection is needed to give a significant improvement in clinical response.

REFERENCES

1. Arcangeli, G., Mauro, F., Nervi, C., and Starace, G.: A critical appraisal of the usefulness of some biological parameters in predicting tumor radiation response of human head and neck cancer. *Br J Cancer* **41**: Suppl. IV, 39–44, 1980.
2. Ash, D.V., Peckman, M.J., and Steel, G.G.: A quantitative study of human tumor response to radiation and misonidazole. *Br J Cancer* **39**:503–509, 1979.
3. Bagshawe, K.D.: Marker proteins as indicators of tumor response to therapy. *Br J Cancer* **41**: Suppl. IV, 186–190, 1980.
4. Bush, R.S.: Conference summary. Comments and conclusions from clinical studies. *Br J Cancer* **41**: Suppl. IV, 323–331, 1980.
5. Catterall, M., Sutherland, I., and Bewley, D.K.: First results of a randomised clinical trial of fast neutrons compared with X or γ-rays in treatment of advanced tumors of the head and neck. *Br Med J* **2**:653–656, 1975.
6. Denekamp, J.: The relationship between the 'cell loss factor' and the response to radiation in animal tumors. *Eur J Cancer* **8**:335–340, 1972.
7. Denekamp, J.: Tumor regression as a guide to prognosis: A study with experimental animals. *Br J Radiol* **50**:271–279, 1977.
8. Denekamp, J.: Experimental tumor systems: Standardization of endpoints. *Int J Radiat Oncol Biol Phys* **5**:1175–1184, 1979.
9. Denekamp, J. ed.: Quantitation of tumor response: A critical appraisal. *Proc. 9th L.H. Gray Conference. Br J Cancer* **41**: Suppl. IV, 1980.
10. Denekamp, J.: Cell kinetics and cancer therapy. W.C. Dewey, ed. C.C. Thomas, pp. 1–162, 1982.
11. Denekamp, J., Fowler, J.F., and Dische, S.: The proportion of hypoxic cells in a human tumor. *Int J Radiat Oncol Biol Phys* **2**:1227–1228, 1977.
12. Denekamp, J., and Joiner, M.: The potential benefit from a perfect radiosensitizer and its dependence on reoxygenation. *Br J Radiol* (in press).
13. Denekamp, J., McNally, N.J., Fowler, J.F., and Joiner, M.C.: Misonidazole in fractionated radiotherapy: Are many small fractions best? *Br J Radiol* **53**:981–990, 1980.
14. Fowler, J.F.: Doses and fractionation schemes to be employed in clinical trials of high LET radiations. In G.W. Barendsen, J.B. Roerse, and K. Breur, eds. *High LET Radiations in Clinical Radiotherapy* pp. 263–266, Binghamton: Pergamon Press, 1979.
15. Glücksmann, A., and Way, S.: On the choice of treatment of individual carcinoma of the cervix uteri based on the analysis of serial biopsies. *J Obstet Gynecol Br Emp* **55**:573, 1948.
16. Henk, J.M., Kunkler, P.B., and Smith, C.W.: Radiotherapy and hyperbaric oxygen in head and neck cancer. *Lancet,* 101–103, 1977.
17. Hewitt, H.B.: The choice of animal tumors for experimental studies of cancer therapy. *Adv Cancer Res* **27**:149–200, 1978.
18. Moench, H.C., and Phillips, T.L.: Carcinoma of the nasopharynx. *Am J Surg* **124**:515–518, 1972.
19. Morrison, R.: The results of treatment of cancer of the bladder—a clinical contribution to radiobiology. *Clin Radiol* **26**:67–75, 1975.
20. Raghavan, D., Gibbs, J., Nogueira Costa, R., et al.: The interpretation of marker protein assays: A critical appraisal in clinical studies and a xenograft model. *Br J Cancer* **41**: Suppl IV, 191–194, 1980.
21. Rasey, J.S., and Nelson, N.J.: Response of an *in vivo–in vitro*8-tumourto X-rays and cytotoxic drugs: Effect of tumor disaggregation method on cell survival. *Br J Cancer* **41**: Suppl. IV, 217–221, 1980.
22. Rockwell, S.: II. *In vivo–in vitro* tumor systems: New models for studying the response of tumors to therapy. *Lab Anim Sci* **27**:831–851, 1977.
23. Scott, O.C.A.: Some observations on the use of transplanted tumors in radiobiological research. *Radiat Res* **14**:643–652, 1961.
24. Sheldon, P.W., and Fowler, J.F.: The effect of recovery from potentially lethal damage on the determination of reoxygenation in a murine tumor. *Br J Radiol* **52**:634–641, 1979.
25. Schukovsky, L.J.: Dose, time, volume relationships in squamous cell carcinoma of the supraglottic larynx. *AJR* **108**:27–29, 1970.
26. Steel, G.G., and Peckham, M.J.: Human tumor xenografts: A critical appraisal. *Br J Cancer* **41**: Suppl. IV, 133–141, 1980.
27. Suit, H., Lindberg, R., and Fletcher, G.: Prognostic significance of extent of tumor regression at completion of radiation therapy. *Radiology* **84**:1100–1107, 1965.
28. Suit, H.D., and Walker, A.M.: Assessment of the response of tumors to radiation: Clinical and experimental studies. *Br J Cancer* **41**: Suppl. IV, 1–10, 1980.
29. Thomlinson, R.H.: An experimental method for comparing treatments of intact malignant tumors in animals and its application to the use of oxygen in radiotherapy. *Br J Cancer* **14**:555–576, 1960.
30. Thomlinson, R.H., Dische, S., Gray, A.J., and Errington, L.M.: Clinical testing of the radiosensitizer Ro-07-0582. III. Response of tumors. *Clin Radiol* **27**:167–174, 1976.
31. Trott, K.R.: Can tumour response be assessed from a biopsy? *Br J Cancer* **41**: Suppl. IV, 163–170, 1980.

32. Urtasun, R., Band, P., Chapman, J.D., Feldstein, M.L., Mielke, B. and Fryer, C.: Radiation and high dose metronidazole (Flagyl) in supratentorial glioblastomas. *N Engl J Med* **294**:1364–1367, 1976.

33. Warenius, H.M., Freedman, L.S., and Bleehen, N.M.: The response of a human tumor xenograft to chemotherapy: Intrinsic variation between tumors and its significance in planning experiments. *Br J Cancer* **41**: Suppl. IV, 128–132, 1980.

CHAPTER 15

Contribution of the Keynote Discussant: Tumor-Cell Survival and the Growth Fraction

Robert F. Kallman, Ph.D.[a]

This paper is presented as a discussion of Chapter 14, *Prediction and Quantification of Tumor Response*, with emphasis on some major kinds of information needed to support such predictions. Indeed, both the fundamental importance and the almost total lack of this information are not widely appreciated.

The neoplastic cells in tumors may be assigned to either of two categories: those in active cycle (P) and those out of cycle (Q). The P compartment contains cells in all phases of the cycle, while cells in the Q compartment are regarded primarily as being in an abnormally prolonged G_1 phase that is frequently termed G_0. It is the conversion of cells in the Q state back to the P state that is usually termed recruitment. While there is considerable inferential evidence suggesting that recruitment occurs (and several models have been developed to describe tumor-cell proliferation kinetics in terms of the transit of cells between these two compartments), it was not until recently that noncycling tumor cells have been shown conclusively to possess the capacity for unlimited proliferation, i.e., clonogenicity.

Clonogenic Q cells have been demonstrated by Barendsen et al.[1] and later by ourselves.[4] In these experiments Q cells are defined operationally as noncycling cells on the basis of their inability to incorporate tritiated thymidine upon continuous or semicontinuous exposure to this DNA precursor. The overall duration of exposure that we have used is at least one standard deviation longer than the mean cell-cycle time of those cells which, on the basis of percent labeled mitosis (PLM) analysis, are readily assignable to the P compartment. In both the Dutch and American experiments, solid tumor systems have been used which are capable of alternate growth *in vivo* and *in vitro* —an absolute requirement of this experimental approach. Solid tumors (the R-1 rhabdomyosarcoma by Barendsen and colleagues, and the EMT6 tumor by ourselves) were grown in syngeneic animals (rats and mice, respectively), and were exposed to ^{3}HTdR semicontinuously by repeated intraperitoneal injection, or continuously by intravenous infusion for 16 and 24 hours, respectively. The tumors were then excised and dispersed into single-cell suspensions which were counted, diluted, plated in culture vessels, and incubated to permit the growth of colonies. Autoradiographs of the cultures were prepared, and the distribution of the ^{3}HTdR (i.e., grain counts) in the colonies was examined and analysed. Because the radioactive label would be excessively diluted by the 15–20 doublings necessary for the formation of macrocolonies, it is virtually impossible to distinguish labeled and unlabeled cells in traditional macroscopic colonies. Therefore, small colonies must be used in these autoradiographic analyses.

[a]Department of Radiology, Stanford University School of Medicine, Stanford, California

With this technique, it is possible to determine whether a given colony arose from a P or a Q cell, i.e., whether the progenitor cell had participated in at least one round of DNA replication during the period of exposure to ^{3}HTdR. An unlabeled colony must have descended from a Q cell. Although it is to be expected that there would be some P cells with cell cycles only slightly longer than the period of ^{3}HTdR infusion, these would be rare. For the EMT6 tumor, the labeling index for all colonies (containing 2–22 cells) scored at 72 hours is typically 0.80 to 0.89. Therefore, approximately 11–20% of the EMT6 colonies arise from unlabeled, or Q, cells. These data provide conclusive proof that cells defined by the experimental conditions as nonproliferating have retained their clonogenic capacity.

The concept of *growth fraction* was introduced by Mendelsohn[5] as a quantitative measurement of the proportion of tumor cells engaged in proliferative activity. Classically, the growth fraction is derived from PLM data. This parameter has been measured in many tumors by many investigators, and it is important to recognize that in virtually all autochthonous tumors, a minority of the cells are in the growth fraction. The EMT6 tumor has a growth fraction of approximately 50%,[6] and yet our microcolony labeling indices are typically 80-90%. This discrepancy between growth fraction and labeling index is, however, only apparent and is probably caused by two factors: (1) Because of a steady flow of cells from P to Q, some of the Q cells present at the end of the 24-hour infusion would have been derived (by aging, maturation, or etc.) from P cells which incorporated ^{3}HTdR and divided earlier during the infusion period. That is, the tumor would contain some new, and therefore labeled, Q cells. (2) P cells which had incorporated label near the beginning of the 24-hour labeling period would have divided at least once, so that the proportion of cells containing ^{3}HTdR (i.e., the proportion of labeled cells) in the suspension might be greater than the proportion of cells incorporating ^{3}HTdR during the incubation. Even though the grain counts of these cells would have been halved by division, such cells would still contain sufficient ^{3}H to be labeled autoradiographically.

Having established that Q cells are potentially clonogenic, it is essential to obtain a better understanding of the factors that can cause the conversion of Q cells to P cells *in vivo*, i.e., the factors which cause recruitment. In designing optimum therapeutic schedules, it is essential to know whether treatment with any of the many possible therapeutic modalities causes recruitment. If recruitment does occur, one must ask when it occurs and how the magnitude and timing of the recruitment are related to dose. The beginnings of informative answers to the question of whether radiation exposure causes recruitment of cells from Q to P are emerging from our experiments in which EMT6 tumors have been irradiated with either 300 or 600 rad and then labeled at increasing times after irradiation, with ^{3}HTdR for a standard 24-hour period. Analysis of labeled and unlabeled microcolonies derived from cells of these tumors reveal systematic changes in colony-labeling indices which can be interpreted as evidence for recruitment.

Although the aforementioned experimental data suggest that Q cells may be recruited in irradiated tumors, these same data also suggest that P and Q cells differ in their radiosensitivity. What do we know about the relative radiosensitivity of P and Q cells? Only brief reflection is necessary to make us aware that this is an extremely important question. While we know that certain chemotherapeutic drugs may be designated as "phase-specific," these are agents which act through interference with DNA synthesis. Many other drugs are denoted as cycle specific, and most of us think of x-rays as cycle specific as well. This concept of the cycle specificity of radiation derives largely from the very extensive investigations of the age-response functions of cells growing exponentially *in vitro*.[2,7]

Quite uniformly, all that we know about such age-response functions suggests that mid-G_1 cells are radioresistant compared with other stages of the cycle; and because noncycling cells tend to be in a state resembling mid-G_1, we might infer that they will be characteristically radioresistant. We acknowledge that plateau-phase cells are a better *in vitro* model of tumor cells *in vivo*, and indeed they do not uniformly support inferences drawn from the age-response functions of exponentially growing cells.[3] But, of course, we rather desperately want to know whether the cells of typical solid tumors in animals confirm the expectations derived from *in vitro* studies. If indeed Q cells are less radiosensitive than P cells (as they are less sensitive to phase-specific chemotherapeutic drugs), then recruitment is a major event to be reckoned with. If, on the other hand, Q cells were found to be more radiosensitive, recruitment would be of only academic interest in understanding radiation action and in scheduling effective radiotherapeutic regimens.

We have attempted to investigate this by performing colony-labeling experiments that are analogous to those in which we have attempted to investigate recruitment. The essential difference between these two kinds of experiments is the order in which tumors are irradiated and labeled. In these differential radiosensitivity experiments, tumors are labeled for 24 hours, then irradiated, and then disaggregated so that the cells can be plated and observed for colony growth. If Q cells were more radioresistant, i.e., if their clonogenic potential were destroyed less than that of P cells, colony-labeling indices should decrease because irradiated P cells would have been rendered nonclonogenic.

TABLE 1. Surviving Fractions (SF) and 3-Day Microcolony ^{3}HTdR Labeling Indices (LI) of RIF-1 Tumor Cells Irradiated *in vivo*

Dose (rad)	SF	Microcolony LI (%) All	Large
0	1.00	88	90
200	0.63	81	83
400	0.69	80	78
600	0.50	91	100
800	0.32	91	98
1000	0.24	95	96

We have obtained some very preliminary data which are intriguing as well as puzzling. Although these data are based upon countless hours of examining carefully prepared autoradiographs, they are not sufficiently adequate to constitute publication as a definitive study. Table 1 lists some of the data that we have at this time.

You can see a rather striking and totally unexpected set of events. If we had done this experiment only with low doses–200 and 400 rad–we would have concluded that Q cells are indeed more radioresistant. The labeling indices have decreased in these dose groups. If, on the other hand, our experiment had been done only with high doses–600–1000 rad–our conclusion would have been just the opposite. The labeling indices of these groups are considerably higher than that shown by the controls. How can we explain these puzzling results?

First, it must be acknowledged that there are some exceedingly dangerous pitfalls to be avoided in this kind of experiment. We must ask some major questions–notably, whether the cells we score in microcolonies would have been capable of truly unlimited growth (i.e., to macrocolonies, had we not fixed them in preparing these autoradiographs). The answer to this is complicated, and we are in the process of investigating this carefully and deliberately. Also, the fact that we have fixed all of these preparations at the same time (namely, after 3 days of incubation) may have introduced another serious artifact–these cells experience significant division delay after irradiation such that the higher the radiation dose, the smaller the 3-day microcolony. This does not appear to be a complication, however, for the ordering of labeling indices tends to be the same for the largest and the smallest possible colony, i.e., the two-celled colony.

If we dare to interpret these data, we might initially be tempted to suggest that these numbers are generated by two extreme kinds of Q cells. One kind of Q cells is more resistant than P cells and the other is more sensitive. After all, there is no reason to think that all Q cells are the same. We regard a P cell that stays in the P compartment as having an essentially infinite lifetime (replicating itself over and over again), but the lifetime of a Q cell is finite. By continuous labeling experiments, we know that Q cells in EMT6 tumors have a maximum lifetime of 3–4 days. It is not unreasonable to suppose that as a Q cell ages, it becomes more and more vulnerable to exogenous insults. This is not to say that old Q cells cannot be clonogenic for, quantitatively, our data certainly indicate that they can. In contrast, young Q cells may be more resilient and their survivability upon irradiation may well be related to their nonparticipation in DNA synthesis.

This line of reasoning may be attractive, and it is consistent with a rather simple interpretation in terms of two quite differently shaped survival curves for P and Q cells. We know that the classical survival curve for a population of growing cells is really a composite of the individual survival curves of numerous cell populations that have different survival parameters due to cell age; and we may invoke the same underlying basis for a single composite survival curve for Q cells. Data, such as the ones I have shown, could well be generated by a Q-cell survival curve that starts with a very broad shoulder so that its low-dose region is above the curve of typical P cells; then, this Q-cell curve might bend over progressively, getting steeper and steeper and crossing the P-cell curve at a dose somewhere between 400 and 600 rad. Certainly, the soundness of this notion can be tested experimentally, and we are making every effort to do so.

The preceding is just one of many different interpretations for data of this kind. As noted at the beginning of this chapter, I chose to offer these observations as a discussant mainly because of their relevance to the chapter. *Prediction and Quantification of Tumor Response*. We must be continually reminded that (1) in predicting tumor responses, most of us are inclined to do so only for the exponentially growing cells, i.e., the P cells; (2) most of us may have suspected that Q cells are of major importance insofar as they might revert to the P state and become clonogenic—if they are recruitable, which they are; and (3) we really know precious little about the ability of Q cells to survive irradiation.

ACKNOWLEDGEMENTS

Original research covered in this paper was supported by USPHS National Cancer Institute grants CA3353, CA25990, and CA10372.

REFERENCES

1. Barendsen, G.W., Roelse, H., Hermens, A.F., Madhuizen, H.T., Van Peperzeel, H.A., and Rutgers, D.H.: Clonogenic capacity of proliferating and nonproliferating cells of a transplantable rat rhabdomyosarcoma in relation to its radiosensitivity. *J Natl Cancer Inst* **51**:1521–1526, 1973.
2. Elkind, M.M., and Whitmore, G.F.: *The Radiobiology of Cultured Mammalian Cells.* New York: Gordon and Breach, 1967.
3. Hahn, G.M., and Little, J.B.: Plateau phase cultures of mammalian cells: An *in vitro* model for human cancer. *Curr Top Radiat Res* **8**:39–83, 1972.
4. Kallman, R.F., Combs, C.A., Franko, A.J., Furlong, B.M., Kelley, S.D., Kemper, H.L., Miller, R.G., Rapacchietta, D., Schoenfeld, D., and Takahashi, M.: Evidence for the recruitment of non-cycling clonogenic tumor cells. *M.D. Anderson Symposium* Feb. 27 – March 2, 1979, (Williams & Wilkins); *Rad Biol in Cancer Research* R.E. Meyn and H.R. Withers, eds. New York: Raven Press, 1980, pp. 397–414.

5. Mendelsohn, M.L.: Autoradiographic analysis of cell proliferation in spontaneous breast cancer of the C3H mouse. III. The growth fraction. *J Natl Cancer Inst* **28**:1015–1029, 1962.
6. Rockwell, S.C., Kallman, R.F., and Fajardo, L.F.: Characteristics of a serially transplanted mouse mammary tumor and its tissue-culture-adapted derivative. *J Natl Cancer Inst* **49**:735–749, 1972.
7. Terasima, T., and Tolmach, L.J.: Variation in several responses of HeLa cells to X-irradiation during the division cycle. *Biophys J* **3**:11–33, 1963.

CHAPTER 16

Effective Tumor-Cell Number and Cell Kinetic Analysis in the Prediction of Tumor Response

Carlo Nervi, M.D.[a]
Giorgio Arcangeli, M.D.[b]

The opportunity of correlating tumor size with the control dose in clinical radiotherapy arises from the necessity of obtaining a maximum of effect with a minimum of complications. The knowledge of the dose-response relationship and, consequently, the possibility of predicting the sterilizing radiation dose may also have an impact upon clinical practice in that an expected poor response to irradiation might justify further treatment by surgery or another form of combined therapies.

Even though patient deaths are mostly related to undetected regional or hematogeneous metastases rather than to local failure, the prediction of cancericidal doses can be theoretically useful at least to confirm the validity of the model employed to quantitate the response. The definition of this model has been one of the major aims of radiobiological investigation during the last decade, and has caused great debates among clinicians. As a matter of fact, the crude transposition of experimental data to clinical practice has been considered inadequate to explain the causes of resistance in the majority of cases.[5] Nevertheless, the introduction in clinical practice of more and more precise parameters and of methods derived from radiobiological research had the effect of transforming radiotherapy into a more rational discipline.

[a]Director, Instituto Medico e di Ricerca Scientifica, Rome, Italy
[b]Head, Division of Radiation Therapy, Istituto Medico e di Ricerca Scientifica, Rome, Italy

One of the most exciting radiobiological analyses in man has been done by Fletcher[3] who was able to correlate tumor-control rate with radiation dose, treatment time, and tumor size for some squamous cell carcinomas and adenocarcinomas. Such a correlation, confirmed by other investigations,[8] supported the validity also in clinical practice of the relationship between tumor-cell number and the radiation dose required to eradicate cancer cells (i.e., dose-response relationship at cellular level).

Clinically, tumor-cell burden is roughly evaluated by means of staging systems. These systems generally take into account the tumor bed and the involvement of particular anatomical structure such as bone or cartilage. However, they often fail when different clinical situations are compared. In fact, the correlation does not hold for tumors of the same T with different histology. For example, in Table 1 the required radiation dose ranges from 35 Gy for neuroblastoma to 80 Gy or above for osteogenic sarcoma. In other instances, the correlation cannot be advanced even for tumors of the same histology but located in different sites (as in Table 2 for T_3 squamous cell carcinoma of the tongue and of the tonsillar fossa). Furthermore, for advanced tumors of the same histology and site, the tumor lethal dose may vary by a factor as much as 1.5.

These discrepancies may well be due to different fractions of hypoxic clonogenic cells, however, a precise criterion of evaluation of these cells *in vivo* as well as their

TABLE 1. Examples of Required Tumor Lethal Doses (95% Tumor-Control Dose Probability)[a]

Dose (Gy)	Tumor	Stage
35	Neuroblastoma	T_1-T_3
40	Seminoma	N^+
45	Skin cancer	T_1
50	Medulloblastoma	T_1-T_3
60–65	Skin cancer	T_2-T_3
70–75	Pharyngeal cancer	T_2
	Cervix cancer	T_1-T_2
	Bladder cancer	T_2-T_3
80 or	Head and Neck cancer	T_3-T_4
above	Breast cancer	T_3-T_4
	Osteogenic sarcoma	

[a]Modified from Rubin et al., 1974

TABLE 2. Failure of Local Control in Relation to Size and Site of Carcinoma[a]

Stage	Tonsillar (%)	Tongue (%)
T_1	6	0
T_2	17	14
T_3	41	21
T_4	67	38

[a]Modified from Fletcher, 1973

TABLE 3. Head and Neck Cancer—Randomized Study[a]

	Stage			
	I	II	III	IV
Before Chemotherapy		24	27	21
After Chemotherapy	26	13	16	17

[a]Nervi et al., 1980

relevance in the complex process of radioresistance has not yet been devised. On the other hand, this explanation is still based on the number of tumor cells (oxygenated or hypoxic) independently from the amount of reoxygenation that can take place during a fractionated radiotherapy course. This could imply that any previous reduction of the cell number will increase the effect of a given radiation dose. In other words, a previous reduction of tumor size would possibly lead to an increase of local control by a subsequent course of radiation.

Such a possibility has been tested by us in a randomized clinical trial where a group of patients with head and neck (H & N) cancer was previously "destaged" by chemotherapy and then irradiated, while the control group was treated only with radiotherapy.[6] Chemotherapy caused a marked reduction of tumor size in most cases, determining a shift in distribution of patients toward the early phases of staging, as shown in Table 3. However, no statistically significant difference in local control or survival could be observed after 4 years among patients with oropharynx and maxillary antrum tumors (Table 4). Better local control and survival in the comparison with the control group were obtained only in patients with intraoral tumors in which a booster dose of 30-35 Gy was given by means of interstitial radium implant. The therapeutic gain in the latter case, rather than to tumor size reduction per se, will be due, possibly, to the better geometry of the lesion achieved by the previous chemotherapy courses at the time of interstitial implant. These observations indicate that chemotherapy does not cause a random reduction of the cancer cells but only of those cells which are sensitive to and/or reached by the drug—implying that only particular cell populations were affected by chemotherapy. Furthermore, some tumors recurred shortly after irradiation, although a complete shrinkage had been achieved by chemotherapy. This suggests that even a crude dose-response relationship

TABLE 4. Head and Neck cancer—Randomized Study Results after 4 Years, all Stages[a]

	Combined Therapy	XRT Alone
Oropharynx	30%	31%
Maxillary antrum	40%	30%
Intraoral	54%	32%
	$P < 0.05$	

[a]Nervi et al., 1980

cannot be applied in circumstances as the tumor-cell number is close to the minimum value. A consequent implication is that the marked effect obtained by chemotherapy and the poor response to the subsequent irradiation might well be due to the kinetic characteristics of the tumor-cell population.

In an attempt to correlate growth dynamics with the response to treatment, an *in vivo* kinetic analysis was also performed in 20 of these H & N patients, before and after treatment, by means of the percent labelled mitosis (PLM) method. The technical procedures as well as the results of this study have already been reported in detail elsewhere.[1,2,6,7]

In this study six cases could not be analyzed because of technical difficulties in specimen preparation or radioautographic procedure. In six other cases no PLM data could be obtained because of the absence or insufficient number of mitoses in the samples examined. In eight cases (1/3 of the total) the PLM data could be fitted by a Barrett simulation model. In six of these the model was able to fit only the first part of the data, the remaining part being poorly fitted due to very scattered points (see Fig. 1 *b*). This indicates that, while the duration of G_2 and S phase could be considered quite reliable, the estimation of the intermitotic time (T_1) was affected by large uncertainties. In the remaining two cases, a satisfactory fit could be obtained for all points (see Fig. 1 *a*).

The reasons for these failures are likely

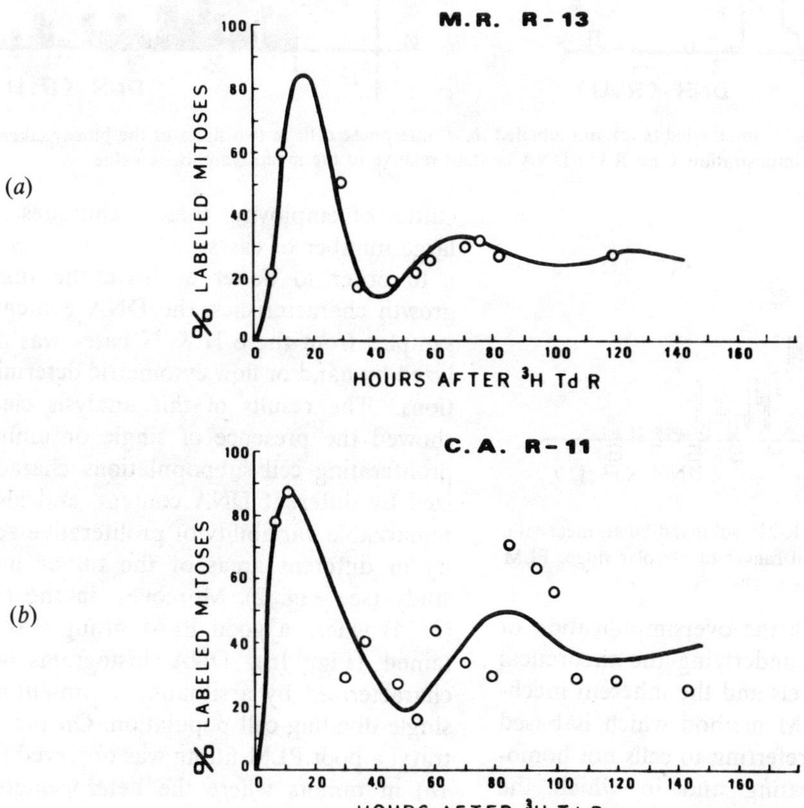

Figure 1. Example of a computer fit (continuous line) according to the Barret simulation model: (*a*) "good fit" (i.e., all PLM data are fitted by the model); (*b*) "bad fit" (i.e., only the first mitotic wave is reproduced by the model).

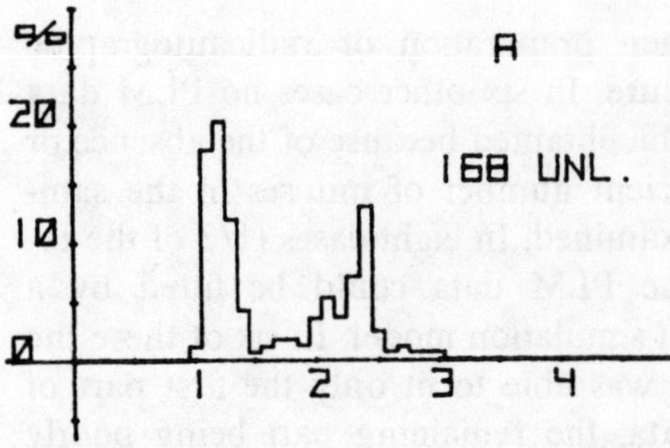

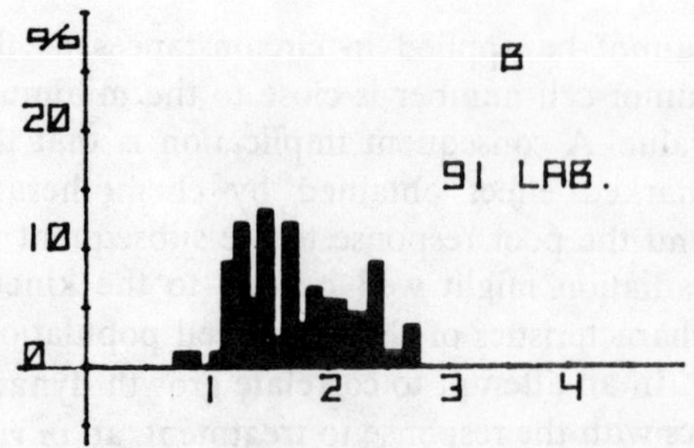

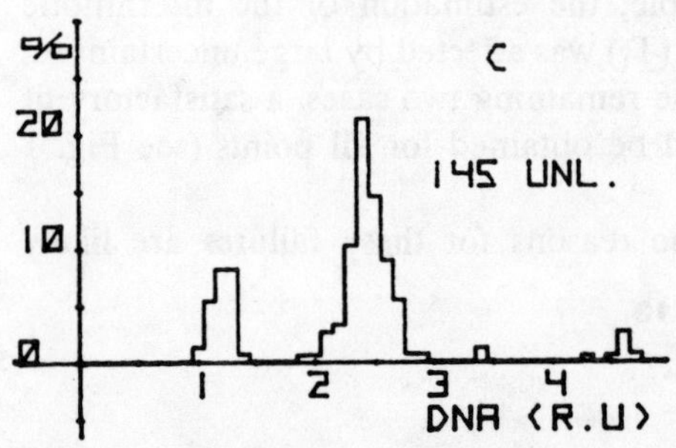

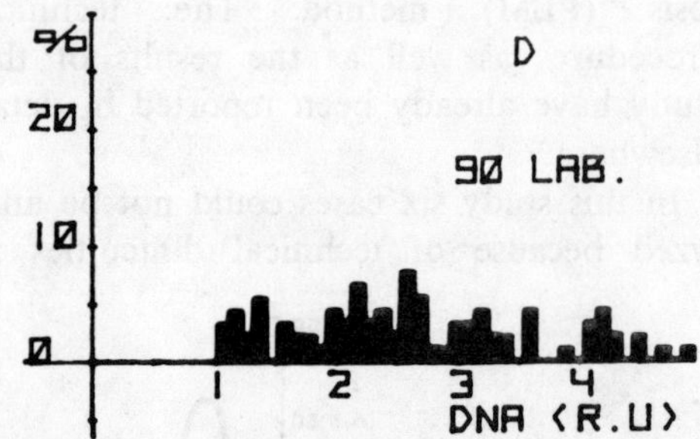

Figure 2. Case C.A. R–11: unlabelled (*a, c*) and labelled (*b, d*) interphase cells in two slides of the biopsy taken 0.5 hours after ^{3}H-TdR administration. Case R.U.: DNA content relative to the mean lymphocite value.

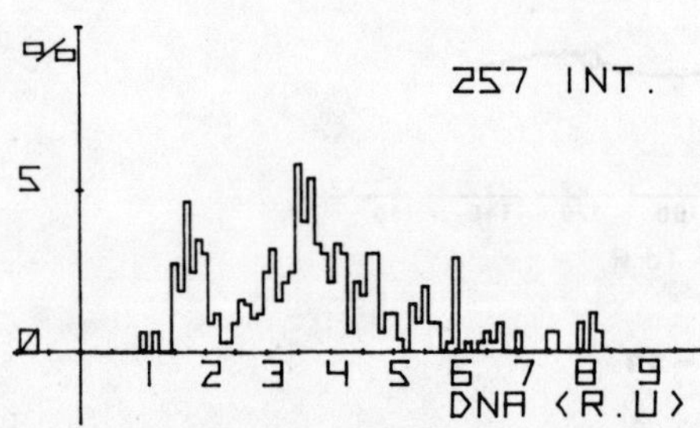

Figure 3. Case F.F. R-21: submandibular metastatic node of squamous cell cancer of alveolar ridge; PLM histogram for interphase cells.

connected to both the oversimplification of the assumptions underlying the theoretical curve fitting models and the inherent mechanism of the PLM method which is based on mean values referring to cells not homogeneously replicating and in which the marker is not homogeneously distributed. However, the fact that the study could not be carried out in 2/3 of the cases demonstrates the scarce feasibility of this kind of investigation and, consequently, the difficulties of employing these techniques in a large number of cases.

In order to better evaluate the tumorgrowth characteristics, the DNA content of samples from these H & N cases was analyzed by hand or flow cytometric determinations.[7] The results of this analysis clearly showed the presence of single or multiple proliferating cell subpopulations characterized by different DNA content, and also a remarkable variability of proliferative activity in different areas of the tumor under study (see Fig. 2). Moreover, in the cases (2/14) where a good PLM fitting was obtained (Fig. 1*a*), DNA histograms were characterized by a situation representing a single dividing cell population. On the contrary, a poor PLM fitting was observed (Fig. 1*b*) in tumors where the heterogeneity of DNA content distribution reflects the presence of mixed populations with different proliferating characteristics. Even more scattered DNA spectra were obtained in the cases where the PLM curve could not be fitted at all (see Fig. 3). In these instances the DNA content of mitotic figures showed a wide spectrum of values pointing to the extreme variability of the tumor proliferative structure.

It has to be stressed that, even in the cases characterized by the presence of a single cell population, the fraction of cells with a DNA content corresponding to the G_1, S, and G_2 phases varied considerably in the several specimens taken at the same time in different areas of the same tumor under study.[7] This can be due to the dispersion of the cycle-phase duration, to the presence of relatively large out-of-cycle compartments, and/or to an intrinsic difference in the cycle structure in different sites.

A further evidence of these proliferative inhomogeneities in human tumors has been obtained with the study of continuous labelling performed on a patient with an advanced, indifferentiated parotid carcinoma with lung metastases ($T_3N_2M_1$). After an intraarterial pulse injection of 1 mCi H^3-TdR, a continuous infusion of 1.5 mCi of the same compound in 300 ml saline was carried out for 8 days. Starting 30 minutes after pulse injection, daily punch biopsies were taken in two opposite sites of the tumor during the 8 days, and then 48 hours and 6 days after the end of infusion. Serial biopsies were also taken during the subsequent irradiation course at times corresponding to 15, 30, and 45 Gy. In order to determine the proportion of labelled interphase cells (LI) and mitoses (LM), 500 to 1000 tumor cells were scored per section in each specimen. All capillary endothelial cells present in the same section were also counted and the relative LI obtained. An average 100 endothelial cells were found in each section. In one site of the tumor, the percentage of LM reached approximately 90% 120 hours after the start of infusion, and then remained around these values, despite some fluctuations (see Fig. 4*a*). In the other specimen a decrease in the labelling level was observed at 168 and 192 hours, despite the continuation of the infusion. The fraction of LI cells in one site also reached 90% after 120 hours, but then dropped to about a 75% level before rising again in spite of infusion disconnection 48 hours before (Fig. 4*b*). In the specimen taken from opposite tumor site, the behavior of LI cells appears to be even less predictable, some fluctuations also being observed during the first 120 hours. After a maximum value of about 80% at 144 hours, a steady decrease in the fraction of labelled cells was observed (Fig. 4*b*).

This was confirmed histologically—168 hours after the onset of infusion, the difference in the labelling between both tumor sites was clearly evidenced (see Fig. 5*a* and *b*). On the contrary, the fraction of the labelled capillary endothelial cells was regu-

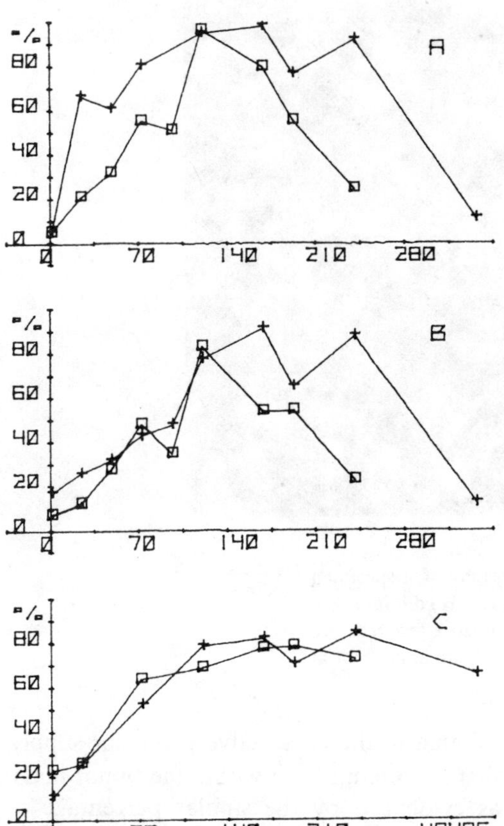

Figure 4. Percent labelled mitoses (*a*), labelled interphases (*b*), and labelled endothelial cells in anterior (+) and posterior (□) part of the tumor (Case M.R.: 168 hours of the continuous ^{3}H-TdR infusion).

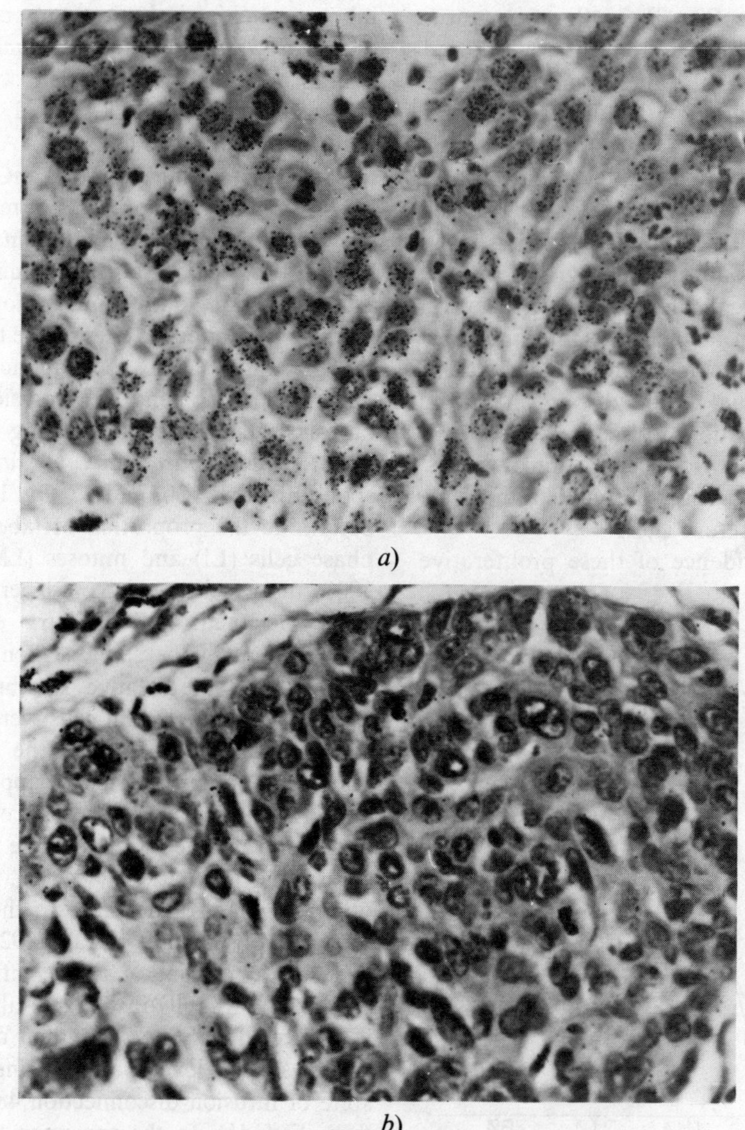

a)

b)

Figure 5. Case M.R.: Autoradiography of a specimen taken after 168 hours of continuous ^{3}HTdR infusion. In (*a*) all cells are labeled, while in (*b*) a few cells are labeled. Note the unlabeled mitotic figure in the central part.

larly distributed throughout the specimens taken from both tumor sites (Fig. 4*c*), their initial LI value (11% and 22%, respectively) being of the same order of that characteristic of the stimulated endothelium.[10] The statistically different labellings in different tumor areas likely reflect a difference in the proliferative activity. In fact, it cannot be attributed to the radioactive precursor supply that is quite uniform within the tumor mass, as evidenced by the similar percentage of the endothelial labelled cells in different tumor areas.

Such differences of proliferative pattern in the same tumor can explain the lack of correlation between cell kinetics parameters

TABLE 5. Cell Kinetics and Radiation Response (Intraoral Cancer, 4 + 4 Patients)[a,b]

Parameter	Control	Failure
Clinical doubling time (days)	29 (13–116)	22 (12–69)
Intermitotic time (hours)	67 (62–73)	68 (52–88)
Growth fraction (%)	43 (31–62)	54 (41–84)
Cell loss (N cells/h/10^4 cells)	54 (40–78)	70 (43–114)
Cells population by DNA content	single and multiple	single and multiple

[a]Values expressed as means and ranges for 3 + 3 patients.
[b]Nervi et al., 1980

and response to irradiation. The data of Table 5 shows that there is a complete overlap between kinetic values characterizing tumors responding or not responding to conventional radiotherapy. No correlation with radiation response could be found even in the few cases characterized by a relatively homogeneous single-cell proliferation.

Until recently, the proliferative pattern of human tumors and, consequently, hypothetical bases for proper treatment scheduling have been obtained only by the labelled nucleoside incorporation method which, as discussed above, is to be considered inadequate to represent the complex process of cell proliferation of human tumors. Recently, reliable techniques for cell dispersal of solid tumors have been introduced. Therefore, flow cytometry may be a promising tool for a better description of the kinetic properties of human tumors and for overcoming at least some of the problems encountered with the PLM method.

Summary

Determination of the dose–response relationship in radiotherapy is required for the optimization of cancer treatment. Tumor-cell number and the pattern of cell proliferation are supposed to be major parameters necessary for a proper definition of the dose-response relationship. In clinical practice it is well known that the result after irradiation is inversely related to the size and extent of a tumor—that is, to the tumor-cell burden. However, in our experience with H & N tumors, a preirradiation reduction of tumor stage and/or size by chemotherapy does not affect the ultimate control of the disease by means of irradiation. Furthermore, no clear correlation can be found between response to treatment and kinetic parameters such as growth rate, generation time, growth fraction, and cell loss. Recently, cytometric analysis of multiple biopsies has been employed in some H & N tumors to better evaluate their cellular and proliferative characteristics. Some major points have been established: (1) multiple clones of cells, recognizable on the basis of their DNA content, are found in solid tumors; (2) the relative fraction of different clones varies throughout the tumor mass, even if some dynamic equilibrium may allow the maintenance of a "mean" tumor behavior; and (3) in cases characterized by a single-cell population, the proliferative activity also varies in different areas of the tumor mass. These observations confirm modern views about human solid tumor heterogeneity, and can explain the observed lack of correlation between response and proliferative parameters obtained with techniques (such as the nucleoside incorporation method) intrinsically unable to reveal proliferative inhomogeneities. The optimization of irradiation requires a precise evaluation of the full set of proliferation parameters in order to completely characterize each individual tumor and, if possible, to establish on these bases an individual treatment.

REFERENCES

1. Bresciani, F., and Nervi, C.: Growth kinetics in human squamous cell carcinoma. In *Growth Kinetics and Biochemical Regulation of Normal and Malignant Cells* B. Drewinko and R.M. Humphrey, eds. Baltimore: William & Wilkins, 1977, pp. 643–661.

2. Bresciani, F., Paoluzzi, R., Benassi, M., Nervi, C., Casale, C., Ziparo, E.: Cell kinetics and growth in squamous cell carcinoma in man. *Cancer Res* **34**:2405–2415, 1974.
3. Fletcher, G.H.: Clinical dose-response curves of human malignant epithelial tumors. *Br J Radiol* **16**:1–12, 1973.
4. Friedman, M.: Clinical studies of the complexities of the recovery and allied phenomena. In *The Biological and Clinical Basis of Radiosensitivity* M. Friedman, ed. Springfield, Mass.: C.C. Thomas, 1974, pp. 389–429.
5. Friedman, M.: Aspects of radiation biology and radiation pathology observed during the treatment of cancer in man. *Br J Radiol* **48**:81–96, 1975.
6. Nervi, C., Arcangeli, G., Badaracco, G., Cortese, M., Morelli, M., and Starace, G.: The relevance of tumor size and cell kinetics as predictors of radiation response in head and neck cancer. A randomized study on the effect of intra-arterial chemotherapy followed by radiotherapy. *Cancer* **41**:900–906, 1978.
7. Nervi, C., Badaracco, G., Morelli, M., and Starace, G.: Cytokinetic evaluation in human head and neck cancer by autoradiography and DNA cytofluorometry. *Cancer* **45**:452–459, 1980.
8. Perez, C.A., Franzska, A.L., Ackerman, L.V., Korba, A., Purdy, J., Powers, W.E.: Carcinoma of the tonsillar fossa. Significance of dose irradiation and volume treated in the control of the primary tumor and metastatic neck nodes. *Int J Radiat Oncol Biol Phys* **1**:817–827, 1976.
9. Rubin, P., Keller, B., and Quick, R.: The range of prescribed tumor lethal doses (PTLD) in the treatment of different human tumors. In *The Biological and Clinical Basis of Radiosensitivity* M. Friedman, ed. Springfield, Mass.: C.C. Thomas, 1974, pp. 435–484.
10. Tannock, I.F., and Hayashi, S.: The proliferation of capillary endothelial cells. *Cancer Res* **32**:77–82, 1972.

CHAPTER 17

Prediction and Quantification of Tumor Response: Prognostic Value of Tumor Pathology

Klaus-Rüdiger Trott[a]

Tumor histopathology has always been an important factor in decision making in radiotherapy. Treatment modality, radiation dosage, prognosis, and treatment effect have been judged according to histopathological criteria before, during, and after radiotherapy.

As a general rule, *before* the start of radiotherapy, a tumor specimen is sent to the pathologist who is to report not only the general diagnosis of cancer but also the exact histopathological classification and grading. The radiosensitivity of tumors with different histology may vary considerably. Lymph nodes affected by lymphomas or seminomas need less than 50% of the dose necessary to control the same lymph nodes affected by squamous cell carcinomas. These differences in radiosensitivity between tumors of different histological classes are well recognized and referred to in the common textbooks of radiotherapy. Experimental data of Barendsen[2] suggest that they may be partly due to differences in cellular radiosensitivity since, in a series of five rat tumors of different histopathology, local tumor response (regrowth delay) correlated in four tumors with the radiosensivity of the derived cell lines; yet Weichselbaum et al.[20] did not find a correlation between the clinical radiosensitivity of several human tumors (e.g., medulloblastoma representing radiosensitive tumors and osteosarcoma and glioblastoma representing radioresistant tumors) and their derived cell lines in their exponential growth phase. More recently, however, they suggested that differences in the capacity to repair potentially lethal damage might explain some of the variability in clinical radiosensitivity of human tumors.[21] Data of Fertil et al.[8] on five different human cell lines displayed the same sequence of radiosensitivity as the tumor types they were derived from. In an extensive review of published survival-curve data, they found a close correlation between the surviving fraction after 2 Gy (the commonly used fractional dose) and the local control dose (TCD-95) of human tumors (to be published). This topic is discussed extensively in Chapter 4.

The differences in clinical radiosensitivity of human tumors of different histopathology are considerable if one compares the extremes: the TCD-50 for fractionated radiotherapy may be as low as 12 Gy in Hodgkin's disease and over 80 Gy in glioblastomas. Yet for the overwhelming majority of human tumors, i.e., for squamous cell carcinomas and adenocarcinomas which together account for over 80% of all human tumors, the difference for tumors of equal size is probably quite small. Usually tumor size determines radiosensitivity more than does tumor histopathology.

The question whether differences in radiosensitivity between different histological

[a]Strahlenbiologisches Institut der Universität München und Abteilung für Strahlenbiologie der GSF Neuherberg, W. Germany.

subgroups or grades can be found within the same histological class is very controversial. Musshoff et al.[12] reported that the local recurrence rate after 40 Gy varied between the different histological types of Hodgkin's disease (Table 1). Accordingly, he recommended different doses for the different histological types: 40 Gy for the lymphocyte predominance, 44 Gy for the nodular sclerosis and the mixed cellularity types, and 46 Gy/5w for the lymphocyte depletion type.

Differences in radiosensitivity are also apparent between various grades of astrocytomas; the local control rate decreases as the tumor dedifferentiates–the anaplastic grade IV being extremely radioresistant.[4] In general, little information on the doses to control tumors locally related to histopathological grading is available although literature on the overall prognostic value of grading is abundant (see, for example, Bloom[3]).

Histopathological grading is usually based on the degree of cell differentiation and cell proliferation as judged from the number of mitoses, cell pleomorphism, cellular differentiation, and structural organization in relation to the tissue of origin. The largest amount of data has been published on carcinoma of the uterine cervix where tumor cells can be divided into three classes:

1. Keratinizing tumor cells
2. Large nonkeratinizing tumor cells
3. Small tumor cells

Some authors[9,13,22] observed a significant correlation between histopathological grading and prognosis. Small cell tumors had the poorest prognosis; large nonkeratinizing tumors had the best prognosis. Yet most other studies could not confirm these results. In a recent review on histopathological types and prognosis of cancers of the uterine cervix, Reagan and Fu[15] concluded that histopathology had no influence on radiosensitivity. Yet on the pattern of tumor infiltration, histopathology is diffuse in anaplastic tumors penetrating deep into the stroma, whereas the large cell nonkeratinizing tumor shows nodular growth without diffuse infiltration into the macroscopically healthy normal tissue but with a regular pushing border. Histopathological grading of squamous cell carcinomas (of the cervix) tells you more about microscopic tumor extension than about tumor radiosensitivity and may therefore be more important for the definition of the treatment volume than for the prescription of radiation dose.[10]

A similar situation may be found in other tumors, too. Most often, however, it is the correlation of tumor anaplasia with the probability of distant metastasis which determines the prognostic value of staging histopathology (as in adenocarcinoma of the prostate with 6% distant metastasis in differentiated stage-C lesions, but over 50% in poorly differentiated stage-C lesions).[14] Best known is the pronounced influence of tumor histopathology on prognosis in breast cancer treated by radical mastectomy[3] which points

TABLE 1. Local Recurrence Rate in Hodgkin's Disease after 40 GY/4 Weeks[a]

Histology	Patients Treated	Local Recurrences
Lymphocyte predominance	13	0
Nodular sclerosis	27	3
Mixed cellularity	23	2
Lymphocyte depletion	15	5
Total	78	10 (13%)

[a] Musshof et al., 1976

to the dependence of microscopic tumor extension and distant spread on the degree of tumor anaplasia.

The observation of histopathological changes in tumor biopsies obtained *during* radiotherapy has only been shown to yield prognostic information in squamous cell carcinomas. The various methods employed by Gusberg (1956), Glücksmann (1974), and Dubrauszky (1966) for quantitating response of carcinoma of the cervix were recently summarized.[18] Their methods consist of counting differentially the number of degenerate cells (Dubrauszky), or differentiating, i.e., either keratinizing cells (Glücksmann) or cells with prominent nucleoli (Gusberg), and comparing them with the number of small, viable, undifferentiated cells. The prognostic value of this simple classification is remarkably good especially in stage III if assessed after a dose of 10 to 20 Gy (see Table 2).

It was suggested that these methods should be adopted to improve the quality of clinical trials with unconventional treatment techniques in carcinoma of the cervix.

These semiquantitative histopathological methods measure the changes in density of viable cells in tumors during radiotherapy which may reflect physiological changes closely related to reoxygenation. Tumors showing rapid decrease in the number of viable cells per microscopic field (and conversely an increase in the number of differentiated, keratinizing, and degenerating cells) may reoxygenate well and therefore have a better prognosis than those tumors in which histopathological morphology does not change appreciably during the first 2 weeks of radiotherapy.[18]

Similar changes have been observed in squamous cell carcinomas of the oral cavity by Cherry et al.[5] and related to prognosis with similar success. The same criteria for good and for poor response were adopted as in carcinoma of the cervix.

Histopathological assessment of tumor response *after* radiotherapy usually adopts the criterion of whether viable tumor tissue is found in the biopsy or not. The presence of viable tumor is generally taken as evidence that radiotherapy was not successful in eradication of the tumor, although Suit et al.[17] showed in mouse adenocarcinomas that in locally controlled tumors viable tumor tissue often persisted for a long time after radiotherapy. In most of our mouse tumors of different histology we find suspect foci of tumor cells in locally controlled fields between 3 and 12 months after irradiation. In various human tumors viable resting tumor was observed surrounded by marked fibrosis many years after radiotherapy; this was taken as evidence that secondary changes in the tumor bed are needed to prevent the quiescent islands of tumor tissue from regrowing into a local recurrence. These islands are commonly regarded as potentially dangerous and often lead to surgical intervention.

Histological persistence of tumor tissue has even been used to quantify tumor response and to compare different treatment modalities. In the treatment of squamous cell carcinomas of the bronchus, Eichhorn et al.[7] compared the effectiveness of photons and neutrons and showed that at autopsy after treatment with neutrons significantly more treatment fields were histologically free of cancer than after cobalt γ-rays. The

TABLE 2. Results after Radiotherapy of Carcinoma of the Cervix (Stage III) According to Histopathological Assessment after a Test Dose

Author	Criterion	Favorable Response	Unfavorable Response
Glücksmann	6 y survival	26/35 (74%)	38/345 (11%)
Dubrauszky	2–3 y rec. free	40/51 (80%)	19/51 (40%)

validity of this end point remains to be established for the different tumor types. Yet, in adenocarcinomas, at least, it appears to be very poor.

In carcinoma of the prostrate, needle biopsies were performed at regular intervals for over 2 years after definite radiotherapy.[6] Positive biopsy rate correlated only with the interval after irradiation; but there was no correlation of biopsy results with prognosis. These data were at large confirmed by Kagan et al.[11] and Perez et al.[14] Also in adenocarcinoma of the uterus, negative tumor histopathology was much better correlated with the interval between preoperative radiotherapy and surgery than with radiation dose (which ranged from 52 Gy to 73 Gy).[23] Similar observations have been reported for adenocarcinomas of the rectum by Rider.[16]

In summary, the clinical observations for adenocarcinomas clearly show that microscopically persistent tumor tissue after definite radiotherapy does not carry a poor prognosis and is no indication for salvage surgery. For other tumors data are less convincing.

The results of preoperative radiotherapy of carcinoma of the bladder T_3 were assessed histologically by Van der Werff-Messing.[19] In 30% of the tumors treated with 40 Gy/4 weeks no tumor was seen in the surgical specimen; their survival rate was over 50% and significantly higher than in another group in which 30% showed no change compared to the preirradiation biopsy (survival rate about 20%). The beautiful quantitative histopathological measurements in Bilharzial bladder after preoperative radiotherapy with 40 Gy by Awwad et al.[1] (1979) show a similar correlation of histologically apparent tumor regression and tumor control. But no correlation could be established between the histopathological classification of radiation damage to tumor cells and prognosis, not even in squamous cell carcinomas of the bladder. The close correlation of histological tumor shrinkage to probability of cure was also apparent in the patients treated by hyperfractionated radiotherapy with 17 fractions of 0.6 Gy per day–a schedule specifically designed for overcoming hypoxia. One may argue that the correlation of tumor regression to local control is not due to more efficient reoxygenation.

Summary

Histopathological analysis of the tumor before, during, and after radiotherapy has been performed and correlated to radiosensitivity and prognosis. In general, the criteria for grading are (1) the degree of cell differentiation *before* radiotherapy, (2) the decrease in density of viable cells per microscopic field *during* radiotherapy, and (3) the persistence of viable tumor *after* radiotherapy. Definite proof of the prognostic value for the individual radiosensitivity remains open but is most likely to exist for squamous cell carcinomas (especially of the cervix) during radiotherapy. The predictive value of histopathological grading with respect to radiosensitivity before radiotherapy appears to be established in a few tumors (e.g., gliomas) but remains controversial in most tumors. Histopathological findings after definite radiotherapy have no prognostic value, with the exception of histologic tumor regression in some tumors after medium-dose preoperative radiotherapy, e.g., of bladder cancer.

REFERENCES

1. Awwad, H., El-Baki, H.A., El-Bolkainy, N., Burgers, M., El-Badawy, S., Mansour, M., Soliman, O., Omar, S., and Khafagy, M.: Preoperative irradiation of T3-Carcinoma in Bilharzial bladder. A comparison between hyperfractionation and conventional fractionation. *Int J Radiat Oncol Biol Phys* **5**:787–794, 1979.
2. Barendsen, G.W.: Variations in radiation response among experimental tumors. In *Radiation Biology in Cancer Research* R.E. Meyn and H.E. Withers, eds. New York: Raven Press, 1980, pp. 333–343.
3. Bloom, H.J.G.: The influence of tumor grade on radiotherapy results. *Br J Radiol* **38**:227–240, 1965.
4. Bouchard, J.: Central nervous system. In *Textbook*

of Radiotherapy G. Fletcher, ed. Philadelphia: Lea and Febiger, 1973.

5. Cherry, C.P., Glücksmann, A., and Walter, L.: The influence of tumor type, persistent precancerous lesions and lymph node involvement on the results of radiotherapy in oral cancers. *Br J Radiol* **40**:612–618, 1967.
6. Cox, J.D., and Stoffel, T.J.: The significance of needle biopsy after irradiation for stage C adenocarcinoma of the prostate. *Cancer* **40**:156–160, 1977.
7. Eichhorn, J.J., and Lessel, A.: Four years' experiences with combined neutron-telecobalt therapy. Investigations on tumor reaction of lung cancer. *Int J Radiat Oncol Biol Phys* **3**:277–280, 1977.
8. Fertil, B., Deschavanne, P.J., Lachet, B., and Malaise, E.P.: In vitro radiosensitivity of six human cell lines. A comparative study with different statistical models. *Radiat Res* **82**:297–309, 1980.
9. Finck, F.M., and Denk, M.: Relationship between histology and survival following radiation therapy. *Obstet Gynecol* **35**:339–343, 1970.
10. Fletcher, G.H.: Cancer of the uterine cervix. *AJR* **111**:225–242, 1971.
11. Kagan, A.R., Gordon, J., Cooper, J.R., Gilbert, H., NuBbaum, H., and Chan, P.: A clinical appraisal of post-irradiation biopsy in prostatic cancer. *Cancer* **39**:637–641, 1977.
12. Musshoff, K., and Slanina, J.: Maligne Systemerkrankungen. In *Strahlentherapie* E. Scherer, ed. Berlin: Springer Verlag, 1976.
13. Ng, A.B.P., and Atkin, N.B.: Histological cell type and DNA value in the prognosis of squamous cell cancer of uterine cervix. *Br J Cancer* **28**:322–331, 1973.
14. Perez, C.A., Walz, B.J., Zivnuska, F.R., Pilepich, M., Prasad, K., and Bauer, W.: Irradiation of carcinoma of the prostate localized to the pelvis: Analysis of tumor response and prognosis. *Int J Radiat Oncol Biol Phys* **6**:555–563, 1980.
15. Reagan, J.W., and Fu, Y.S.: Histologic types and prognosis of cancers of the uterine cervix. *Int J Radiat Oncol Biol Phys* **5**:1015–1020, 1979.
16. Rider, W.D.: Radiation for rectal cancer. *Can Med Assoc J* **117**:1119–1120, 1977.
17. Suit, H.D., and Gallager, H.S.: Intact tumor cells in irradiated tissue. *Arch Pathol* **78**:648–651, 1964.
18. Trott, K.R.: Can tumor response be assessed from a biopsy? *Br J Cancer* **41**: Suppl. IV, 163–170, 1980.
19. von der Werff-Messing, B.: Preoperative irradiation followed by cystectomy to treat carcinoma of the urinary bladder category T3NX, 0-4MO. *Int J Radiat Oncol Biol Phys* **5**:394–401, 1979.
20. Weichselbaum, R.R., Epstein, J., Little, J.B., and Kornblith, P.L.: In vitro cellular radiosensitivity of human malignant tumors. *Eur J Cancer* **12**:47–51, 1976.
21. Weichselbaum, R.R., Nove, J., and Little, J.B.: X-ray sensitivity of human tumor cells in vitro. *Int J Radiat Oncol Biol Phys* **6**:437–440, 1980.
22. Wentz, F.M., and Lewis, G.C.: Correlation of histologic morphology and survival following radiation therapy. *Obstet Gynecol* **26**:228–232, 1965.
23. Wilson, J.F., Cox, J.D., Chabazian, C.M., and del Regato, J.A.: Time dose relationships in endometrial adenocarcinoma: Importance of the interval from external pelvic irradiation to surgery. *Int J Radiat Oncol Biol Phys* **6**:597–600, 1980.

CHAPTER 18

Empirical Clinical Means of Predicting Tumor Response

Giorgio Arcangeli, M.D.[a]
Carlo Nervi, M.D.[b]

The prognostic value of tumor regression during and by the end of radiotherapy has been debated for many years. Radiotherapists have often attempted to correlate tumor regression with the final outcome of the disease, the general feeling being that early tumor regression is indicative of a high probability of tumor control while tumor persistence at the end of treatment generally indicates failure.

However, Table 1 shows the results of several recent studies in which an attempt has been made to correlate final local tumor control with regression at various intervals from the beginning of treatment.

Post-treatment Assessment

Let us consider the last two columns of Table 1. Complete local control was achieved in 74% of head and neck (H & N) cancers and in 69% of those uterine cervix cancers that showed complete tumor clearance, but only in 12% of H & N cancers that showed tumor persistence by 30 to 180 days after the end of treatment. Thus, tumor clearance and persistence are seen to be useful clinical predictors of local outcome. Unfortunately, an indicator of the prognosis at this time cannot influence the treatment policy in an individual treatment.

[a]Head, Division of Radiation Therapy, Istituto Medico e di Ricerca Scientifica, Rome, Italy
[b]Director, Istituto Medico e di Ricerca Scientifica, Rome, Italy

Tumor Regression at the Completion of Treatment

Most results are presently based on tumor regression. Local tumor control was obtained in 57% of H & N cancers and in 65% of uterine cancers that showed complete tumor shrinkage, and in 27% of H & N cancers and 39% of uterine cancers that still showed tumor persistence. Thus, tumor clearance or persistence at the end of irradiation is clearly not a reliable guide in predicting the curability of these types of cancers. However, tumor persistence in *advanced* tumors of H & N clearly indicates a bad prognosis, as in only 11% of these cases a complete local control was achieved. A predictor at the end of treatment, however reliable, could only partially influence the treatment policy.

Tumor Regression during Treatment

Let us now examine the results during the course of irradiation. At first glance, tumor clearance can be considered a good predictor only in uterine cervix cancer in which 84% of tumors that showed complete regression were completely sterilized. In contrast, a complete control was obtained in only 62% of H & N tumors when tumor regression was complete and 43% when incomplete. However, if only early H & N tumors are considered, 82% of those that showed complete regression during irradiation were locally controlled, compared with 50% of

TABLE 1. Local Tumor Control in Relation to Tumor Regression

Reference	Site	During Treatment		End of Treatment		30-180 Days after Treatment	
		TC[a]	TP[b]	TC	TP	TC	TP
Sobel et al., 1976	H & N	5/11	63/135	46/68	23/159	140/199	2/96
Suit et al., 1965	H & N	–	–	19/36	10/16	–	–
Barkley and Fletcher, 1977	H & N	–	–	137/249	46/117	–	–
Dawes, 1980							
All stages	H & N	–	–	–	–	230/300	36/221
early tumors		–	–	–	–	92/99	3/8
Mantyla et al., 1979							
All stages	H & N	18/26	24/67	44/77	8/27	–	–
early tumors		14/17(82%)	15/30(50%)	32/49	6/9	–	–
advanced tumors		4/9	9/37	12/18(43%)	2/18(11%)	–	–
TOTAL	H & N	23/37(62%)	87/202(43%)	246/430(57%)	87/319(27%)	370/499(74%)	38/317(12%)
Marcial and Bosch, 1970*	cervix	102/121	–	145/231	–	47/68	–
Grossman et al., 1973†	cervix	–	–	193/304	86/222	–	–
TOTAL	cervix	102/121(84%)	–	338/517(65%)	86/222(39%)	47/68(69%)	–
TOTAL	H&N + cervix	125/158(79%)	87/202(43%)	584/947(62%)	173/541(32%)	417/567(74%)	38/317(12%)

[a] TC = tumor clearance.
[b] TP = tumor persistence.
*Results expressed as 3-years' survival. The original results observed at the end of external radiotherapy or at radium application have been arbitrarily assigned to the "During Treatment" group. The results observed within 30 days after radium have been assigned to the "End of Treatment" group.
†Results expressed as 5-years' cancer-free survival. The results expressed as "excellent" or "good" have been arbitrarily grouped in TC; those originally expressed as "fair" and "poor" have been grouped on TP.

persisting tumors. This means that, at least in some instances, tumor persistence or clearance may be useful predictors. A reliable indication of the prognosis at this time could be useful in determining the choice of surgical treatment (when possible) or of continued radiotherapy.

An earlier indicator of prognosis in an individual treatment would also be very useful for determining whether a change to using high LET radiation–particular radiation fractionation schedules, radiation combined with hypoxic-cell sensitizers, hyperthermia, or antineoplastic drugs–is worthwhile considering the associated risks of (neuro)toxicity and/or the use of particularly time-consuming techniques. The optimum would be the identification of poorly responding tumors before treatment. Unfortunately no biological property is known at present to be a clear-cut predictor of radiation response.[1,2]

Tumor Regression at the Beginning of Irradiation

It was decided to test the possibility of employing tumor regression, scored at 10 days after an initial large single dose of 8–10 Gy, as a predictor of the final outcome of a subsequent conventional course of radiation. The rationale for this approach is based on several, not mutually exclusive, observations:

1. Marked tumor shrinkage after (an) initial large radiation dose(s), other than resulting from high relative radiosensitivity, could result in *extensive reoxygenation* because of the reduced intercapillary distance and may cause greater sensitivity to subsequent treatment.[5,7]
2. A marked initial tumor response could reflect an *increased cell killing* after a relatively large radiation fraction.[7]
3. The response to single radiation doses suggest a relationship between radiosensitivity and the initial process of cell removal.[5]

In other words, extensive tumor shrinkage after an initial large radiation dose could be of considerable value not only in predicting a favorable prognosis, but also in determining (because of reoxygenation) a better response to the remaining radiotherapy.

Some preliminary clinical observations using this approach have been recently published.[1,2] In this chapter the study has been extended to other groups of tumors including those characterized by a slow response to radiation (i.e., prostate cancer, melanoma, sarcoma).

Table 2 shows the results obtained in all groups of tumors. It is clear that the tumors which regressed most after the initial dose of 8 to 10 Gy had the highest probability of local control by the subsequent conventional fractionation radiotherapy while the tumors which regressed least were most likely not to be responsive to subsequent radiation.

In Figure 1 the shrinkage trends of all tumors under study are shown in terms of observed shrinkage curves. After the initial fractional dose, 46 tumors (52%) shrank less than 10% of the initial volume, 14 (16%) shrank between 10 and 30%, and 28 (31%) shrank more than 30%. Following the subsequent conventional fractionation radiotherapy, complete local response within 30 to 60 days after the completion of treatment was achieved in 26% of tumors of the first group, in 43% of tumors of the second group by the end of treatment or a few days later, and in 86% of tumors of the third group within the treatment time.

An analysis of the data of the first group of tumors shows a difference between prostate, sarcoma, and melanoma tumors in comparison with the other cases (Table 2). In fact, the probability of complete response is statistically different ($p < 0.05$) for the two sets of data. Accordingly, these particular tumors, showing a slower regression rate, were excluded from further statistical analy-

TABLE 2. Local Tumor Control in Relation to % Shrinkage after an Initial Large Dose

Site	No.	Shrinkage (10%)	Shrinkage (10–30%)	Shrinkage (30%)
H & N	20	0/7	2/4	7/9
Lung (nonoat)	15	1/7	1/2	5/6
Prostate	12	[6/10][a]	[2/2][a]	–
Breast	10	0/2	0/2	6/6
Bladder	10	0/5	0/2	3/3
Colo-rectal (postop. recurr.)	10	0/4	1/2	3/4
Melanoma (nodes)	6	[2/6][a]	–	–
Sarcoma (soft tissues)	5	[3/5][a]	–	–
TOTAL	88	12/46(26%)	6/14(43%)	24/28(86%)
TOTAL less [ ][a]		1/25(4%)	4/12(33%)	

[a] [ ] = slowly responding tumors.

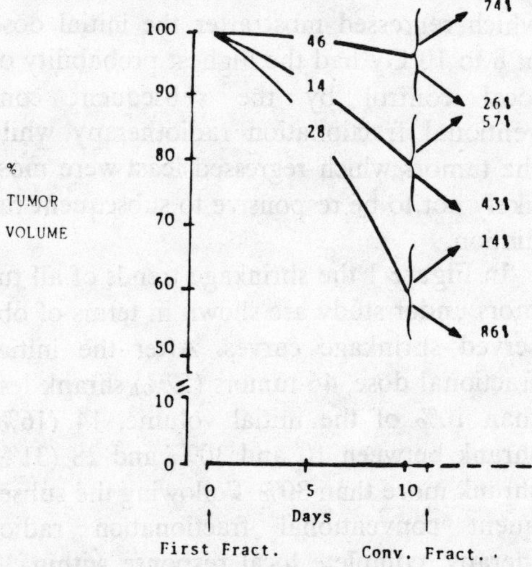

Figure 1. Tumor shrinkage 10 days after an initial large dose: 46 tumors shrank less than 10%, 14 between 10 and 30%, and 28 more than 30%; ↗ = % tumor persistence or recurrence and ↘ = % tumor clearance after a subsequent course of conventional fractionation.

sis. First a χ^2 test was applied to ascertain whether the complete response could have been random in all groups—this probability was less than 0.005. Furthermore, as in Figure 2, the data were examined by plotting the percent tumors locally controlled as a function of the shrinkage after the initial fractional dose. According to the method of Snedecar and Cochran,[10] an arbitrary score of 0, 1, or 3 was assigned to tumors characterized by an initial shrinkage of less than 10%, between 10 and 30%, or more than 30%, respectively. This approach shows that increasing shrinkage correlates with increasing control rate—the probability of achieving a complete response in "poorly responding" tumors is only 4%, whereas a marked initial response corresponds to a complete tumor clearance in more than 85% of the cases. A linear regression line has been fitted to each set of data indicating that there is a significant correlation ($p < 0.0005$) between initial tumor shrinkage and ultimate cure probability. Therefore, the prediction, in our experience, becomes more reliable with increasing tumor regression rate.

The problem now is whether it is possible to increase the value of prediction from tumor regression at the beginning of irradiation in slowly responding tumors.

Figure 3 shows the correlation of complete local control with the initial tumor regression scored in 10 prostate carcinomata, 10 days after a dose of 10 Gy combined with a single administration of 2 g/m² misonidazole and followed by a conventional course of radiotherapy. The rationale of this approach is based on the hypothesis that a large number of hypoxic cells in a tumor relates to the efficiency of cell removal or to

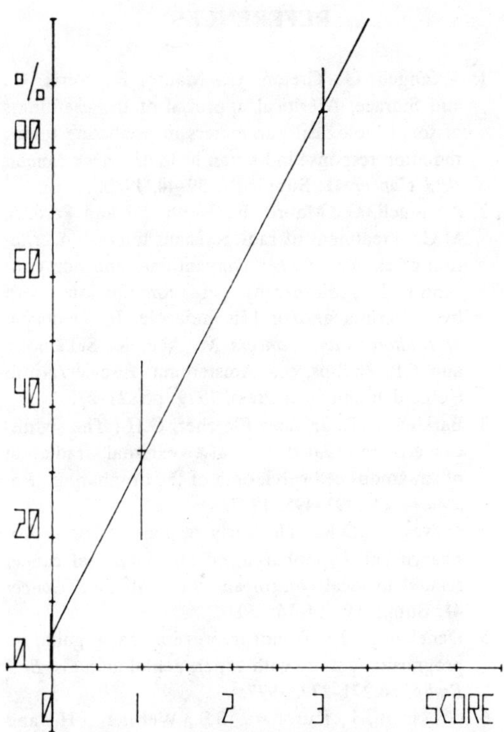

Figure 2. Percent of tumors controlled as a function of the shrinkage observed 10 days after an initial large dose. An arbitrary score of 0, 1, or 3 was assigned to tumors showing an initial shrinkage $< 10\%$, 10 to 30%, or $> 30\%$, respectively. A linear regression line has been fitted to each set of data, indicating that there is a significant correlation ($p < 0.0005$) between the initial tumor shrinkage and the ultimate cure probability. Prostate, melanoma, and sarcoma tumors have been excluded from this analysis (see text).

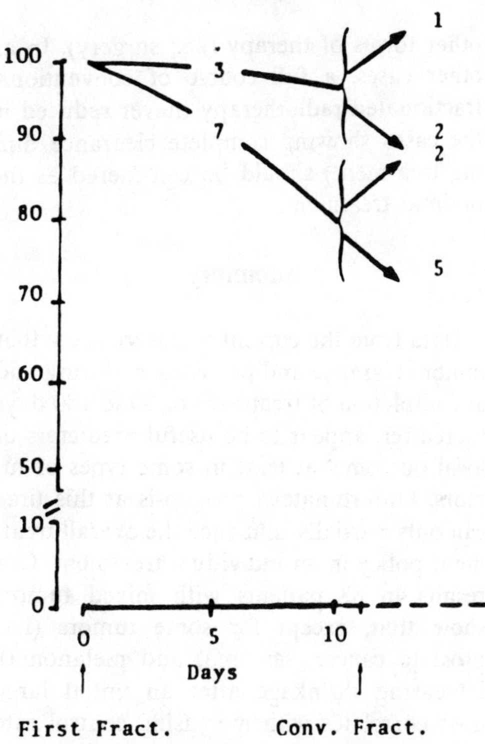

Figure 3. Tumor shrinkage in 10 prostatic carcinomata, 10 days after an initial dose of 10 Gy combined with a single administration of 2 g/m² misonidazole (three tumors shrank less than 10% and seven between 10 and 30%); ↗ = number of tumors persisting or recurring and ↘ = number of tumors cleared after a subsequent course of conventional fractionation.

the cell-cycle time and, hence, to the rate at which cell death after irradiation is expressed.[5]

Unfortunately, the number of cases is still insufficient for a statistically significant indication. Nevertheless, seven out of ten tumors showed a shrinkage between 10 and 30%, and only three remained unaffected after the "test" dose of radiation and misonidazole. Of the first group of seven tumors, five had complete clearance by the end of the subsequent conventional irradiation, and two showed only some transient shrinkage. Of the second group of three tumors, two were completely cleared several days after the completion of irradiation, and one remained unaffected by the treatment. This suggests that in some of these tumors a significant number of hypoxic cells is present and responsible for their slow regression rate during irradiation, even though the concomitant role of other mechanisms cannot be excluded. Hence, the regression rate after an initial large dose of radiation and misonidazole could be a useful parameter for predicting the final tumor outcome, although further studies along these lines are necessary before a routine application of this approach to radiotherapy. From this point of view, tumors that do not respond to an initial large dose of radiation and misonidazole would be the best candidates for special radiation fractionation schedules, combination of radiation with other agents, other types of radiation (i.e., high LET), or other forms of therapy (i.e., surgery). In all other cases, a full course of conventional fractionated radiotherapy (never reduced in the cases showing complete clearance during treatment) should be considered as the optimal treatment.

Summary

Data from the current literature show that tumor clearance and persistence, during and at completion of treatment or 30 to 180 days thereafter, appear to be useful predictors of local outcome, at least in some types of tumors. Unfortunately, prognosis at this time can only partially influence the overall treatment policy in an individual treatment. Our results in 88 patients with mixed tumors show that, except for some tumors (i.e., prostate cancer, sarcoma, and melanoma), increasing shrinkage after an initial large dose correlates with increasing control rate after a subsequent course of conventional radiotherapy. Therefore, the prediction, in our experience, becomes more reliable with increasing tumor regression rate. In some slowly responding tumors (i.e., prostate cancer) there is evidence that the regression rate after an initial large radiation dose and misonidazole could be a useful parameter for predicting the final tumor outcome after a subsequent course of conventional radiotherapy. Tumors showing no response to an initial large radiation dose and misonidazole would be the best candidates for special radiation fractionation schedules, multimodality treatments, or other forms of therapy.

ACKNOWLEDGEMENT

Supported by the G. & L. Shenker Research Foundation

REFERENCES

1. Arcangeli, G., Creton, G., Mauro, F., Nervi, C., and Starace, A critical appraisal of the usefulness of some biological parameters in predicting tumor radiation response in human head and neck cancer. *Br J Cancer* **41**: Suppl. IV, 39–44, 1980.
2. Arcangeli, G., Mauro, F., Nervi, C., and Pardini, M.C.: Treatment of radioresistant tumors: A criterion of choice between conventional and non-conventional radiotherapy in combination with hyperthermia and/or Misonidazole. In *Treatment of Radioresistant Cancers* M. Abe, K. Sakamoto, and T.L. Phillips, eds. Amsterdam: Elsevier/North Holland Biomedical Press, 1979, pp. 21–27.
3. Barkley, H.T., Jr., and Fletcher, G.H.: The significance of residual disease after external irradiation of squamous cell carcinoma of the oropharynx. *Radiology* **124**:493–495, 1977.
4. Dawes, P.J.D.K.: The early response of oral, oropharyngeal, hypopharyngeal and laryngeal cancer related to local control and survival. *Br J Cancer* **41**: Suppl. IV, 14–16, 1980.
5. Denekamp, J.: Tumor regression as a guide to prognosis: A study with experimental animals. *Br J Radiol* **50**:271–279, 1977.
6. Grossman, I., Kurohara, S.S., Webster, J.H., and George, F.W., III: The prognostic significance of tumor response during radiotherapy in cervical carcinoma. *Radiology* **107**:411–415, 1973.
7. Holsti, L.R., Salmo, M., and Elkind, M.M.: Unconventional fractionation in clinical radiotherapy. *Br J Cancer* **37**: Suppl. III, 307–310, 1978.
8. Mantyla, M., Kortekangas, E., Valavaara, R.A., and Nordman, E.M.: Tumor regression during radiation treatment as a guide to prognosis. *Br J Radiol* **52**:972–977, 1979.
9. Marcial, V.A., and Bosch, A.: Radiation-induced tumor regression in carcinoma of the uterine cervix: Prognostic significance. *AJR* **108**:113–123, 1970.
10. Snedecar, G.W., and Cochran, W.G.: *Statistical Methods* 6th ed. Ames, Iowa: Iowa State University Press, 1967, pp. 246–248.
11. Sobel, S., Rubin, P., Keller, B., and Poulter, C.: Tumor persistence as a predictor of outcome after radiation therapy of head and neck cancers. *Int J Radiat Oncol Biol Phys* **1**:873–880, 1976.
12. Suit, H., Lindberg, R., and Fletcher, G.H.: Prognostic significance of extent of tumor regression at the completion of radiation therapy. *Radiology* **84**:1100–1107, 1965.

CHAPTER 19

The Prognostic Significance of the Clinical Status of a Tumor at the Completion of Irradiation

Gilbert H. Fletcher, M.D.[a]
H. Thomas Barkley, M.D.[b]

At the Curie Foundation in the 1920s weekly observations were made of the regression of tumors, especially tumors of the skin or of the mouth and throat. It was recognized by Coutard and later by Baclesse that exophytic tumors regressed rapidly and had a better prognosis than infiltrating or ulcerating ones. From these observations the concept arose that a fast regression rate of a tumor mass, leaving clinically no residual disease at the completion of irradiation, carries a favorable prognosis. Baclesse in the 1940s made the observation about breast cancer, always an infiltrative tumor, that small masses disappeared faster than large masses and had a better prognosis.

The significance of those two closely linked parameters, i.e., clinical variety and tumor size, on the predictability of the ultimate outcome cannot be considered in general terms, but must be assessed within different clinical and pathologic frameworks. Separate guidelines for treatment must also be determined for specific presentations. In this essay we review and discuss clinical data rather than offer possible explanations for different rates of regression.

[a]Professor, Division of Radiotherapy, The University of Texas System Cancer Center, M. D. Anderson Hospital and Tumor Institute, Houston, Texas

[b]Associate Radiotherapist and Associate Professor of Radiotherapy, Department of Radiotherapy, The University of Texas System Cancer Center, M. D. Anderson Hospital and Tumor Institute, Houston, Texas

Squamous Cell Carcinomas of the Upper Respiratory and Digestive Tracts

Because of the early clinical disappearance of exophytic lesions like those of the tonsillar fossa and supraglottic larynx (which often have completely regressed by the fourth week of radiotherapy), the tendency had been to keep the total dose lower for this type of lesion than for lesions that have not regressed. Until the mid-1960s, it was the practice at M. D. Anderson Hospital (MDAH) to treat 1-1½ weeks beyond the week in which the lesion had clinically disappeared (Baclesse's rule of thumb). Therefore, some T_2 and T_3 tumors of the tonsillar fossa and supraglottic larynx did not receive more than 6000 rad in 6 weeks because no tumor was visible or palpable by the fourth to the fifth week.

In a study comparing 5-FU and irradiation (6000 rad in 6 weeks) with irradiation alone (7000 rad in 7 weeks), it was found that tumors treated by 5-FU and 1000 rad per week regressed during treatment more rapidly than did those treated by 1000 rad per week alone (see Fig. 1); however, the difference in control rates favored irradiation only (see Table 1).[7,8] Obviously, although the adjuvant chemotherapy pro-

TABLE 1. Results at 5 Years in Randomized Series of Pharyngeal Wall Lesions[e]

Treatment	Stage T3	Stage T4	No. of Patients	No Evidence of Disease	Primary Uncontrolled	DM[d]	Unk	ID
5FU[a] + ^{60}Co 6000 rad	3	9	12	1	8	2	1	0
^{60}Co 7000 rad	5	11	16[b]	5[c]	4	1	1	2

[a] 60 mg/kg of 5FU intravenously in 5 days; 19 patients received radiation treatment after 5FU; 9 patients received 5FU during second week of radiation treatment.
[b] 3 patients died from complications.
[c] 1 patient salvaged by surgical excision of residual disease.
[d] DM = distant metastases; Unk = unknown; ID = intercurrent disease.
[e] From Fletcher, G. H. et al., 1967.

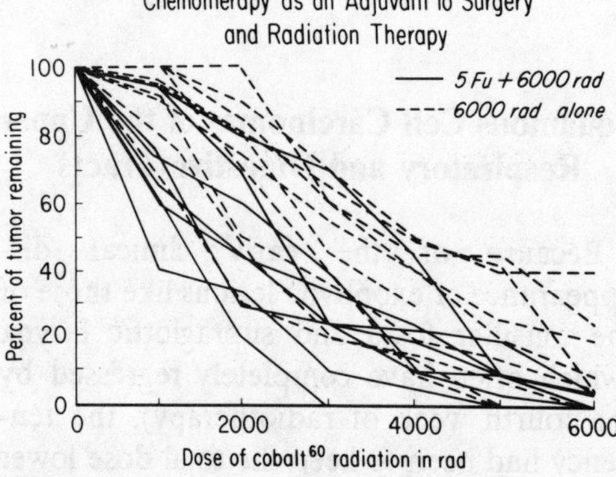

Figure 1. Regression rates of T_3 and T_4 squamous carcinomas of the posterior and lateral pharyngeal wall. After receiving 1000 rad per week, at 6 weeks the tumors in both groups had received 6000 rad alone or with 5-FU. The null hypothesis (that there is no difference in the regression of the tumor in the two groups) is rejected at the levels of 0.03 for 1000 rad, 0.06 for 2000 rad, 0.08 for 3000 rad, 0.07 for 4000 rad, 0.11 for 5000 rad, and 0.04 for 6000 rad (Mann-Whitney rank test for nonparametric distribution) (From Fletcher GH, 1963)

duced a faster regression, it was not as effective in terms of tumor control as the extra 1000 rad given in the seventh week of irradiation. This result prompted an analysis in the early 1960s of the meaning of the regression rate of squamous cell carcinoma of the oropharynx. No correlation was found between the clinical status at the end of treatment and the ultimate outcome.[13] Following the analysis, the total dose was no longer gauged according to the rate of regression but according to the initial size of the tumor, so that T_2 and T_3 tumors, even those that regressed rapidly, were given 7000 rad in 7 weeks.

A recent analysis has been done, considering as residual disease not some tautness or a rubbery feel which is always present in tumors that involve the glossopalatine sulci or base of the tongue, but only hard infiltration with or without ulceration. Under these rigid criteria a correlation has been found between a favorable outcome with no clinical evidence of disease at the end of treatment and a poor outcome with clinically residual disease at the end of treatment (see Table 2).[1]

Separating the clinical material into two periods—one from 1948 through 1965 and one from 1966 through 1970—one sees that the patients without clinically residual disease at the end of treatment had fewer failures in the second period than in the first period (Table 2). By and large, in the second period, tumor doses for the rapidly regressing T_2 and T_3 lesions had been increased by 500 rad. Because the dose-response curves for squamous cell carcinomas are rather steep for T_2 and T_3 lesions of the supraglottic larynx and T_3 and T_4 tumors of the tonsillar fossa (see Fig. 2), a dose increment of 500 rad produces significantly higher control rates (see Fig. 3 and Table 3). The control rate of the slowly regressing tumors remained the same throughout both periods because these tumors had always re-

TABLE 2. Clinical Evaluation of the Status of the Primary Lesion at the End of Treatment Related to Failure Rates in Squamous Cell Carcinomas of the Oropharynx—All Stages, 1948-1970 (Analysis, 1976)[c]

	Status at End of Irradiation			
	Residual Present		No Residual Present	
	1948–1965	1966–1970	1948–1965[a]	1966–1970[a]
Recurrence at Primary Site	61%(49/80)	60%(22/37)	37%(60/161)[b]	18%(16/88)[b]

[a] Approximately 500-rad higher total dose in the period 1966–1970.
[b] $p < 0.01$.
[c] From Barkley, H.T., and Fletcher, G. H., 1977.

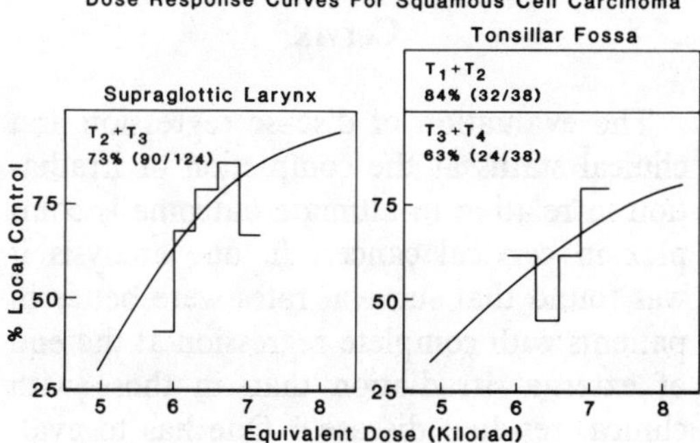

Figure 2. Dose-response curves for two stage-groupings of squamous cell carcinomas of the head and neck (Poisson model). Histograms show estimated local control rates for two stage-groups in 300-rad intervals. Equivalent doses in 6-weeks treatment time are used. (Adapted from Thames H.D. et al, 1980.)

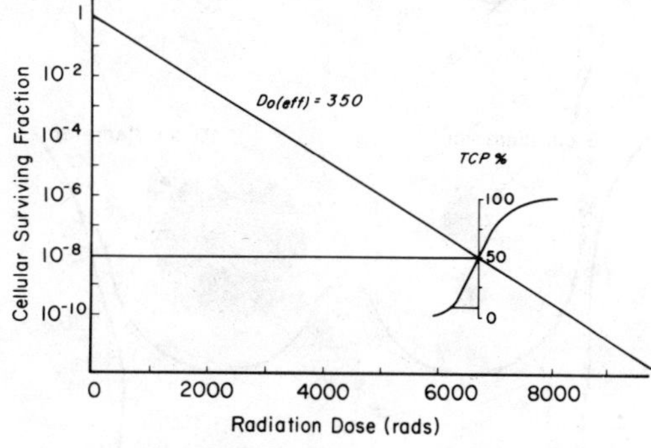

Figure 3. Diagram illustrating the relationship between D_o (eff) with fractionated irradiation and the tumor control probability (TCP).

Using statistical methods, one can demonstrate that, with fractionated irradiation, $3 \times D_o$ (eff) (approximately 1000 rad for 200 rad fractions) can theoretically increase the probability of tumor control (TCP) from 10 to 90%.[15] Clinically it has been shown that, with an increase of approximately 500 rad, control was increased from 50 to 80% for tonsillar fossa tumors[11] and from 70 to 87% for supraglottic larynx tumors.[6] (From Fletcher, G.H., 1981)

ceived a high total dose which was not increased after 1966. For slowly regressing infiltrative lesions, as shown in an analysis of results in squamous cell carcinoma of the base of the tongue, at least 7500 rad is needed.[12]

Breast

At MDAH only breast tumors with grave signs have been treated by irradiation alone. In breast cancer local control is a function not only of the size of the tumor, but also of associated features such as peau d'orange, satellite nodules, etc. Recurrences on the chest wall may develop at or beyond the margins of the radiation fields, making it almost impossible to quantitate rigidly the correlation of tumor regression during treatment with the ultimate outcome.

The general impression is that control correlates principally with the size of the tumor. A tumor mass in excess of 10 cm in diameter has virtually never regressed completely at the end of a protracted irradiation of 70 days, despite doses of 9000 to 10,000 rad; whereas a smaller mass, up to 5 cm in diameter, has usually completely regressed with smaller doses prior to the end of treat-

TABLE 3. Control Rates by Periods

	Tonsillar Fossa[a] T_3 + Selected T_4		Supraglottic Larynx[b] T_2 + Exophytic T_3
1954–early 1960s	50%(8/16)	1954–1963	70%(38/54)
Early 1960s–June 1968[c]	81%(47/58)	1964–1972[c]	87%(52/60)

[a] From Schukovsky, L.J., and Fletcher, G.H., 1973.
[b] From Fletcher, G. H., 1980.
[c] Approximately 500-rad higher dose in second period.

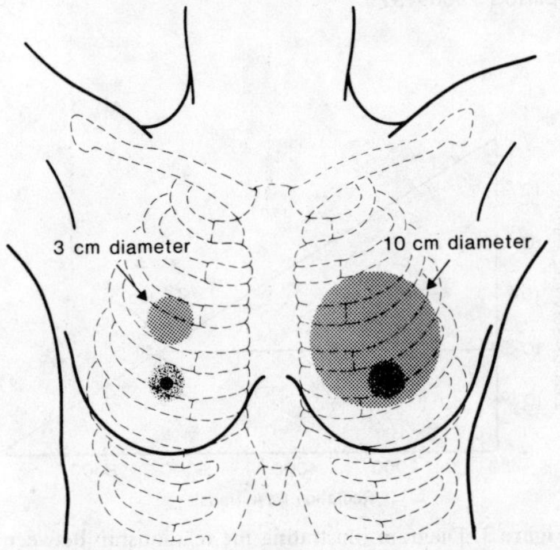

Figure 4. Probability of control correlated with irradiation dose and volume of cancer in adenocarcinoma of the breast from data from the Curie Foundation.[2]

Dose (rad)	*Volume*	*Control*
7000–8000/8–9 weeks	2–3 cm primary	65%
	> 5 cm primary	30%
8000–9000/8–10 weeks	> 5 cm primary	56%

Because of the early disappearance of the mass in the breast, relatively small doses were given resulting in a failure rate of 35%.

ment (see Fig. 4). However, the fact that a mass is palpable at the completion of treatment does not necessarily mean that there is active disease. We know of several cases in which a mastectomy is performed because of a persistent mass, and only amorphous hyaline material is found in the surgical specimen. Conversely, the disappearance of a small mass at 5 weeks with 5000 rad or at 8 weeks with 6000 rad must not preclude a boost with either an interstitial implant or with external beam through a reduced portal.

Cervix

The evaluation of disease regression and clinical status at the completion of irradiation in relation to ultimate outcome is complex in cervical cancer. In one analysis it was found that survival rates were better in patients with complete regression at the end of external irradiation than in those with clinical residual disease.[10] One has to evaluate separately the primary lesion and parametrial infiltration. Lesions of the uterine cervix are essentially of two clinical varieties: exophytic lesions on the exocervix and lesions of the endocervix that infiltrate the myometrium and can reach considerable dimensions (see Fig. 5). In exophytic lesions of the exocervix, 4000 rad in 4 weeks always produces a complete regression of the disease, making possible an effective intracavitary gamma-ray therapy application. In lesions of the endocervix that invade the myometrium, producing a barrel-shaped type of lesion (Fig. 5) if there is marked shrinkage after 4000 rad in 4 weeks, a maximalized intracavitary gamma-ray therapy—primarily intrauterine gamma-ray therapy of no less than three insertions, each 2 weeks apart—produces high control rates.[6]

The bulk of parametrial infiltration is not reflected in the stage. When parametrial disease of a nonmassive nature reaches the pelvic wall, there is usually a softening of the induration at the end of external irradiation; whereas if parametrial disease is rock-hard and massive, it is usually present at the end of treatment (usually external irradiation alone to doses of 6000 to 7000 rad). Although, as would be expected from the lesser bulk of tumor, the rate of ultimate control is higher in the less massive parametrial infiltrations than in the rock-hard indurations present at the completion of treatment, this does not always mean that the latter patient will not be cured.[3] Over a number of months the palpatory findings can change to rubbery, but still firm, pelvic fibrosis. Thus, it is the initial bulk of the disease, rather than its regression rate, that should be the guide to treatment and prognosis.

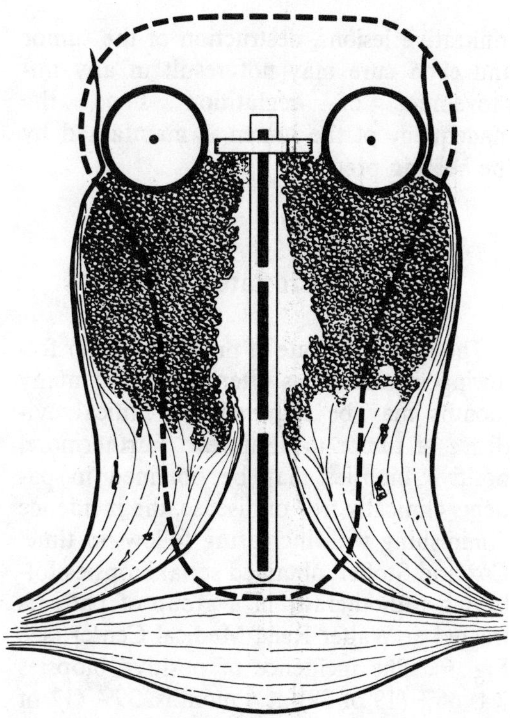

Figure 5. In the bulky lesions of the endocervix, tumor cells deep in the myometrium are beyond the zone of adequate dosage because of the pear-shaped isodose distribution of the radium system, unless considerable shrinkage has taken place by the time of the intracavitary gamma-ray therapy. (From Fletcher, G.H., 1980).

Lung and Esophagus

Each facet of regression can be illustrated by bronchogenic carcinoma due to its wide variety of histologic categories, cellular kinetics, growth characteristics, and volume. Unfortunately, in only a small percentage of patients can tumor extent be reliably identified from x-rays since the associated shadows caused by atelectasis, consolidation, or pneumonitis cannot be separated. In those situations where volume can be identified, there is evidence that regression is related to increasing dose and survival is related to extent of regression. In small cell carcinoma, characterized by faster turnover time and a high proportion of cells in the proliferating pool, response to radiation is prompt and, judged by subsequent x-rays, often complete. Despite this apparent response, however, a reduction in dose below about 5000 rad results in equally rapid recurrence. For intermediate-turnover-time squamous carcinoma and long-turnover-time adenocarcinoma, regression rates are functions of their individual turnover times and are proportional to the total dose given. The influence of site and growth pattern is also frequently seen; e.g., a patient with an exophytic squamous carcinoma arising in a main bronchus may have complete relief of atelectasis within 3 weeks of beginning radiation therapy, while after a similar amount of radiation there may be no change in the chest film of a patient with adenocarcinoma arising in a more peripheral site and obstructing a main bronchus by extrinsic pressure.

Cancer of the esophagus, on the other hand, being overwhelmingly squamous in origin, has regression characteristics that depend on the type of growth, as in cancer of the oropharynx. Relief of dysphagia is seen promptly in those patients with a primarily exophytic tumor, shrinkage of which by doses in the range of 3000 rad in 10 fractions (noncurative) leaves an adequate lumen. In those patients with circumferential infiltrative lesions, destruction of the tumor and even cure may not result in any improvement of deglutition since the inadequacy of the lumen is maintained by the healing process.

Prostate

The regression rate of prostatic cancer following irradiation is often slow, and many months may be required for clinical evidence of tumor to disappear. Furthermore, positive biopsies may be obtained in patients clinically free of disease, the incidence diminishing with increasing follow-up time. Cox and Stoffel[4] obtained serial biopsies following radiotherapy in a group of patients treated at Walter Reed Medical Center (see Fig. 6). The incidence of positive biopsies was 66% (19 of 29) at 4 months, 39% (12 of 31) at 10 months, 31% (8 of 26) at 16 months, and 19% (7 of 37) at 30 months. Those data suggest that complete regression in some prostate carcinomas may require 3 years or more, and yet local control rates are high. While the high local control rates may reflect, in part, a slow recurrence pattern, it is clearly wrong to base treatment or prognosis on regression rate in this cancer.

The long natural history of this disease suggests that the tumor cells are often slowly proliferating and have a long turnover time; and with most cell types, death following irradiation is predominantly due to lysis during mitosis, although some nonviable cells may complete several divisions before lysis occurs. Therefore, the slow regression rate frequently observed in patients with prostatic carcinoma is not unexpected.

Discussion

In squamous cell carcinomas of the mouth and throat, the correlation between clinical disappearance of disease at the completion of treatment and permanency of control is disturbed both by geographical misses—caused by extension of the disease clinically not recognizable initially—and by the frequent appearance of another primary tumor at the periphery of the initially treated area. This is particularly true in tumors of the faucial arch which is an anatomical site known for multicentric lesions. The ability to predict control from a clinically complete regression varies from one anatomical site to another. For instance, if there is a complete regression of a T_3 tumor of the tonsillar fossa after a tumor dose of 7000 rad, one can predict a high probability of control; whereas for a similarly staged tu-

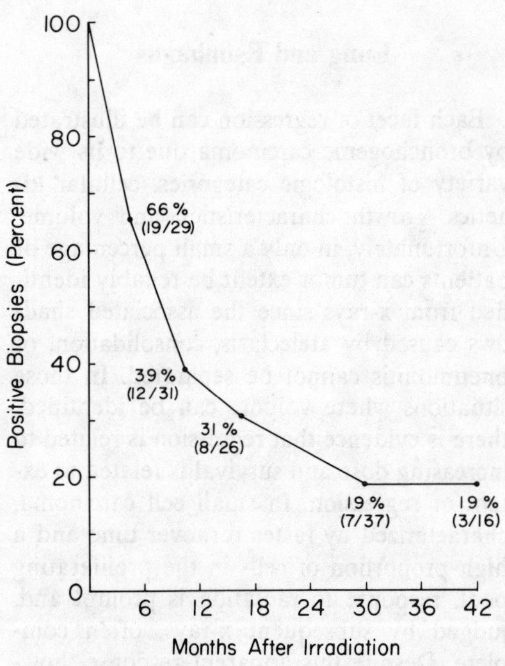

Figure 6. Between August 1970 and March 1973, 38 patients with cancer of the prostate were treated with radiation therapy at Walter Reed Medical Center (median follow-up interval = 48 months). Gradual disappearance of palpable tumor was noted in all patients, although two patients developed palpable evidence of local recurrence. Serial biopsies obtained in 33 patients showed no correlation with the clinical findings. The incidence of positive biopsies diminished with increasing follow-up time. (Adapted from Cox, J.D., and Stoffel, T.J., 1977.)

mor on the posterior pharyngeal wall, despite fairly early flattening of the tumor and 7000 rad tumor dose, success is less predictable. A possible explanation is that malignant clonogens on the prevertebral fascia may stay hypoxic.

If one chooses to treat cancer of the breast with irradiation alone, the size of the mass(es) in the breast and axilla is the determining parameter.

The regression rate in squamous cell carcinomas of the uterine cervix is significant not only on a biological, but also on a physical, basis since intracavitary gamma-ray therapy is more effective after the disappearance of masses that reduce the effectiveness of the radioactive system by pushing the radioactive sources away from the deep infiltrating disease.

There are two important guidelines. First, one must not stop irradiation after a tumor has completely regressed. In head and neck carcinomas and modest-sized adenocarcinomas of the breast, if the tumor has regressed completely during external irradiation that encompasses a wide area around the tumor, a boost must be given. Table 4 is a mathematical model showing that in a tumor with 10^7 clonogens, although the subclinical level is reached with at most 10^5 clonogens, it requires at least $5D_0$ (eff) to bring to a low probability the survival of one clonogen.

Second, the lack of disappearance of tumor at the completion of treatment does not mean that the patient will not be cured. In large breast cancers, some soft tissue sarcomas, chondrosarcomas, and sometimes in nodular sclerosing Hodgkin's disease, large residual masses may be devoid of surviving malignant clonogens; the slow regression may merely reflect the rate at which the mass resolves. When there is clinically residual disease at the completion of treatment, the final total dose is limited by the tolerance of the normal tissues. Prohibitively high and severe complications must be avoided. Unnecessary biopsies of slowly regressing tumors may lead to subsequent necrosis and should be discouraged.

Summary

A sweeping generalization concerning the relationship of regression rate and clinical status at the end of treatment to ultimate outcome is unrealistic for different clinical contexts and is not useful in treatment planning. Valid conclusions can be:

TABLE 4. Number of Cells Killed with Successive Equal Dose Fractions Where Each Fraction Reduces Survival to 10%[a,b]

Number of Dose Fractions	Accumulated Dose (rad)[a]	No. of Viable Cells Irradiated	No. of Cells Killed	No. of Cells Surviving
1	500	100,000,000	90,000,000	10,000,000
2	1000	10,000,000	9,000,000	1,000,000
3	1500	1,000,000	900,000	100,000
4	2000	100,000	90,000	10,000
5	2500	10,000	9,000	1,000
6	3000	1,000	900	100
7	3500	100	90	10
8	4000	10	9	1

[a] It is assumed for this example that each dose fraction of 500 rad reduces cell survival to 10% (it is not a recommended treatment regimen).

[b] From Fletcher, G.H., 1980.

1. A fast regression of a tumor carries a good prognosis but must not be a reason to diminish the total dose within tolerance.
2. Clinical residual disease at the end of treatment is not a certain indicator of the presence of viable tumor cells and does not mean that the lesion will not be controlled.

ACKNOWLEDGEMENT

This investigation was supported in part by Grants CA06294 and CA05654 from the National Cancer Institute, Department of Health, Education and Welfare, U.S.A.

REFERENCES

1. Barkley, H.T., Jr., and Fletcher, G.H.: The significance of residual disease after external irradiation of squamous cell carcinoma of the oropharynx. *Radiology* **124**:493–495, 1977.
2. Calle, R., Fletcher, G.H., and Pierquin, B.: Les bases de la radiotherapie curative des epitheliomas mammaires. *J Radiol Electrol Med Nucl* **54**:929–938, 1973.
3. Castro, J.R., Issa, P., and Fletcher, G.H.: Carcinoma of the cervix treated by external irradiation alone. *Radiology* **95**:163–166, 1970.
4. Cox, J.D., and Stoffel, T.J.: The significance of needle biopsy after irradiation for stage C adenocarcinoma of the prostate. *Cancer* **40**:156–160, 1977.
5. Fletcher, G.H.: *Textbook of Radiotherapy* 2nd ed. Philadelphia: Lea & Febiger, 1973, p. 713.
6. Fletcher, G.H.: *Textbook of Radiotherapy* 3rd ed. Philadelphia: Lea & Febiger, 1980.
7. Fletcher, G.H., Suit, H.D., Howe, C.D., Samuels, M., Jesse, R.H., Jr., and Villareal, R.U.: Clinical method of testing radiation sensitizing agents in the squamous cell carcinomas. *Cancer* **16**:355–362, 1963.
8. Fletcher, G.H., Suit, H.D., Lindberg, R.D., Howe, C.D., Samuels, M.L., and Smith, J.P.: Chemotherapy as an adjuvant to surgery and radiation therapy. In *UICC Monograph Series* vol. 10, 9th International Congress. Berlin: Springer-Verlag, 1967, pp. 177–184.
9. Fletcher, G.H., Withers, H.R., and Peters, L.J.: Boost in radiotherapy: Rationale and technique. In *Proceedings of a Symposium on Electron Beam Therapy* Florence C.H. Chu and John S. Laughlin, eds., Memorial Sloan-Kettering Cancer Center, New York, 1981, pp. 107–112.
10. Marcial, V.A., and Bosch, A.: Radiation-induced tumor regression in carcinoma of the uterine cervix: Prognostic significance. *AJR* **108**:113–123, 1970.
11. Schukovsky, L.J., and Fletcher, G.H.: Time-dose and tumor volume relationships in the irradiation of squamous cell carcinoma of the tonsillar fossa. *Radiology* **107**:621–626, 1973.
12. Spanos, W.J., Jr., Schukovsky, L.J., and Fletcher, G.H.: Time, dose and tumor volume relationships in irradiation of squamous cell carcinomas of the base of the tongue. *Cancer* **37**:2591–2599, 1976.
13. Suit, H., Lindberg, R., and Fletcher, G.H.: Prognostic significance of extent of tumor regression at completion of radiation therapy. *Radiology* **84**:1100–1107, 1965.
14. Thames, H.D., Jr., Peters, L.J., Spanos, W., and Fletcher, G.H.: Dose response of squamous cell carcinomas of the upper respiratory and digestive tracts. *Br J Cancer* **41**:25–38, 1980.
15. Withers, H.R., and Peters, L.J.: Biologic aspects of radiation therapy. In Fletcher GH: *Textbook of Radiotherapy* 3rd ed., Philadelphia: Lea & Febiger, 1980, pp. 103–180.

CHAPTER 20

Contribution of the Discussion Initiator

Stanley B. Field, B.Sc., Ph.D.[a]

The preceding papers have all addressed the question: Which factors may be useful in predicting tumor radiosensitivity?

There are three separate periods when a prognosis may be made, i.e., before, during, or after treatment. The prognosis underlies decisions as to further treatment and can also help in early assessment of clinical trials. The following information is available to the therapist:

1. Tumor site and staging
2. Tumor size, giving regression or regrowth rate
3. Histology
    a. Histological type
    b. Grading
    c. Extension

There was general agreement that larger tumors, especially if endophytic, carry a worse prognosis than smaller or exophytic lesions, even if the histologies are similar. As an example, Dr. Fletcher compared the resistance of lesions of the postpharyngeal wall (endophytic) with the more sensitive tumors of the tonsillar fossa (exophytic). Also, Dr. Nervi pointed out that, in his experience with tumors of the head and neck, reduction in tumor bulk by chemotherapy did not render the tumors more sensitive to radiotherapy. There was some discussion on this point and general agreement with Dr. Nervi's findings.

[a]Head, Department of Biology, Medical Research Council, Cyclotron Unit, Hammersmith Hospital, London, England

Drs. Fletcher and Arcangeli indicated that rapid regression during therapy points to a good prognosis, especially for carcinoma of the cervix. This was supported in the discussion by Dr. Dische. Perhaps the finding is the result of differences in hypoxia and extent of reoxygenation as suggested by Dr. Denekamp on the basis of animal experiments. Dr. Fletcher discussed the difference between regression during treatment either leading to greater tumor sensitivity or providing the means for an improved treatment plan. With other tumors, e.g., bronchogenic or esophageal carcinomata, the correlation between regression and sterilization is poor. Dr. Fletcher also showed no correlation between tumor status at the end of treatment and the final outcome for tumors of the esophagus. However, in a recent examination of lesions of the tonsillar fossa using improved and rigid criteria for tumor detection, such a correlation was found. Perhaps the new imaging technology could help here, and careful tumor measurement might lead to useful information on a variety of lesions. Certainly it was felt that the absence of detectable tumor mass was *not* an indication to stop before the prescribed end of treatment. An important point made by Dr. Fletcher was that we cannot make broad generalizations: each tumor type must be considered separately. Dr. Arcangeli, following a method devised by Holsti and Elkind, showed that the rate of regression after a single dose of 8 to 10 Gy was a useful indicator of the response to subsequent conventional radiotherapy. This raises the question of how general such an approach could be made. The longer the wait after treatment before making an assessment, the more accurate the assessment is expected to be. A late determination would still be useful if another form of treatment, such as hyperthermia, were envisaged.

Dr. Nervi considered the possible role of a range of kinetic parameters, including tumor growth rate, generation time, growth fraction, cell loss, and DNA content. Even with the use of flow cytometry he felt that no useful correlations were yet possible. There was general agreement on this point.

Dr. Trott pointed out that only 1% or less of tumor cells survive the first one third of treatment. One may well ask how histology can possibly help radiotherapy during or after treatment. Even so, histological changes in squamous cell carcinoma, especially cervical tumors, do appear to correlate with the final result, although this is not in routine clinical usage. Can electron microscopy or cytochemistry be of additional value?

Various other potentially important prognostic factors have been discussed recently, e.g., low hemoglobin levels can lead to tumor hypoxia and radioresistance as proved by Dr. Bush and his colleagues. Additional useful information may be obtained from the use of improved methods in tumor localization and measurement, serum levels of tumor markers, and kinetic parameters. It is also important to take note of tumor heterogeneity since failure is due to the most resistant components.

At a more mechanistic level it is established that D_o and D_q and other important radiobiological parameters vary with cell type and radiation conditions. Methods to derive these parameters in clinical practice include volume measurements together with mathematical models and may employ the techniques of tumor regrowth or growth of tumors as xenografts or in culture. Many questions have yet to be asked and answered concerning these techniques, and new and better methods need to be devised.

CHAPTER 21

Keynote Address: Normal Tissue Radioresistance in Clinical Radiotherapy

H. Rodney Withers, M.D., Ph.D.[a]
H.D. Thames, Ph.D.[b]
L.J. Peters, M.D.[c]
G.H. Fletcher, M.D.[c]

During the past 25 years there has been an impressive increase in our understanding of the biology of radiotherapy. Relationships between dose and cell killing; the role of repair mechanisms in single and multifraction treatments using high and low LET radiations; the influence on tumor responses of oxygen, hypoxic-cell sensitizers, and reoxygenation; effects of division-cycle-related variations in radiosensitivity and tissue kinetics on radiation responses; and the interaction of radiation with drugs or hyperthermia are some of the more obvious areas in which there have been great strides.

There remain, however, many phenomena of which we are relatively ignorant. Consider, for example, one normal tissue—the alimentary tract. We do not understand the acute swelling and dysfunction in salivary glands after relatively low doses of radiation, and why irradiation of the abdomen causes vomiting, why bowel obstruction is more likely in bowel bound by adhesions, or the reason for the edema of bowel wall long after completion of radiotherapy. We do not understand the acute transudation through capillary walls after irradiation nor the decrease in interstitial pressure during irradiation. These are some examples of the many phenomena which we do not understand and which may not necessarily have a basis in cell killing.

Two other unresolved problems are of particular importance to the radiotherapist: the increase in normal tissue injury with increase in volume irradiated and the pathobiology and radiobiology of late effects of radiation. The pathobiology of the volume effect remains shrouded in mystery and will not be further discussed here. We will direct our attention to other aspects of the late responses of normal tissues.

Pathobiology of Late Effects

The belief that "late" effects of radiation result from vascular injury is so old that its origin is obscure. Several observations must have made it seem a reasonable premise: erythema develops early, suggesting that blood vessels are "radiosensitive"; and in old radiation fields, surface telangiectasis is often obvious. Histologically, small arteries in heavily irradiated tissues are degenerate, and the intimal thickening is sometimes sufficient to completely occlude the lumen. In experimental animal systems a wide variety of anatomical and functional changes has been observed in irradiated blood ves-

[a]Department of Radiation Oncology, University of California, Los Angeles, Calif., Center for Health Sciences, Los Angeles, Calif. 90024
[b]Department of Biomathematics, University of Texas, M.D. Anderson Hospital, Houston, Texas 77030
[c]Division of Radiotherapy, University of Texas, M.D. Anderson Hospital, Houston, Texas 77030

sels.[10,11,20,24,29,31,32,38,41,42,45–47,51,52,59,66] However, it has never been established that these vascular changes actually *cause* late effects, and on the basis of known radiobiology, it is now more reasonable to assume that they do not, and that vascular damage is merely one form of late injury which commonly coexists with the other changes resulting from slow depletion of parenchymal and/or stromal cells after radiation.[60,72,75]

Radiation-induced cell death is generally the result of interference with the reproductive integrity of the cell,[30] and hence is expressed only if the cell attempts division—and even then not necessarily in the first division cycle after irradiation.[57] Therefore, the rate at which radiation injury becomes manifest is a reflection of the turnover kinetics of the target cells of the tissue, responses appearing quickly in rapidly turning-over tissues and slowly in cell populations that turn over slowly. It is most reasonable, therefore, to regard acute and late effects to be analogous in having as their pathobiological basis the depletion of parenchymal or supporting cells, and different only in the rate at which the target cells express radiation lethality.[60,72,76]

If it is depletion of parenchymal or stromal cells, not injury to the vasculature, that leads to acute and late tissue injury, which cells are critical to the "survival" of various organs? There are sufficient data on which to make reasonable assumptions regarding the target cells for most slowly developing injuries. This is a broad subject, and only four examples will be discussed here to illustrate the logical appeal of the concept. It has been discussed in other publications.[40,60,72,76]

NERVOUS SYSTEM

In the brain, spinal cord, and peripheral nerves, the predominant radiopathological effect is demyelination. Unmyelinated neurones centrally and in the autonomic system are not affected at clinical dose levels. These observations imply that oligodendrocytes centrally[36,75] and Schwann cells in peripheral nerves (which are the cells responsible for myelination and also undergo slow turnover), are the primary target cells whose slow depletion leads to characteristic functional and structural changes.[12,62,75]

PITUITARY

Damage to the pituitary becomes apparent slowly (over years) after its incidental irradiation during radiotherapy, but is limited to those functions related to the anterior lobe.[48] This suggests that the critical cells are the secretory cells of the anterior pituitary because, if the essential lesion was damage to blood vessels, both lobes of the gland should be affected. It is interesting to note also that the nerve supply from the hypothalamus to both lobes is unmyelinated, and therefore, unresponsive to radiation.

KIDNEY

Histologically, it is possible, after doses within a certain range, to see focal regeneration of complete renal tubules, and it is reasonable to assume that these are clonally derived and that the target for radiation nephritis is the epithelium of the renal tubule, or some subpopulation thereof. If one cell or more survives, the whole tubule will repopulate and the nephron will survive. Arterial and glomerular changes are minor at a time when tubule damage is extensive, and the arteriolar changes, if they develop, appear later and in kidneys in which tubule depletion is permanent.

The concept of renal tolerance being determined by the renal tubule cell explains why the function of the organ is easily compromised by radiation. Rather than considering the kidney to be a large number of cells capable of restoring renal function, it should be regarded as consisting of a large number of independent entities (tubules), each consisting of as few as perhaps 10^3 epithelial cells. If each tubule contains so few cells, and if tubules survive independently with no capacity to repopulate one another, reducing cell survival to 10^{-4} would leave only about 10% of the tubules capable of reconstructing themselves. Thus, relatively little cellular depletion is necessary to destroy renal function because of the compartmentalization of the target cells and their subsequent limited capacity for reconstruction through repopulation.

CONNECTIVE TISSUES

The atrophy and thickening of the collagen in the dermis, for example, can be easily understood in terms of depletion of fibroblasts with consequent lack of turnover of collagen, that which remains becoming cross-linked, thickened, and degenerate. Lack of fibroblasts also explains the lack of contraction and the slow healing of necrotic ulcers because it is the transformation of fibroblasts to myofibroblasts which is necessary for wound contraction.

Comparison of Acute and Late Responses

KINETICS OF DEVELOPMENT OF INJURY

The division of radiation effects into early and late is arbitrary. There is a vague zone of separation between them, most acute effects having subsided by 1–2 months after the end of a 6-week course of radiation and most late effects becoming apparent after that. Within each generic group there is a spectrum of rates of development of measurable responses, especially within the late-effects group. Not only is the rate of expression of late injury more variable between the various slowly proliferating tissues, but also for a given "late-effects" tissue there is a wider spread in the distribution of times to appearance of the effect, which is consistent with the random distribution of target-cell-division cycle times.

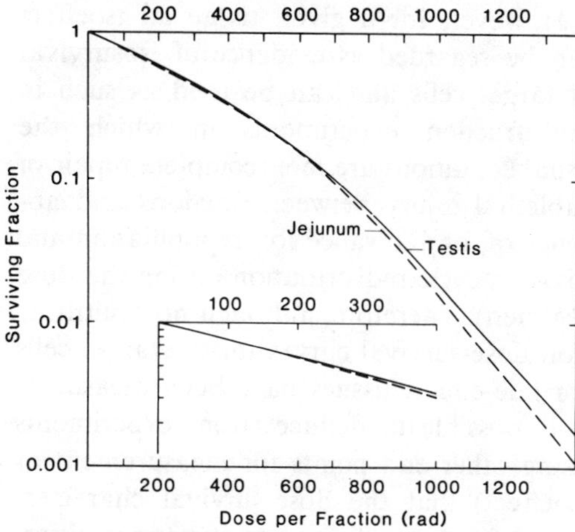

Figure 1. Single-dose survival curves for jejunal crypt cells and the stem cells of the spermatogenic epithelium, derived from multifraction experiments on the assumption of equal effect per fraction[55] Although these tissues show very different responses to radiation, the dose-survival characteristics of the stem cells are almost identical.

THE RELATIONSHIP OF CELLULAR RADIOSENSITIVITY TO TISSUE RESPONSE

Differences in the severity of injury in various organs exposed to the same dose of radiation may result from true differences in cellular radiosensitivity or may merely reflect differences in the expression of injury by cells of similar radiosensitivity. Recently, it has become apparent that the radiosensitivity of the stem cells of jejunal crypts and spermatogenic epithelium are indistinguishably different from one another (see Fig. 1), despite the remarkable differences in the kinetics of their responses.[54,56] Thus, within 10 to 14 days after a 1000-rad single dose, the jejunal mucosa of the mouse has returned to normal while the testis is still losing weight, and the sperm count will remain severely depressed for months and may never return to normal during its lifetime.[43] Thus, many factors, such as stem-cell number, division-cycle and amplification-compartment kinetics, cell-loss rate and regeneration capacity, as well as cellular radiosensitivity, enter into the radiation response of a tissue.

However, for a given tissue an isoeffect can be regarded as evidence of isosurvival of target cells and can be used as such in multifraction experiments in which the usual conditions are met (complete repair of sublethal injury between fractions and absence of, or allowance for, repopulation and division-cycle redistribution during the dose regimen). Therefore, although no multifraction dose-survival curves for the target cells for late-effects tissues have been measured, it is possible to deduce (from experiments using other end points for measurement of isoeffect) that the dose-survival characteristics of target cells for late effects are different from those for the target cells of acute responses. The major difference between the responses of rapidly and slowly responding tissues is that injury to slowly responding tissues is more sensitive to the effects of dose fractionation.

CLINICAL AND LABORATORY OBSERVATIONS

It has been noted clinically[1-5,13,25,26,28,39,44,49,50,53,58] and experimentally[6,7,15,18,23,33,35,58,73] that increasing the size of dose per fraction leads to a divergence in the acute and late responses, the late responses becoming relatively more severe. It has also been noted in other studies that for equal acute responses, the late responses to neutrons is more severe than that for x-rays.[37,73] Both of these observations, at first, seem consistent with the target cells for late injury having a greater capacity for repair of sublethal injury than the cells involved in acute responses; but this is not so.

TARGET CELL RADIOSENSITIVITY—EARLY AND LATE RESPONDING TISSUES

A general statement which explains the differences in the fractionated dose responses of early and late reacting tissues is that the ratio, β/α (parameters of the linear-

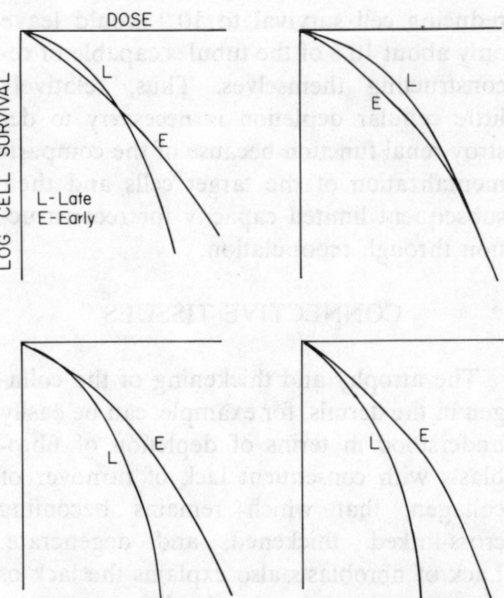

Figure 2. Four examples of dose-survival curves in which the ratio (β/α) of cell killing by accumulated sublethal injury to cell killing by single-hit events is greater for late-responding tissues (L) than for early-responding tissues (E). The derivation, in mathematical terms, of the general significance of the ratio β/α to the relationship between acute and late injury on which the curves are based[55] is summarized in the Appendix.

quadratic dose-survival curve), is greater for late than for acute reactions[55,56] (see also Appendix). In other words, accumulation of sublethal radiation injury plays a greater role in killing the target cells for late effects than it does in killing those for acute effects. Theoretical dose-survival curves illustrating this general statement are shown in Figure 2. (Because we do not know in absolute terms the relative numbers of target cells or the extent to which they must be depleted for the various acute and late effects, it is not possible to select one pair of configurations as being the most appropriate.)

Early and late multifraction radiation responses are modelled in terms of cell survival in Figure 3 using the single dose-survival curves of Figure 2(*a*). The early (*E*) and late (*L*) multifraction curves differ in their relative "effective" slopes, depending upon the size of dose per fraction—the variation being greater for cells of the late-effects tissue. These survival-curve patterns are consistent with the observations of dissociation between acute and late effects with variations in dose-fractionation patterns which involve changes in the size of dose per fraction.

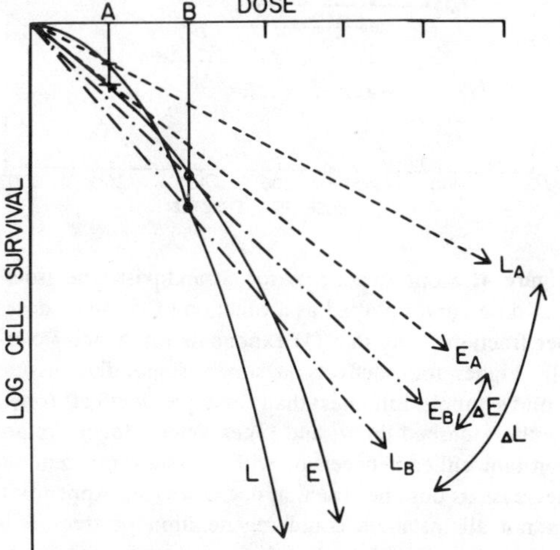

Figure 3. Hypothetical single- (full lines) and fractionated- (dashed lines) dose-survival curves for the target cells of tissues which respond to radiation early (*E*) or late (*L*) Fig. 2*a*). These curves are consistent with experimental data (Figs. 4 to 7) and illustrate a radiobiological basis for the clinical observation that late injury increases more, relative to early response, as the size of dose per fraction increases. For a series of doses of *A* rad, the effective survival curves for the cells whose depletion leads to early and late injury are E_A and L_A, respectively, and for multiple doses of *B* rad, are E_B and L_B. The relative increase in effectiveness of the *B* rad regimen is greater for the cells of the slowly responding tissue (ΔL) than for those of the acutely responding tissue (ΔE). A similar divergence between acute and late responses with increase in size of dose per fraction would be seen if the survival curves for the target cells for acute and late injury were related to one another in the ways shown in the other three panels of Figure 2.

If it is assumed that tumors constitute an acutely responding tissue and that late-responding normal tissues are dose limiting, there is a potential therapeutic gain to be exploited from dose fractionation. To optimize such a therapeutic gain, it is necessary to define the shapes of dose-survival curves (Figs. 2 and 3) more precisely. The two important parameters, from a clinical viewpoint, are the initial slopes of the survival curves and, more importantly, the ranges of dose over which the curves begin bending appreciably from their initial exponential slope. Furthermore, if late effects determine the tolerable total dose, the most important single parameter to be determined is the region of initial flexure of the survival curve for the target cells for late effects, as it is with doses in that region, or below, that the greatest difference between acute and late responses will be achieved in a fractionated dose regimen.[69] This can be appreciated from study of Figures 2 and 3.

Analysis of Experimental Data

To substantiate the claim that the β/α ratio is greater for the killing of the target cells for late- than for early-responding tissues, various experimental data will be compared.

Much of the experimental data on acute and late tissue responses relate to doses too high to be of much clinical interest. Available data on acute and late normal tissue responses to doses ranging up to 600 rad have been analyzed by four different methods (see Fig. 4 to 7 and Table 1) in the hope of identifying directions in which progress may be made in maximizing the therapeutic ratio through dose fractionation. Because evaluable end points of tissue response require large decrements in cell survival and therefore large single doses, the data represented in Figures 4 to 8 are derived from multifraction experiments using doses per fraction that approach the range of clinical interest. In no such experiments can equal effect per fraction be guaranteed because it is impossible to ensure complete repair of sublethal damage, lack of repopulation, and constancy of division-cycle distribution in the target cells surviving previous dose(s). Nevertheless, most of the data analyzed were from experiments planned to allow full repair of sublethal damage between dose fractions with a minimum of perturbation from other phenomena.

TABLE 1. Sources of Data and Involved Organs for Figures 4, 5, 6 and 7

Curve	Tissue	Reference
1	Skin	Douglas[16]
2	Skin	Fowler[27]
3	Skin	Hopewell[32]
4	Spinal Cord	van der Kogel[61]
5	Spinal Cord	White[65]
6	Kidney	Caldwell[9]
7	Colon	Withers[7]
8	Jejunum	Thames[65]
9	Spleen	Withers[68]
10	Lung	Field[21,22]
11	Testis	Thames[56]
12	Kidney	Hopewell[34]
13	Lung	Wara[64]
14	Skin	Withers[73]
16	Spinal Cord	van der Kogel[62]
17	Skin	Berry[67]
18	Skin	Howes[35]
19	Multiple	Withers[68]
20	Skin	Field[23]
21	Skin, Lung	Dutreix[18;19]
22	Gut	Wambersie[63]
23	Oral mucosa	Peters (personal comm.)

LOG-LOG ISOEFFECT CURVE EXPONENTS

Figure 4 shows estimated values for the exponent for fraction number in Strandqvist-type isoeffect-dose curves plotted for ranges of dose per fraction for a variety of rapidly and slowly responding tissues. In general, the exponents for late effects are higher than those for early effects and remain so to lower doses per fraction. This finding is equivalent to a higher β/α ratio for late effects (see Appendix). These data are more of historical than practical quantitative importance[71] but indicate that increasing dose fractionation is more important in reducing late than acute effects, and that this greater sparing continues to the lowest doses tested.

INCREMENTAL DOSE PER FRACTION FOR ISOEFFECT

In Figure 5 data from multifraction isoeffect experiments are plotted by a method[68] based on that of Dutreix et al.[19] The maximum value of D_s at which a curve for ΔD_r reaches zero defines the region of flexure of the single-dose-survival curve. This is of great clinical relevance. In Figure 5 the values for ΔD_r for late effects are higher than those for acute effects at low values of D_s, but no data exist which define the intercept with the abscissa for the curves for late effects. Nevertheless, the plots in Figure 5 suggest that, relative to acute effects, the values for ΔD_r for late effects would reach zero at lower values of D_s, and hence that the single-dose-survival curve for the target cells for late injury may be presumed to diverge from exponential (or near exponential) at lower doses than the curves for cells of acutely responding tissues. This is consistent with the comparative survival curves presented in Figures 2 and 3 and with the

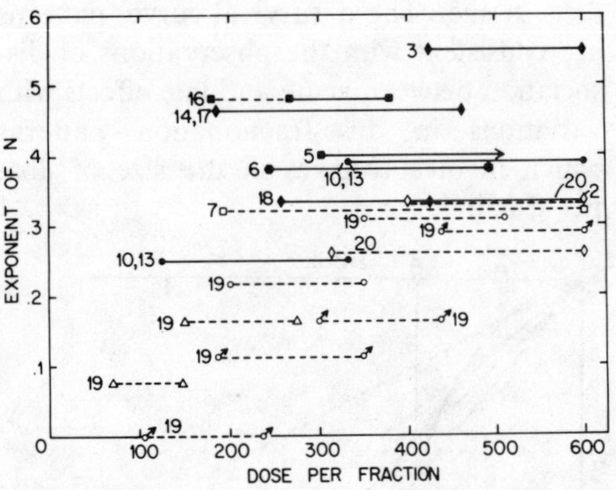

Figure 4. Slope exponents for Strandqvist-type isoeffect-dose curves plotted as a function of range of doses per fraction. Note that (1) exponents for N are generally higher for isoeffects in slowly responding tissues (solid symbols, full lines) than for acute isoeffects (open symbols, dashed lines); and (2) exponents for N are not constant either between or within tissues and tend to decrease as dose per fraction decreases (see Appendix). In not all instances could regeneration of stem cells during the experimental multifraction regimens be excluded—this would be most likely to occur in acutely responding tissues and would raise the value for the exponent. Such repopulation occurring more in the acutely responding than late-responding tissues, especially when large numbers of small dose fractions were used, would tend to minimize the difference between the fractionation reponses of the acutely and slowly responding tissues. For sources of data see Table 1.

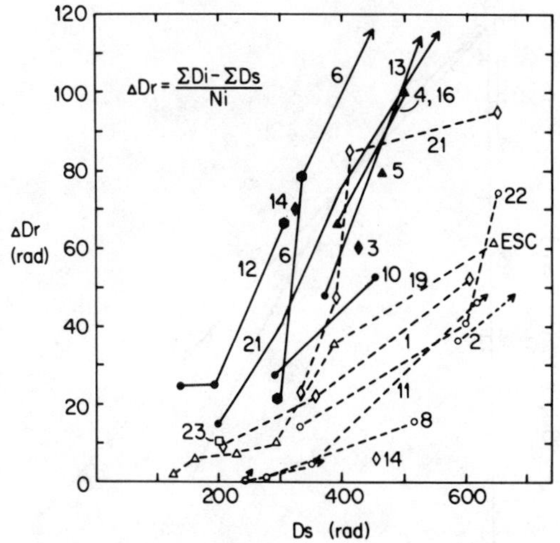

Figure 5. ΔD_r plotted as a function of D_s, where ΔD_r is the incremental dose per fraction required for an isoeffect when N_i fractions, each of D_i, replace a regimen of fewer $N_s s$ doses, each of D_s. For example, if a regimen of 25 × D_s were to be replaced by a regimen of 30 fractions, the new fractional dose would be (25/30 × D_s + ΔD_r). Comparisons based on this modification of a D_r plot[19] are meaningful only when ΔD_r values for a given D_s were derived from the same change in fractionation pattern (i.e., the same ratio of N_i/N_s). Although this was not always the case, differences in N_i/N_s ratio, where they existed, were small enough that the general patterns of curve positions and shapes are valid even though the ΔD_r values at given D_s values are not always precisely comparable in different tissues.

At least between doses of 200 and 600 rad, dose fractionation leads to more sparing (i.e., a greater incremental dose for an isoeffect) in tissues which respond slowly to radiation (solid symbols, solid lines) than in those which show an early response (open symbols, dashed lines). The value of D_s at which ΔD_r is not detectably different from zero is the dose at which the single-dose-survival curve begins to diverge measureably from its initial exponential slope: The data suggest that this occurs at lower doses in tissues developing late responses than in those responding early. The intercepts of the curve with the D_s abscissa would be shifted to the left, to lower doses, if more repopulation occurred during regimens using multiple small fractions than in those using fewer large fractions.

At low doses, e.g., 0–300 rad, the values for ΔD_r, especially those for early responses, approach, or may be, zero, but none of the data is sufficiently accurate or precise to differentiate between two-component or linear-quadratic survival curve models. (For sources of data see Table 1.)

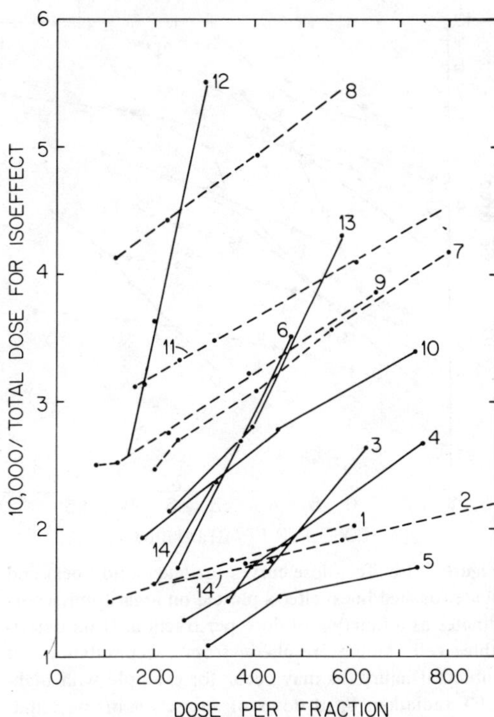

Figure 6. Inverse of total isoeffect dose as a function of dose per fraction—an F_e plot of the Douglas and Fowler type. Full lines are for data from slowly responding tissues, dashed lines from acutely responding tissues. Since the total doses for the various isoeffects range up to > 9000 rad, the ordinate is scaled, for convenience, as 10,000/total dose except in the case of line 9, for endogenous spleen colonies, where the ordinate represents 2500/total dose. Note that the curves for late effects are steeper and their intercepts lower than for acute effects; this is consistent with the fact that the β/α ratios in a linear-quadratic model for the single-dose-survival curves are higher for late than for acute effects. Although highly suggestive of it, these data do not prove conclusively a higher β for the survival curve for the target cells for late injury because the isoeffects for various tissues do not represent identical decrements in target-cell survival. Nevertheless, with so many tissues represented in the figure, it is likely that the numbers of target cells in the two general types of tissue are in some cases roughly equal. (For sources of data see Table 1.)

higher β/α ratio for late effects (see Appendix).

The practical implication of curves of the type shown in Figure 5 may also be appreciated by reference to Figure 3. Assuming once again that tumors are a typical early-responding tissue, the therapeutic ratio would vary at doses between the zero-dose intercepts of the ΔD_r curves for early and late responding tissues since these would represent the regions of flexure in the single-dose-survival curves for the target cells of

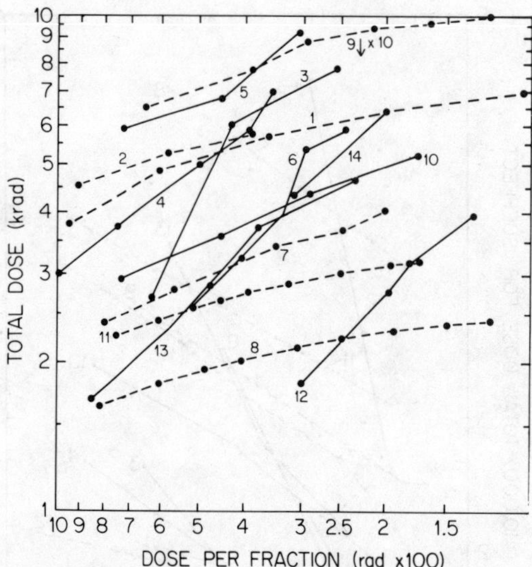

Figure 7. Isoeffect-dose curves for late (solid lines) and acute (dashed lines) effects plotted on logarithmic coordinates as a function of dose per fraction. If no detectable cell killing resulted from accumulation of sublethal injury (as may occur for example with high-LET radiation, or at doses of sparsely ionizing radiation low enough that insufficient unrepaired sublethal injury accumulates to cause lethality), the lines would be horizontal. Conversely, the steeper the line over a certain dose range, the greater the potential for reducing cell killing over that dose range by dividing the dose into smaller fractions to allow for repair of sublethal injury. Note that (1) the curves for late effects rise more steeply than those for acute effects over a wide dose range and especially between 600 and 200 rad (there being few data below 200 rad); and (2) if regeneration were to occur during the course of the fractionated dose regimen, it would cause the curves to rise more steeply as the dose/fraction decreased (and therefore number of fractions and overall treatment duration increased). Regeneration was not excluded in all experiments, but would affect the response of acutely reacting tissues more than slowly responding tissues to reduce the difference between the slopes of the two different sets of curves.

The sources of data are given in Table 1. The curves 8 and 11 represent data taken from single-dose-survival curves generated from multifraction experimental data using a linear quadratic model. Curve 9 is displaced upward by one decade for convenience of presentation. A conclusion from the steeper slopes for late effects is that the β/α ratio is greater for the target cells for late effects (see Appendix). The same conclusion is reached from analysis of the F_e plot (Fig. 6) for reasons explained in the Appendix.

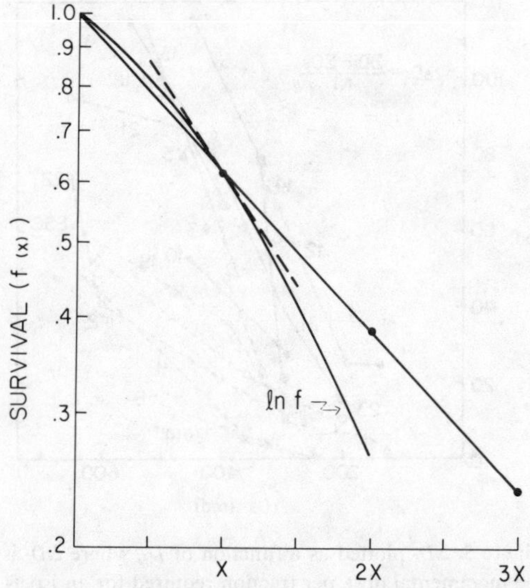

Figure 8. The steepness of the response to the single dose *x*—i.e., the slope of the tangent to the dose-survival curve (dashed line), *dlnf/dx*—is always greater than the steepness of the multifraction response to repeated doses of the same size—i.e., (*lnf*)/*x* (solid line). The ratio of (*lnf*)/*x* to *dlnf/dx*, when subtracted from 1, gives the number -of-fractions exponent of the Strandqvist-type plot. That exponents are always greater for late responses implies that the ratio of these slopes is always greater for late responses, independently of choice of survival model. Equality occurs when killing is predominantly single-hit, on the initial linear segment, of the dose-survival curve.

tumors (acute responses) and for late effects, respectively. The therapeutic ratio would increase as dose per fraction was reduced and would be maximal when doses per fraction were equal to, or less than, the intercept with the abscissa of the ΔD_r curve for late effects.[69]

F_e PLOTS

In Figure 6 isoeffect doses for acute and late injuries are plotted (as their inverse) as a function of dose per fraction in the manner proposed for acute skin reactions by Douglas and Fowler.[17] The ratio of the slope of the line to its intercept at zero dose is independent of level of effect and equals the ratio β/α of linear-quadratic survival model parameters. The curves for late effects are steeper and their extrapolated intercepts lower than for acute effects so that the β/α ratio is greater for late than for acute effects. As shown in the Appendix, this conclusion is equivalent to that reached from other isoeffect representations[55] and is consistent with the more rapid increase in severity of late injuries with increase in size of dose per fraction noted clinically.

Because the levels of cell survival corresponding to the various isoeffects in Figure 6 are not the same, the predicted intercepts and slopes of these F_e curves cannot be correlated with one another in a significant way. Nevertheless, among the many tissues represented it is not unlikely that some target-cell numbers are roughly equal and thus that the apparently larger slopes (β) for late effects have some significance.

ISOEFFECT VS. DOSE PER FRACTION

Isoeffect doses from multifraction experiments for various end points are presented as a function of dose per fraction on logarithmic coordinates in Figure 7. Since fraction number, as used in present-day Strandqvist-type curves, is not a good index of dose per fraction when different isoeffects are considered, and since dose per fraction is the important variable, this new type of plot (Fig. 7) is more "correct," and in this respect resembles F_e plots. The curves for late effects are steeper than those for acute effects showing in a quantitative manner the greater degree of sparing which occurs in slowly responding tissues when doses per fraction are reduced. Again, the steeper slope for late effects implies a larger β/α ratio for late-effect target cells (see Appendix). As also illustrated by earlier figures, the fractionation response, especially for late effects, is not well quantified at low doses. Also, if regeneration occurred during the course of multifraction experiments, it is likely to have affected the acutely responding tissues more than those responding slowly, and this would raise the total dose for large numbers of small doses, reducing the difference between acute- and late-effects curves. Thus, the real differences are not less than those observed.

Conclusions

Late effects of radiation injury in normal tissues are most likely the result of division-cycle-related death of slowly dividing parenchymal and/or stromal cells. This concept simplifies the understanding of dose-response relationships and suggests directions for research in reducing late effects.

If late injury in normal tissues is not the result of vascular injury, but of death of slowly proliferating cells, slow regeneration of survivors is possible. In view of this, long-established policies regarding retreatment of previously irradiated areas may deserve review. Consider as a model the response of the kidney proposed earlier. If the dose from a first course of treatment were low enough that no nephrons were eliminated, slow regeneration of the tubular epithelium would restore the organ to normal, and retreatment at some later time with the same dose may be possible. Since the loss of nephrons would be expected to follow a typical sigmoid relationship with dose, there would be a threshold dose below which no nephrons were lost followed by a relatively narrow dose range over which there would be a rapid destruction of the organ. Therefore, the potential for retreatment would be essentially independent of dose below a certain threshold but above that threshold would be sharply dose dependent. Also, if the time between treatment courses were shortened, the extent of regeneration would be limited and the tolerance of the organ, even if relatively low doses had been given, would be reduced in an interval-dependent manner. Similarly, skin after low doses may, with time, restore itself to complete normality with respect to radiation tolerance, whereas after higher doses such restoration may never occur because of the excessive depletion of target cells (fibroblasts) by the first course. It seems reasonable to extrapolate these considerations to other slowly responding tissues and to encourage further investigation of the phenomenon of "remembered" dose.[8,14]

Multifraction dose-responses in human and experimental animal tissues show that the "target" cells in early- and late-responding tissues differ in their dose-survival relationships, the ratio β/α of linear-quadratic model parameters being greater for the slowly proliferating cells of which the slowly responding tissues are comprised.[55] The differences between the dose-fractionation effects in acute- and late-responding tissues is not readily explained in terms of differences in repair of potentially lethal damage but may be determined by division-cycle-related variations in radiosensitivity—most target cells in slowly responding tissues being, presumably, in early G_1.

If tumor cells respond like the cells of rapidly proliferating normal tissues, and slowly responding normal tissues determine the total doses that may be given in radiotherapy, then the therapeutic ratio will vary with the size of dose per fraction. If the effects of proliferation of clonogenic tumor cells are ignored, the optimum dose per fraction would be any dose within the initial exponential region of the dose-survival curve for the target cells for late effects.[69] If the survival curve for slowly responding cells were continuously bending (as predicted by a linear-quadratic survival-curve formula), the optimum dose per fraction would be vanishingly small, but for practical purposes would be within the range at which it is impossible to detect deviation from linearity in the low-dose region. These considerations have obvious implications for hyperfractionation.

While the optimum dose per fraction may be predictable from the shapes of dose-survival curves, other factors, such as regeneration, division-cycle redistribution, and in the case of the tumors, reoxygenation, need to be considered; but these affect primarily the selection of an optimal rate at which dose fractions should be repeated. Also, of course, the practical logistics of treatment enter into the definition of optimal rate.

Summary

It is more logical to view the late structural and functional effects of radiation as the result of direct parenchymal depletion than as changes secondary to vascular damage. The dose-survival characteristics of the "target" cells in late-effects tissues are different from those for the "target" cells in acutely responding tissues. (The accumulation of sublethal injury with increasing dose assumes more importance in the killing of the target cells for late effects than it does in the stem cells of acutely responding tissues.) Thus, the "sparing" effect of dose fractionation is greater for late than for acute effects, suggesting that hyperfractionation may increase the therapeutic ratio by sparing late-effects tissues relative to acutely responding tumors.

ACKNOWLEDGMENTS

We are grateful to Dr. John Hopewell who kindly provided recent additional unpublished data on pig kidney responses to multiple doses of radiation. This work was supported by U.S.P.H.S. Grants Ca 11138 (now 29644), Ca 6294, Ca 29026, and Ca 11430 awarded by the National Cancer Institute.

Appendix

Let f(x) denote the surviving fraction of target cells after single dose x. Thus, the dose-survival curve is ln f(x), and effect E is related to total dose D = Nx given in N fractions by

$$E = -N\, lnf(x) \qquad \text{(A1)}$$

Early and late effects E are illustrated schematically in Figure 3.

LOG-LOG ISOEFFECT CURVES

By differentiating (A1) implicitly with respect to N, and recalling that x = D/N and E is held constant, we find

$$d\,E/dN = 0 = -lnf - N\,(d\,lnf/dx)\,(d\,(D/N)/(dN))$$
$$= -lnf - N\,(d\,lnf/dx)\,(N^{-1}\,dD/dN - N^{-2}D).$$

We multiply by N/D and compute

$$(lnf)/x + (d\,lnf/dx)\,(d\,ln\,D/d\,ln\,N - 1) = 0$$

whence the slope of the isoeffect plot is

$$dln\,D/d\,ln\,N = 1 - \left(\frac{lnf}{x}\right)\Big/\left(\frac{d\,ln\,f}{dx}\right). \qquad \text{(A2)}$$

For example, for the linear-quadratic model we find

$$dlnD/dlnN = \beta x/(\alpha + 2\beta x). \qquad \text{(A3)}$$

Thus, the consequence of larger isoeffect slopes for late effects is

$$(\beta/\alpha)_L\ (1 + 2\,(\beta/\alpha)_E x) > (\beta/\alpha)_E\ (1 + 2\,(\beta/\alpha)_L x)$$

which is equivalent to

$$(\beta/\alpha)_L > (\beta/\alpha)_E. \qquad \text{(A4)}$$

Finally, by comparing (A2) and Figure 8, we see that

slope of isoeffect plot

= 1 − (slope of response to fractionated doses x/ slope of response to single dose x). (A5)

INCREMENTAL DOSE PER FRACTION FOR ISOEFFECT (δD_r)

Clearly δD_r goes to zero as the ratio of slopes of responses to fractionated and acute doses goes to 1 (see Fig. 5 and (A5)), and increases as this ratio increases. That is, δD_r increases as the β/α increases (see (A4)).

F_e PLOTS

By manipulation of (A1) we find

$$1/D = lnf(x)/Ex.$$

which, when differentiated with respect to x, gives

$$\frac{d}{dx}\left(\frac{1}{D}\right) = \frac{1}{Ex}\left[\frac{lnf}{x} - \frac{dlnf}{dx}\right].$$

For the intercept we find by l'Hôpital's rule

$$\lim_{x\to 0}\left(\frac{1}{D}\right) = -\frac{dlnf}{dx}\Bigg|_{x=0} /E$$

Therefore, the ratio of slope to intercept in the F_e plot is

$$\text{slope/intercept} = x^{-1}\left[1 - \left(\frac{lnf}{x}\right)\Big/\left(\frac{dlnf}{dx}\right)\right]$$
$$\left(\frac{dlnf}{dx}\right)\Big/\left(\frac{dlnf}{dx}\right)_{x=0}. \qquad \text{(A6)}$$

For the linear-quadratic model it may be verified that slope/intercept = β/α. Thus, the slope-intercept ratio contains the slope of the isoeffect plot (A2) as a factor.

ISOEFFECT DOSE VS. DOSE PER FRACTION

For the isoeffect plot of Figure 7, we differentiate the relationship D = -Ex/lnf(x) to find

$$\frac{dlnD}{dlnx} = 1 - \left(\frac{dlnf}{dx}\right)\Big/\left(\frac{lnf}{x}\right),$$

or in terms of the reversed direction of the abscissa in Figure 7

$$\frac{dlnD}{d(-ln\,x)} = \left(\frac{dlnf}{dx}\right)\Big/\left(\frac{lnf}{x}\right) - 1. \qquad \text{(A7)}$$

In each of the relations equations (A2), (A6), and (A7), the crucial variable is the ratio of slopes of responses to fractionated and acute doses, as pictured in Figure 8.

REFERENCES

1. Andrews, J.R.: Dose time relationships in cancer radiotherapy. A clinical radiobiology study of extremes of dose and time. *AJR* **93**:56–74, 1965.
2. Arcangeli, G., Friedman, M., and Paoluzi, R.: A quantitative study of late radiation effect on normal skin and subcutaneous tissues in human beings. *Br J Radiol* **47**:44–50, 1974.
3. Atkins, H.L.: Massive single dose weekly fractionation technique in treatment of head and neck cancer. *AJR* **91**:50–60, 1964; Massive dose technique in radiation therapy of inoperable carcinoma of the breast. *AJR* **91**:80–89, 1964.
4. Bates, T.D., and Peters, L.J.: Dangers of the clinical use of the NSD formula for small fraction numbers. *Br J Radiol* **48**:773, 1975.
5. Bennett, M.R.: The treatment of Stage III squamous carcinoma of the cervix in air and hyperbaric oxygen. *Br J Radiol* **51**:68, 1978.
6. Berry, R.J., Wiernik, G., and Patterson, T.J.S.: Skin tolerance to fractionated X-irradiation in the pig—how good a predictor is the NSD formula? *Br J Radiol* **47**:185–190, 1974.
7. Berry, R.J., Wiernik, G., Patterson, T.J.S., and Hopewell, J.W.: Excess late subcutaneous fibrosis after irradiation of pigskin consequent upon the application of the NSD formula. *Br J Radiol* **47**:277–281, 1974.
8. Brown, J.M., and Probert, J.C.: Early and late radiation change following a second course of irradiation. *Radiology* **115**:711–716, 1975.
9. Caldwell, W.L.: Time-dose factors in fatal post-irradiation nephritis. In *Cell Survival After Low Doses of Radiation,* T. Alper, ed. Bristol, J. Wiley, 1975, pp. 328–332.
10. Casarett, G.W.: Similarities and contrasts between radiation and time pathology. In *Advances in Gerontological Research*. B. Strehler ed.,New York: Academic Press, 1964, pp. 109–163.
11. Casarett, G.W.: Aging. In *Radiation Effect and Tolerance of Normal Tissues (Basic Concepts in Radiation Pathology)* Frontiers of Radiation Therapy and Oncology, vol. 6, J. Vaeth, ed. New York: S. Karger, 1972, pp. 479–485.
12. Cheng, V.S.T., and Schulz, M.D.: Unilateral hypoglossal nerve atrophy as a late complication of radiation therapy of head and neck carcinoma: A report of four cases and a review of the literature and peripheral and cranial nerve damages after radiation therapy. *Cancer* **35**:1537–1544, 1975.
13. Chu, F.C.H., Glicksman, A.S., and Nickson, J.J.: Late consequences of early skin reactions. *Radiology* **94**:669–672, 1970.
14. Denekamp, J.: Residual radiation damage in mouse skin 5 to 8 months after irradiation. *Radiology* **115**:191–195, 1975.
15. Denekamp, J.: Early and late reactions in mouse feet. *Br J Cancer* **36**:322–329, 1977.
16. Douglas, B.G.: The response of mouse skin to multiple small doses of radiation. In *Cell Survival After Low Doses of Radiation*, T. Alper, ed. Bristol, J. Wiley, 1975, pp. 342–350.
17. Douglas, B.G., and Fowler, J.F.: The effect of multiple small doses of x-rays on skin reactions in the mouse and a basic interpretation. *Radiat Res* **66**:401–426, 1976.
18. Dutreix, J., and Wambersie, A.: Cell survival curves deduced from non-quantitative reactions of skin, intestinal mucosa and lung. In *Cell Survival After Low Doses of Radiation: Theoretical and Clinical Applications,* T. Alper, ed., Bristol: J. Wiley, 1975, pp. 335–341.
19. Dutreix, J., Wambersie, A., and Bounik, C.: Cellular recovery in human skin reactions: Application to dose fraction number overall time relationship in radiotherapy. *Eur J Cancer* **9**:159–167, 1973.
20. Fajardo, L.F., and Stewart, J.R.: Pathogenesis of radiation-induced myocardial fibrosis. *Lab Invest* **29**:244–257, 1973.
21. Field, S.B., and Hornsey, S.: Repair in normal tissues and the possible relevance to radiotherapy. *Strahlentherapie* **153**:371–379, 1977.
22. Field, S.B., Hornsey, S. and Kutsutani, Y.: Effects of fractionated irradiation on mouse and lung and a phenomenon of slow repair. *Br J Radiol* **49**:700–707, 1976.
23. Field, S.B., Morris, C., Denekamp, J., and Fowler, J.F.: The response of mouse skin to fractionated x-rays. *Eur J Cancer* **11**:291–299, 1975.
24. Fike, J.R., and Gillette, E.L.: ^{60}Co and negative pimeson irradiation of microvasculature. *Int J Radiat Oncol Biol Phys* **4**:825–828, 1978.
25. Fletcher, G.H., Barkley, H.T., and Schukovsky, L.J.: Present status of the time factor in clinical radiotherapy. Part II. The nominal Standard Dose Formula. *J Radiol Electrol* **55**:745–751, 1974.
26. Fletcher, G.H., and Schukovsky, L.J.: The interplay of radiocurability and tolerance in the irradiation of human cancers. *J Radiol Electrol* **56**:383–400, 1975.
27. Fowler, J.F., Denekamp, J., Delapeyre, C., Harris, S.R., and Sheldon, P.W.: Skin reactions in mice after multifraction X-irradiation. *Int J Radiat Biol* **25**:213–223, 1974.
28. Gauwerky, F., and Langheim, F.: Der Zeitfaktor bei der strahleninduzierten subkutanen fibrose. *Strahlentherapie* **154**:608–614, 1978.
29. Glatstein, E.: Alterations in rubidium-86 extraction in normal mouse tissues after irradiation. An estimate of long-term blood flow changes in kidney, lung, liver, skin and muscle. *Radiat Res* **53**:88–101, 1973.
30. Gray, L.H.: In *British Empire Cancer Campaign Report,* p. 143, 1954.
31. Hirst, D.G., Denekamp, J., and Travis, E.L.: The response of mesenteric vessels to irradiation. *Radiat Res* **77**:259–275, 1979.

32. Hopewell, J.W.: The importance of vascular damage in the development of late radiation effects in normal tissues. In *Radiation Biology in Cancer Research.* R.E. Meyn and H.R. Withers, eds. New York: Raven Press, 1980, pp. 449–459.
33. Hopewell, J.W., Forte, J.L., Young, C.M.A., and Wiernik, G.: Late radiation damage to pig skin. *Radiology* **130**:783–788, 1979.
34. Hopewell, J.W., and Wiernik, G.: Tolerance of the pig kidney to fractionated X-irradiation. In *Radiobiological Research and Radiotherapy,* vol. I. Vienna, International Atomic Energy Agency, 1977, pp. 65–73.
35. Howes, A.E., and Brown, J.M.: Early and late response of the mouse limb to multifractionated X-irradiation. *Int J Rad Oncol Biol Phys* **5**:13–22, 1979.
36. Hubbard, B.M., and Hopewell, J.W.: Changes in the neuroglial cell populations of the rat spinal cord after local X-irradiation. *Br J Radiol* **52**:816–821, 1979.
37. Hussey, D.H., Gleiser, C.A., Jardine, J.H., Raulston, G.L., and Withers, H.R.: Acute and late normal tissue effects of 50 MeV $_{d/Be}$ neutrons. In *Radiation Biology in Cancer Research,* R.E. Meyn and H.R. Withers, eds. New York: Raven Press, 1980, pp. 471–488.
38. Jolles, H., and Harrison, R.G.: Enzymatic processes and vascular changes in the skin radiation reaction. *Br J Radiol* **39**:12–18, 1966.
39. Kim, J.H., Chu, F.C.H., and Hilaris, B.: The influence of dose fractionation on acute and late reactions in patients with postoperative radiotherapy for carcinoma of the breast. *Cancer* **35**:1583–1586, 1975.
40. Kimeldorf, D.J.: Radiation-induced alterations in odontogenesis and formed teeth. In *Pathology of Irradiation* C.C. Berdjis, ed. Baltimore: Williams & Wilkins, 1971, pp. 278–289.
41. Law, M.P., and Thomlinson, R.H.: Vascular permeability in the ears of rats after X-irradiation. *Br J Radiol* **51**:895–904, 1978.
42. Lindop, P.J.A., Jones, A., and Bakowska, A.: The effect of 14-MeV electrons in the blood vessels of the mouse ear lobe. In *Time and Dose Relationships in Radiation Biology as Applied to Radiotherapy.* V.P. Bond, H.D. Suit, and V. Marcial, eds. Brookhaven National Laboratory Report BNL-5032 (C-57), 1970, pp. 174–180.
43. Meistrich, M.L., Hunter, N.R., Suzuki, N., Trostle, P.K., and Withers, H.R.: Gradual regeneration of mouse testicular stem cell after exposure to ionizing radiation. *Radiat Res* **74**:349–362, 1978.
44. Montague, E.D.: Experience with altered fractionation in radiation therapy of breast cancer. *Radiology* **90**:962–966, 1968.
45. Moustafa, H.T., and Hopewell, J.W.: Blood flow changes in pig skin after single doses of X-rays. *Br J Radiol* **52**:138–144, 1979.
46. Phillips, T.L.: An ultrastructural study of the development of radiation injury in the lung. *Radiology* **87**:49–54, 1966.
47. Phillips, T.L., Benak, S., and Ross, G.: Ultrastructural and cellular effects of ionizing radiation. In *Frontiers of Radiation Therapy and Oncology* vol. 6, J. Vaeth, ed. New York: S. Karger, 1972, pp. 21–43.
48. Samaan, N.A., Maor, M., Sampiere, V.A., Congin, A., and Jesse, R.H.: Hypopituitrism after external irradiation of nasopharyngeal cancer. In *Recent Advances in Diagnosis and Treatment of Pituitary Tumors* J.A. Linfoot, ed. New York: Raven Press, 1979, pp. 315–330.
49. Sause, W.T., Stewart, J.R., Plenk, H.P., and Leavitt, D.D.: Late skin changes following twice-weekly electron beam radiation to post-mastectomy chest walls. *Int J Rad Oncol Biol Phys* **7**:1541–1544, 1981.
50. Singh, K.: Two regimes with the same TDF but differing morbidity used in the treatment of Stage III carcinoma of the cervix. *Br J Radiol* **51**:357–362, 1978.
51. Stearner, S.P., and Christian, E.J.B.: Long-term vascular effects of ionizing radiations in the mouse: Capillary blood flow. *Radiat Res* **73**:553–567, 1978.
52. Stearner, S.P., Yang, V.V., and Devine, R.L.: Cardiac injury in the aged mouse: Comparative ultrastructural effects of fission spectrum neutrons and gamma rays. *Radiat Res* **78**:429–447, 1979.
53. Stell, P.M., and Morrison, M.D.: Radiation necrosis of the larynx. *Arch Otolaryngol* **98**:111–113, 1973.
54. Thames, H.D., and Withers, H.R.: Test of equal effect per fraction and estimate of initial clonogen number in microcolony assays of survival after fractionated irradiation. *Br J Radiol* **53**:1071–1077, 1980.
55. Thames, H.D., and Withers, H.R.: Changes in early and late radiation responses with altered dose-fractionation: Implications for dose-survival relationships. Submitted to *Int J Radiat Oncol Biol Phys.* **8**:219–226, 1982.
56. Thames, H.D., Withers, H.R., Mason, K.A., and Reid, B.O.: Dose-survival characteristics of mouse jejunal crypt cells. Submitted to *Int J Rad Oncol Biol Phys.* **7**:1591–1597, 1981.
57. Thompson, L.H., and Suit, H.D.: Proliferation kinetics of X-irradiated mouse L-cells studied with time-lapse cinematography. *Int J Radiat Biol* **15**:347–354, 1969.
58. Turesson, I.: Fractionation and dose rate in radiotherapy. Ph.D. thesis, University of Göteborg, 1978.
59. Ullrich, R.L., and Casarett, G.W.: Interrelationship between the early inflammatory response and subsequent fibrosis after radiation exposure. *Radiat Res* **72**:107–121, 1977.
60. van den Brenk, H.A.S.: Radiation effects on the pulmonary system. In *Pathology of Irradiation,*

C.C. Berdjis, ed. Baltimore: Williams & Wilkins, 1971, pp. 569–591.

61. van der Kogel, A.J.: Radiation tolerance of the rat spinal cord: Time dose relationships. *Radiology* **122**:505–509, 1977.
62. van der Kogel, A.J.: Mechanisms of late radiation injury in the spinal cord. In *Radiation Biology in Cancer Research*, R.E. Meyn and H.R. Withers, eds. New York: Raven Press, 1980, pp. 461–470.
63. Wambersie, A.J., Dutreix, J., Guelette, J., and Lellouch, J.: Early recovery for intestinal stem cells as a function of dose per fraction evaluated by survival rate after fractionated irradiation of the abdomen of mice. *Radiat Res* **58**:498–515, 1974.
64. Wara, M.W., Phillips, T.L., Margolis, L.W., and Smith, V.: Radiation pneumonitis: A new approach to the derivation of time-dose factors. *Cancer* **32**:547–552, 1973.
65. White, A., and Hornsey, S.: Radiation damage to the rat spinal cord: The effect of single and fractionated dose of x-rays. *Br J Radiol* **51**:515–523, 1978.
66. White, D.C.: The histopathologic basis for functional decrements in late radiation injury in diverse organs. *Cancer* **37**:1126–1143, 1976.
67. Withers, H.R.: Isoeffect curves for various proliferative tissues in experimental animals. In *Proceedings of Conference on Time-Dose Relationships in Clinical Radiotherapy.* Madison: Madison Printing and Publishing Co., 1975(a), pp. 30–38.
68. Withers, H.R.: Lethal and sublethal cellular injury in multifraction irradiation. *Eur J Cancer* **11**:581–583, 1975(b).
69. Withers, H.R.: Response of tissues to multiple small dose fractions. *Radiat Res* **71**:24–33, 1977.
70. Withers, H.R., and Mason, K.A.: The kinetics of recovery in irradiated colonic mucosa of the mouse. *Cancer* **34**:896–903, 1974.
71. Withers, H.R., and Peters, L.J.: Biological basis of radiotherapy. In *Textbook of Radiotherapy* G.H. Fletcher, ed. Philadelphia, Lea & Febiger, 1980, pp. 103–180.
72. Withers, H.R., Peters, L.J., and Kogelnik, H.D.: The pathobiology of late effects of irradiation. In *Radiation Biology in Cancer Research* R.E. Meyn and H.R. Withers, eds. New York: Raven Press, 1980, pp. 439–448.
73. Withers, H.R., Thames, H.D., Flow, B.L., Mason, K.A., and Hussey, D.H.: The relationship of acute to late skin injury in 2 and 5 fraction/week γ-ray therapy. *Int J Radiat Oncol Biol Phys* **4**:595–601, 1978.
74. Withers, H.R., Thames, H.D., Hussey, D.H., Flow, B.L., and Mason, K.A.: RBE of 50 MV (Be) neutrons for acute and late skin injury. *Int J Radiat Oncol Biol Phys* **4**:603–608, 1978.
75. Zeman, W., and Samorajski, T.: Effects of irradiation on the nervous system. In *Pathology of Irradiation* C.C. Berdjis, ed. Baltimore: Williams & Wilkins, 1971, pp. 213–277.
76. Zeman, W., and Solomon, M.: Effects of radiation on striated muscle. In *Pathology of Irradiation* C.C. Berdjis, ed. Baltimore: Williams & Wilkins, 1971, pp. 171–185.

CHAPTER 22

Contribution of the Keynote Discussant

Jack F. Fowler, D.Sc., Ph.D., M.Sc., F. Inst. P.[a]

Dr. Withers has said many wise things with which I agree. He pointed out phenomena we do not understand, such as swelling, vomiting, adhesions, transudation (which may not necessarily have a basis in cell killing), and the increase in normal tissue injury with volume irradiated.

Dr. Withers argued that late injuries cannot have as a common cause radiation damage to blood vessels because they occur in different normal tissues at different times and at different dose levels.

I agree with this conclusion and can quote the results from our laboratory of Fiona Stewart on bladder and David Hirst on arterioles in the mouse mesentery. In the bladder, radiation injury did not occur until the expected time required for turnover of the epithelium of the wall, and then at 9–10 months, vascular damage was also seen. This contrasts with the early appearance of vascular damage (at 6 weeks to 6 months) in the mesentery where no parenchymal damage resulted from this early vascular expression of injury.

Thus, it seems clear that the timing of radiation injury depends upon the turnover time of the irradiated parenchymal cells. This still leaves a "snowball" effect as a possible contribution of vascular damage which may begin as secondary damage and progress to cause yet more parenchymal damage. In this circular process it will be difficult to distinguish the chicken from the egg.

[a]Gray Laboratory of the Cancer Research Campaign, Mount Vernon Hospital, Northwood, Middlesex, England

Dr. Withers went on to discuss the effect of size of each dose fraction in multiple-fraction radiotherapy, using the "log cell kill per Gy" as a simple concept for visualizing changes in fractionation. From the observation that late effects increase more steeply with dose per fraction than early effects, he shows that the ratio of final-to-initial slopes of the relevant dose-response curves are greater for late than for early damage. The cell-survival curves bend downward more sharply for late than for early damage. This fact represents a warning and possibly a promise. The range of dose over which the survival curve begins to bend downward from their initial slope is important in radiotherapy. If late effects determine the tolerance dose, then each dose fraction should not exceed the dose at which the survival curve for target cells for late effects bends down. It is at just such doses per fraction that optimum sparing of late tissues may be found. If tumors are typically early-responding tissues, some therapeutic gains may therefore be obtained.

It is important to obtain data which will tell us at what dose per fraction the survival curves for late-reacting tissues begin to bend away from their initial exponential region at low doses per fraction. Isoeffect experiments with multiple doses, each of small size relevant to radiotherapy, are still too seldom done. Dose per fraction is a more important variable to plot than fraction number. Based on shapes of survival curves at low doses, it seems possible that very small doses per fraction may turn out to give the best therapeutic ratio, but the intervals between fractions depend on other factors such as reoxygenation and repopulation.

Dr. Withers finally pointed out that "remembered-dose" experiments can test the hypothesis that vascular damage is not the main cause of late injury. If retreatment with radiation, long after a first treatment, requires a large dose, then the parenchymal cells have replenished themselves, leaving little other latent damage. The "remembered dose" should depend upon the time interval as long as the relevant cells have not fully repopulated. If results are not consistent with this model, then the hypothesis will not be correct. The valuable point is that the hypothesis *can* be tested.

Furthermore, multifraction experiments can be done to investigate the curve shapes at low doses per fraction to explore the idea that therapeutic gains can be obtained by choosing the smallest possible sizes of dose per fraction. Dr. Withers' paper is therefore very constructive and stimulating, and I urge you to study it carefully.

CHAPTER 23

Response of Normal Tissues: Implications for Clinical Radiotherapy

Stanley B. Field, B.Sc., Ph.D.[a]
Adam Michalowski, Doc. Dr. Hab. Med.[b]

In all cancer therapy the limiting factor is the response of critical normal tissues. Animal tissues often closely resemble those in man, both anatomically and physiologically, and respond to radiation in a similar way. It is therefore rational to study the response of animal tissues to different types of anticancer agents with a view to cautious extrapolation to man. One justification for this approach is the similarity between mouse and man in the lowest doses of radiation required to produce a measurable response in various normal tissues (see Table 1).

A gain in understanding of the response of human tissue to irradiation has been a major contribution made by the radiation biologist. This has been particularly true for the use of new treatment modalities. One example is fast neutrons, aspects of which will be discussed briefly below. The hope is always that a deeper understanding will lead to new and successful treatment modalities.

It is now generally accepted that tissue reaction is primarily determined by the radiobiological response of the cells of the tissue. Therefore, the concepts derived from cell-survival curves are of paramount importance. Since most types of cells die at division (although not necessarily at the first attempt), the timing of a tissue reaction will depend, to a first approximation, on the normal proliferation characteristics of the tissue. For example, changes in the gut will be manifest after hours or a few days, whereas a reaction in the bladder or liver may take months or years to develop. But tissues may also be classified in another way which will be discussed below.

Of great importance in radiotherapy is tissue response to fractionated treatments. The following factors have been shown to be important:

1. Repair of sublethal damage
2. Repair of potentially lethal damage

TABLE 1. A Comparison of "Threshold Doses" in Mouse and Man for Damage to Various Tissues[d]

	Mouse[a]	Man[b]
Bone marrow	600	300
Small intestine	900	1400–1850[c]
Lung	1000	1000–1150
Kidney	1300	900–1100
Spinal Cord	2000	1600–1950
Esophagus	2000	1750–2050

[a] Values for mice are approximate threshold doses in rad to produce death, or in the case of spinal cord, paraplegia.

[b] Values for man are normal standard doses (ret) likely to cause between 25 and 50% complications.

[c] This value is probably high because the rapid proliferation of the intestinal cells is not adequately allowed for in the Ellis formula.

[d] From Fowler and Denekamp, 1976.

[a]Head, Dept. of Biology, M.R.C. Cyclotron Unit, Hammersmith Hospital, London, England
[b]Dept. of Biology, Hammersmith Hospital, M.R.C. Cyclotron Unit, London, England

TABLE 2. $D_2 - D_1$ Values for Various Tissues

Tissues	Species	End Point	$D_2 - D_1$ (rad)	Reference
Skin	Pig	Radiodermatitis	500–700	Fowler[21]
	Rat	Radiodermatitis	890	Field[19]
	Mouse	Radiodermatitis	500	Denekamp[5]
	Mouse	Epidermal clones	350	Withers[58]
			570	Denekamp[5]
Esophagus	Mouse	LD50	560	Hornsey and Field[27]
			850	Phillips and Ross[44]
Gastrointestinal tract	Mouse	LD50	450	Hornsey and Vatistas[31]
		Macrocolony assay	400	Withers and Elkind[59]
Cartilage	Rat	Growth stunting	400	Dixon[8]
			350	Kember[35]
Lung	Mouse	LD50 (both lungs)	400–500	Field and Hornsey[15]
			350	Phillips and Margolis[43]
Spinal Cord	Rat	ED50	950	White and Hornsey[57]
			600	van der Kogel[53]
Testis	Mouse	Clonal assay	300[a]	Withers et al.[61]
Hemopoietic tissues	Mouse	Spleen nodules	100	Till and McCulloch[51]
Endothelial cells	Rat	Stimulated dermal blood vessels	300	Reinhold and Buisman[46]
		Colonies in granuloma pouch	180	van den Brenk et al.[52]
		Cell counts in mesentery	700	Hirst et al.[26]

[a] Decreases with increasing time between fractions.

3. Other slower repair processes
4. Repopulation of surviving cells
5. Reassortment of cells in their mitotic cycle.

These factors have been shown to occur to different extents in different tissues so that the effect of dose fractionation is tissue dependent. There may, in addition, be other factors which will eventually come to light.

Repair of Sublethal Damage

Accumulation and repair of sublethal damage (SLD) has been well documented.[12] In general SLD is less for cells *in vitro* than for the cells of most tissues *in vivo*. This may be due to the greater intercellular contact between cells in solid tissues. In spheroids, for example, the capacity for accumulation and repair of sublethal damage is increased over the same cells grown individually.[10] In some tissues the repair of sublethal damage (i.e., $D_2 - D_1$) is very large, as in skin, intestine, and spinal cord; but in others (e.g., the hemopoeitic system) it is much less. Table 2 gives values for repair between two large doses ($D_2 - D_1$) in a range of normal tissues.

Repair of Potentially Lethal Damage

Repair of potentially lethal damage

(PLD) has been demonstrated with cells *in vitro* and also with experimental tumors.[24,45,50] It is normally manifest by an increase in D_o of the survival curve which occurs during an interval after irradiation before cells are called upon to divide. Techniques are not yet available for measuring PLD in normal tissues, but there is no reason to believe it will not occur, especially in organs such as liver or kidney in which stimuli for proliferation unmask latent radiation injury.

Slow-Repair Processes

Two types of slow repair have been identified, one similar to repair of PLD and the other to repair of SLD. Van den Brenk et al.[52] and Reinhold and Buisman[47] investigated the response of capillary endothelium to irradiation. The technique used by both groups was to stimulate cell proliferation in these otherwise slowly dividing tissues at various times after treatment. They observed a slow-repair process with a half-time of about 1 week. Curtis,[3] using chromosome abnormalities as the end point for damage to mouse liver, also observed very slow repair manifest by a steady disappearance of the abnormalities, although McKay et al.[38] believe that there is no repair of chromosome damage in liver of Chinese hamsters. This type of repair may be analogous to repair of PLD but with a much longer time course. A second type of slow-repair process has been demonstrated to occur between two dose fractions in mouse lung. It is thought not to be due to cell proliferation.[2,18] In rat spinal cord, however, late proliferation almost certainly does play a role.[54,57] Slow repair may have a number of important implications in late damage to normal tissues and in residual injury after irradiation.[28]

Repopulation

Following irradiation cells undergo a period of mitotic delay after which there may be renewed proliferation. Tissue damage is repaired in this way, often rendering radiation decreasingly effective as the period of protraction of the treatment is increased. It is known, at least in some tissues (e.g., skin and intestine) that cell proliferation after irradiation is stimulated by homeostatic control in response to the presence of dying cells or to products of cell lysis.

Reassortment

Since cell sensitivity varies throughout the mitotic cycle, a dose of radiation will preferentially kill the sensitive cells, leaving mostly those in the resistant phases as survivors. After irradiation the remaining resistant cells are at first delayed and then move toward the more sensitive phase. Thus, a second dose will be more effective if given some time after the first treatment than if given immediately after. This process is in competition with the repair processes, all of which render the population less sensitive with time after a first irradiation. In addition mitotic delay is not constant for cells at all stages of the cell cycle, and the net effect of irradiation is to cause a temporary accumulation of cells in the G_2 phase. This process adds to the partial synchrony of the population caused by preferentially killing the sensitive cells. All these processes combined cause the sensitivity to a second treatment to vary with time, the pattern depending on the kinetics of the various phenomena for each tissue. The effect of reassortment becomes extremely complicated with many fractions or with irradiation at low dose rates and cannot be predicted with any certainty.

Multifraction Irradiation

Radiotherapists need to know the relationship between the total dose, number of fractions, and overall treatment time for a given degree of normal tissue damage. Various isoeffect formulae have been suggested for this purpose. Whether or not these formulae are accurate over the therapy range of treatment times and number of fractions is the subject of much debate. It is even more dubious whether these relationships may be extrapolated beyond the therapy range.

The most commonly used formula has the form

$$TD = N^{\alpha} T^{\beta} \qquad (1)$$

where TD is the total dose given in N fractions in an overall treatment time of T days.

Ellis[13] suggested $\alpha = 0.24$ and $\beta = 0.11$ for tolerance to vascularized connective tissue, but the formula has been the subject of much discussion and modification.[14,34,36,42] It remains a useful "rule of thumb."

The question may be posed: What are the factors responsible for N and for T? The N factor, being related to the number of dose fractions, is thought to be primarily influenced by repair of sublethal damage. Since this is usually complete in a few hours, it is theoretically possible to give several fractions per day without changing the N factor. Extensive repair of sublethal damage will normally be consistent with a large exponent for N–i.e., a large sparing by fractionation. Tissues showing little repair of SLD will have a small exponent for N and show little sparing by fractionation. If repair of potentially lethal damage occurs in normal tissues *in situ*, it will also cause the N factor to be increased.

The T factor is more difficult to explain with certainty. In rapidly proliferating tissues it is probably due to cellular repopulation, in which case a power function (such as $T^{0.11}$) is unlikely to be universally applicable. In slowly proliferating tissues T may be due to slow repair for which a power function would be more appropriate.

Much effort has been directed at establishing knowledge about these factors in normal animal tissues. Several groups of workers have measured isoeffect curves and repair between small doses in various normal tissues.[4,7,9,11,16,18,20,27,47,54,56,57] Much work has also been done on repopulation and the T factor (see Denekamp and Fowler[6] for a review). In general it is found that α lies between 0.2 and 0.4 for different tissues, but there are indications that it is reduced for very large numbers of fractions. The factors controlling T are less well documented. For low LET radiation the N factor is by far the most important; for high LET radiation this will not be the case, but effects of fractionation are not so large.

Predictions for New Treatment Modalities: Fast Neutrons

Animal studies on normal tissues can give essential information about new treatment modalities. This may be illustrated in the examples from research with fast neutrons. It is well established that relative biological effectiveness (RBE) increases with decreasing dose per fraction, and that RBE varies with tissue and neutron energy.[17] It is known that for skin the RBE is the same for four animal species, including man, enabling extrapolation to be made from animal results with confidence. Such data have been used to calculate the equivalent doses of x-rays given in the early Californian trial of Neutron Therapy.[49] We also now have a reasonable understanding of RBE in terms of the various tissue repair processes.

Recently much progress has been made in understanding the results of fractionated photon and neutron irradiation of the central nervous system. It is well established that the isoeffect curves for photons are significantly steeper for spinal cord and brain than for skin, a best fit to equation (1) being given by $\alpha = 0.38$, $\beta = 0.02$ (see Fig. 1).[29,55] The use of this "modified Ellis formula" provides a satisfactory explanation of why treatment of brain tumors using high doses, but given in many fractions, is well toler-

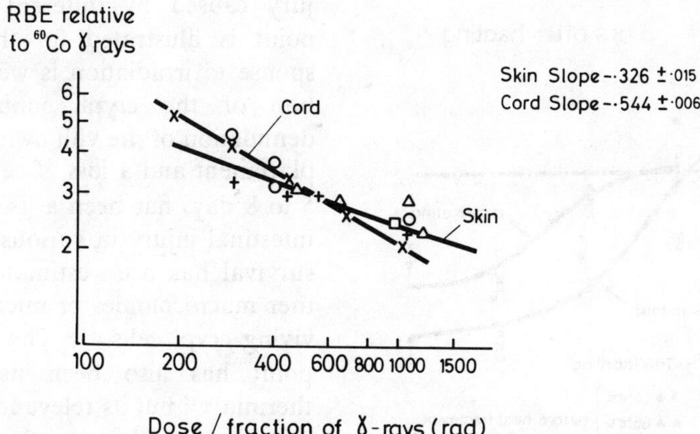

Figure 1. Isoeffect curve for x-ray-induced CNS damage in rats, including progressive radiculopathy in lumbar cord, myelopathy, and vascular injury in cervical cord and brain damage. The data are normalized to 10 fractions by dividing the total dose in N fractions D_N by D_{10}, and the effect of different overall treatment times is corrected by $T^{0.02}$.[29]

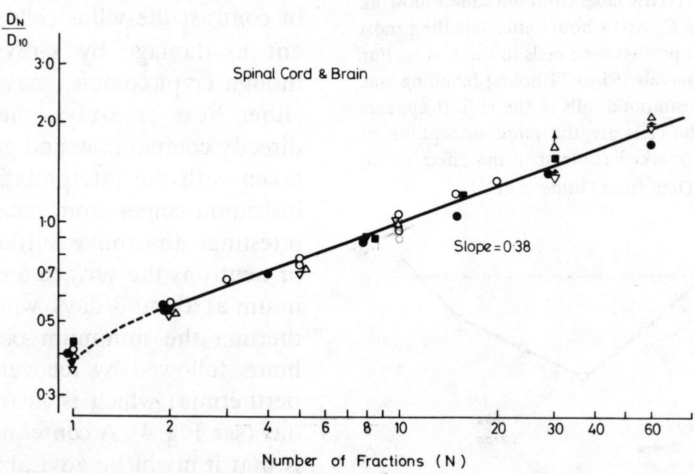

Figure 2. RBE relative to dose/fraction of γ-rays for acute skin damage (neutrons of Ed = 16 MeV) and damage to spinal cord (neutrons of Ed = 16 and 22 MeV). (Data from Hornsey, personal communication.)

ated.[29,48] However, the isoeffect curve for neutron irradiation of CNS has a very small value of α, as is the case for most tissues, so that the RBE as a function of dose per fraction increases more steeply for CNS than for other tissues (see Fig. 2). Thus, for small doses per fraction the RBE for CNS is particularly high. With the Hammersmith cyclotron the RBE is approximately 5.3 at the level of 180 rad photons.[25] Therefore, great care must be taken in predicting the tolerance dose for neutrons on the CNS. The use of factors derived for other tissues (or worse, a constant RBE of 3 as is sometimes adopted) can lead to the prediction of an overdose.[37] Using the modified formula, Halnan and Hornsey[25] derived a tolerance dose for neutron damage to cervical cord of approximately 850 rad, and Hornsey et al.[30] derived a tolerance dose for brain of 1100 rad—both values being in good agreement with clinical findings.

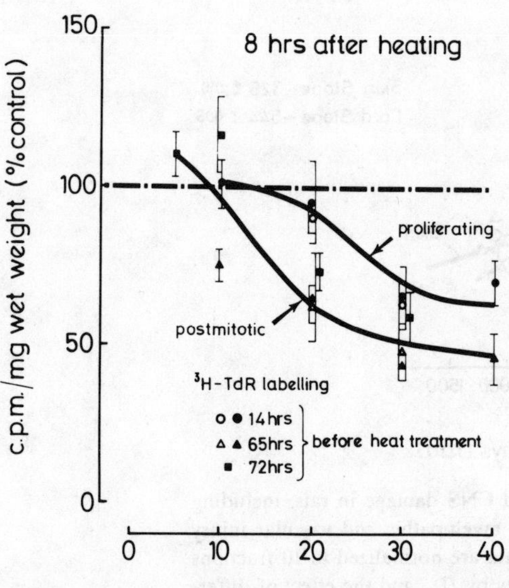

Figure 3. Loss of ³H-TdR label from intestine following hyperthermia at 43°C. At 14 hours after labelling most of label was in the proliferating cells in the crypts. For the longer time intervals (65 to 72 hours) labelling was primarily in the postmitotic cells in the villi. It appears that the postmitotic cells are the more susceptible to thermal injury, in marked contrast to the effect of ionizing radiation. (Data from Hume et al.[33])

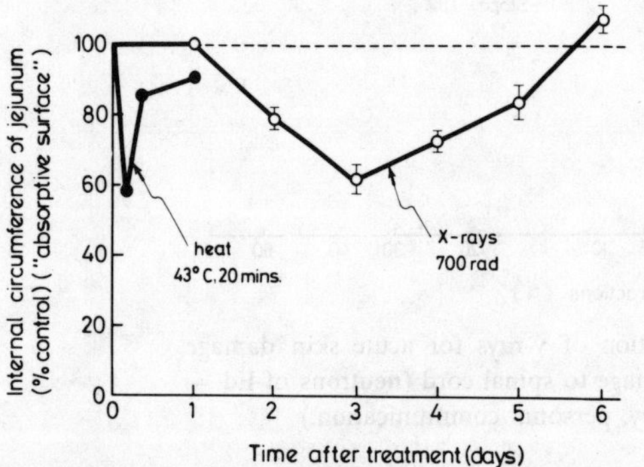

Figure 4. Changes in "absorptive surface" of mouse jejunum after hyperthermia or x-rays.

Choice of Tissue End Points

It was pointed out above that after irradiation most cell types die if they attempt mitosis. With other modalities this might not be the case. It is therefore not necessarily possible to directly compare tissue injury caused by different modalities. The point is illustrated for the intestine. Response to irradiation is well known; depletion of the crypt population leads to denudation of the villi owing to a lack of replacement and a loss of cell cover. LD50 at 5 to 8 days has been a useful end point for intestinal injury in various species, and cell survival has been estimated by scoring either macrocolonies or microcolonies of surviving crypt cells.[59,60] The microcolony end point has also been used after hyperthermia[32,41] but its relevance is questionable. After heating there is a loss of villi within a few hours[32] which is not seen after irradiation, and recent experiments by Hume et al.[33] indicate that the postmitotic cells on the villi are more sensitive to heat injury than the dividing cells in the crypts (see Fig. 3). In contrast the villus cells are highly resistant to damage by x-rays. Therefore, although crypt colonies may be counted after either heat or x-rays, the results are not directly comparable, and great care must be taken with the interpretation. A further illustration comes from measurements of the intestinal absorbtive surface.[40] After x-rays or neutrons the surface area reaches a minimum at about 3 days, whereas after hyperthermia the minimum occurs after a few hours followed by recovery (with mild hyperthermia) which is nearly complete in 1 day (see Fig. 4). A consequence of this result is that it might be advisable for any patient receiving hyperthermia to the abdomen to avoid having food pass along the intestine for a day after heating since this would cause further wear on the already damaged lining and may greatly impair absorption.

Early and Late Damage–Tissue Classification

It has long been accepted that, because irradiated cells die at mitosis, rapidly proliferating tissues show damage early and slowly proliferating tissues respond long af-

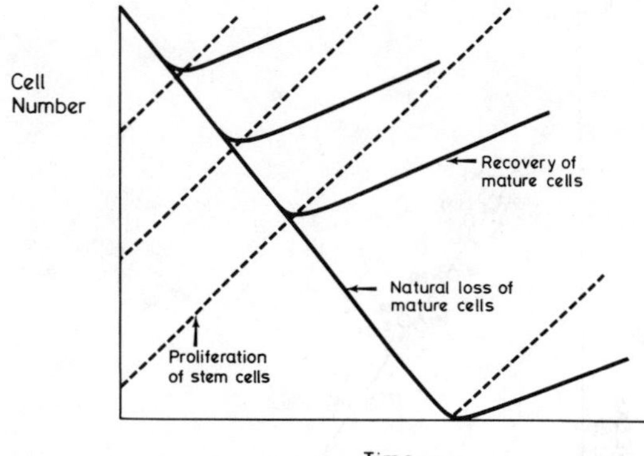

Figure 5. The solid lines show the natural loss of mature cells in an irradiated type-A population. A depleted stem cell population will cease replacing the mature cells until adequate repopulation has taken place.

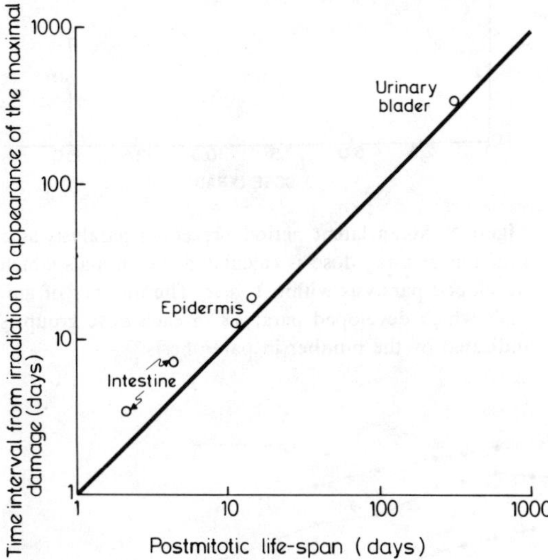

Figure 6. The interval between irradiation and appearance of maximal injury as a function of the life span of the postmitotic cells. The solid line is drawn at 45°.

ter irradiation. Michalowski, however, has suggested a further refinement of this simple concept. Two basic types of tissue are defined. In type A there exists a defined stem cell compartment. These cells proliferate and feed into the differentiating compartment. Mature postmitotic cells are eventually lost by natural processes. Irradiation will depopulate the stem cell compartment. It is postulated that the outflow from the mature compartment is unaffected and that there is no cytocidal effect on mature cells (which therefore immediately begin to be depleted). Tissue damage will result from inadequacy in the mature cell compartment, but is not directly affected by depletion of the stem cells. Thus, the timing of loss in tissue function or of observable injury will be dependent on the life span of the mature cells. It will be relatively independent of dose size, although small reactions which are produced by small doses will reach a peak slightly earlier than after larger doses due to earlier repopulation (see Fig. 5). Timing of the maximum response will be dose independent, as has been well established in tissues such as intestine, epidermis, and bone marrow.

Figure 6 shows that, for a range of type-A tissues, the timing of maximal response is equal to the postmitotic life span. Note that the slowly proliferating bladder epithelium is included in this category.

Type-B tissues contain cells for which there is no histological evidence of differences in degree of differentiation. The cells all look alike and all appear to be capable of proliferation. In contrast with type A, overt tissue damage will be dependent on *all* cells in type-B tissues. Type-B tissues may contain, at any time, a small fraction of cells with a fairly short cycle time or a larger fraction with a much longer cycle time. In either case the initial response to radiation will result from the natural loss of quiescent cells accompanied by the radiation-induced loss of proliferating cells. The latter will be dose dependent so that the total loss will occur faster with increasing dose (see Fig. 7). But as cells are lost, the homeostatic control mechanisms will operate to restore the tissue to its full cell complement. This will involve accelerated proliferation leading to an avalanche effect as more cells attempt to divide and die as a result. In this case the larger doses will cause the avalanche to occur earlier (Fig. 7). Thus, for type-B tissues, the timing of injury will be dose dependent–i.e., larger doses showing injury earlier. Examples where this occurs are shown in Figure 8

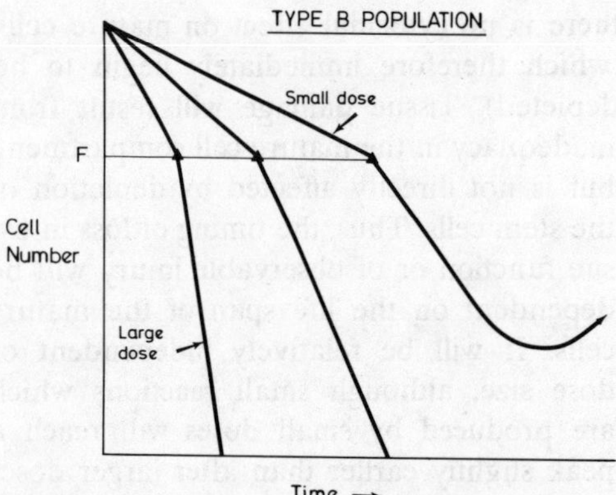

Figure 7. Loss of cells due to irradiation of a type-B population. A larger dose will initially produce a greater loss than a smaller dose. The subsequent avalanche, resulting from the irradiated population attempting to replace the lost cells by cell division (schematically depicted as starting at F), will occur more rapidly with larger doses.

for mouse spinal cord damage and Figure 9 for skin contraction.

Tissues falling into categories A and B are given in Table 3. In general those with long turnover times fall into group B, but this is not always the case–a notable exception being bladder epithelium.

The differences between tissue types A and B have important clinical implications.

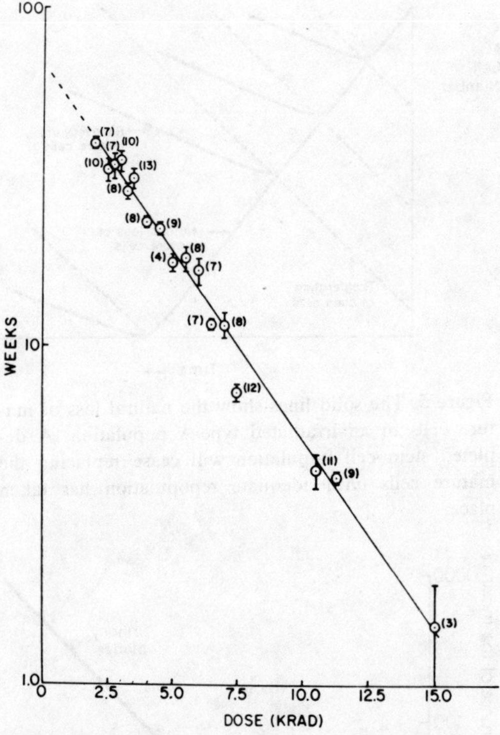

Figure 8. Mean latent period preceding paralysis as a function of x-ray dose is calculated for animals which developed paralysis within 1 year. The number of animals which developed paralysis in each dose group is indicated by the number in parenthesis.[23]

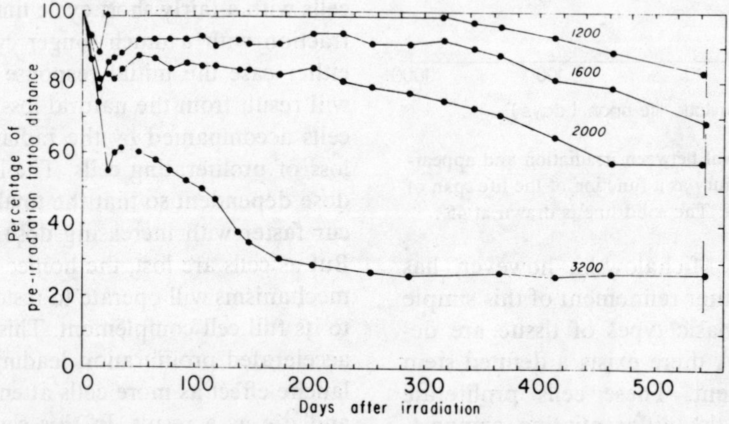

Figure 9. Time course of decrease in the distance between tattoo marks in mouse skin after single exposures of x-rays. Numbers in the figure represent the dose in rad, and vertical bars (shown only for final points) are the standard deviations for each point. The figure shows the early effect of the larger doses and the late occurrence of contraction after small doses. (Data from Masuda, personal communication.)

TABLE 3. Tissue Classification for Proliferative Organization and Type of Radiation Response[a]

Type-A Populations	Type-B Populations
Epidermis	Dermis
Epithelial lining of the digestive and urinary tracts	Stromal connective tissues
Erythro- and granulopoietic tissues	Endothelium
	Neuroglia
	Mesothelium
	Liver parenchyma
	Kidney parenchyma

[a]With the exception of stromal connective tissues and mesothelium, each tissue has been classified on the basis of radiobiological evidence.

Type-A tissues respond at a time characteristic of the tissue. After this time it is unlikely that any further consequence of irradiation will ensue. In contrast, the response of type-B tissues occurs later with decreasing dose so that the possibility of serious late consequences can never be excluded. In addition, type-B tissues are likely to respond dramatically to some unrelated trauma, e.g., that due to an infection or mechanical injury. Such recall phenomena are well known in radiotherapy.

Summary

Cancer therapy is limited by the response of normal tissues. In rodents and larger animals normal tissues often closely resemble those in man, both anatomically and physiologically. It is therefore relevant to study the response of animal tissues to treatments envisaged in the clinic. Such studies give information on the various repair processes which control the effects of fractionation, residual injury, and RBE. This has been illustrated by recent results on CNS.

It is proposed that normal tissues fall broadly in two categories. Category A has cells which either proliferate or perform tissue-specific functions. In category B all cells are capable of doing both. The manifestations of radiation response in these two types of tissue are different.

With radiation most cells die at mitosis. Other modalities may lead to 'intermitotic' death (direct cytocidal effect) resulting in a different time course (e.g., postmitotic cells in the intestine are more sensitive to hyperthermia than the cells in the crypts and are lost within a few hours of treatment). Therefore, for any study the tissue end points chosen must depend on the modality under investigation.

REFERENCES

1. Alper, T.: Hypothesis. Elkind recovery and "sublethal damage": a misleading association. *Br J Radiol* **50**:459–467, 1977.
2. Coultas, P.G., Ahier, R.G., and Field, S.B.: Cell proliferation in normal and irradiated mouse lung. *Radiat Res* **85**:516–528, 1981.
3. Curtis, H.J.: Biological mechanisms of delayed radiation damage in mammals. In *Current Topics in Radiation Research* vol. III, Ebert and Howard, eds. Amsterdam: 1967, pp. 139–174.
4. Denekamp, J.: Changes in the rate of repopulation during multifraction irradiation of mouse skin. *Br J Radiol* **46**:381–387, 1973.
5. Denekamp, J., Ball, M.M., and Fowler, J.F.: Recovery and repopulation in mouse skin as a function of time after irradiation. *Radiat Res* **37**:361–370, 1969.
6. Denekamp, J., and Fowler, J.F.: Cell proliferation kinetics and radiation therapy. In *Cancer: A Comprehensive Treatise* vol. 6, F.F. Becker, ed. New York: Plenum Press, 1976, pp. 101–137.
7. Denekamp, J., and Harris, S.R.: The response of mouse skin to multiple small doses of radiation. In *Cell Survival After Low Doses of Radiation: Theoretical and Clinical Implications,* T. Alper, ed. Institute of Physics and J. Wiley, New York: 1975, pp. 342–350.
8. Dixon, B.: The effect of radiation on the growth of vertebrae in the tails of rats. II. Split doses of X-rays and the effect of oxygen. *Int J Radiat Biol* **15**:215–226, 1969.
9. Douglas, B.G., and Fowler, J.F.: The effect of multiple small doses of X-rays on skin reactions in the mouse and a basic interpretation. *Radiat Res* **66**:401–426, 1976.

10. Durand, R.E., and Sutherland, R.M.: Effects of intercellular contact on repair of radiation damage. *Exp Cell Res* **71**:75–80, 1972.
11. Dutreix, J., Wambersie, A., and Bounik, C.: Cellular recovery in human skin reactions: Applications to dose, fraction number, overall time relationship in radiotherapy. *Eur J Cancer* **9**:159–167, 1973.
12. Elkind, M.M., and Sutton, H.: Radiation response of mammalian cells grown in culture. I. Repair of X-ray damage in surviving Chinese hamster cells. *Radiat Res* **13**:556–593, 1960.
13. Ellis, F.: Dose, time and fractionation: A clinical hypothesis. *Clin Radiol* **20**:1–7, 1969.
14. Ellis, F., and Sorenson, A.: A method of estimating biological effect of combined intercavity low dose-rate radiation with external radiation in carcinoma of the cervix uteri. *Radiology* **110**:681–686, 1974.
15. Field, S.B., and Hornsey, S.: Damage to mouse lung with neutrons and X rays. *Eur J Cancer* **10**:621–627, 1974.
16. Field, S.B., and Hornsey, S.: The response of mouse skin and lung to fractionated X-rays. In *Cell Survival after Low Doses of Radiation: Theoretical and Clinical Implications* T. Alper, ed. Institute of Physics and J. Wiley, New York, 1975, pp. 362–368.
17. Field, S.B., and Hornsey, S.: Aspects of OER and RBE relevant to neutron therapy. In *Advances in Radiation Biology*, vol. 8, J.T. Lett and H. Adler, eds. New York: Academic Press, 1979, pp. 1–49.
18. Field, S.B., Hornsey, S., and Kutsutani, Y.: Effects of fractionated irradiation on mouse lung and a phenomenon of "slow repair." *Br J Radiol* **49**:700–709, 1976.
19. Field, S.B., Jones, T., and Thomlinson, R.H.: The relative effects of fast neutrons and X-rays on tumour and normal tissue in the rat. II. Fractionation: Recovery and reoxygenation. *Br J Radiol* **41**:597–607, 1968.
20. Field, S.B., Morris, C., Denekamp, J., and Fowler, J.F.: The response of mouse skin to fractionated X-rays. *Eur J Cancer* **11**:291–299, 1975.
21. Fowler, J.F., Bewley, D.K., Morgan, R.L., and Silvester, J.A.: Experiments with fractionated X-irradiation of the skin of pigs. II. Fractionation up to five days. *Br J Radiol* **38**:278–284, 1965.
22. Fowler, J.F., and Denekamp, J.: Radiation effects on normal tissues. In *Cancer: A Comprehensive Treatise* vol. 6, F.F. Becker, ed. New York: Plenum Press, 1976, pp. 139–180.
23. Geraci, J.P., Thrower, P.D., Jackson, K.L., Christensen, G.M., Parker, R.G., and Fox, M.S.: The relative biological effectiveness of fast neutrons for spinal cord injury. *Radiat Res* **59**:496–503, 1974.
24. Hahn, G.M., and Little, J.B.: Plateau phase cultures of mammalian cells. *Curr Top Radiat Res* **8**:39–83, 1972.
25. Halnan, K.E., and Hornsey, S.: RBE values for neutron therapy. *Int J Radiat Oncol Biol Phys,* **7**:601–604, 1981.
26. Hirst, D.G., Denekamp, J., and Hobson, B.: Proliferation studies of the endothelial and smooth muscle cells of the mouse mesentery after irradiation. *Cell Tissue Kinet* **13**:91–104, 1980.
27. Hornsey, S., and Field, S.B.: The effects of single and fractionated doses of X-rays and neutrons on the oesophagus. *Eur J Cancer* **15**:491–498, 1979.
28. Hornsey, S., and Field, S.B.: Slow repair and residual injury. In *Radiation Biology in Cancer Research. 32nd Annual Symposium on Fundamental Cancer Research* (Houston) 1980, pp. 489–499.
29. Hornsey, S., Morris, C.C., and Myers, R.: The relationship between fractionation and total dose for x-ray induced brain damage. *Int J Radiat Oncol Biol Phys,* **7**:393–396, 1981.
30. Hornsey, S., Morris, C.C., Myers, R., and White, A.: RBE for damage to the CNS by neutrons. *Int J Radiat Oncol Biol Phys,* **7**:185–189, 1981.
31. Hornsey, S., and Vatistas, S.: Some characteristics of the survival curve of crypt cells of the small intestine of the mouse. *Br J Radiol* **36**:795–800, 1963.
32. Hume, S.P., Marigold, J.C.L., and Field, S.B.: The effect of local hyperthermia on the small intestine of mouse. *Br J Radiol* **52**:657–662, 1979.
33. Hume, S.P., Marigold, J.C.L., and Michalowski, A.: The effect of local hyperthermia on the non proliferative, compared with proliferative, epithelial cells of the mouse intestinal mucosa. *Radiat Res* In press.
34. Kellerer, A.M.: Grundlagen der Ellis-Formel. *Strahlentherapie* **153**:384, 1977.
35. Kember, N.F.: Cell survival and radiation damage in growth cartilage. *Br J Radiol* **40**:495–505, 1967.
36. Kirk, J., Gray, W.M., and Watson, E.R.: Cumulative radiation effect. I. Fractionated treatment regimes. *Clin Radiol* **22**:145, 1971.
37. Laramore, G.E., Blasko, J.C., Griffin, T.W., and Groudine, M.T.: Fast neutron teletherapy for advanced carcinomas of the oropharynx. *Int J Radiat Oncol Biol Phys* **5**:1821–1827, 1979.
38. McKay, L.R., Shaw, S.M., and Brooks, A.L.: Metaphase chromosome aberrations in the Chinese hamster liver *in vivo* after either acute or fractionated ^{60}Co irradiation. *Radiat Res* **57**:187–194, 1974.
39. Masuda, K.: Personal communication, 1980.
40. Meder, J., and Michalowski, A.: Changes in the absorptive surface of mouse jejunum as a measure of acute radiation effect. In preparation.
41. Merino, A., Peters, L.J., Mason, K.A., and Withers, H.R.: Effect of hyperthermia on the radiation response of the mouse jejunum. *Int J Radiat Oncol Biol Phys* **4**:407–414, 1978.
42. Orton, C.G., and Ellis, F.: A simplification in the use of the NSD concept in practical radiotherapy. *Br J Radiol* **46**:529–537, 1973.
43. Phillips, T.L., and Margolis, L.: Radiation pathol-

ogy and the clinical response of lung and oesophagus. In *Frontiers of Radiation Therapy and Oncology*, vol. 6, J.M. Vaeth, ed. Basel: S. Karger, 1972, pp. 254–273.

44. Phillips, T.L., and Ross, G.: Time-dose relationships in the mouse oesophagus. *Radiology* **113**:435–440, 1974.
45. Phillips, R.A., and Tolmach, L.J.: Repair of potentially lethal damage in X-irradiated HeLa cells. *Radiat Res* **29**:413–432, 1966.
46. Reinhold, H.S., and Buisman, G.H.: Radiosensitivity of capillary endothelium. *Br J Radiol* **46**:53–57, 1973.
47. Reinhold, H.S., and Buisman, G.H.: Repair of radiation damage to capillary endothelium. *Br J Radiol* **48**:727–731, 1975.
48. Salazar, O.M., Rubin, P., Feldstein, M.L., and Pizzutiello, R.: High dose radiation therapy in the treatment of malignant gliomas: Final report. *Int J Radiat Oncol Biol Phys* **5**:1733–1740, 1979.
49. Sheline, G.E., Phillips, T.L., Field, S.B., Brennan, J.T., and Raventos, A.: Effects of fast neutrons on human skin. *Am J Roentgenol Rad Ther Nucl Med* **111**:31–41, 1971.
50. Shipley, W.U., Stanley, J.A., Courtenay, V.D., and Field, S.B.: Repair of radiation damage in Lewis lung carcinoma cells following *in situ* treatment with fast neutrons and X-rays. *Cancer Res* **35**:932–938, 1975.
51. Till, J.E., and McCulloch, E.A.: Early repair processes in marrow cells irradiated and proliferating *in vivo*. *Radiat Res* **18**:96–105, 1963.
52. van den Brenk, H.A.S., Sharpington, C., Orton, C., et al.: Effects of X-irradiation on growth and function of the repair blastema (granulation tissue). II. Measurements of angiogenesis in the Selye pouch in the rat. *Int J Radiat Biol* **25**:277–289, 1974.
53. van der Kogel, A.J.: Radiation tolerance of the spinal cord: Dependence on fractionation and extended overall times. In *Radiobiological Research and Radiotherapy* vol. I. Vienna: IAEA, 1977, pp. 83–90.
54. van der Kogel, A.J.: Radiation tolerance of the rat spinal cord: Time–dose relationships. *Radiology* **122**:505–509, 1977.
55. van der Kogel, A.J.: *Late Effects of Radiation on the Spinal Cord.* Doctoral thesis. Rijswijk, The Netherlands: Radiobiological Institute of the Organisation for Health Research TNO, 1979.
56. Wambersie, A., Dutreix, J., Guelette, J., and Lellough, J.: Early recovery for intestinal stem cells, as a function of dose per fraction evaluated by survival rate after fractionated irradiation of the abdomen of mice. *Radiat Res* **58**:498–515, 1974.
57. White, A., and Hornsey, S.: Radiation damage to the rat spinal cord: The effect of single and fractionated doses of x-rays. *Br J Radiol* **51**:515–523, 1978.
58. Withers, H.R.: The dose survival relationship for irradiation of epithelial cells of mouse skin. *Br J Radiol* **40**:187–194, 1967.
59. Withers, H.R., and Elkind, M.M.: Radiosensitivity and fractionation response of crypt cells of mouse jejunum. *Radiat Res* **38**:598–613, 1969.
60. Withers, H.R., and Elkind, M.M.: Microcolony survival assay for cells of mouse intestinal mucosa exposed to radiation. *Int J Radiat Biol* **17**:261–267, 1970.
61. Withers, H.R., Hunter, N., Barkley, H.Y., Jr., and Reid, B.O.: Radiation survival and regeneration characteristics of spermatogenic stem cells of mouse testis. *Radiat Res* **57**:88–103, 1974.

CHAPTER 24

Late Effects of Various Dose-Fractionation Regimens

Ingela Turesson, M.D. Gustaf Notter, M.D.[a]

During the last 10 years normal tissue reactions after different dose-fractionation regimens have been discussed intensely. Numerous experimental dose-effect curves for different normal tissue end points have been presented as reviewed by Field and Michalowski.[7] But there is still a lack of *clinical* dose-response curves for early and late normal tissue reactions for various fractionation schedules. In clinical practice it is very difficult to establish dose-response curves. At present, the human data comprise dose-incidence curves for bladder complications[9] and for laryngeal necrosis.[10] However, valuable clinical observations on normal tissue reactions for various dose-fractionation regimens have been presented.[1,2,4] These reports mainly concern skin and subcutaneous tissue. They all describe a lack of correlation between acute and late tissue response. Some of them have also pointed out the danger of using the NSD formula for small numbers of fractions, i.e., for a large dose per fraction.

However, a very important consequence of adoption of the NSD formula[6] is that it has focused attention on the necessity of calculating isoeffect doses in radiotherapy. Ellis' formula also stimulated us, 8 years ago, to start a series of prospective fractionation studies on human skin. In these studies we have stipulated the following experimental conditions:

- Only one area should be used for evaluation of the radiation effect.
- The patient should serve as his or her own control if possible.
- The absorbed dose should be checked for each dose fraction.
- The acute reaction should be monitored twice a week until it has declined.
- The late reaction should be monitored at least every fourth month up to 5 years and then twice a year.

We have used the CRE (Cumulative Radiation Effect) formula proposed by Kirk et al.[8] which is merely a generalization of the NSD formula.

Our conclusions are that for early skin reactions the CRE (or NSD) formula predicts equivalent dose levels with better than 7% reliability for doses per fraction between 1.0 and 7.3 Gy, and for a number of fractions between 4 and 50 if the overall treatment time is limited to 4 weeks or less.[11,12]

Based upon recent clinical investigations, we are able to generalize the applicability of the formula to an overall treatment time of more than 4 weeks provided that irradiation is avoided during pronounced skin reactions. During this phase, about 30 to 45 days after commencement of irradiation, it may be assumed that the proliferation rate in the skin epithelium is increased (Hopewell, personal communication).[5] This may be the reason why we have found a higher sensitivity than predicted by the CRE (or NSD) formula to daily fractions for overall treatment times of 5 to 6 weeks (see Fig. 1). It is

[a]Department of Radiotherapy, University of Göteborg, Sahlgrenska Hospital, Göteborg, Sweden

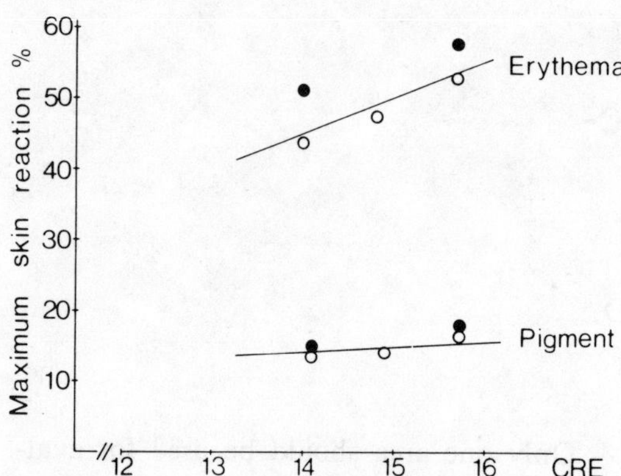

Figure 1. The acute erythema and pigmentation as a function of CRE. The solid lines are based on various fractionation schedules limited to overall times of 4 weeks or less. The solid circles represent fractionation schedule 5 × 1.8 Gy per week–25 and 30 fractions given within 5 and 6 weeks, respectively. The open circles represent fractionation schedule 2 × 3.6 Gy per week–10, 11, and 12 fractions given within 5, 5.5, and 6 weeks, respectively.

also in agreement with the acute pig skin reactions reported by Berry et al.[3] and Withers et al.[16]

However, the acute reaction in normal tissue is not the main problem in radiotherapy. It can be eliminated by modifying the fraction size and the interval between fractions, or by including an interval to allow for repopulation of surviving cells. The late effects on normal tissue are of most relevance in curative radiotherapy. By implication, a model that predicts equivalent late reactions is required. Such a model must be very exact, as for curative purpose the total dose is limited by an accepted degree of risk for complications, and a misjudgement in dose of about 5 to 10% might be disastrous.

This chapter presents the results concerning the late reactions which allow us to (1) characterize the correlation between acute and late effects, (2) construct dose-response curves for acute and late effects within a limited dose range, and (3) calculate a preliminary correction factor for the CRE formula for late effects.

Final conclusions can only be drawn after a follow-up period of 5 years.

Patients and Methods

PATIENTS

The skin reaction was studied in the parasternal region of patients operated upon for breast carcinoma. In most studies the patients were irradiated on two bilateral fields with different dose schedules. Each patient thus served as her own control.

A comparison of different fractionation schedules was also performed between groups of patients irradiated unilaterally in the parasternal region.

RADIATION PROCEDURE

Electron beams of 12 and 13 MeV, and x-rays of 200 kV, HVL 1.2 mm Cu, were used. The field size was 5 × 12 cm². Each dose fraction was checked with TL dosimeters.

EARLY SKIN REACTIONS

The skin erythema and pigmentation were measured by reflectance spectrophotometry, as described earlier.[11,12] The reproducibility of this method in determination of the acute skin erythema in four series spread over several years is shown in Table 1. The four dose schedules were predicted to give the same biological effect. It is evident that the dosimetry and the spectrophotometry method used are reliable, and that the applied RBE values of 1.18 and 1.0 are reasonable for the 200 kV x-rays and the electron beams, respectively.

The good reproducibility of the model enables conclusions to be drawn from relatively small series of patients (about 25–35 patients), and permits construction of dose-response curves by combining different series of patients. Moreover, the long follow-up required for late reactions results in natural loss of patients. By adding different series, more reliable results can be obtained.

LATE SKIN REACTIONS

The development of telangiectasia was

TABLE 1.

Year of Investigation	Total dose (Skin Surface)	Radiation Quality	RBE	^{60}Co-equivalent dose (Skin Surface)	Maximum erythema (95% Conf.)
1974	16 X 235 R	x-rays hvl: 1.2 mm^3	1.18	16 X 2.54 Gy	49.3 ± 3.5
1978	16 X 2.15 Gy	Hvl: 1.2 mm^3	1.18	16 X 2.54 Gy	51.4 ± 2.1
1974	4 X 675 R	x-rays hvl:1.2 mm^3	1.18	4 X 7.29 Gy	50.4 ± 3.5
1977	4 X 7.29 Gy	electron beam 12 MeV	1.0	4 X 7.29 Gy	52.4 ± 3.5

TABLE 2. Scoring System for Late Reactions in Human Skin

Relative Score	Absolute Score
0 = No difference in telangiectasia	0 = No telangiectasia
1 = Minimal difference in telangiectasia	1 = Minimal telangiectasia
2 = Distinct difference in telangiectasia	2 = Distinct telangiectasia
3 = Very marked difference	3 = Very marked telangiectasia

registered every 3–4 months on an arbitrary scale comprising both a *relative* score of the difference in reaction between two fields in the same patient and an *absolute* score (see Table 2). Scoring of the difference in telangiectasia–i.e., the relative score–is the most sensitive method and is possible when the patient is her own control. But the absolute score is necessary for comparison between various series and for patients irradiated unilaterally only. A photograph is also taken at each control, both during the acute phase and during the follow-up.

FRACTIONATION SCHEDULES

In one study, the dose per fraction was varied between 1.0 and 7.3 Gy, the frequency between 1 and 15 fractions per week, and the total number of fractions between 4 and 50, within an overall treatment time of 3–4 weeks.

In a second study, the fractionation schedules of 5 × 1.8 Gy per week and 2 × 3.6 Gy per week with irradiation during 5–6 weeks were compared.

Results

The development of telangiectasia after one and five fractions per week for CRE is shown in Figure 2. The series includes 27 patients irradiated bilaterally. The influence of the individual differences is thus minimized. The curves "score ≥ 1" include all patients with any degree of telangiectasia: minimal, distinct, or very marked. The curves "score ≥ 2" include the patients with distinct or very marked telangiectasia. The curves "score = 3" include only patients with very marked telangiectasia.

After 5 years 50% of the patients were completely free from telangiectasia after five fractions per week, compared with only 17% of the patients treated with one fraction per week. Moreover, no patient had very marked telangiectasia after five fractions per week, compared with 50% of the patients after one fraction per week.

However, the telangiectasia has a very slow time course, and only the curves for score ≥ 1 had flattened out after 4 years and allowed final conclusions. It is possible that

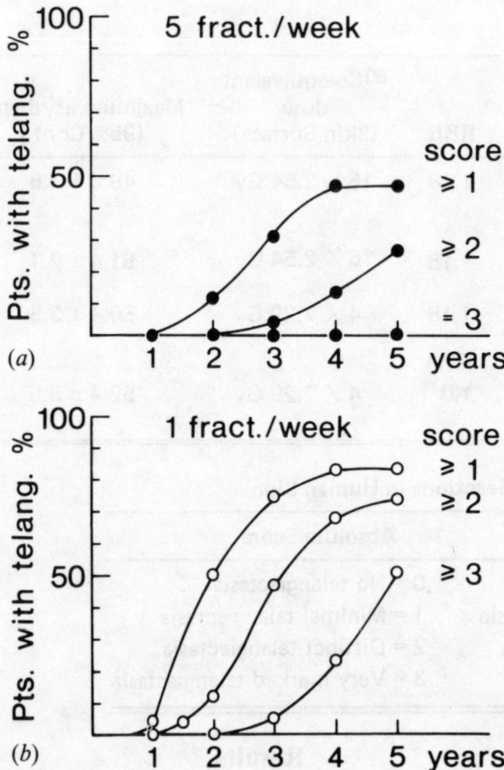

Figure 2. The development of telangiectasia after (*a*) five fractions per week (16 × 2.54 Gy within 22 days) and (*b*) one fraction per week (4 × 7.29 Gy within 22 days) for CRE 15. The acute reactions were identical (see Turesson and Notter, 1976).

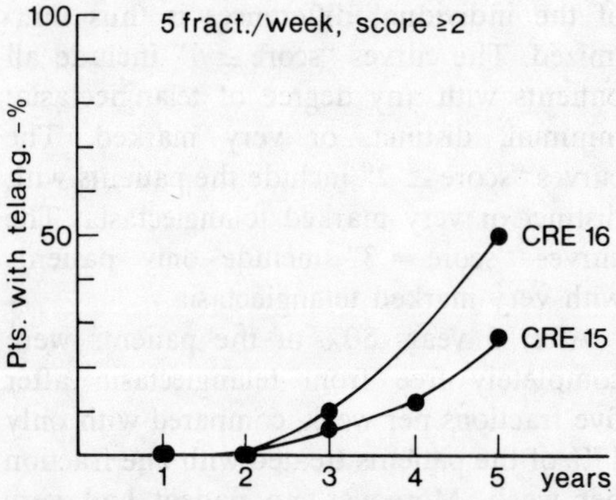

Figure 3. The development of telangiectasia after 5 fractions per week for CRE 15 and CRE 16.

all patients who had developed minimal telangiectasia will also develop very marked telangiectasia if the follow-up is long enough. The slow time course for late effects therefore may result in an inherent source

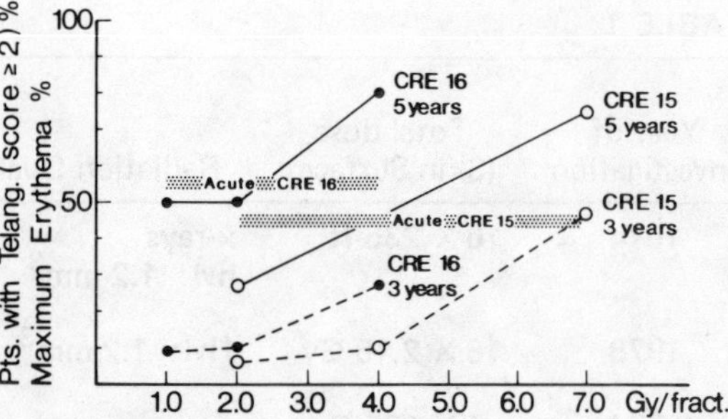

Figure 4. The percent of maximum acute erythema and number of patients with telangiectasia as a function of dose per fraction at 3 and 5 years for CRE 15 and CRE 16. Doses per fraction of 1, 2, 4, and 7 Gy correspond to 15, 5, 2, and 1 fraction per week, respectively.

of error in clinical and experimental studies if the follow-up is too short.

On the other hand, a score of 1 represents a very small and therefore uncertain effect. More reliable conclusions can be drawn when distinct telangiectasia has developed, i.e., when the curves "score ≥ 2" have flattened out. But this end point requires more than 5 years follow-up within this dose range which means that some patients will probably be lost to follow-up.

Figure 3 shows the proportion of patients with telangiectasia at two dose levels—CRE 15 and 16—after five fractions per week of about 2 Gy. At 5 years there is a significant difference.

In Figure 4 the results of follow-up of the patients thus far is summarized. The acute reactions and the incidence of telangiectasia with a score of ≥ 2 at 3 and 5 years for two CRE levels are plotted against the dose per fraction (the dose per fraction plotted here was rounded off for simplicity).

As stated above for acute reactions, the CRE formula predicts equivalent dose levels between 1 and 7 Gy per fraction, provided irradiation during pronounced reactions is avoided.

Concerning late reactions a dose per fraction above 2 Gy results in more pronounced reactions than predicted by the CRE (NSD) formula or by the acute reactions. Below 2 Gy per fraction there is no sparing of late reactions relative to the acute reactions, and

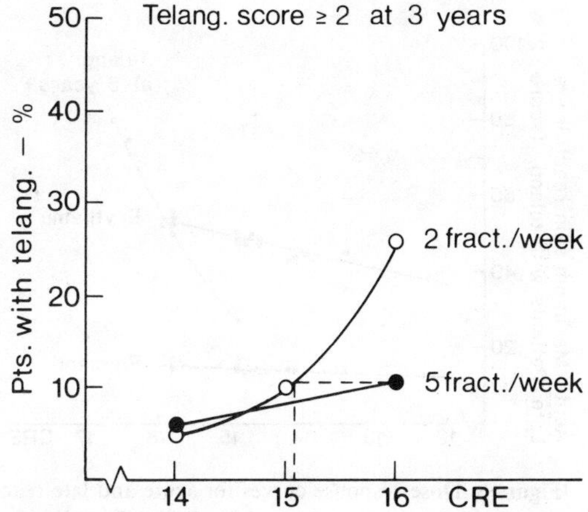

Figure 5. Number of patients with telangiectasia at 3 years. The solid circles represent fractionation schedule 5 × 1.8 Gy per week–25 and 30 fractions within 5 and 6 weeks, respectively. The open circles represent fractionation schedules 2 × 3.6 Gy per week–10, 11, and 12 fractions within 5, 5.5, and 6 weeks.

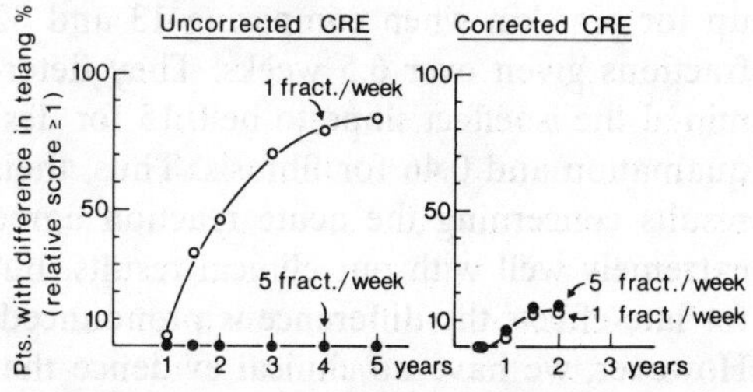

Figure 6. Percent of patients with difference in telangiectasia (i.e., a relative score ≥ 1 when five fractions per week were compared with one fraction per week). The total doses were calculated according to (*a*) the uncorrected formula (16 × 2.54 Gy compared with 4 × 7.29 Gy within 22 days) and (*b*) the corrected formula (16 × 2.54 Gy compared with 4 × 6.63 Gy within 22 days).

the CRE formula is valid. However, it is evident that for late reactions the CRE and (NSD) formulae have to be corrected for doses per fraction above 2 Gy.

Discussion

It is important to express the higher incidence of telangiectasia in terms of absorbed dose which should also allow correction of the CRE (NSD) formula for late effects. A very preliminary correction, calculated from the dose-effect curves of five and two fractions per week after 3 years follow-up, is presented in Figure 5. Changing from 1.8 Gy to 3.6 Gy per fraction at an effect level of CRE 16 should be corrected for by 6%—i.e., a change from 3.6 Gy to 3.4 Gy per fraction. The same correction was valid for score ≥ 1 and score ≥ 2.

It must be emphasized that the configurations of the dose-response curves are such that the correction depends on the effect level. No difference in late effects could clinically be distinguished for CRE 14 after 3 years follow-up. The weakness in this study is the low dose level, and the question is whether this correction is enough at higher dose levels.

However, from observations in patients irradiated with 2.6 Gy and 4.5 Gy per fraction to CRE 19 and 21 we conclude that a correction of the CRE formula by about 5% is reasonable when changing from dose fractions of about 2 Gy to 4 Gy.

We have also repeated an earlier study comparing five fractions and one fraction per week with a dose reduction of 10% for the once-a-week irradiation (see Fig. 6). In judging early trends the difference in telangiectasia between the two fields was scored (see Table 2). For example, when we used the uncorrected CRE formula about 50% of the patients demonstrated more telangiectasia at 2 years after one fraction compared to five fractions per week. No patient showed more telangiectasia after five fractions per week. However, after the dose reduction the same number of patients had more severe reactions after five fractions as after one fraction per week. So far, with only a limited follow-up of 2 years, the correction of the CRE formula by about 10% when changing from about 2–7 Gy per fraction seems reasonable. We have earlier postulated this correction from experimental data published in the literature.[13] The correction factor was correlated to the dose per fraction.

Since then more experimental data on late effects have been published by van der Kogel[14] and White and Hornsey[15] which

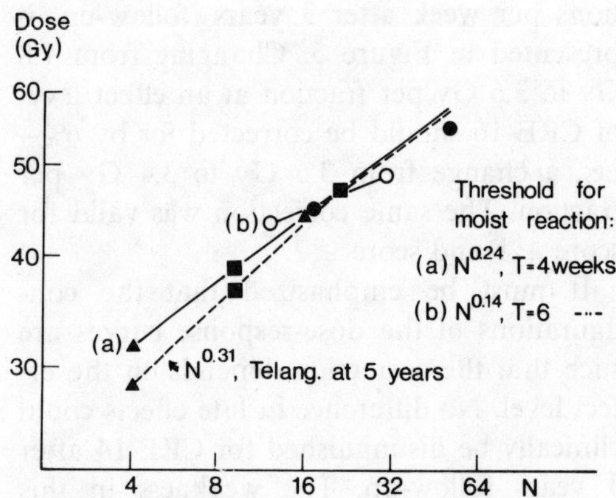

Figure 7. Isoeffect doses as a function of the number of fractions for acute and late reactions in human skin. Solid triangles = 4 to 16 fractions; solid squares = 9 to 21 fractions; solid circles = 17 to 50 fractions in bilateral parasternal irradiation; and open circles = 12 to 30 fractions in unilateral parasternal irradiation.

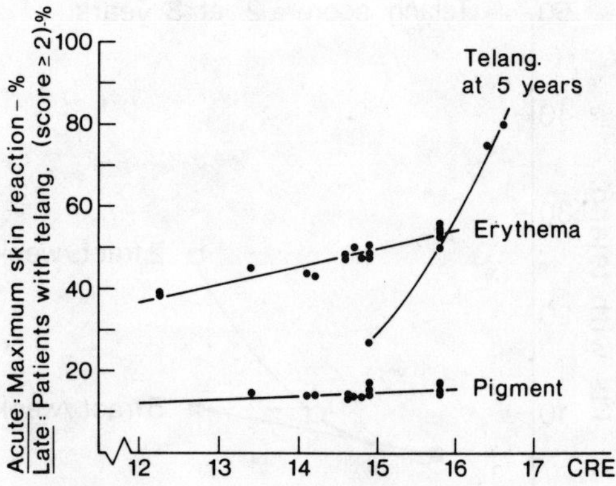

Figure 8. Dose-response curves for acute and late reactions in human skin as a function of CRE. The dose-response curve for telangiectasia is valid for five fractions per week of about 2 Gy.

agree rather well with our correction factor. An important point is that White and Hornsey report a much longer latent period after smaller doses per fraction (i.e., for 15 and 30 fractions) than after single doses or a few large fractions.

Most commentators have described the importance of the dose per fraction in terms of an exponent for N, i.e. the number of fractions. Figure 7 summarizes the isoeffect doses as a function of fraction number for the early and late skin reactions in our clinical studies, for comparison with results published in the literature. For acute reactions we found that the slope 0.24 for N is valid between 4 and 50 fractions if the overall treatment time is limited to 4 weeks. Between 12 and 30 fractions the slope for N became 0.14 when the overall treatment time was 6 weeks.

For late effects the correction corresponds to a slope of 0.31 between 4 and 30 fractions, i.e., from about 7–2 Gy per fraction. However, we found no reason to abandon the exponent 0.24 for doses per fraction below 2 Gy or for a number of fractions above 30.

The isoeffect slope between 12 and 30 fractions given within 6 weeks was 0.14 for the acute reaction and 0.31 for telangiectasia at 5 years (calculated from the results in Figures 1 and 5, respectively). Withers et al.[16] used almost the same experimental setup for pig skin when comparing 13 and 32 fractions given over 6.5 weeks. They determined the isoeffect slope to be 0.15 for desquamation and 0.46 for fibrosis. Thus, their results concerning the acute reaction agree extremely well with our clinical results, but for late effects the difference is pronounced. However, we have no clinical evidence that our correction factor is too small.

A few words about skin reactions as end points. Dose-response curves for the acute and late effects in our investigations are presented in Figure 8. Erythema is significantly correlated to CRE and is useful as an acute end point up to CRE 16. Above that effect level there is a risk of moist desquamation. On the other hand, pigmentation is not correlated to dose in this range. Compared with the acute reactions, the dose-incidence curve for telangiectasia at 5 years (valid for five fractions per week of about 2 Gy) is much steeper, indicating the degree of accuracy required in clinical dosage.

Summary

These clinical investigations of various dose-fractionation regimens on human skin show that:

– The late reactions cannot be predicted from the early reactions.
– The dose-response curves for late reactions are much steeper than for early reactions.
– Equivalent doses for various fractionation schedules concerning late effects can be calculated by means of a corrected CRE (NSD) formula; the correction must be considered preliminary because further follow-up is needed.

A clinical fractionation study of this type requires:

– Extremely careful dosimetry
– Study of the same anatomical region
– Very long follow-up
– Studies at different effect levels

Skin reaction is the only end point we have studied systematically for different fractionation regimens. Our experience with the CRE formula as a model for calculating isoeffect doses for different fractionation schedules in routine clinical use can be summarized as follows:

– The CRE formula has been used prospectively since 1972 in all patients.
– CRE-equivalent weekly doses to 5 × 2.0 Gy per week has been used. (Although the fractionation schedule is changed, the overall treatment time is still the same).
– The CRE range was 18 to 21 for curative radiotherapy on carcinomas.
– No irradiation was applied during pronounced acute reactions.

No unexpected complications have been observed under these conditions.

REFERENCES

1. Arcangeli, G., Freidman, M., and Paoluzi, R.: A quantitative study of late radiation effect on normal skin and subcutaneous tissues in human beings. *Br J Radiol* **47**:44–50, 1974.
2. Bates, T.D., and Peters, L.J.: Danger of the clinical use of the NSD formula for small fraction numbers. *Br J Radiol* **48**:773, 1975.
3. Berry, R.J., Wiernik, G., and Patterson, R.J.S.: Skin tolerance to fractionated X-irradiation in the pig–how good a predictor is the NSD formula? *Br J Radiol* **47**:185–190, 1974.
4. Chu, F.C.H., Glicksman, A.S., and Nickson, J.J.: Late consequences of early skin reactions. *Radiology* **96**:669–672, 1970.
5. Denekamp, J.: Changes in the rate of proliferation in normal tissues after irradiation. In *Radiation Research: Biomedical, Chemical, and Physical Perspectives* O.F. Nygaard, H.I. Adler, and W.K. Sinclair, eds. New York: Academic Press, 1975, pp. 810–825.
6. Ellis, F.: Fractionation in radiotherapy. In *Modern Trends in Radiotherapy*, Vol. 1, T.J. Deely and C.A.P. Wook, eds. London, Butterworths, 1967, pp. 34–51.
7. Field, S.B., and Michalowski, A.: Endpoints for damage to normal tissues. *Int J Radiat Oncol Biol Phys* **5**:1185–1196, 1979.
8. Kirk, J., Gray, W.M., and Watson, E.R.: Cumulative radiation effect. I. Fractionated treatment regimes. *Clin Radiol* **22**:145–155, 1971.
9. Morrisson, R.: The results of treatment of cancer of the bladder–a clinical contribution to radiobiology. *Clin Radiol* **26**:67–75, 1975.
10. Stewart, J.G., and Jackson, A.W.: The steepness of the dose response curve both for tumour cure and normal tissue injury. *Laryngoscope* **85**:1107–1111, 1975.
11. Turesson, I., and Notter, G.: Skin reactions after different fractionation schedules give the same cumulative radiation effect. *Acta Radiol Ther* **14**:475–484, 1975.
12. Turesson, I., and Notter, G.: Control of dose administered once a week and three times a day according to schedules calculated by the CRE formula, using skin reaction as a biological parameter. *Radiology* **120**:399–401, 1976.
13. Turesson, I., and Notter, G.: The response of pig skin to single and fractionated high dose-rate and continuous low dose-rate ^{137}Cs-irradiation. III. Re-evaluation of the CRE system and the TDF system according to the present findings. *Int J Radiat Oncol Biol Phys* **5**:1773–1779, 1979.
14. van der Kogel, A.J.: Late effects of radiation on the spinal cord. Thesis, Rijswijk, Netherlands, 1979.
15. White, A., and Hornsey, S.: Radiation damage to the rat spinal cord: The effect of single and fractionated doses of x-rays. *Br J Radiol* **51**:515–523, 1978.
16. Withers, H.R., Thames, H.D., Flow, B.L., Mason, K.A., and Hussey, D.H.: The relationship of acute to late skin injury in 2 and 5 fractions per week γ-ray therapy. *Int J Radiat Oncol Biol Phys* **4**:595–601, 1978.

CHAPTER 25

Changing Concepts in the Tolerance of Radioresistant and Radiosensitive Normal Tissues and Organs

Philip Rubin, M.D.[a]
Henry Keys, M.D.[b]
Colin Poulter, M.D.[c]

There are no radiation tolerance doses *per se* for normal tissues and organs in this combined modality era. The concepts of radioresistance and/or radiosensitivity can no longer be viewed in isolation in both a biologic and clinical sense. The vast radiation biology and pathology literature[25,41] built upon numerous laboratory experiments both *in vivo* and *in vitro* is gradually being supplanted–and after decades of clinical practice. Late effects in patients are occurring after the delivery of "safe" doses below threshold levels. The additive effects of multiagent chemotherapy, prior to, during, or after a course of radiation has altered set patterns of radiation response, and untoward reactions occur at different times and in an unpredictable fashion.[51] In a similar manner, the innovations in the radiation armametarium[40]–such as high LET radiation (neutrons), hyperthermia, and hypoxic-cell radiosensitizers–when added to or mixed with conventional photons, are producing unexpected late effects. The increase in second malignancies and leukemia is also of concern to oncologists combining different modes, i.e., chemotherapy and radiation.[38]

[a]Professor and Chairman, Department of Radiation Oncology, University of Rochester Cancer Center, Rochester, New York
[b]Assistant Professor, Department of Radiation Oncology, University of Rochester Cancer Center, Rochester, New York
[c]Associate Professor, Department of Radiation Oncology, University of Rochester Cancer Center, Rochester, New York

The concept of treatment optimization by adding two or more modes implies increasing cure rates. However, it must be accomplished without increasing toxicity or, alternately, maintaining cure rates but decreasing toxicity. The focus in reporting results has tended to stress an increase in response rates rather than better therapeutic ratios. Often the immediate or early known tumor effects are reported before late effects can occur or be analyzed. In this presentation, a brief review of "classic concepts" in radiation resistance and radiation sensitivity of normal tissues and organs will be offered, and then unique reactions and complications will be surveyed in a variety of vital tissues.

True vs. Apparent Radioresistance of Cells

The concept of cellular radioresistance or radiosensitivity is based upon *in vitro* measurements of cloning before and after irradiation. The radiation characteristics of mammalian cells is defined in terms of D_q and D_o–the shoulder and slope of the survival curve.[25] The longer the shoulder and the shallower the slope–increase in the D_q and D_o–the greater the degree of radioresistance in that larger radiation doses are required for the same degree of cell kill.

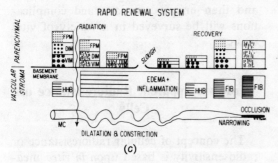

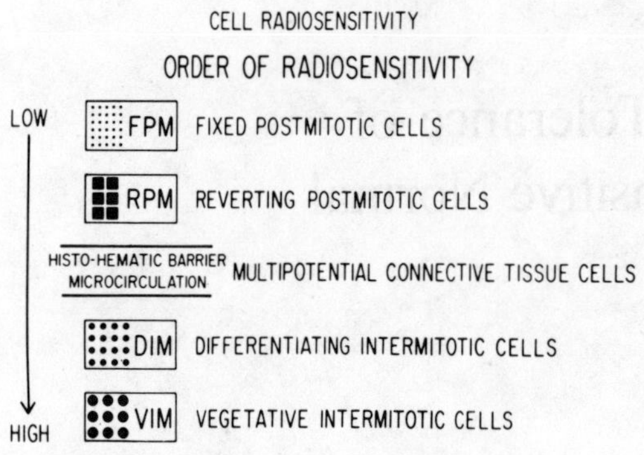

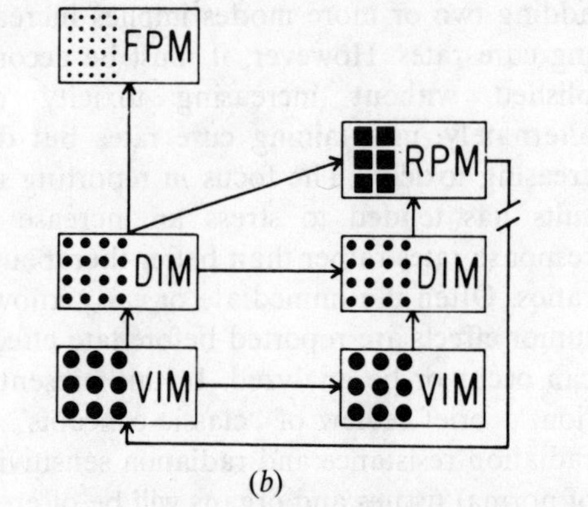

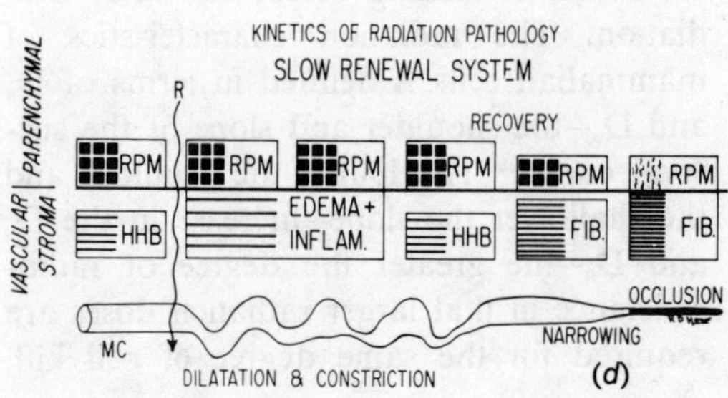

Figure 1. The concept of relative radiation sensitivity and radioresistance is shown based on the criterion of cell death previously described and defined by Casarett and rests on the mitotic behavior and potential of cells. Thus, vegetative (VIC) and differentiating into mitotic cells (DIM) are more radiosensitive than reverting postmitotic (RPM) or fixed postmitotic (FRM) cells which are more radioresistant. (*a*) Cell radiosensitivity and resistance is shown in reference to the histo-hematic barrier microcirculation consisting of multipotential connective tissue cells which are considered to be at the center of the scale of reference cells. (*b*) Tissues are generally organized in two patterns and according to their cell kinetics in maturation. On the left-hand side, most epithelial linings are illustrated for epidermal and epithelial surfaces having a stem cell compartment and a mature functioning cell which is a mixed postmitotic cell. On the right-hand side, there are tissues that have a large capacity for regeneration and have reverting postmitotic cells best illustrated by the liver. (*c*) The cell kinetics of the events in rapid renewal systems is shown following irradiation with the predominant effect on the radiosensitive component–mainly the intermitotic cell or stem cell–with a delay to onset of symptoms according to the cell-cycle length. Recovery is also a function of surviving cells. A different response is taking place in the vasculo-connective tissue stroma, referred to as the histo-hematic barrier (HHB), with the initial response being edema and inflammation, with changes in the microcirculation (MC) of dilatation and constriction with gradual resolution leading to fibrosis (FIB) and a build-up of the histo-hematic barrier with narrowing and occlusion of the microcirculation, which in turn, if complete, leads to necrosis and destruction of all cells as a later event. Thus, there are two periods of expression of radiation injury. (*d*) The cell kinetics of the slow renewal system differ in that there is very little change following irradiation in the acute or early stage. The dominant events in the histo-hematic barrier and microcirculation are similar to those in rapid renewal systems. However, the latent period for change is long and is only seen in the chronic or late period where the histo-hematic barrier and fibrosis coupled with changes in the microcirculation leading to occlusion result in severe tissue and cellular necrosis. The events in the kidney are a clear illustration of these types of changes. (Data from Rubin and Casarett, 1968.)

Phenomena that increase the capacity of cells to repair or repopulate following radiation add to the "radioresistance" of tissues as compared to reoxygenation or reassortment or recruitment that tend to increase this radiosensitivity.[13] A listing of cells by their D_o value is often considered their in-

herent or essential radiosensitivity in a radiobiologic sense and rests upon measuring response in a normal environment or media. Conditional radiosensitivity refers to environmental changes such as changes in oxygen levels with photon radiation that in turn alter cell response. In addition, a concept of relative radiation resistance is based upon criterion of cell death previously described and defined by Casarett[41] and rests on the mitotic behavior and potential of cells. Thus, vegatative (VIC) and differentiating intermitotic cells (DIM) are more radiosensitive than reverting postmitotic (RPM) or fixed postmitotic (FRM) cells which are more radioresistant (see Fig. 1).

Relative Radioresistance of Tissues[41]

The relative radioresistance of tissues is determined largely by the radiosensitivity of its parenchymal cells, and in the case of an organ containing a variety of different cells, the relative radiosensitivity of the organ is determined by its most radiosensitive cells. The response is further conditioned by the fine vasculature, the fibroconnective tissue, and the relative oxygenation of the tissue during irradiation. The radiation sensitivity of the microvasculature is in between VIC and DIM cells versus RPM and FPM cells. The various types of tissue and organs are listed in their order of decreasing radiosensitivity based upon direct radiation effect or hypoplasia of cells (see Table 1).

There is much room for argument regarding the relative precise order of different tissues and organs, especially with different criteria used; but in the case of *in vitro* tissue and organs, damage to the microcirculatory apparatus can occur after moderate dose schedules in a longer period of time or can appear more rapidly with larger doses in a short time. The expression of radiation injury occurs earlier for rapidly renewing tissues with short cell cycles versus slow renewal tissues with very long cell cycles and small fractions of actively dividing cells.

Concept of Tissue and Organ Recovery and Replacement Fibrosis[41]

The term recovery is used in a general way relating to the degree to which a tissue or organ returns to its preirradiation normal functional and morphologic status. Repair processes are typical or primary processes, i.e., healing by primary intention or atypical or secondary processes–healing by secondary intention. Primary repair processes include the cellular concept of repair of sublethal damage measured as the D_q or repopulation by surviving stem cells (homeotypic regeneration), or by transformation of different cells not regularly engaged in the production of cells of the kind lost (heterotypic transformation). For example, a radiation response to depletion of bone marrow stem cells within the bone stimulates a heterotypic transformation of cells lining the Haversian canals in cortical bone which form new bone marrow cells.[42,44]

Secondary repair processes are those by which tissue cells are killed by irradiation and replaced by fibrosis. The lost parenchymal cells are often associated with microcirculatory damage and injury to the interstitial connective tissue which promotes a replacement fibrosis.[41] This set of events deserves much more study and has been neglected in all *in vitro* as well as many *in vivo* systems. As in any scar formation, replacement fibrosis usually involves a decrease in the original functional capacity and resilience, owing to replacement of more specialized cells and tissue by inferior tissue. Furthermore, this fibrotic tissue often tends to degenerate progressively and to break down more easily than normal tissue under further insults, leading to neurosis. Histopathologically, a permanent residual damage occurs after irradiation, but also includes such changes as genetic mutations, chromosomal aberrations, and other intracellular

TABLE 1. Organs in Decreasing Order of Relative Radiosensitivity Based on Relatively Direct Organ Effect (Parenchymal Hypoplasia)[a]

Organs	Relative Radiosensitivity	Chief Mechanisms of Parenchymal Hypoplasia
Lymphoid organs Bone marrow (and blood) Testes Ovaries Intestines	High	Destruction of parenchymal cells, especially the vegetative or differentiating intermitotic cells that are precursors to the mature parenchymal cells
Skin and other organs with epidermoid linings (cornea, oral cavity, esophagus, rectum, vagina, uterine cervix, urinary bladder, ureters, etc.)	Fairly high	Destruction of vegetative and differentiating intermitotic cells of stratified epithelium
Optic lens, stomach		Destruction of proliferating epithelial cells
Fine vasculature	Medium	Damage of endothelium, plus some inflammatory reaction to destruction of associated, dependent, sensitive parenchymal cells
Growing cartilage		Destruction of proliferating chondroblasts, plus some damage of fine vasculature and connective tissue elements
Growing bone		Destruction of connective tissue cells and chondroblasts or osteoblasts, plus some damage of fine vasculature
Mature cartilage or bone Salivary glands Respiratory organs Kidneys Liver Thyroid Adrenal Pituitary	Fairly low	Hypoplasia secondary to damage of fine vasculature and connective tissue elements with relatively less contribution by direct effects on parenchymal tissues
Muscles Brain Spinal cord Heart muscle	Low	Hypoplasia secondary to damage of fine vasculature and connective tissue elements with little contribution by direct effects on parenchymal tissues

[a] Data from Rubin and Casarett, 1968.

defects, as well as permanent hypoplasia, fibroatrophy, and an increase in the histohematic barrier and reduction in the reserve functional and regenerative capacity of tissues.

Histopathologic Sequence of Events[41]

The clinical pathologic course of events is illustrated in the indicated diagrams and shows the relationship between reparable

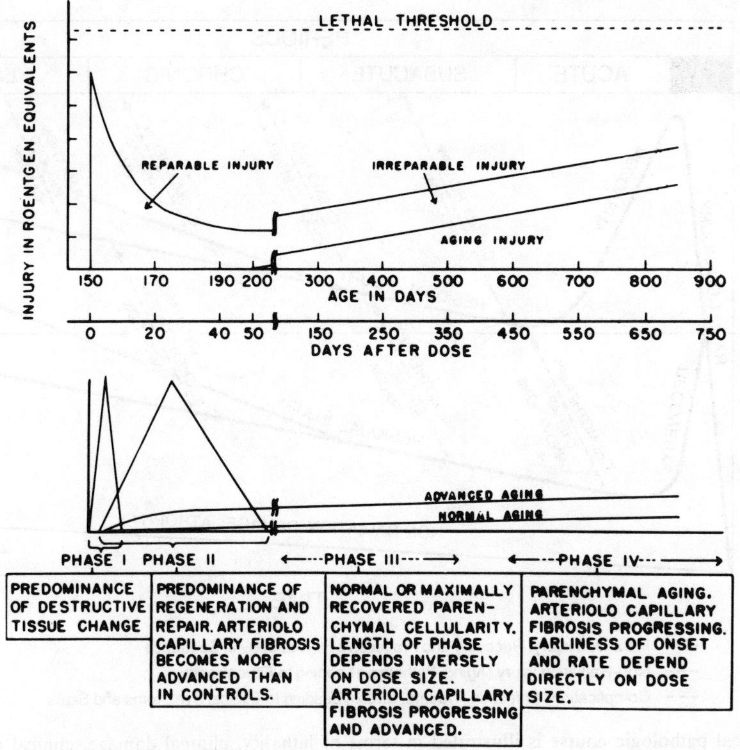

Figure 2. The clinical pathologic course of events is illustrated showing the relationship between reparable and irreparable components of radiation injury and temporal phases in the histopathologic sequence of reversible and irreversible effects. (Data from Casarett, 1963.)

and unreparable components of radiation injury and temporal phases in the histopathologic sequences of reversible and irreversible effects (see Figs. 2 and 3).

At no time is there a silent histopathologic period, although the degree or rate of progression may vary considerably. With electron microscopy, early cellular lesions can be identified that may not be recognized on a light microscopy level. This is well illustrated by rapid changes identified in alveolar type-II cells immediately after irradiation seen ultrastructurally but not appreciated on routine histopathologic level.

Furthermore, the addition of more stress or insult to organs by other modalities and innovations combined concurrently with irradiation or added later to tissues that have sustained radiation treatment may precipitate clinically significant complications during an otherwise clinically "silent" period. The trauma or infection with surgery, the additivity of chemotherapeutic agents (both cycle and phase-specific agents), and the effects of treatment innovations previously mentioned may dramatically alter radioresistant tissues and organs or change this tolerance. The concept of tissue or organ senescence[6] following chemotherapy is essential to comprehending the "unexpected" late effects that are gradually becoming better understood. All normal cells and tissues have limited regenerative capacities–the feature that distinguishes a normal cell from a transformed cell. Radiation therapy and chemotherapy use up these tissue reserves and lead to stem cell depletion or premature tissue senescence.

Dose-Limiting Organs and Tissues in Radiation Oncology

The categorization of organs and tissues

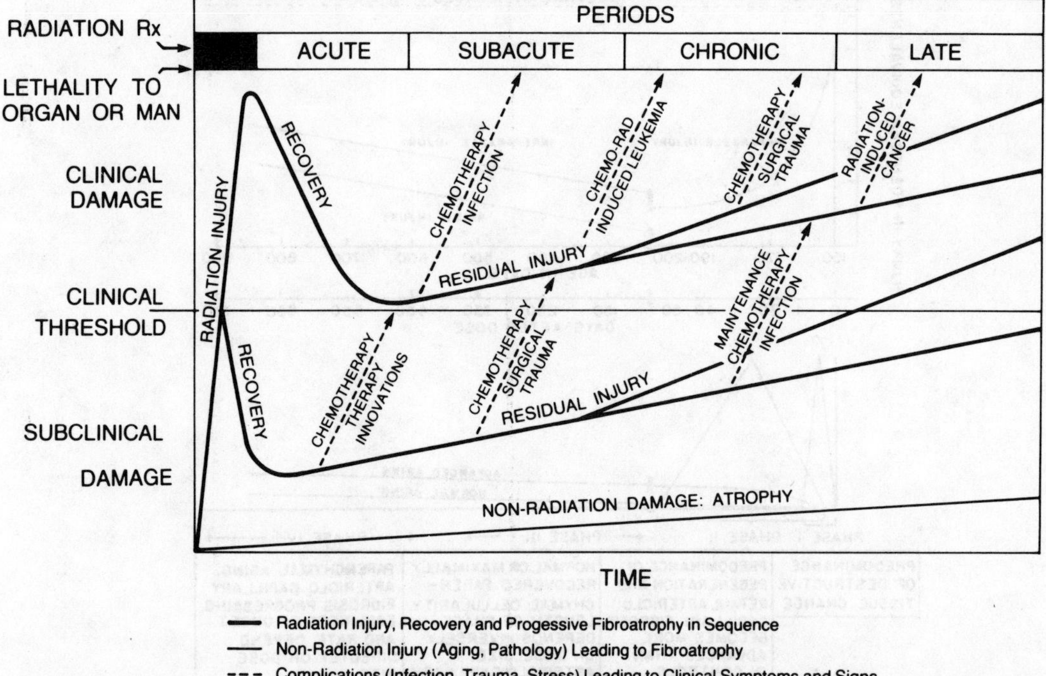

Figure 3. The clinical pathologic course is illustrated in terms of lethality, clinical damage, clinical threshold, and subclinical damage on one scale and time on the other. The sequence of events following a high or low dose is illustrated by two lines which are parallel to the aging or nonradiation damage or atrophy that occurs normally in tissues. There are many events that can change the level of residual injury in the slope of the line, such as surgical trauma, infection, and, more important, chemotherapeutic agents and new radiation therapy innovations. These are major factors influencing the changing concepts in tissue and organ radiosensitivity and radioresistance.

into three classes was done to define the relative dose limitations of each organ in radiation treatment.[43] This is an arbitrary organization and stresses the vitalness of the organ or tissue for survival versus severe morbidity with injury. It is an attempt to define the life threatening and severe complications from more moderate or perhaps reversible injuries. The first category applies to class-I organs (see Table 2) in which radiation lesions are fatal or result in severe morbidity. The second category applies to class-II organs (see Table 3) in which radiation lesions result in moderate to mild morbidity and, in exceptional circumstances, fatality; permanent sequelae, however, are generally compatible with survival. The third category applies to class-III organs (see Table 4) in which radiation lesions result in mild, transient, reversible effects or in no morbidity. The tolerance dose consists of minimal tissue tolerance dose ($TTD_5\Sigma_5$) which is defined as that dose associated with a 5% rate of complications occurring within 5 years of treatment; maximal tissue tolerance dose is the dose associated with a 50% complication rate over the same time span ($TTD_{50}\Sigma_5$) (see Fig. 4).

The concept of normal standard dose (NSD) of Ellis[14] was basically designed to be applied to normal tissues and organs. Recent literature in experimental systems shows it needs to be modified for early versus late effects and may not be an accurate predictor. However, for various critical normal organs, it is desirable to think in terms of NSD, and where data is lacking it can be utilized as a guide whenever applying unfamiliar or unique fractionation regimens or split courses in clinical practice. That is, a

TABLE 2. Class-I Organs: Fatal/Severe Morbidity[a]

Organ	Injury	$TD_{5/5}$	$TD_{50/5}$	Whole or Partial Organ (Field size or length)	Reference
Bone marrow	Aplasia, pancytopenia	250	450	Whole	Bond et al.
		3000	4000	Segmental	Rubin et al.
Liver	Acute and chronic hepatitis	2500	4000	Whole	Ingold et al., 1965
		1500	2000	Whole strip	Kraut et al., Tefft
Stomach	Performation, ulcer, hemorrhage	4500	5500	100 cm	Friedman, 1952
Intestine	Ulcer, perforation, hemorrhage	4500	5500	400 cm	Friedman, 1952
		5000	6500	100 cm	Roswit et al.
					Palmer
Brain	Infarction, necrosis	5000	6000	Whole	Kramer et al., 1972
Spinal cord	Infarction, necrosis	4500	5500	10 cm	Phillips and Buschke, 1969
Heart	Pericarditis and pancarditis	4500	5500	60%	Wara et al., 1973
					Newton
					Stewart and Fajardo
		7000	8000	25%	Lindgren
Lung	Acute and chronic pneumonitis	3000	3500	100 cm	Gish et al.
					Lokick et al.
		1500	2500	Whole	Wara et al., 1973
Kidney	Acute and chronic nephrosclerosis	1500	2000	Whole (strip)	Kraut et al., Tefft
		2000	2500	Whole	Kunkler et al.
					Luxton and Kunkler
Fetus	Death	200	400	Whole	Ruch

[a]Data from Rubin et al., 1975.

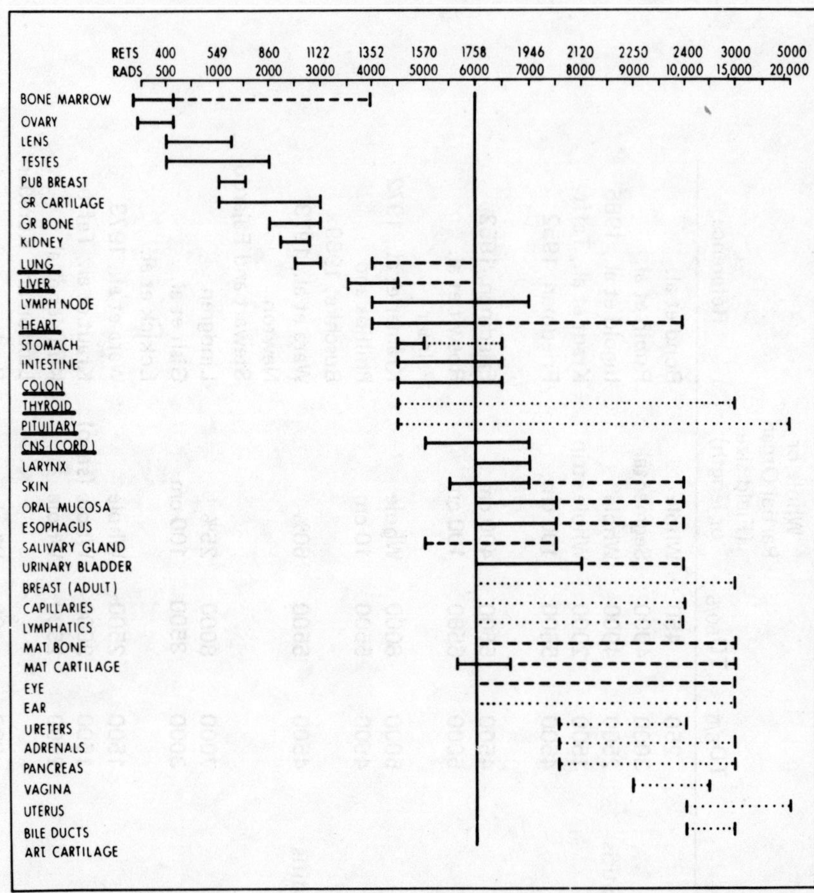

Figure 4. Each line plotted is a linear display of the tolerance dose for each of the organs listed. The tolerance dose can be read in rad at the top of the diagram and starts with the minimum tissue tolerance ($TTD_5\Sigma_5$) which is defined as the dose associated with a 5% rate of complications occurring within 5 years of treatment; the end of the line is the maximum tissue tolerance dose which is the dose associated with 50% complication rate over the same time span ($TTD_{50}\Sigma_5$). The ret gradations are hypothesized based on conventional delivery of radiation in radiation therapy practice consisting of 200 rad/day, 1000 rad/week to total doses shown. The solid lines refer to whole organ irradiation, the dash lines to partial organ irradiation, and the dotted lines are estimations based upon experimental rather than human data. (Data from Rubin and Casarett, 1968.)

direct translation from rad at conventional fractionation schedules of 200 rad per day, 1000 rad per week will yield a ret dose that can be utilized as a "guide" for unorthodox fractionation schemes rather than relying upon the total rad dose alone. An illustration can be found from spinal cord complications data that have occurred after delivery of a seemingly safe rad dose within spinal cord tolerance. If a ret dose were used, it may have avoided overdosage;[29] however, these calculated ret doses are extrapolations and will need to be modified as experience is documented. As stated from animal experiments, NSD formula is different for early and late events and modification for each normal system may be required.[53]

Changing concepts in normal tissue and organ radioresistance will be illustrated by reexamination of some of the tenets presented by Rubin and Casarett in their

TABLE 3. Class-II Organs: Moderate/Mild Morbidity[a]

Organ	Injury	$TD_{5/5}$	$TD_{50/5}$	Whole or Partial Organ (Field Size or Length)
Oral cavity and pharynx	Ulceration, mucositis	6000	7500	50 cm
Skin	Acute and Chronic dermatitis	5500	7000	100 cm
Esophagus	Esophagitis, ulceration	6000	7500	75 cm
Rectum	Ulcer, stricture	6000	8000	100 cm
Salivary glands	Xerostomia	5000	7000	50 cm
Bladder	Contracture	6000	8000	Whole
Ureters	Stricture	7500	10,000	5–10 cm
Testes	Sterilization	100	200	Whole
Ovary	Sterilization	200–300	625–1200	Whole
Growing cartilage, bone (child)	Growth arrest, dwarfting	1000 1000	3000 3000	Whole 10 cm
Mature cartilage, bone (adult)	Necrosis, fracture, sclerosis	6000 6000	10,000 10,000	Whole 10 cm
Eye				
retina		5500	7000	Whole
cornea		5000	>6000	Whole
lens		500	1200	Whole or part
Endocrine Glands				
thyroid	Hypothyroidism	4500	15,000	Whole
adrenal	Hypoadrenalism	>6000	–	Whole
pituitary	Hypopituitarism	4500	20,000–30,000	Whole
Peripheral nerves	Neuritis	6000	10,000	10 cm
Ear				
Middle	Serous otitis	5000	7000	Whole
Vestibular	Meniere's syndrome	6000	7000	Whole

[a]Data from Rubin et al., 1975.

monograph, *Clinical Radiation Pathology* published in 1968. A series of so-called or classified radioresistant structures are much more vulnerable than previously thought only a decade later. This is due to the ability to deliver larger depth doses with megavoltage irradiation without limitations posed by skin reactions, to the widespread use of combination chemotherapy and radiation therapy in this multimodal era, and to innovations in radiation treatment introduced this past decade. It is apparent from the linear display of dose-response curves that there has been a shift of many of the radioresistant organs into a more radiosensitive category. This assumes 6000 rad/6 weeks is at the tolerance of vasculo-connective tissue stroma and is the dividing line between radiosensitive and radioresistant organs. Thus, the following organs no longer fit the radioresistant category and will be discussed in more detail: (1) lung; (2) heart; (3) liver; (4) colo-rectum; (5) CNS, brain, spinal cord; and (6) endocrine glands: thyroid and pituitary.

LUNG

In our original classification of relative radiosensitivity of tissues, respiratory epithelia was considered to be one of the more radio-

TABLE 4. Class-III Organs: Mild/No Morbidity[a]

Organ	Injury	$TD_{5/5}$	$TD_{50/50}$	Whole or Partial Organ (Field Size or Length)
Muscle (child)	Atrophy	2000–3000	4000–5000	Whole
Muscle (adult)	Fibrosis	6000	8000	Whole
Lymph nodes and Lymphatics	Atrophy, sclerosis	5000	>7000	Whole node
Large Arteries and viens	Sclerosis	>8000	>10,000	10 cm
Articular Cartilage	None	>50,000	>500,000	Joint surface (m.m.)
Uterus	Necrosis, Perforation	>10,000	>20,000	Whole
Vagina	Ulcer, Fistula	9000	>10,000	Whole
Breast (Child)	No Development	1000	1500	Whole
Breast (Adult)	Atrophy, Necrosis	>5000	>10,000	Whole

[a] Data from Rubin et al., 1975.

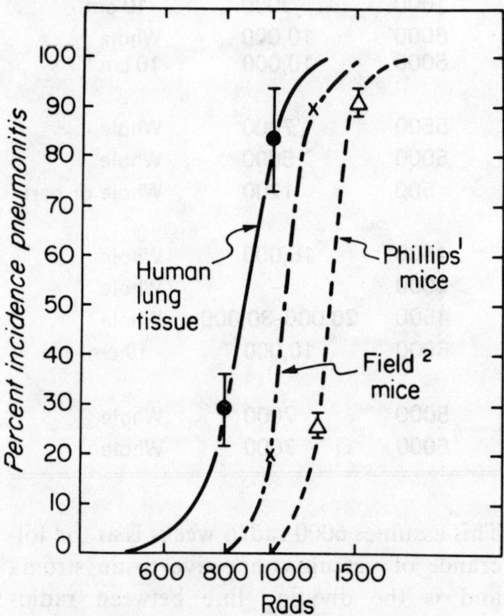

Figure 5. The incidence of radiation pneumonitis is a very steep dose-response curve and illustrates the sensitivity of the lung. There is a parallelism between the human data derived from the hemi-body irradiation experience from the Ontario Cancer Institute and the induction of radiation pneumonitis in mice from two different investigators. (Data from Fryer et al, 1978.)

resistant tissues. The reactions occurred usually in the postirradiation period weeks to months after the completion of a fractionated course of therapy. Recent evidence from both the clinical and laboratory arena suggest this is perhaps one of the most radiosensitive of all organs and, depending upon the dose/time factors, it is even more dose limiting than bone marrow when large field irradiation is used.

The most precise dose-effect data has emerged from the half-body irradiation program for palliating overt metastases from Toronto. In a careful series of studies, the following facts have emerged: Lethal radiation pneumonitis can occur with single doses of 700–800 rad and become uniformly fatal at 900–1000 rad indicating a very steep dose-response curve[20,23] (see Fig. 5). Correction for increased lung transmission with supervoltage radiation is essential, particularly for patients treated with telecobalt units.[53] Although this event can be reversible, it usually appears 3 months after irradiation is given and is most often progressive and fatal.[20] A parallel exists between animal dose-effect curves and human data.[23]

In the laboratory, dramatic early changes are seen in alveolar type-II cells[35] and have been correlated with the rapid release of surfactant identified in alveolar lavage specimens at 1 hour, 1 day, and 1 week.[45] The predictive value of these findings for fatality and later interstitial septal fibrosis is under study. The ultrastructural lesions are only detectable by electron microscopy; there are

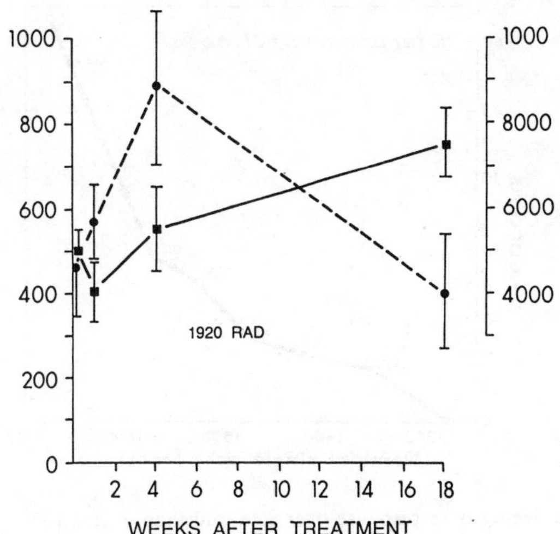

Figure 6. This illustrates the early release of surfactant following irradiation which continues to rise up to 4 weeks and to some degree is mirrored in the first week by the remaining surfactant in lung measured as animal phospholipid phosphorus. (●) = mmoles phospholipid phosphorus/2 lungs lavage. (■) = mmoles phospholipid phosphorus/2 lungs tissue homogenate.

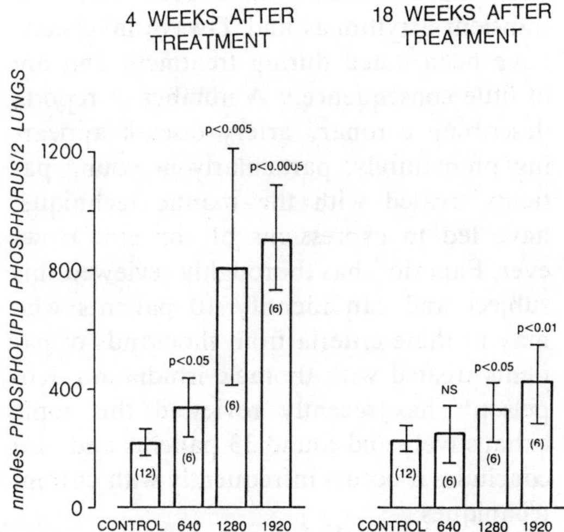

Figure 7. The marked increase of released surfactant measured by alveolar lavage shows a dramatic difference between 600 and 1200 rad suggesting a very deep dose response; this could be used as a biochemical marker to predict for lethality which occurs much later in the manifestation of an acute pneumonitis. These findings, when compared with Figure 5, suggest that alveolar surfactant levels may predict for later effects; this may be the first biochemical marker to predit for late radiation effects.

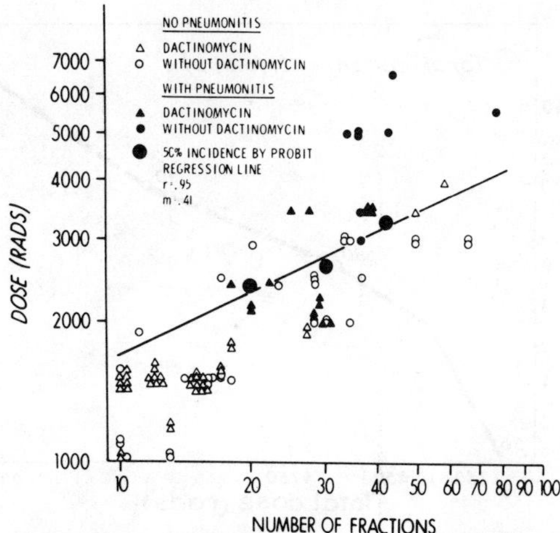

Figure 8. Dactinomycin D produces radiation pneumonitis with much lower doses of radiation. There is a 1000 to 2000 rad difference between the radiation dose producing pneumonitis with and without dactinomycin. (Data from Wara et al., 1973.)

no changes seen by light microscopy or clinical function studies until months later[33] (see Figs. 6 and 7).

A large number of drugs have been identified which produce pulmonary complications and include bleomycin, busulfan, chlorambucil, cyclophosphamide, melphalan, and BCNU.[57] One of the most intensively studied agents is BCNU which has resulted in severe, late pulmonary toxicity and lethality and was discovered unfortunately in surviving brain tumor patients kept on prolonged maintenance drug schedules for months to years.[2] An increase in late pulmonary reactions has been identified when bleomycin, actinomycin D, and adriamycin have been added to radiation schedules.[10] The modification in dose has been plotted by Phillips and Wara[56] (see Fig. 8) for children receiving radiation and actinomycin D for Wilms' tumor. The masking of radiation lesions by prednisone has been recognized when MOPP programs were combined with intensive chest irradiation for Hodgkin's disease patients. Sudden stoppage of prednisone leads to fulminating pneumonopathy, and careful tapering of steriods is required. When treating the whole of both lungs and the mediastinum, further dose modification is required.[7]

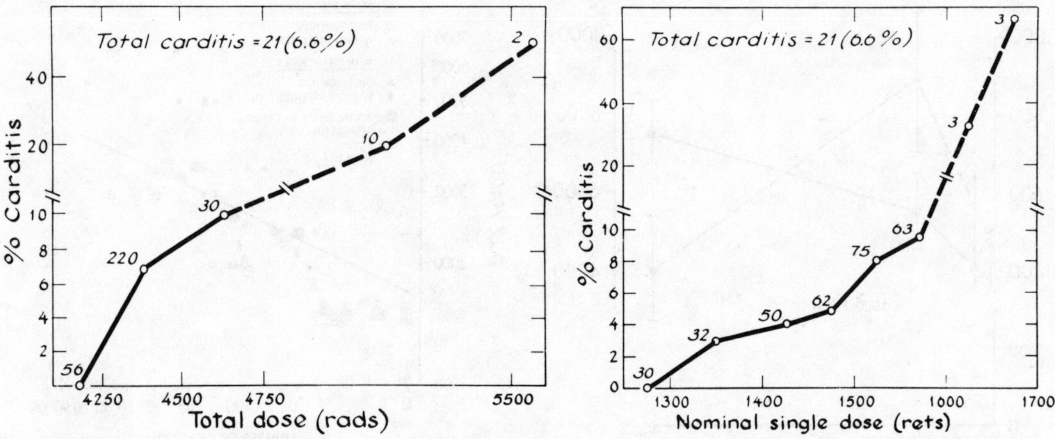

Figure 9. The heart, once considered radioresistant, shows a deeper dose response over 2000 rad than over a 1000-rad range. When the ret is used, correcting for fractionation and time, the dose-response curve appears to be even steeper. (Data from Stewart et al, 1971.)

Thus, the entire concept of pulmonary tolerance to radiation has been altered from a relative radioresistance to extreme radiosensitivity.

HEART

The heart has long been considered a radioresistant structure, particularly when compared to the lungs, as experimentally induced lesions required exceedingly large doses to produce recognizable injury.[34] It was in 1967 that Cohn *et al.* described the clinical and pathologic features of patients with evidence of radiation-induced pericarditis following treatment of thoracic tumors. At the same time, Stewart[50] and Fajardo[18] noted the onset of an acute pericarditis after the completion of a course of mantle irradiation, often associated with pericardial effusion and sometimes with signs of tamponade. Most patients recovered but a few developed chronic constrictive pericarditis hearts. From their dose-response data, it is evident that the effects are both volume and dose dependent (see Fig. 9).

The risk was greatest when the entire pericardium was included. If the entire heart received less than 3000 rad the incidence was 19%, whereas above 3000 rad the complication occurred in 50% of patients of whom 36% required treatment (Table 5). With subcarinal shielding at 1500–2000 rad, this has occurred in 2/400 patients or 0.025%.

The development of cardiac myopathies following irradiation have been rare, but transient arrythmias and T-wave inversions have been noted during treatment and are of little consequence.[41] A number of reports describing coronary artery disease appearing prematurely, particularly in young patients treated with the mantle technique, have led to expressions of concern. However, Fajardo[17] has thoroughly reviewed this subject and can identify 10 patients who may fit these criteria from thousands of patients treated with thoracic irradiation. Kopelson[30] has recently reviewed this topic exhaustively and found 33 patients and also concludes it occurs infrequently with current techniques.

By contrast, the list of cardiotoxic chemotherapeutic agents is increasing and includes actinomycin D, MOPP, VP-16-213, mithramycin, cyclophosphamide, mitomycin C, imidazole carboxamide, and the anthracycline derivatives–adriamycin, dacmorubicin, and rubidazone.[16] Eltringham has gleaned the literature and presented an analysis of the role each of these agents has

TABLE 5. Radiation Pericarditis as a Function of Dose to the Whole Pericardium[b]

	Radiation Dose (rad)			
	⩽599	600–1500	1501–3000	>3000
Pericardial irradiation	198	42	123	14
Pericarditis[a]	14 (7)	5 (12)	23 (19)	7 (50)
Pericarditis requiring treatment[a]	3 (1.5)	4 (9.5)	8 (6.5)	5 (36)

[a]Number of patients in group; percentage of total number in parentheses.
[b]Data from Stanford University Medical Center; Carmel and Kaplan, 1976.

TABLE 6. Dose of Adriamycin and Incidence of Cardiomyopathy in Adults[a]

Total dose (mg/m²)	Number at Risk	Cardiomyopathy	Frequency (%)
<450	738	0	0
451–550	26	0	0
501–550	32	3	9
551–600	15	3	20
>600	37	15	41
Total >550	52	18	35
Total <550	796	3	0.4

[a]Data from Lefrak et al., 1973; Eltringham, 1979.

had in producing cardiac complications.[15] Of all of these agents, adriamycin is the most toxic, and it is evident it has produced more severe cardiac cripples in the 5 years of its existence than has occurred with use of radiation therapy in 5 decades. The exact molecular lesion is unknown, but is believed to be interference with myocardial DNA-dependent RNA synthesis at the nuclear and/or mitochondrial level which would affect functional and structural proteins.[3] This is expressed as direct damage to myocytes which are lost, causing large diffuse particles of fibrosis to appear. The incidence of cardiomyopathy is dose related; Lenaz and Page[32] have recommended that a dose of 550 mg/m² not be exceeded in adults, and Gilladoga[24] suggests 500 mg/m² in children (see Table 6).

Of concern to radiation oncologists are the additive effects of adriamycin and radiation which are time independent. That is, adriamycin has the capability of producing "recall phenomenon" of latent subclinical radiation changes in small intramyocardial vessels and myocytes even as late as 10 years after radiotherapy. The meticulous work of Billingham[3] with endocardial biopsies in humans identified a variety of anthracycline-induced damage to myocytes by electron microscopy. Doses as low as 180 mg/m² of adriamycin produced recognizable myocyte lesions, and at 240 mg/m² (see Fig. 10) virtually all patients had subclinical disease. The pathology score for cardiac damage increased for a given dose of adriamycin when the heart had been previously irradiated. Of greatest concern is the wide range of elapsed times between the administration of radiation and adriamycin—i.e., 1

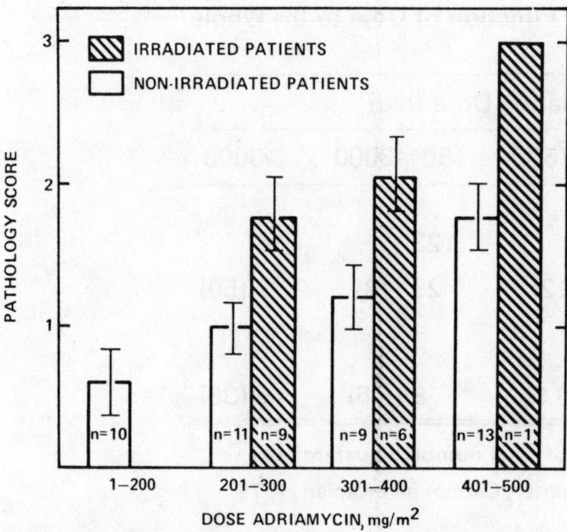

Figure 10. Subclinical pathology is present in both irradiated and nonirradiated patients with adriamycin. Although 500 mg/m² is considered a safe dose, it is apparent that changes can be seen with doses as low as 100 to 200 mg/m². The effect is increased when irradiation is used and even greater pathologic changes are noted. (Data from Billingham, 1979.)

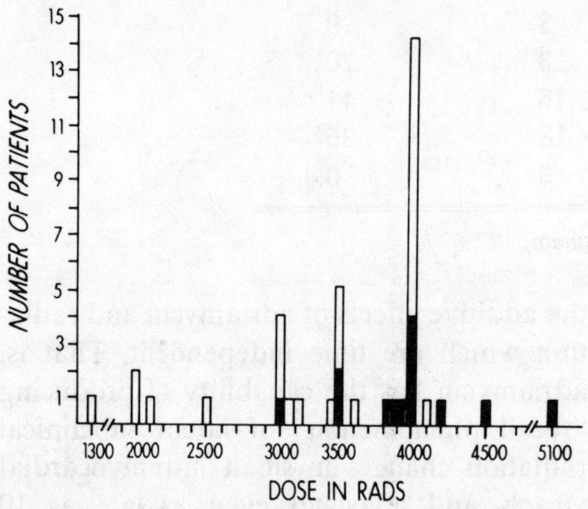

Figure 11. This bar graph illustrates a threshold for radiation hepatopathy at 3000 rad with a major increase in incidence between 3500 and 4000 rad reaching the $TTD_{50}\Sigma_5$ level; above 4500 rad it can be expected to universally occur when the whole liver is irradiated with conventional fractional doses of 200 rad daily. (Data from Ingold, et al., 1965.)

year to 14 years–that resulted in enhanced effects. Once irreversible damage occurs due to adriamycin cardiotoxicity, it leads to a 50% mortality in adults with resultant heart failure.

Further experimental studies *in vivo* and *in vitro* have established the additive nature of these two modes. The Eltringham[15] New Zealand rabbit heart model predicts reasonably accurately for late effects in man. The correlated histopathology and electron micrographs by Fajardo[18] have illustrated the alteration in spatial myofibers, capillary damage, and myocardial fibrosis. As in lung, a vulnerability of pediatric patients to combined therapy modes has been noted for cardiomyopathies as compared to adults.

LIVER

The liver was long thought to be a radioresistant structure, and it was with the introduction of megavoltage techniques in treating the upper abdomen in lymphomas and ovarian cancer patients that the concept of tolerance doses changed. Experimental data indicated very large doses of radiation were required to produce histopathologic damage well beyond the range employed clinically.[41] The reports by Ingold et al.[25] of a radiation hepatopathy manifested a few months after the completion of radiation therapy as a tender hepatomegaly, ascites without jaundice associated with an abnormal alkaline phosphatase, and BSP retention, came as a surprise. This occurred with fractional daily doses when total doses greater than 3000 rad were used (see Fig. 11), particularly above 3,500 and 4000 rad, to ablate localized lymphomas. The concentrated dose/time schedules used in abdominal strip techniques further reduced the "safe threshold" dose to 1500–2000 rad as compared with doses reported by Wharton *et al.*[58] for acute and chronic radiation hepatitis. As more rapid dose delivery schedules appeared in Hodgkin's disease, such as 2000 rad in 10 days with 2000 rad fractions, abnormal enzyme levels and thrombocytopenia appeared.[49] Thin shield (50% transmission) techniques protracting the same radiation dose over 4–5 weeks have reduced the possibility of this late effect. Again, the use of a total rad dose is not as reliable as the use of a ret dose when different fractionation and time/dose schedules are used.

The increasing incidence and nature of

hepatic dysfunction in the pediatric age group became evident with similar or even lower radiation doses when the entire liver or the entire right lobe of the liver was irradiated and combined with actinomycin D (AMD) and vincristine (VCR) in Wilm's tumor patients.[8] Contrasting patients treated for right-sided tumors versus left-sided tumors or unirradiated patients, evidence accumulated that both hepatic and marrow toxicity were increased. Liver irradiation interfered with the normal metabolism and excretion of AMD and VCR, increasing blood levels and slowing turnover times. A peripheral sequestration of platelets occurs in the region of the radiation-damaged, fine hepatic venules and may be the mechanism for the veno-occlusive lesion that characterizes this hepatitis. Further drug effects due to elevated levels acting on the bone marrow can intensify this platelet depression. Their findings clearly point to an increased incidence of radiation hepatopathy in patients treated by radiation and drugs versus drugs alone with striking elevations in LDH and SGOT values. Fortunately, this lesion is reversible with prednisone, further suggesting vasculitis as the underlying mechanism (see Fig. 12).

GASTRO-INTESTINAL COLON

The gastro-intestinal tract has long been known to be radiosensitive since "intestinal deaths" were described following whole-body irradiation once the dose exceeded 1000 rad.[5] A variety of investigations in animals reported alterations in fat absorption, protein leakage, and electrolyte imbalance when large segments of bowel have been exposed to radiation.[41] In those clinical settings requiring large-field intestinal irradiation, daily doses are kept to fractional doses of 150 rad or less or large abdominal fields are divided into strips to allow daily doses greater than 200 rad to be given. Dose delivery can be protracted at a lower dose rate by attenuation filters in beams to take advantage of the large shoulder of the intestinal epithelial survival curve, allowing for repair of sublethal damage.[59]

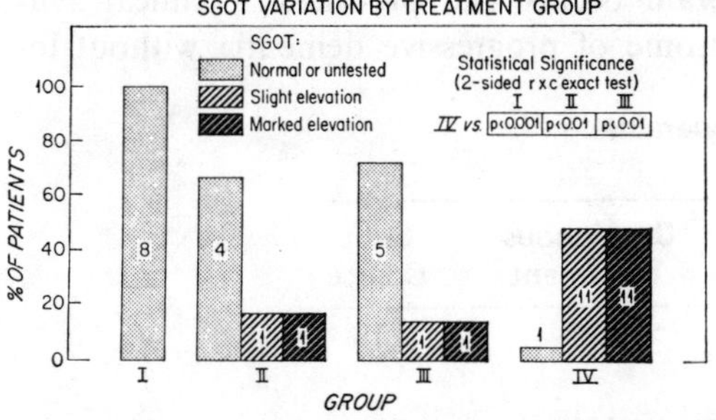

Figure 12. The marked elevation in enzymes in group IV refers to those patients who had their liver irradiated and also received chemotherapy. The liver irradiation slows the usual metabolic process which detoxifies these agents, resulting in greater liver damage as well as an indirect effect on the blood marrow. (Data from Cassady et al. 1979.)

Although most experimental systems investigating intestinal mucosa have studied early mucosal damage and have widely employed regenerating crypt counting techniques,[58] these readily quantifiable changes do not correlate with the late severe or life-threatening damage that occurs with radiation injury of bowel.[48] The basic late lesion is a vascular endothelial proliferation, subendothelial lipid deposits, collagenization, and thrombosis of vessels. Associated necrosis of smooth muscle in the muscularis mucosa next to occluded vessels can lead to perforation and obstruction. Therefore, the early measurable mucosal events do not predict for later injury, and an absence of intestinal symptoms during irradiation does not mean late damge will not occur.[39]

Recorded radiopathologic injury indicates at comparable doses the incidence of small bowel injury is 2–3 times higher than that reported for colon.[22] The incidence of severe injury is 30–40% at 5000 rad for small intestines versus 10% for transverse colon. Rectal injury below 5000 rad is rare and reaches the 5% level at 5500 rad.[22] Doses as high as 6000 rad, if delivered in longer periods of time with smaller daily fractions of 150–180 rad, are considered reasonably safe for treating pelvic neoplasms.[21] It is for this reason that current cooperative group protocols for

treating irradiation or in a split-course fashion so that this dose would be achieved in 7 to 10 weeks.[12] Unfortunately, these seemingly safe radiation schedules have proved disastrous when combined with seemingly well-tolerated chemotherapy agents such as 5FU and CCNU, in maintenance programs. Despite the absence of acute effects during radiation therapy and the subsequent administration of chemotherapy, late fistualization and necrosis have occurred in 29%, 6 months to 2 years later in a series of patients so treated by Danjoux & Catton.[12] The concept of stem cell senescence[6] is a likely explanation for this unfortunate set of events. With fractionated or split-course radiation therapy followed by maintenance chemotherapy, the reserve regenerative capacity of intestinal epithelia and the endothelial cells of microcirculation may be used up. The colo-rectum, considered a relatively radioresistant structure, has proved to be vulnerable to combined modality treatment, as is confirmed in the discontinued ECOG advanced rectal cancer study (see Table 7).

BRAIN, SPINAL CORD, AND PERIPHERAL NERVES

The assumption that the central nervous system is resistant to irradiation has lead to the delivery of high doses for malignant gliomas. A dose-response curve is emerging for photon irradiation utilizing median survival ranging from 5000 to 7000 rad based on reports from recently completed cooperative group studies of the Brain Tumor Surgical Adjuvant Group by Walker[55] and an RTOG pilot study of Salazar and Rubin[46] where doses above 7000 and 8000 rad of photons have been tolerated. Walker, Strike, and Sheline[55] in an exhaustive review and reanalysis of literature of radiation effects on the brain for delayed reactions, have provided new guidelines in neurorets for high-dose radiation and for combining radiation and chemotherapy (see Fig. 13). In contrast, the results of Catterall et al.[9] with neutron brain radiation have been fraught with late brain damage to potential survivors in that tumor sterilization or considerable antitumor effects have been found at autopsy. Evidence of diffuse brain damage to normal brain occurs and produces a clinical syndrome of progressive dementia without lo-

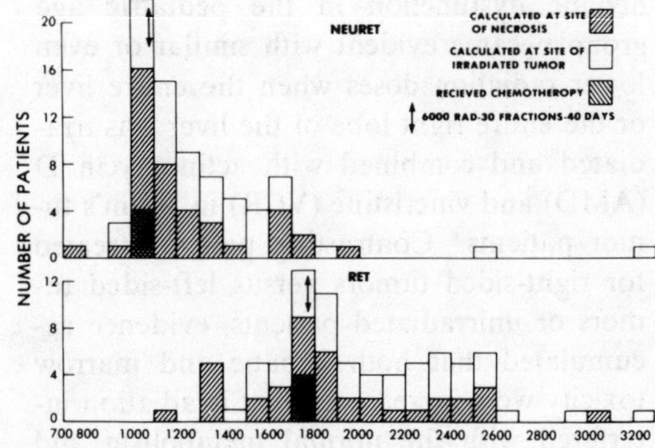

Figure 13. Number of reported instances of necrosis at various ret or neuret doses. (Data from Sheline *et al.*, 1980.)

TABLE 7. EST 3276: Rectum (Inoperable)—Late Complications[b]

	Overall	Continuous Treatment	Split Course
Chemo-radiotherapy		69%	21%
Radiotherapy			
Treatment Reactions[a]	23% (7 of 30)	43% (3 of 7)	57% (4 of 7)
Chemotherapy Toxicity	48% (10 of 21)	60% (6 of 10)	40% (4 of 10)

[a] Primarily bowel obstruction
[b] Data from E.C.O.G. study, Danjoux and Catton, 1979.

calizing signs. Attempts at mixing photons and neutrons are in progress to capture the benefits of both forms of radiation without the untoward effects.

The exact mechanism of neutron injury to the brain is not fully understood. Several biologic factors may be important to account for these effects and include the lipid content, oxygen metabolism, the relationship of blood vasculature with nervous tissue, and certain vulnerable zones such as the hypothalmus and brain stem. The presence of tumors with a high-hydrogen content, as in fat, may lead to a 15–20% increase in absorbed dose for neutrons. Since the brain is composed largely of lipids, this component may be responsible for an increase in neutron energy absorption. Increased vascular damage by neutrons may occur when blood vessels are located in a high-fat environment.

Peculiar encephalopathies have occurred with combinations of safe doses of radiation and chemotherapy (particularly with methotrexate) in childhood leukemias. Low to moderate doses of 2000–2400 rad to the cranial content when combined with systemic and intrathecal methotrexate yield a high encephalopathy as compared to the modalities above.

The spinal cord has always been considered more vulnerable to radiation since Boden's observations of spinal cord injury in 1948. Based upon Boden's data[4], rather low tolerance doses were predicted when applying a line with the same slope as Strandquist's to cases reported. More recently, Kramer[31] and Phillips[37] concluded that the maximum acceptable dose was 5000 rad in 5 weeks with conventional fractions of 200 rad. The use of larger fractions leads to a series of radiation myelopathies, particularly with split-course treatment to lung. The NSD should be used as a guide when unique fractionation is used. The 5% incidence occurs between 1300 and 1500 rets, depending on level and length of spinal cord segment. Based on van der Kogel and Barendsen's observations[53] in rat spinal cord irradiation, the slope was found to be 0.44, not 0.33, higher than that predicted by the Ellis formula. This has been further confirmed by Hornsey[26] in neutron therapy experiments. Split-course irradiation was widely adopted following Abramson and Cavanaugh's[1] report of a successful increase in median survival for lung cancer. The total dose/total time equation was less for split-course schedules than continuous-dose schedules, i.e., 4000 rad in 5 weeks versus 5000 rad for 5 weeks, respectively. Again, this has proved to have disastrous consequences, and the value of a ret dose guide versus a rad dose guide to tolerance now unfortunately rests on firm data. The same proved to be true for lung fibrosis in our experience and with the recent RTOG study in that the total rad dose per total time was not an accurate guide.[29]

Mention should be made of hypoxic-cell radiosensitizers and peripheral-nerve neurotoxicity as an illustration of a radiation innovation leading to a new toxicity in a tissue considered radioresistant. A specific and selective effect occurs in myelin sheaths and has been well described in a sequential fashion in a series of ultrastructural studies.[11]

ENDOCRINE GLANDS

Endocrine glands have been considered to be among the most radioresistant structures and rarely limit the dose of radiation. The thyroid gland requires massive rad dose well beyond doses commonly used for cancericidal therapy. Ablative of the normal thyroid gland doses from I^{131} therapy have been in excess of 10,000 rad to as high as 30,000 to 50,000 rad. The thyroid gland is frequently irradiated in adult head and neck cancers and receives doses of 5000 to 6000 rad with relative impunity.

The development of overt hypothyroidism in Hodgkin's disease patients again came as a surprise. The incidence from Stanford is 20% for recognizable symptoms

TABLE 8. Hypopituitarism Following Incidental Pituitary Irradiation Delivered for Tumors of the Head and Neck[a]

Sex	Age	Primary Disease	Estimated Pituitary Dose	Interval of Radiation of Hypopituitarism	Pituitary Function Tests	Tests
M	45 years	Ca of Nasopharynx	6000 rad	8 years	PBI decreased, urinary gonadotrophins decreased; urinary 17-OHCS decreased; response to metyrapone ±	Bradley
M	39 years	Ca of 1 maxillary sinus	6500 rad	7 years	PBI decreased; TSH decreased, rise following TRH injection; urinary gonadotrophins decreased; growth hormone decreased, no response to insulin; plasma cortisol decreased, no response to insulin, rise following vasopressin injection	Larkins and Martins
F	12 years	Ca of nasopharynx	9000 rad	11 years	Growth retardation, amenorrhea; BMR decreased; PBI normal; urinary 17 KS and 17 OHCS decreased	Tan and Kunarathnam
M	8 months	Retinoblastoma	4000 rad	7 years	Growth hormone decreased; other pituitary functions normal	Grumbach et al.;
M	6 years	Midbrain tumor	5060 rad	7½ years	Growth hormone decreased other pituitary functions normal	
M	4 years	Medulloblastoma	4500 rad	6 years	Growth hormone decreased; other pituitary functions normal	
M	4½ years	Embryonal rhabdomyosarcoma of nasopharynx	7500 rad	5½ years	Growth hormone decreased, no response to insulin and arginine stimulation; other pituitary functions normal	Fuks et al.;

[a] Data from Fuks et al., 1976.

as weight gain, sluggishness, drowsiness, and depressed thyroid hormone levels to as high as 44% for laboratory evidence of compensated hypothyroidism with elevated TSH levels in presence of normal thyroxine levels. There is evidence that the iodine burden after lymphangiography may be a cofactor in these patients. The tolerance dose is below 4000 rad to avoid this problem.

The normal pituitary gland likewise requires huge radiation doses to effect ablation in the range of 20,000–30,000 rad in order to produce detectable changes in end-organ secretion within 1 year's time. This has been achieved by precise high-dose delivery techniques such as Bragg peak proton and stripped nuclei beams and stereotactic yttrium implants into the sella turcica. The finding of hypopituitarism in long-term survivors of pediatric brain tumors after moderate doses of 5000 rad suggest a greater radiosensitivity than previously recognized. The hypothalmus and pituitary need shielding in children if high dose radiation therapy is applied in brain tumors (see Table 8).

Summary

The concepts of normal tissue and organ tolerance to radiation are undergoing change. It is evident in reviewing clinical radiation pathology writings of Casarett and this author that with the introduction of megavoltage irradiation, combined drug–radiation regimens, unusual and unorthodox fractionation, innovations in radiation (such as high-LET neutron beams), hyperthermia, and hypoxic-cell radiosensitizers, so-called radioresistant tissues and organs are becoming vulnerable. Late effects of a severe and life-threatening nature are appearing in unexpected circumstances. Careful pilot studies need to be done, and, in favorable patients, adjuvant chemotherapy and radiotherapy programs require adequate follow-up to be sure they are safe. Optimization of treatment needs to be directed to reducing toxicity as well as increasing curability. The following includes new dictums and guidelines in the combined modality era:

1. Radiation therapy and chemotherapy can be additive even when "safe" schedules are given and can lead to late effects despite intervals up to months or years between time of administration of these modes.
2. Whole-organ irradiation reduces the total dose that can be tolerated as compared to irradiation of part of an organ.
3. When using unorthodox fractionation, calculate the total rad dose in ret, particularly with large fractional doses, since it is a more reliable guide than total rad doses.
4. There are major differences in tolerance for pediatric versus adult tissues and organs, and dose reduction should be done for younger age groups.
5. Reliable measures, parameters, and indices of early or acute damage that predict for late effects are essential to future investigators in this combined modality era.

REFERENCES

1. Abramson, N., and Cavanaugh, P.J.: Short-course radiation therapy in carcinoma of the lung: A second look. *Radiology* **108**:685–687, 1973.
2. Aronin, P.A., Mahaley, M.S., Jr., Rudnick, S.A., Dudka, L., Donohue, J.R., Selker, R.G., and Moore, P.: Prediction of BCNU pulmonary toxicity in patients with malignant gliomas: An assessment of risk factors. *N Engl J Med* **303**:183–187, 1980.
3. Billingham, M.E.: Endomyocardial changes in anthracycline-treated patients with and without irradiation. *Front Radiat Ther Oncol* **13**:67–81, 1979.
4. Boden, G.: Radiation myelitis of the cervical spinal cord. *Br J Radiol* **21**:464, 1948.
5. Bond, V.P.: The role of infection in illness following exposure to acute total body irradiation. *Bull NY Acad Med* **33**:359, 1957.
6. Botnick, L.E., Hannon, E.C., and Hellman, S.: Late effects of cytotoxic agents on the normal tissue of mice. *Front Radiat Ther Oncol* **13**:36–47, 1979.

7. Carmel, R.J., and Kaplan, H.S.: Mantle irradiation in Hodgkin's disease: An analysis of technique, tumor irradication and complications. *Cancer* **37**:2813–2825, 1976.
8. Cassady, J.R., Carabell, S.C., and Jaffe, N.: Chemotherapy-irradiation related hepatic dysfunction in patients with Wilm's tumor. *Front Radiat Ther Oncol* **13**:147–160, 1979.
9. Catterall, M., Bloom, H.G.J., Ash, D.V., Walsh, L., Richardson, A., Uttley, D., Gowing, N.F.C., Lewis, P., and Chaucer, B.: Fast neutrons compared with megavoltage x-rays in the treatment of patients with supratentorial blioblastoma: A controlled pilot study. *Int J Radiat Oncol Biol Phys* **6**:261–266, 1980.
10. Chan, P.Y.M., Kagan, A.R., Byfield, J.E., Rao, A.A., Gilbert, H.A., and Nussbaum, H.: Pulmonary complications of combined chemotherapy and radiotherapy in lung cancer. *Front Radiat Ther Oncol* **13**:136–144, 1979.
11. Conroy, P.J., von Burg, R., Passalacqua, W., Penney, D.P., and Sutherland, R.M.: Misonidazole neurotoxicity in the mouse. *Int J Radiat Oncol Biol Phys* **5**:983–992, 1979.
12. Danjoux, C.E., and Catton, G.E.: Delayed complications in colo-rectal carcinoma treated by combination radiotherapy and 5-Fluorouracil—Eastern Cooperative Oncology Group (E.C.O.G.) Pilot Study. *Int J Radiat Oncol Biol Phys* **5**:311–316, 1979.
13. Elkind, M., and Whitmore, G.F.: *Radiobiology of Cultured Mammalian Cells* New York: Gordon & Breech, 1967.
14. Ellis, F.: The relationship of biological effect to dose-time-fractionation in radiotherapy. *Curr Top Radiat Res* **4**:359–397, 1968.
15. Eltringham, J.R.: Cardiac response to combined modality therapy. *Front Radiat Ther Oncol* **13**:161–174, 1979.
16. Eltringham, J.R., Fajardo, L.F., Stewart, J.R., and Klauber, M.R.: Investigation of cardiotoxicity in rabbits from adriamycin and fractionated cardiac irradiation: Preliminary results. *Front Radiat Ther Oncol* **13**:21–25, 1979.
17. Fajardo, L.F., and Stewart, J.R.: Coronary artery disease after radiation. *N Engl J Med* **286**:1265–1266, 1972.
18. Fajardo, L.F., Stewart, J.R., and Cohn, K.E.: Morphology of radiation-induced heart disease. *Arch Pathol* **86**:512, 1968.
19. Fertil, B.D., and Malaise, E.P.: Inherent cellular radiosensitivity as a basic concept for human tumor radiotherapy. *Int J Radiat Oncol Biol Phys,* **7**: 621–630, 1980.
20. Fitzpatrick, P.J., and Rider, W.D.: Half-body radiotherapy. *Int J Radiat Oncol Biol Phys* **1**:197–207, 1976.
21. Fletcher, G.: *Textbook of Radiotherapy* 2nd ed. Philadelphia: Febiger, 1973, pp. 620–664.
22. Friedman, M.: Calculated risks of radiation injury to normal tissue in the treatment of cancer of the testis. In *Proceedings of Second National Cancer Conference* 1952, pp. 390–400.
23. Fryer, C.J.H., Fitzpatrick, P.J., Rider, W.D., and Poon, P.: Radiation pneumonitis: Experience following a large single dose of radiation. *Int J Radiat Oncol Biol Phys* **4**:931–936, 1978.
24. Gilladoga, A.C., Tan, C.T., Phillips, F.C., Sternberg, S.S., Tang, C., Wollner, N., and Murphy, M.L.: Cardiac status of 40 children receiving adriamycin over 495 mg/m² and animal studies. *Proc Am Assoc Cancer Res* **15**:107, 1974.
25. Hall, E.J.: *Radiobiology for Radiologists,* 2nd ed. New York: Harper & Row, 1978.
26. Hornsey, S., Morris, C.C., Myers, R., and White, A.: Relative biological effectiveness for damage to the central nervous system by neutrons. *Int J Radiat Oncol Biol* **7**:185–190, 1981.
27. Ingold, J.A., Reed, G.B., Kaplan, H.S., and Bagshaw, M.A.: Radiation hepatitis. *AJR* **93**:200–208, 1965.
28. Kaplan, H.S.: *Hodgkin's Disease* 2nd ed. Cambridge, Mass: Harvard University Press, 1972.
29. Keller, B., Salazar, O., and Rubin, P.: Radiation toxicity in the treatment of lung cancer: Radiation myelitis—an analysis of time-dose factors. To be published.
30. Kopelson, G., and Herwig, K.J.: The etiologies of coronary artery disease in cancer patients. *Int J Radiat Oncol Biol Phys* **4**:895–908, 1978.
31. Kramer, S., Southard, M.E., and Mansfield, C.M.: Radiation effects and tolerance of the central nervous system. *Front Radiat Ther Oncol* **6**:332, 1972.
32. Lefrak, E.A., Pitha, J., Rosenheim, S., and Gottlieb, J.A.: A clinicopathologic analysis of adriamycin cardiotoxicity. *Cancer* **32**:302–314, 1973.
33. Moosavi, H., McDonald, S., Rubin, P., Cooper, R., Stuard, I.D., and Penney, D.P.: Early radiation dose response in lung: An ultrastructural study. *Int J Radiat Oncol Biol Phys* **2**:921–932, 1977.
34. Moss, A.J., Smith, D.W., Michaelson, S., and Shriner, B.F.: Radiation technique for the production of localized necrosis in the intact dog. *Proc Soc Exp Biol Med* **112**:903–905, 1963.
35. Penney, D.P., and Rubin, P.: Specific early fine structural changes in lung following irradiation. *Int J Radiat Oncol Biol Phys* **2**:1123–1132, 1977.
36. Penney, D.P., Shapiro, D.L., Rubin, P., and Finkelstein, J.: Long-term effects of radiation on the mouse lung and potential induction of radiation pneumonitis. *Int J Radiat Oncol Biol Phys,* to be published.
37. Phillips, T.L., and Busky, F.: Radiation tolerance of the thoracic spinal cord. *AJR* **105**:659, 1969.
38. Rosner, F., Grunwald, H.W., and Zarrabi, M.H.: Acute leukemia as a complication of cytotoxic chemotherapy. *Int J Radiat Oncol Biol Phys* **5**:1705–1708, 1979.

39. Rubin, P.: Radiation toxicology: Quantative radiation pathology for predicting effects. *Cancer* **39**:729–736, 1977.
40. Rubin, P., ed.: The radiation oncology research program. *Int J Radiat Oncol Biol Phys* New York: Pergamon Press, May 1979.
41. Rubin, P., and Casarett, G.W.: *Clinical Radiation Pathology,* vols. I and II. Philadelphia: W.B. Saunders, 1968.
42. Rubin, P., and Casarett, G.W.: A direction for clinical radiation pathology. *Front Radiat Ther Oncol* **6**:1–16, 1972.
43. Rubin, P., Cooper, R.A., Jr., and Phillips, T.L., eds.: *Radiation Biology and Radiation Pathology Syllabus* Chicago: American College of Radiology, 1975.
44. Rubin, P., and Scarantino, C.W.: The bone marrow organ: The critical structure in radiation-drug interaction. *Int J Radiat Oncol Biol Phys* **4**:3–23, 1978.
45. Rubin, P., Shapiro, D.L., Finkelstein, J.N., and Penney, D.P.: The early release of surfactant following lung irradiation of alveolar type II cells. *Int J Radiat Oncol Biol Phys* **6**:75–77, 1980.
46. Salazar, O.M., Rubin, P., Feldstein, M.L., and Pizzutiello, R.: High dose radiation therapy in the treatment of malignant gliomas: Final report. *Int J Radiat Oncol Biol Phys* **5**:1733–1740, 1979.
47. Schenken, L.L., Burholt, D.R., Hagemann, R.F., and Kovacs, C.J.: Combined modality oncotherapies. Cell kinetic approaches for avoidance of gastrointestinal toxicity. *Front Radiat Ther Oncol* **13**:82–101, 1979.
48. Schultz, H.P., Glatstein, E., and Kaplan, H.S.: Management of presumptive or proven Hodgkin's disease of the liver: A new radiotherapy technique. *Int J Radiat Oncol Biol Phys* **1**:1–18, 1975.
49. Sheline, G.E., Wara, W.M., and Smith, V.: Therapeutic irradiation and brain injury. *Int J Radiat Oncol Biol Phys* **6**:1215–1228, 1980.
50. Stewart, J.R., Cohn, K.E., Fajardo, L.F., Hancock, E.W., and Kaplan, H.S.: Radiation-induced heart disease. A study of 25 patients. *Radiology* **89**:302, 1967.
51. Vaeth, J.M., ed.: Radiation effect and tolerance, normal tissues. *Front Radiat Ther Oncol* **6**, 1972.
52. Vaeth, J.M., ed.: Combined effects of chemotherapy and radiotherapy on normal tissue tolerance. *Front Radiat Ther Oncol* **13**, 1979.
53. van der Kogel, A.J., and Barendsen, G.W.: Late effects of spinal cord irradiation with 300 kV x-rays and 15 MeV neutrons. *Br J Radiol* **47**:393–398, 1974.
54. Van Dyk, J., Keane, T.J., Kan, S., Rider, W.D., and Fryer, C.J.H.: Radiation pneumonitis following large single dose irradiation: A re-evaluation based on absolute dose to lung. *Int J Radiat Oncol Biol Phys* **7**:461–468, 1981.
55. Walker, M.D., Strike, T.A., and Sheline, G.E.: An analysis of dose-effect relationship in the radiotherapy of malignant gliomas. *Int J Radiat Oncol Biol Phys* **5**:1725–1732, 1979.
56. Wara, W.M., Phillips, T.L., Margolis, L.W., and Smith, V.: Radiation pneumonitis: A new approach to the derivation of time-dose factors. *Cancer* **32**:547, 1973.
57. Weiss, B.R., and Muggia, F.M.: Cytotoxic drug-induced pulmonary disease: Update. 1980. *Am J Med* **68**:259–266, 1980.
58. Wharton, J.T., Declos, L., Gallagher, S., and Smith, J.P.: Radiation hepatitis induced by abdominal irradiation with the cobalt 60 moving strip technique. *AJR* **117**:73, 1973.
59. Withers, H.R., and Elkind, M.: Microcolony survival assay for cells of mouse intestinal mucosa exposed to radiation. *Int J Radiat Oncol Biol Phys* **17**:261–267, 1970.

CHAPTER 26

Contribution of the Keynote Discussant

Maurice M. Tubiana, M.D.[a]

Normal tissue damages and in particular late effects in critical normal tissues constitute the limiting factor for clinical radiotherapy as well as for combination treatment by radiotherapy and chemotherapy. Their study is therefore of paramount importance. Furthermore, whereas the studies of the effect of ionizing radiation on murine tumors have been of little use for the understanding of their effect on human tumors, the study of the effects on normal tissue has been of great clinical value.

The first five chapters of Part III covered various facets of this problem and have brought interesting and original data. However, the topic is so large that all of its aspects cannot be discussed in a 2-hour session. Therefore, I shall attempt to stress a few points not presented which may be of clinical relevance.

The first is the role of *host factors*. The most obvious is age. It is well known, for example, that the bone marrow tolerance of elderly patients to extended field irradiation is much lower than that of younger adults or children. Their tolerance to combinations of radiotherapy and chemotherapy is also much reduced, although wide variations are observed among patients of a same age, for example 55 or 60 years. The most probable explanation is a reduction in the pool of hemopoietic stem cells, but this has not yet been substantiated by clinical data. Despite the clinical interest of such studies, few investigations have been devoted to elucidate the causes of these differential responses.

Other factors, such as sex, intercurrent disease, in particular inflammatory reactions and infections, are also of importance for the reaction of normal tissue. Moreover, intrinsic differences in radiosensitivity have been observed which might be of genetic origin.[1,8] In some diseases, such as ataxia telangictasia, DNA repair after X-irradiation is perturbed; more recently an increased radiosensitivity has been observed in cells from patients with hereditary diseases involving a reduced cellular content of glutathion.[5] However, such conditions are extremely rare and it is not yet known to what extent genetic constitutions could explain the differences in normal tissue damage observed among patients.

The previous chapters have shown that irradiation of normal tissues causes a progressive depletion of the stem cell compartment that explains most of the late effects. However, it should be stressed that besides the decrease in cell number there is also a reduction in the *proliferative potential* of the surviving stem cells.[9,10,14,15,18] In fact if the stem cells had an unlimited proliferative capacity, regeneration after irradiation would always be complete after sufficiently long delays. This is not so. *In vitro*, the growth curve of surviving irradiated cells is often slower than that of normal cells, and when they are cloned the size of the colonies tend to be more heterogeneous and, on the average, smaller.

Nontransformed fibroblasts, *in vitro*, undergo only a finite number of mitoses. Irradiation reduces their capacity for further reproduction, and the life span of the surviving clones was found to be reduced when the cells had received 6 Gy or more. In ad-

[a]Institut Gustave-Roussy, Villejuif, France

dition the reduction in life span was greater when the cells were older at the time of irradiation.[11]

Bone marrow is a critical tissue for both radiotherapy and chemotherapy. Thus, its hemopoietic stem cells have been extensively studied. When normal bone marrow is transferred into a lethally irradiated mouse to bring about repopulation and when hemopoietic cells from this mouse are transferred 2 weeks later into another preirradiated mouse, they are less effective in restoring hemopoiesis than were cells from the primary donor. When further serial transplantations are carried out, there is a progressive decline in the repopulating ability of CFU-S, in spite of the fact that the transplanted bone marrow had never been irradiated. This decrease in the self-renewal ability of CFU-S is also demonstrated by counting the number of CFU-S in the individual spleen colonies produced by bone marrow after various numbers of passages.[15,17,18] Irradiation enhances this decline in repopulating ability of hemopoietic stem cells. In experiments in which mice are irradiated, a high proportion of surviving CFU-S also have a low capacity for CFU-S production, and there is no improvement in this capacity during follow-up.[23] When the bone marrow of an irradiated mouse is grafted into irradiated mice, its growth lags behind that of a graft of similar size originating from a normal mouse. This demonstrates a qualitative defect in the irradiated CFU-S. The same is observed for the bone marrow of a mouse treated with drugs such as busulfan. However, the toxic effect of drugs on the proliferative capacity of stem cells varies widely among antimitotic drugs.[9] In the future it might be advisable in combined treatments to favor those drugs which have the least effect on the proliferative potential of hemopoietic stem cells.

The sequellae observed after irradiation of experimental animals and in patients suggest that both the quantative effect (depletion of the stem cell pool) and the qualitative defect of bone marrow are of importance. In mice, 6 months after total body irradiation at 500 rad, the number of bone marrow nucleated cells and the number of circulating leukocytes are normal, but the number of multipotential stem cells is still reduced; the regeneration of the stem cell pool is not yet completed in spite of a higher than normal fraction of stem cells in proliferation. Eighteen months after irradiation the observed contrast between an increased rate of stem cell proliferation and an increased number of bone marrow cells on the one hand, and leukopenia on the other hand, demonstrates the existence of a granulopoiesis defect, probably intramedullary death.[4]

Six months after a subtotal irradiation of 500 rad, with one limb shielded, the number of multipotential stem cells is only slightly below normal in the irradiated bone marrow, but the proliferative activity of the CFU-S is higher than normal. This suggests that hemopoiesis is not as effective as in normal mice. Eighteen months after irradiation the numbers of CFU-S and of nucleated cells are significantly decreased in both irradiated and protected areas which demonstrates that the early recovery was not definitive and that the importance of the hemopoietic defect increases with time. After higher doses (1950 rad delivered in 13 sessions), the hemopoietic activity of the irradiated territories never recovers completely; the number of stem cells (CFU-S and CFC-G) fluctuates, decreasing again after 1 year of follow-up following a temporary rise.[4]

In patients, after irradiation, regeneration of bone marrow is never total. For example, a total body irradiation delivering a dose of only 1 Gy, performed a few months after a total body irradiation of 4 Gy, caused a very severe aplasia, whereas such a dose given to previously unirradiated patients causes only a slight depression of the number of circulating cells.[21] It has also been observed that after a course of radiotherapy the depression observed in the hemopoietic activity of irradiated territories is long lasting and exists even a decade after irradiation. Furthermore, in some patients submitted to extended-field irradiation, studies carried out with ^{59}Fe demonstrated the existence of an ineffective erythropoiesis.

In recent years, it has been shown that proliferation and differentiation of normal cells are controlled by *humoral factors*. The role of these factors in the expression and repair of the normal tissue damages deserves to be studied, as such factors in the future might be used to enhance normal tissue recovery. In order to substantiate this point of view let us summarize a few pertinent data.

We have shown in 1959 that during a course of radiotherapy the depression of hemopietic activity occurring in irradiated territories is compensated by a stimulation of the nonirradiated hemopoietic tissues.[19] Moreover, this stimulation occurs before any decrease in the production of circulating blood cells. This observation suggested the existence of long-range stimulators regulating hemopoiesis. Furthermore, local regeneration after irradiation depends not only upon the absorbed dose, but also upon the amount of irradiated hemopoietic tissue. When only 20 or 30% of the bone marrow is irradited, the activity of the irradiated areas remains low for many years, probably because the increase in cell proliferation in unirradiated tissues is sufficient to maintain a normal number of circulating blood cells. When the volume of the irradiated bone marrow is large ($>60\%$) even after doses as high as 4000 rad in 4 weeks, a regeneration is observed which is documented by radioactive iron uptake, bone marrow biopsies, and culture of progenitor cells.[12] This regeneration is probably due to the intense stimulation of hemopoiesis throughout the body, caused by the inability of the unirradiated tissues to achieve a sufficient cell production.

A series of experimental data confirmed and expanded these findings. In a normal mouse most of the CFU-S are quiescent and an *in vivo* administration of radioactive thymidine kills only a very small and undetectable percentage of them. On the other hand the committed progenitor cells and the recognizable differentiated cells are actively proliferating, and a third to a half of them die due to incorporation of radioactive thymidine in their DNA. During the hours following an intravenous injection of one mCi of radioactive thymidine into a mouse, two indirect effects are observed: (1) a rapid decrease in the number of CFU-S probably due to differentiation and (2) the entry into S phase of most of the CFU-S.[22]

Some drugs acting on cells in S phase, such as hydroxyurea or cytosine arabinoside, also induce differentiation of CFU-S and trigger into proliferation previously quiescent CFU-S.

After subtotal irradiation the study of the shielded bone marrow or spleen shows similar data. In the protected leg, 15 minutes after exposure, the number of CFU-S is considerably reduced, probably due to differentiation; during the following 8 hours, most of the CFU-S are triggered into proliferation.[3,7]

These two sets of data suggest the presence of long range factors after irradiation. One of these is probably released by committed progenitors or more differentiated cells and induces the differentiation of CFU-S, probably in order to compensate for the depletion of the maturing compartments. Another long-range factor triggers quiescent CFU-S into proliferation. These factors have been extensively studied by E. Frindel et al. at Villejuif.[6] By an *in vitro* method, they demonstrated that a humoral factor is released by the irradiated bone marrow which significantly increases the proportion of CFU-S in S phase of normal bone marrow. The amount of factor secreted is a function of the x-ray dose; when the latter is too large there is no secretion showing that the factor is probably secreted only by viable cells.[2] The duration of the release is short (only a few hours), and a reirradiation does not provoke additional secretion.[2] Drugs like cytosine arabinoside are also able to induce the secretion of these factors.

The fact that during iterative partial body irradiation the proportion of multipotential stem cells in S phase is only temporarily increased suggests that the secretion of stimulating factors is also only temporary.[3] Therefore, stimulators, once they are purified, might be of clinical interest for stimulating the activity of unirradiated areas.

Bone marrow also secretes an inhibitor, and the proliferation kinetics of hemopoiesis is probably regulated by such humoral factors—inhibitors and stimulators—as well as by short-range factors.

In summary, many factors are involved in the late effects on normal tissues: depletion of the irradiated tissue of stem cells, partial loss of proliferative capacity of some of the surviving stem cells, vascular and bed effects, and perturbation of the regulating mechanisms. A better understanding of these phenomena may help to reduce the severity of the sequellae observed in patients.

REFERENCES

1. Arlett, C., and Harcourt, S.: Survey of radiosensitivity in a variety of human cell strains. *Cancer Res* **40**:926–932, 1980.
2. Croizat, H., and Frindel, E.: Study of a CFU-S stimulating factor liberated by bone marrow cells after total or partial body irradiation. *Exp Hematol* **8**:185–191, 1980.
3. Croizat, H., Frindel, E., and Tubiana, M.: Abscopal effect of irradiation on hematopoietic stem cells of shielded bone marrow. Role of migration. *Int J Radiat Biol* **30**:347–358, 1976.
4. Croizat, H., Frindel, E., and Tubiana, M.: Long term radiation effects on the bone marrow stem cells of C_3H mice. *Int J Radiat Biol* **36**:91–99, 1979.
5. Deschavanne, P., Malaise, E.P., and Revesz, L.: Radiation survival of glutathione deficient human
6. Frindel, E., Croizat, H., and Vassort, F.: Stimulat-
fibroblast in culture. *Br J Radiol* **54**:361–362, 1981.
ing factors liberated by treated bone marrow. In vitro effect on CFU kinetic. *Exp Hematol* **4**:56–61, 1976.
7. Gidali, J., and Lajtha, L.G.: Regulation of haemopoietic stem cell turnover in partially irradiated mice. *Cell Tissue Kinet* **5**:147–157, 1972.
8. Hanawalt, P.C., and Cooper, P.K.: DNA repair in bacteria and mammalian cells. *Ann Rev Biocehm* **48**:783–856, 1979.
9. Hellman, S., and Botnick, L.E.: Stem cell depletion: An explanation of the late effects of cytotoxins. *Int J Radiat Biol* **2**:181–184, 1977.
10. Hendry, J.H., and Lajtha, L.G.: The response of hemopoietic colony-forming units to repeated doses of x-rays. *Radiat Res* **52**:309–315, 1972.
11. Laublin, G., Deschavanne, P.J., and Malaise, E.: Effects of ionizing radiations on the life-span of non-transformed human fibroblasts. *Int J Radiat Biol* **36**:281–288, 1979.
12. Morardet, N., Parmentier, C., and Flamant, R.: Etude par le fer 59 des effets de la radiotherapie etendue des hématosarcomes sur l'érythropoiese. *Biomedecine* **18**:228–234, 1973.
13. Patt, H.M., and Maloney, M.A.: Evolution of marrow regeneration as revealed by transplantation studies. *Exp Cell Res* **71**:307–312, 1972.
14. Perman, V., Cronkite, E.P., Bond, V.P., and Sorensen, D.K.: The regenerative ability of haematopoietic tissues following lethal X-irradiation. *Blood* **19**:724–737, 1962.
15. Pozzi, L.V., Andreozzi, U., and Silini, G.: Serial transplantation of bone marrow cells in irradiated isogenic mice. *Curr Top Radiat Res* **8**:259–302, 1973.
16. Rubin, P., Landman, S., Mayer, E., Keller, B., and Ciccio, S.: Bone marrow regeneration and extension after extended field irradiation in Hodgkin's disease. *Cancer* **32**:699–711, 1973.
17. Schofield, R.: The relationship between the spleen colony-forming cell and the haemopoietic stem cell. *Blood Cells* **4**:7–25, 1978.
18. Siminovitch, L., Till, J.E., and McCulloch, E.A.: Decline in colony-forming ability of marrow cells subjected to serial transplantation into irradiated mice. *J Cell Comp Physiol* **64**:23–31, 1964.
19. Tubiana, M., Bernard, C.I., and Lalanne, C.: Modification de l'érythropoïése aprës radiothérapie pelvienne. *Acta Radiol* **52**:321–335, 1959.
20. Tubiana, M., Frindel, E., Croizat, H., and Parmentier, C.: Effects of radiations on bone marrow. *Pathol Biol* **27**:326–334, 1979.
21. Tubiana, M., Lalanne, C.M., and Surmont, J.: Total body irradiation for organ transplantation. *Proc R Soc Med* **54**:1143–1150, 1961.
22. Vassort, F., Wintherholer, M., Frindel, E., and Tubiana, M.: Kinetics parameters of bone marrow stem cells using in vivo suicide. *Blood* **41**:789–796, 1973.
23. Wu, Chu-Tse, and Lajtha, L.G.: Haemopoietic stem cells kinetics during continuous radiations. *Int J Radiat Biol* **27**:41–50, 1975.

CHAPTER 27

Keynote Address: A Critical Look at Empirical Formulae in Fractionated Radiotherapy

Jack F. Fowler, D.Sc., Ph.D., M.Sc., F. Inst. P.[a]

In the beginning was the cube root formula, followed by Strandqvist's data[21] which did not disagree significantly, as pointed out by Cohen.[6] The total dose in "daily" fractionated radiotherapy was assumed to be proportional to the cube root of overall time in days. Strandqvist and Cohen plotted the "tolerance dose" against overall time on a log-log graph and drew straight lines whose slope was the exponent of overall time–a slope of 0.33[6] being equal to the cube root relationship. Biology, however, abhors straight lines–or at least most radiobiologists do–and many arguments have developed about the extent to which biological and clinical results can be represented by such relationships without misleading amounts of error.

In the early 1960s experimental work in the skin of pigs demonstrated the separate factors of time and fraction number.[10] Later, the NSD formula proposed by Ellis,[8] which was derived from clinical observations and Strandqvist's and Cohen's straight log-log plots, agreed roughly with the pig skin results, although the log-log plot for pig skin was steeper for a few large fractions and shallower for many small fractions than the average slope of 0.24 chosen by Ellis as the exponent of fraction number. This divergence, although not statistically significant at the time, was pointed out by Liversage[15] and later by others when reliable clinical data became available.[3,7] The most important discrepancy was that a few large fractions cause more damage to normal tissues than would be predicted either by the NSD formula or by the early reactions in the same tissues.

However, several years passed before such discrepancies emerged (as they now have), and during this time ingenious but quantitatively small modifications of the NSD rule of thumb took root, especially CRE[14] and TDF.[16]

The NSD formula, being obviously a simplification and probably an oversimplification, has stimulated much work to disprove it, and has therefore been useful as a catalyst in the field. In addition, for modest changes of fractionation with no change of the type of tissue or volume treated, NSD has helped to avoid wrong doses that might have been given to patients if no such rule of thumb had been available. It remains useful for acute skin and mucosal reactions, but for late reactions in skin and other organs it should be restricted to between 8 to 10 and 25 to 30 fractions and to overall times shorter than 6 weeks. For small numbers of large fractions, the change of tolerance dose with fraction number is steeper than 0.24, being closer to 0.4. The divergences from NSD, TDF, or CRE now documented include (1) dissociation between acute and late radiation injury, (2) time factor in fractionated radiation, and (3) fraction size or number effect.

[a]Director, Gray Laboratory, Mount Vernon Hospital, Northwood, Middlesex, England

Dissociation Between Acute and Late Radiation Injury

More severe late damage has been reported than would be expected from the level of acute injury or from the NSD or CRE formulae when (1) a small number of large fractions were used or when (2) unusually prolonged overall times were used. The first discrepancy has been reported sporadically in the literature but with increasing conviction.[1-4,17,22-24] Nevertheless, a few clinical trials are still in progress using large doses per fraction, and we await their results with interest.

The Time Factor in Fractionated Irradiation

The avoidance of acute reactions by prolongation but the nonavoidance of late injury by the same means is entirely as predicted from simple cell kinetics. The tissues that suffer late injury cannot be expected to proliferate significantly during the few weeks of radiotherapy (as the acutely reacting skin and mucosa do), especially if radiation doses are well spread apart, e.g., only one or two fractions per week. There is now good evidence for the dissociation caused by a few large doses or by overprolongation,[13,23] although the simple picture of late injury being insensitive to overall time is complicated by the phenomenon of "slow repair" observed in lung[9]—but not in bladder[20] or spinal cord[25] of experimental animals.

In any case, the time factors cannot be as predicted by the NSD or CRE formulae and cannot be the same for both late and acute injury. It is because the time factors are on the average smaller than the "fraction number" or "repair" factors in normal tissue injury that it has taken so long to demonstrate significant divergencies. For late damage they are smaller than the exponent of 0.11 in the Ellis[8] formula.[18,19,26]

From a cell kinetics point of view, very long overall treatment times should be avoided so that tumor cells do not over proliferate. The use of several weeks as an overall time in radiotherapy is because acute normal tissue injury can be avoided and perhaps because reoxygenation can occur in the tumor.

The Fraction-Size or Number Effect

There may be a dose per fraction above which serious normal tissue injury is more likely for a given expectation of cure of tumors. There is, however, no agreement about this. The increasing evidence that large doses per fraction do cause undue normal tissue damage was mentioned above. Nevertheless, doses of 500 to 700 rad per fraction are sometimes used at one or two fractions per week, and clinical trials using 400 rad per fraction at two or three fractions per week are still in progress. The empirical formulae give no warning that such regimes may cause undue late injury, but the consciousness is growing that this may be so and such warnings should now be discussed. The exponent of fraction number appears to be greater than 0.24 for a few large fractions but becomes lower at large numbers of small fractions.[11,12]

It makes kinetic sense, as mentioned above, to treat tumors with a short overall time provided that acute injury to normal tissues is avoided and provided that hypoxic cells are dealt with in some way other than reoxygenation requiring several weeks to accomplish. This would probably be better done by using several small fractions per day (allowing several hours between them for Elkind repair to occur) than by using a few large fractions. Clinical evidence, as always, takes a long time to obtain.

One reason for wanting to use a few large fractions would be that the tumor-cell survival curve has a large shoulder, as has been alleged for malignant melanoma cells, for example. This leads into tumor and therapeutic ratio considerations but does not diminish the warnings about the possibly larger normal tissue damage than would be expected from the predictions of NSD, TDF, or CRE if a few large doses are used.

If, on the other hand, tumors are radioresistant due to fast proliferation instead of to large cell-survival shoulders, a large "dose per day" would indeed be needed. This would be better given by several small doses per day, including logically weekends, or by continuous irradiation. It should be noted that Turesson and Notter found, in experiments on pig skin, that Liversage's continuous-irradiation, dose-rate formula fitted their results better than the CRE dose-rate formula.[22,23]

Conclusions

NSD, TDF, and CRE do not work for less than 8 to 10 fractions nor for overall times exceeding about 6 weeks. In such cases, severe late damage has been reported clinically although acute reactions, especially to skin and mucosa, were acceptable as predicted by the formulae.

The evidence has accumulated gradually that a small number of large fractions can show this "dissociation" between moderate acute but severe late injury to normal tissues.

The evidence has also been hard to find—although more predictable from simple tissue kinetics—that unusually prolonged schedules will avoid acute injury but will not avoid late damage.

The time factors employed in the empirical formulae cannot, of course, be correct, but they are not large and have not been as misleading as the fraction-number factor when restricted to overall times of 6 weeks or less.

These formulae were intended for use when modest alterations to existing fractionated schedules were contemplated, such as the completion of an interrupted schedule, a change from five to three fractions per week, or a change from one schedule to the other where the volume irradiated is not altered. It is wrong to stretch the use of such formulae to very nonstandard fractionations or to techniques involving boosts or shrinking fields. Within the limitations of 8 or 10 to 25 or 30 fractions and no longer than 6 weeks overall time, it also appears that the exponent of N should be 0.3 to 0.4 for a few large doses for skin, spinal cord, lung, and kidney (although possibly lower for larger numbers of small fractions). The exponent of time should be less than 0.11 for late injury and cannot be a constant.

NSD, TDF, and CRE enabled the separation to be made between overall time and fraction number—something which had not been done before. The fact that significant contrary data has taken so long to accumulate indicates that, within certain limits, they were more useful than having no such formulae available. These formulae, although increasingly limited in usefulness as our knowledge expands, have stimulated much valuable work which has clarified the discrepancies.

Summary

Empirical formulae can at best work over a limited range only. It has now been shown, from clinical data, that the Ellis NSD formula applies well only to early injury in skin and mucosa. Late damage in these tissues cannot be represented by ret doses for fewer than 8–10 fractions nor for more than 6 weeks overall time, although within these limitations it is a useful approximation for early reactions.

Other organs, in which the dose-limiting response occurs many months after irradiation, show a smaller dependence of tolerance dose on overall time (the exponent of T being 0–0.06 instead of 0.11) and a larger dependence on fraction number (the exponent of N being closer to 0.4 than 0.24). A few large dose fractions are more damaging than the conventional NSD formula suggests.

The reasons for choosing a long overall time in radiotherapy are to allow reoxygenation and, historically, to avoid acute reactions. However, late reactions are not spared by prolongation and if hypoxic cells are eliminated by some other means, the optimum overall times in radiotherapy would become shorter with a better chance of killing tumor cells.

REFERENCES

1. Andrews, J.R.: Dose-time relationships in cancer radiotherapy. A clinical radiobiology study of extremes of dose and time. *AJR* **93**:56–74, 1965.
2. Arcangeli, G., Friedman, M., and Paoluzi, R.: A quantitative study of late radiation effect on normal skin and subcutaneous tissues in human beings. *Br J Radiol* **47**:44–50, 1974.
3. Bates, T.D., and Peters, L.J.: Dangers of the clinical use of the NSD formula for small fraction numbers. *Br J Radiol* **48**:773, 1975.
4. Bennett, M.B.: The treatment of Stage III squamous carcinoma of the cervix in air and hyperbaric oxygen. *Br J Radiol* **51**:68, 1978.
5. Caldwell, W.: Tolerance of skin and kidneys to conventional or split course fractionation. In *Proceedings of the Conference on Time-Dose Relationships in Clinical Radiotherapy* Madison, Wisconsin: University of Wisconsin, 1975, pp. 38–42.
6. Cohen, L.: Fractionation in radiotherapy. Ph.D. Thesis, University of Witwatersrand, 1955.
7. Dutreix, J.: Isoeffect total dose as a function of the number of fractions for skin, intestine and lung. In *Proceedings of the Conference on Time-Dose Relationships in Clinical Radiotherapy* Madison, Wisconsin: University of Wisconsin, 1975, pp. 21–30.
8. Ellis, F.: Dose, time and fractionation: A clinical hypothesis. *Clin Radiol* **20**:1–7, 1969.
9. Field, S.B., Hornsey, S., and Kutsutani, Y.: Effects of fractionated irradiation on mouse lung and a phenomenon of slow repair. *Br J Radiol* **49**:700–707, 1976.
10. Fowler, J.F., Morgan, R.L., Silvester, J.A., Bewley, D.K., and Turner, B.A.: Experiments with fractionated x-ray treatment of the skin of pigs. I. Fractionation up to 28 days. *Br J Radiol* **36**:188–196, 1963.
11. Hopewell, J.W., Foster, J.L., Young, C.M.A., and Wiernik, G.: Late radiation damage to pig skin. The effects of overall treatment time and number of fractions. *Radiology* **130**:783–788, 1979.
12. Hopewell, J.W., and Wiernik, G.: Tolerance of the pig kidney fractionated X-irradiation. In *Radiobiological Research and Radiotherapy*, vol. I. Vienna: IAEA, 1977, pp. 63–65.
13. Howes, A.E., and Brown, M.J.: Early and late response of the mouse limb to multifractionated X-irradiation. *Int J Radiat Oncol Biol Phys* **5**:13–21, 1979.
14. Kirk, J., Gray, W.M., and Watson, E.R.: Cumulative radiation effect. I. Fractionated treatment regimes. *Clin Radiol* **22**:145–155, 1971.
15. Liversage, W.E.: A critical look at the ret. *Br J Radiol* **44**:91–100, 1971.
16. Orton, C.G., and Ellis, F.: A simplification in the use of the NSD concept in practical radiotherapy. *Br J Radiol* **46**:529–537, 1973.
17. Peters, L.J., and Withers, H.R.: Morbidity from large dose fractions in radiotherapy. *Br J Radiol* **53**:170–171, 1980.
18. Phillips, T.L., Margolis, L.W., and Ross, G.: Radiation pathology and clinical response of lung and oesophagus. In *Frontiers of Radiation Therapy and Oncology*, J.H. Vaeth, ed. Basel: Karger, vol. 6, 1972, pp. 254–273.
19. Phillips, T.L., and Ross, G.: A quantitative technique for measuring renal damage after irradiation. *Radiology* **109**:457–462, 1973.
20. Stewart, F.A.: The effects of hyperthermia and ionizing radiation on bladder, skin and an experimental tumour in mice. Ph.D. Thesis, University of London, 1979.
21. Strandqvist, M.: Studien über die kumulative Wirkung der Röntgenstrahlen bei Fraktionierung. *Acta Radiol*, (supple 55), 1–318, 1944.
22. Turesson, I., and Notter, G.: Skin reactions after different fractionation schedules giving the same CRE. *Acta Radiol Ther Phys Biol* **14**:475–484, 1976.
23. Turesson, I., and Notter, G.: Late skin reactions after different fractionation schedules giving the same CRE in patients. *Proc Eur Assoc Radiol*, 1979, and personal communication.
24. Watson, E.R., Halnan, K.E., Dische, S., Saunders, M., Cade, I., McEwen, J.B., Wiernik, G., Perrins, D.J.D., and Sutherland, I.: Hyperbaric oxygen and radiotherapy: A medical Research Council trial in carcinoma of the cervix. *Br J Radiol* **51**:879–887, 1978.
25. van der Kogel, A.J.: Late effects of radiation on the spinal cord: Dose-effect relationships and pathogenesis. Thesis, TNO Radiobiological Inst. Rijswijk, Netherlands, 1979.
26. Withers, H.R.: Isoeffect curves for various proliferative tissues in experimental animals. In *Proceedings of Conference on Time-Dose Relationships in Clinical Radiotherapy*, Madison, Wisconsin: University of Wisconsin, 1975, pp. 30–38.
27. Withers, H.R., Flow, B.L., Huchton, J.I., Hussey, D.H., Jardine, J.H., Mason, K., Raulston, G.L., and Smathers, J.B.: Effect of dose fractionation on late and early skin responses to gamma rays and neutrons. *Int J Rad Oncol Biol Phys* **3**:227–233, 1977.

CHAPTER 28

Contribution of the Keynote Discussant

Lester J. Peters, M.D.[a]

Dr. Fowler has reviewed the historical development of the clinical isoeffect formulae and has discussed the major pitfalls that may result from their uncritical application. Reappraisal of the clinical basis of all the formulae shows that the data on which they are based are totally inadequate to support the mathematical edifices built upon them.[1] However, the data have long been submerged by impressive formulae and tabulations which convey a degree of precision and reliability that has turned out to be unwarranted. Specifically, as Dr. Fowler has pointed out, clinical results using a few large dose fractions calculated to be equivalent to a standard regimen have yielded, in most cases, an excessive incidence of late radiation complications.

This clinical experience is perfectly consistent with the results of many detailed radiobiological studies in animals which have shown that the exponent for *N* (number of dose fractions) is significantly greater for late responses (i.e., skin contracture, nephrosclerosis, spinal cord necrosis, and lung fibrosis), than for acute skin reactions (see Chapter 21). Likewise, the exponent of *T* (overall time of treatment) for late effects is lower than for acute reactions determined by rapid cell renewal systems, explaining why excessively protracted treatments are also associated with an increased incidence of late complications.

At first sight it would seem a relatively trivial matter to change the exponents of the formulae–to "get them right" for prediction of late effects (see Chapter 24). However, as more is known about the shape of cellular radiation dose-response curves, it is becoming increasingly apparent that no one set of exponents is "right" over an extended range.[2] Further, as Dr. Fowler has implied, the appropriate exponent for fractionation depends on the *size* of dose per fraction rather than the *number* of dose fractions. This has major significance when the total tolerance dose for different tissues and volumes varies appreciably.

The standard practice of radiotherapy has evolved to its present level of sophistication on a well-documented and clinically appreciated proportionality between acute and late reactions. This proportionality enables the vigilant radiotherapist to modify the dose given to patients who show untoward acute reactions. However, it is absolutely critical for us as therapists to realize that when significant changes to our base of experience are made, this proportionality will most likely no longer hold. Figure 1 depicts some of the ways in which the relationship between acute and late reactions for regular daily treatment is perturbed by alterations in fractionation or radiation quality. If one moves to a regimen causing relatively *more* acute toxicity, the change is self-protective; much more insidious is the change to regimens where acute reactions are relatively *less* severe. No one would dispute that in many clinical situations, results of standard radiotherapy are less than optimal, and it is not surprising that altered fractionation is frequently suggested either as a way of improving the clinical results or of reducing the physical and emotional effort expended by patients undergoing radiotherapy. These are laudable aims, but must be tempered with caution when the size of dose per frac-

[a]Division of Radiotherapy, M.D. Anderson Hospital, and Tumor Institute at Houston, Houston, Texas

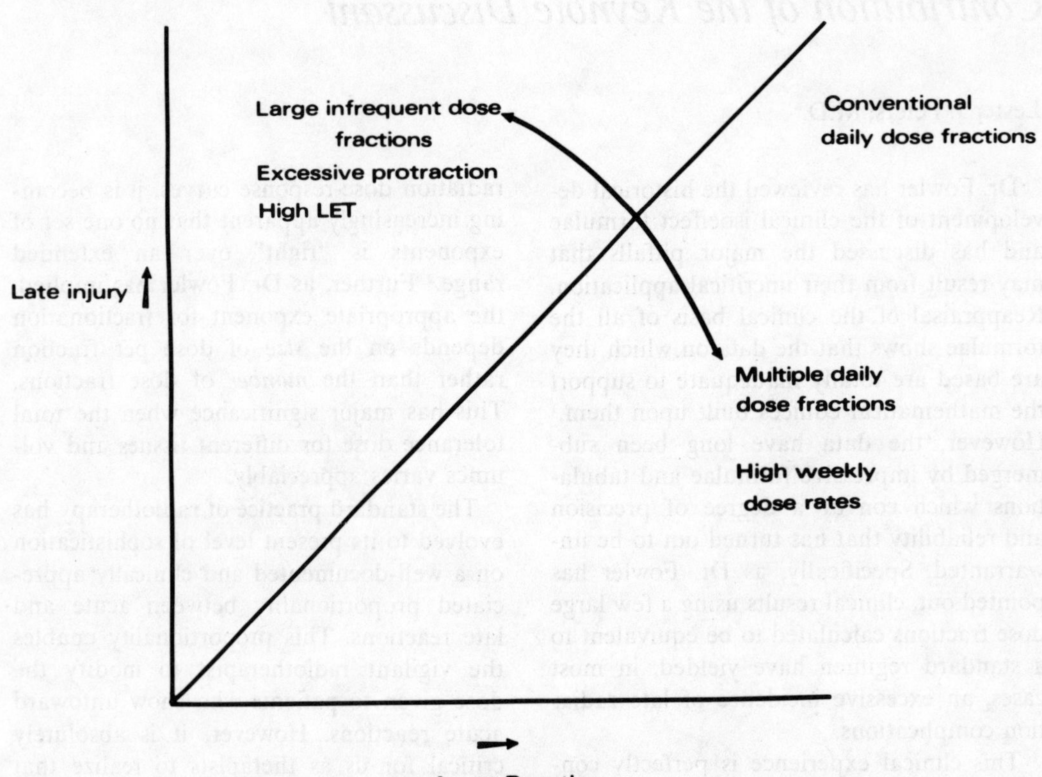

Figure 1. With conventional daily fractions of 200 rad, a given acute reaction is associated with a predictable level of late injury. This proportionality does not hold when significant changes in dose fractionation (or in radiation quality) are made. The most insidious changes are those which reduce the acute reaction for a given level of late injury.

tion is significantly increased. There is nothing intrinsically wrong with using large dose fractions in situations where the clinical results appear to indicate a therapeutic gain, e.g., in malignant melanomata. The important fact to take into account is that doses calculated on the basis of NSD or TDF will be too high, and the therapist should allow for a margin of safety by reducing the calculated dose until there is an opportunity to appraise the late effects of the new regimen.

One of the reasons for the popularity of the isoeffect formulae, especially the TDF tables, is that clinicians have found it reassuring to have a scientific basis for modification of treatment schedules imposed by some external factor, i.e., a break in treatment. The formulae in current use are quite satisfactory for most of these applications since only small extrapolations are usually made from standard treatment regimens, and it matters hardly at all what exponents are used. In fact, the amended dose schedules obtained from the formulae usually agree with clinical intuition. The risk inherent in using the formulae is that the therapist will observe that the predictions for small adjustments in treatment are safe and will therefore assume that large extrapolations are permissible, oftentimes resulting in excess morbidity.

The empirical formulae (particularly the NSD) have also become popular in the reporting of clinical results, to accommodate differences in treatment regimens in different eras and at different institutions. It is obviously necessary to reduce diverse treatament regimens to a common denominator for data reporting. However, I submit that there is a danger in reporting cure rates or complications as a function of ret since the impression is conveyed that *any* regimen giving the same ret value will yield comparable results. This is clearly not the case: It has already been stressed that the NSD exponents are inappropriate for late effects, and the heterogeneity of most tumor types (excluding skin) is such that it is impossible to confidently assign exponents for tumor control. To me, a more prudent way of reporting is to normalize the dose regimens used to an equivalent dose appropriate to the median fractionation schedule actually used. For example, if most patients were treated say in 30 fractions over 6 weeks, but some, for various reasons were treated with different a dose fractionation, then there would be less error in normalizing all doses to a 6-week equivalent dose than in extrapolating them far beyond the area of clinical experience to derive notional single doses.

In summary, the empirical isoeffect formulae should be valued for what they are—i.e., easy ways of making reasonably safe adjustments to radiotherapy regimens over relatively small ranges, with separate consideration being given to dose fractionation and overall time. My fear is that they are being overextended and that radiotherapy by formulae is displacing clinical observation and judgement.

REFERENCES

1. Fletcher, G.H., and Barkley, H.T.: Present status of the time factor in clinical radiotherapy. 1. The historical background of the recovery exponents. *J Radiol Electrol Med Nucl* **55**:443, 1974.
2. Douglas, B.G., and Fowler, J.F.: The effect of multiple small doses of x-rays on skin reactions in the mouse and a basic interpretation. *Radiat Res* **66**:401, 1976.

CHAPTER 29

Multifractionated Irradiation: Biological Bases

J. Dutreix, M.D.[a]
A. Wambersie, M.D.[b]

Multifractionated irradiation is usually understood as an irradiation with several fractions per treatment day. In comparison with standard treatment, it implies a change in one or several factors of the time-dose distribution–namely, fraction size, overall time, and number of treatment days (see Fig. 1 and Table 1). These changes are intended to bring in some practical advantages and/or eventually some radiobiological benefit.

Number of Treatment Days

The reduction of the number of treatment days has obviously some practical advantages (see Table 2). For an outpatient it means fewer visits to the radiotherapy department, but the longer stay each treatment day may outweigh this advantage.

The reduction of the number of treatment days can bring a more obvious advantage when an adjuvant therapy is associated to the irradiation, with chemical or physical sensitizers or possibly with chemotherapy.

Multifractionation is currently used with hypoxic-cell sensitizers to solve the problem raised by the toxicity of these drugs. Clinical experience has shown that the total dose of misonidazole which can be safely administered to patients is restricted to approximately 20 g. If this amount of drug were shared between all fractions of a conventionally fractionated treatment, the blood concentration should not reach the level required for an actual sensitization. The usual dose per treatment is 2 g and the total acceptable dose is exhausted in 10 treatments. With a 2-g treatment the serum concentration reaches a peak (5 mg/1) at approximately 2–4 hours and remains above 80% of the peak for 6 hours. During this time, two or three radiation fractions can be delivered so that all the radiation treatment can be done under sensitizer by reducing the number of treatment days.

Thus, multifractionated irradiation allows a better use of the tissue saturation by the toxic drug.

The problem raised by hyperthermia is of a different nature. The duration of the hyperthermic application is usually 1 hour, and it is not commonly resumed 5 times per week. Radiosensitization by hyperthermia is efficient several hours before and after heating so that three fractions can be delivered at each heat application and all the radiation treatment can be done with a reasonable number of heat applications. Multifractionated irradiation is actually used by Arcangeli et al.[2] for association to hyperthermia: three fractions of 1.6 Gy are delivered at 4-hour intervals, before, during, and after the thermal application of 1-hour heating at 42°C.

Some biological problems are raised by this kind of combined treatment. More data

[a]Institut Gustave-Roussy, Villejuif, France, Universitê de Paris-Sud, France
[b]Cliniques Universitaires St. Luc, Brussels, Belgium, Universitê Catholique de Louvain, Belgium

TABLE 1. Examples of Multifractionated Irradiation

Daily Dose (Gy)	Interval (hours)	Total Dose (Gy)	Overall Time	Reference
2 × 1.50[a]	8	60	3 weeks[b]	Fletcher[12]
1.50[c]	–	60[c]	6 weeks	(breast Ca)
2 × 2.23[a]	4–6	35.7	10 days[b]	Choi[5]
2.35[c]	–	37.6[c]	22 days	(metastatic T.)
3 × 1.00[d]	8	84	Split course[e]	Littbrand[14]
1 × 2.00[c]	–	65[c]	2 × 3 weeks + 2 weeks rest	(bladder)
3 × 1.45[a,f]	8	30	7 days	Simpson[15]
3 × 0.65[d]	8			(glioblastoma)
3 × 0.50[d]	8	40	28 days[e]	
5 × 0.75	3	75	Split course	Cosset and Eschwege[6]
5 × 0.70	3	56	2 × 2 weeks + 2–3 weeks rest	
8 × 0.9	2	72	Split course 2 × 5 days + 2 weeks rest	Castera[4]
17 × 0.6	1	40	Split course 2 × 2 days + 1 week rest	Awwad et al.[3]

[a] Conventional fraction size.
[b] Reduced overall time.
[c] Conventional irradiation, second arm of the clinical trial.
[d] Reduced fraction size.
[e] Conventional overall time.
[f] Concentrated irradiation.

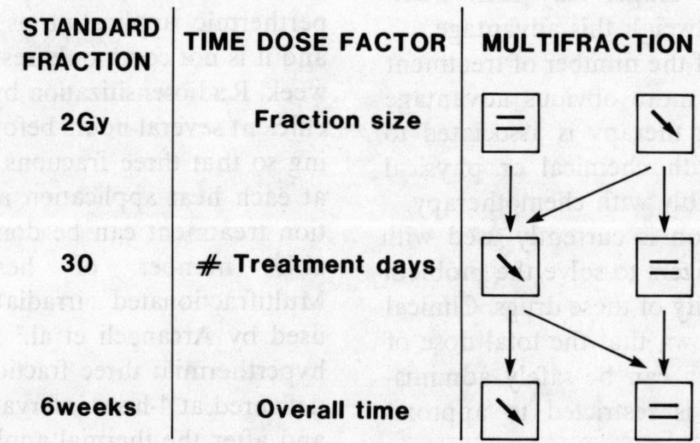

Figure 1. Alteration of the standard time-dose factor by multifractionation. The values for standard fractionation are given for comparison. Several types of schedules are applied to multifractionated irradiation, as indicated in the last column.

TABLE 2. Multifractionation

Reduced Number of Treatment Days

- Fewer patient visits (but longer stay)
- Better use of adjuvant therapy
  - Sensitizers
  - Hyperthermia

Reduced Overall Time

- Shorter hospital stay
- Less delay before surgery
- Faster symptomatic relief
- Increased efficiency on fast growing tumors

TABLE 3. Thermal Enhancement Ratio (TER) as a Function of the Time Interval Between Heat Application (42.4°C for 1 Hour) and Irradiation[b]

	Time Interval (hours)	TER Skin	TER Tumor[a]
Preheating	6	1.2	1.2
	3	1.2	1.5
	2	1.3	1.5
	0	1.7	1.9
Postheating	0	1.85	1.9
	2	1.15	1.5
	3	1.05	1.5
	6	1.0	1.2

[a] Fibrosarcoma tumor in WHT mice.
[b] Data from Stewart and Denekamp, 1976.

are needed on the variation of the TER (thermal enhancement ratio) and on the difference in sensitization of the tumor and normal tissues with the time interval between heat and radiation (see Table 3). Furthermore, the possible interference on the TER of subsequent irradiations at an interval of a few hours requires some investigation.

Overall Time

Multifractionated irradiation allows a reduction of the overall time without using the large fractions considered detrimental by most radiotherapists. Various treatment sequences have been used with large differences in the fraction size and number of daily fractions (Table 1).

Fletcher[12] has used two fractions of 1.5 Gy with the intent of shortening to one-half the overall time for inflammatory breast cancer.

Simpson,[15] by using three daily fractions of 1.5 Gy, shortens the full treatment (30 Gy) to 7 days, while by using 3 daily fractions of 0.5 the overall time is kept at the conventional value of 28 days.

Some authors use a large daily fraction number with reduced fraction size. In the protocol used at Gustave-Roussy Institute for head and neck tumor,[6] five daily fractions of 0.75 Gy are delivered five times per week in two series of 2-week treatments separated by 2–3 weeks of rest (total dose = 75 Gy); for extended tumors of the chest or abdomen, the fraction size is reduced to 0.7 Gy and the total dose to 56 Gy.

Castera[4] uses eight daily fractions of 0.9 Gy at 2-hour intervals for head and neck tumors, and the full treatment (72 Gy) is delivered in two series of 5 days at 2-week intervals.

Awwad,[3] by using 17 daily fractions of 0.6 Gy, carries out a preoperative irradiation of bladder carcinoma in two series of 2-treatment days at 1-week intervals.

The reduction of the overall time has some practical advantages:

1. It shortens the hospital time for the patient.
2. It shortens the delay of surgery due to preoperative treatment.

It may also cause some radiobiological benefit. In principle, it would be advisable to minimize the repopulation taking place during the treatment time when it is slower for normal tissue than for tumor, e.g., for fast-growing tumors. On the other hand, it would be detrimental in the opposite situation for which a weekly dose of 10 Gy is considered to be a major factor of tolerance with conventionally fractionated irradiation.

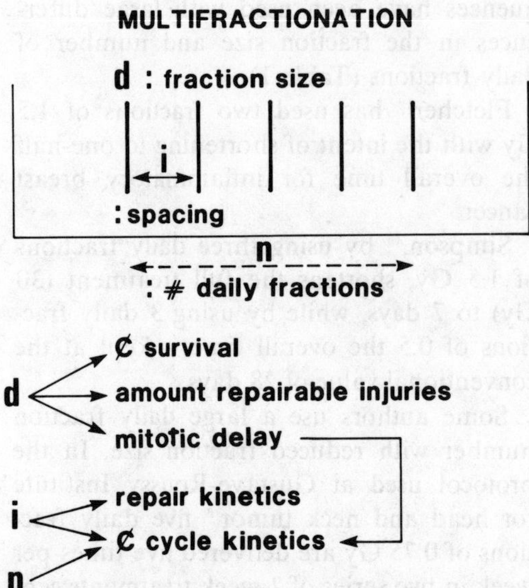

Figure 2. Biological processes affected by the physical parameters of the multifractionated irradiation.

Cell Survival in Multifractionated Irradiation

The size, spacing, and number of the daily fractions involve major biological processes (see Fig. 2).

To fraction size are related (1) cell survival resulting from each fraction and (2) the amount of potentially repairable cell injuries left after each fraction; the actual repair between subsequent fractions depends on the time interval.

The distribution of the cells in the cycle may vary during the course of the daily irradiation on account of progression of surviving cells in the cycle and of mitotic delay; it can cause a variation of the radiosensitivity at the subsequent daily fractions.

Thus, cell survival at the end of a treatment day depends on several biological mechanisms. The possibility of a differential effect between tumor and normal tissue is open to discussion.

In most of multifractionated irradiations the fraction size is similar or close to the usual fraction size of a standard irradiation, say approximately 2 Gy. If a time interval longer than 3 hours is provided between the fractions, we can expect an almost full repair of sublethal injuries so that at each subsequent fraction the cell-survival curve has recovered its initial shape—ignoring the possible variation related to the cell-cycle distribution. In this respect the situation is the same as for a conventional fractionated irradiation.

However, the time necessary to approach a full repair of sublethal injuries is still debated.[18] In a clinical study on human skin early reaction (desquamation), we observed that the repair of sublethal injuries was almost complete after a 2-hour interval between two doses of 1.9 Gy.[8] (We also observed an almost full repair when a dose of 7.5 Gy was delivered in 8 hours with 16 fractions of 0.46 Gy at 30 minute intervals). However, Notter (in a private communication) observed for somewhat larger doses that the repair was not complete at 4 hours—two fractions of 3.5 Gy at 4-hour intervals being equivalent to two fractions of 4 Gy at 24-hour intervals.

The possibility of differential effect between tumor and normal tissue could arise from a slower repair of the tumor cells. However, there is no direct evidence of such a possibility.

Nevertheless, it is suggested by some experiments carried out on hyperthermia that the decrease of the TER with the time interval between irradiation and heat application is faster for normal tissues than for tumor (Table 3).[16]

If the mechanism of radiosensitization by heat is the impairment of repair of sublethal injuries, the TER should be directly related to the amount of sublethal injuries still unrepaired at the moment of heat application. Thus, a difference between two tissues of the variation of the TER as a function of time after irradiation should reflect a difference in the kinetics of the spontaneous repair.

The repetition of irradiation at a short interval should cause a differential effect. For instance, if 3 hours after a first fraction the repair of sublethal injuries is complete for normal cells and only partial for tumor cells,

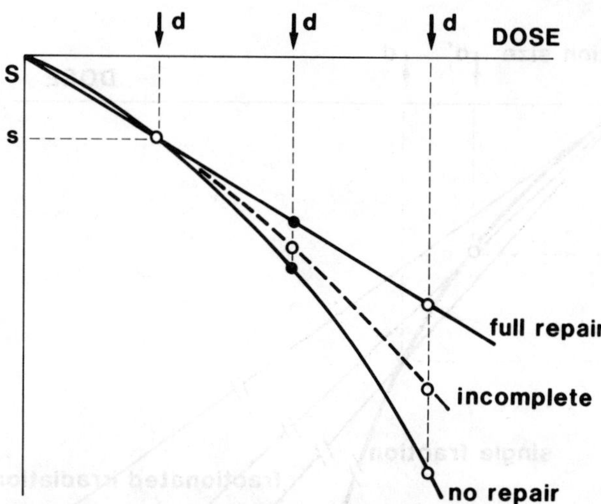

Figure 3. Daily cell survival in multifractionated irradiation–role of cell repair. The cell-survival curve labelled "no repair" is the single-dose cell-survival curve (usual semilog plot). If the interval between fractions is large enough for a full repair between the n daily fractions of size d ($n = 3$), the cell survival for each treatment day is s^n, s being the survival for a dose d assuming a negligible repopulation during the daily irradiation and no change in radiosensitivity. An incomplete repair leads to an intermediate value. Multifractionation could cause a differential effect between two tissues if their repair between fractions is different.

the cell killing produced by a second fraction would be the same as for the first fraction for normal cells and larger for tumor cells.

The differential effect could be amplified if several fractions are delivered during the time necessary for a full repair of tumor cells (see Fig. 3).

The fraction size can be smaller than usual (say 2 Gy) when a large number of daily fractions is used. The question of a possible therapeutic benefit by reducing the fraction size is still discussed.

The effect to reducing the fraction size depends on the shape of the cell-survival curve. A fraction of size d leads to a survival s. If this dose is repeated at intervals long enough to achieve a full repair of sublethal injuries–and disregarding any other biological mechanism such as repopulation and/or cycle redistribution–the survival S for a total dose D varies along the exponential the slope of which is defined by the point of coordinates (d,s). If the irradiation is carried out with smaller fractions d', a total dose D leads to a survival S' higher than S; similarly, for achieving the same survival S a larger dose D' ($> D$) is necessary for smaller fractions.

On account of the initial slope of the single-dose curve which is observed for most biological systems,[1] as the fraction size decreases, D' increases to a maximum value D *max*, defined by the initial tangent to the single-dose curve (see Fig. 4).

Some quantitative data are available to assess the total increase necessary when the fraction size is reduced. Some data have been obtained for human skin desquamation[10,18] and a formula expressing the single-dose survival curve has been proposed by Douglas et al.[7] From this one can compute the additional dose to be applied, for instance, when fractions of 2 Gy are replaced by smaller fractions.

Radiobiological data have been assessed for intestinal mucosa in mice on LD 50/5[13,21] and for lung on LD50/180.[9,11] We found that the cell-survival curve for intestinal mucosa was the same as for skin desquamation. The shoulder of the cell-survival curve for lung is broader, so that the effect of

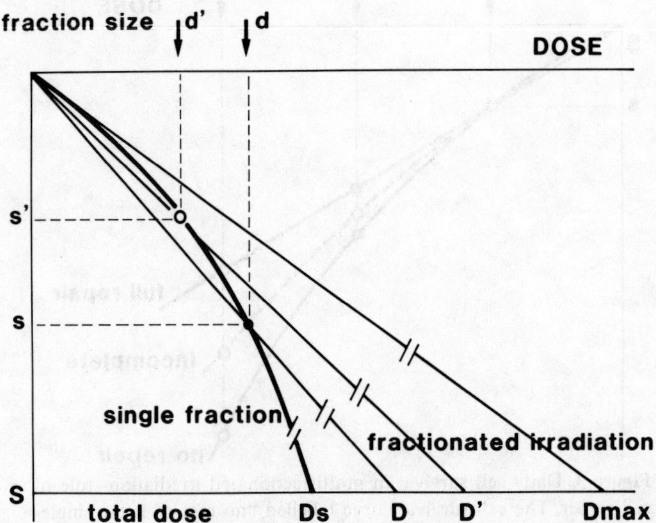

Figure 4. Role of the fraction size. When the fraction size *d* is reduced, the total dose *D* necessary to achieve a given cell survival *S* increases. The additional dose depends on the shape of the single-dose-survival curve. Thus, an alteration of the fraction size can cause a differential effect between two tissues. (For simplicity, we assume a full repair between fractions and no change in radiosensitivity).

reducing the fraction size is larger for lung than for skin or intestine and the additional dose is larger (see Table 4).

Thus, a reduction of the fraction size brings about a relative protection of lung with respect to the two other tissues. For instance, when the fraction size is reduced from 2 to 0.5 Gy, the total dose must be increased by 14% for the skin reaction and by 25% for lung. If the total dose is adjusted to obtain the same skin reaction, the change in fraction size leads to a dose reduction of 10% for lung. A therapeutic benefit of reducing the fraction size can only be expected if the additional dose is larger for normal tissues than for the tumor. When considering the skin desquamation the benefit is doubtful or at least very small since the additional dose is not large for this reaction (Table 4).

TABLE 4. Additional Dose (%) required when 2 Gy Fractions are replaced by Fractions of Smaller Size *d*

	d(Gy)			
	1	0.5	0.2	→0
Skin[a]	9	14	16	19
Intestine[b]				
Lung[c]	15	25	35	–

[a] Data from Douglas, 1975.
[b] Computed from experimental data, Wambersie et al., 1974.
[c] Computed from experimental data, Dutreix and Wambersie, 1974.

The situation may be very different for late reactions if the additional dose is larger than for early reactions. This is suggested by experimental studies and clinical findings. Turesson and Notter[20] have found a discrepancy between the isoeffect dose for early and late skin reactions: the smaller the fraction size (in the range 2.43–7.29 Gy) the less severe the late reactions. Clinical observations at our Institute–and at several other centers–lead to the conclusion that the reduction of the fraction size from 3 to 2 Gy causes a significant therapeutic benefit. The possibility of increasing the benefit with smaller fraction size is worth investigating.

It must be considered, however, that the reduction of the fraction size could be detrimental for some tumors. For instance, Turesson and Notter[19] found that 3 × 1.0 Gy was more efficient than 2.4 Gy for skin reaction while the control of the Ca of the breast was less.

The effect of multifractionation on hypoxic cells should depend on the fraction size and the interval between fractions. If the size of the fractions is the same as for standard fractionation, say 2 Gy, one may fear that reoxygenation would be less complete when the interval is reduced from 1 day to a few hours. However, reoxygenation is a fast mechanism, and a significant reoxygenation can occur within a few hours. The kinetics of reoxygenation may differ according to the tumor type, and more data are needed for assessing the actual risk associated to the reduction of the interval between fractions. Using smaller fractions should allow a larger reoxygenation since the number of the sequences offered to reoxygenation is increased in proportion to the fraction number. Furthermore, the repair of sublethal damage has been reported to be delayed under hypoxic condition for some tumors,[17] so that, mentioned above (Fig. 3), the repetition of fractions at a short interval should increase the cell killing of hypoxic cells.

In conclusion, multifractionation has several practical advantages and some practical inconveniences.

The possibility of a radiobiological benefit, however, is still open to discussion. It may arise from differences in the contribution of sublethal injuries, in the kinetics of their repair, and from differences in the cell-cycle kinetics between tumor and normal tissues. The differential effect could arise from the effect on these biological processes of the alteration of the fraction size, the number and spacing of daily fractions, and the overall time.

Radiobiological data suggest a possibility but do not bring any evidence of a therapeutic benefit; the clinical studies now in progress should provide the final judgment on the question of multifractionation.

REFERENCES

1. Alper, T.: Cell survival after low doses of radiation. Bristol: J. Wiley, 1975.
2. Arcangeli, G., Barocas, A., Mauro, F., Nervi, C., Spano, M., and Tabocchini, A.: Multiple daily fractionation (MDF) radiotherapy in association with hyperthermia and/or misonidazole: Experimental and clinical results. *Cancer* **45**:2707–2711, 1980.
3. Awwad, H.K., Abd, El Baki, H., El Bolkainy, M.W., Burgers, M.V., El Badaway, S., Mansour, M.A., Soliman, O., Omar, S., and Khafagy, M.: Preoperative irradiation of T3 carcinoma in Bilharzial Bladder: A comparison between hyperfractionation and conventional fractionation. (To be published).
4. Castera, D., Legros, M., and Mouillet, J.: Etude de la radiothérapie hyperfractionnée chez 56 patients atteints de tumeurs de la tête et du cou. *J Radiol Electro Med Nucl* **59**:611–614, 1978.
5. Choi, C.H., and Suit, H.D.: Evaluation of rapid radiation treatment schedules utilizing two treatment sessions per day. *Radiology* **116**:703–707, 1975.
6. Cosset, J.M., and Eschwege, F.: L'irradiation hyperfractionnée. In *Actualités Carcinologiques* G. Mathe and B. Hoerni, eds. Paris: Expansion Scientifique Française, 1979, pp. 87–90.
7. Douglas, B.G., Fowler, J.F., Denekamp, J., Harris, S.R., Ayres, S.E., Fairman, S., Hill, S.A., Sheldon, R.W., and Stewart, F.A.: The effect of multiple small fractions of x-rays on skin reactions in the mouse. In *Cell Survival after Low Doses of Radiation,* T. Alper, ed. Bristol: J. Wiley, 1975, pp. 351–361.
8. Dutreix, J.: Current techniques in the use of non-standard fractionation. In *High Energy Photons and Electrons,* S. Kramer, N. Suntharalingam, and G.F. Zinninger, eds. New York: J. Wiley, 1975, pp. 115–128.
9. Dutreix, J., and Wambersie, A.: Isoeffect total dose as a function of the number of fractions for skin, intestine and lung. *Proceeding of the Conference on Time-Dose Relationships in Clinical Therapy,* W.L. Caldwell, and D.D. Tobert, eds. University of Wisconsin, 1974, pp. 21–30.
10. Dutreix, J., and Wambersie, A.: Cell survival deduced from nonquantitative reactions of skin, intestinal mucosa and lung. In *Cell Survival after Low Doses of Radiation* T. Alper, ed. Bristol: J. Wiley, 1975, pp. 335–341.
11. Field, S.B., and Hornsey, S.: The response of mouse skin and lung to fractionated x-rays. In *Cell Survival after Low Doses of Radiation,* T. Alper, ed. Bristol: J. Wiley, 1975, pp. 335–341.
12. Fletcher, G.H., Barkley, H.T., and Shukovsky, L.J.: Present status of the time factor in clinical radiotherapy. II. The nominal standard dose formula. *J*

Radiol Electrol Med Nucl **55**:745–741, 1974.

13. Gueulette, J.: Tolerance de la muqueuse intestinale a une irradiation fractionnée par 60 Cobalt. Importance relative du nombre de fractions et de l'étalement. Thesis, Université Catholique de Louvain, 1977.
14. Littbrand, B., Edsmyr, F., and Revesz, L.: A low dose fractionation scheme for the radiotherapy of carcinoma of the bladder. *Bull Cancer* **62**:241–249, 1975.
15. Simpson, W.J.: In *Time and Dose Relationships in Radiation Biology as Applied to Radiotherapy.* Discussion. In *Proceedings of the NCI-AEC Conference* (Carmel, California, September 1969). Brookhaven National Laboratory, p. 301.
16. Stewart, F., and Denekamp, J.: Fibrosarcoma regrowth delay: X-rays and hyperthermia. Gray Laboratory Report, 1976, pp. 63–64.
17. Suit, H.D., and Urano, M.: Repair of sublethal radiation injury in hypxoic cell of C_3H mouse mammary carcinoma. *Radiat Res* **37**:423–434, 1969.
18. Turesson, I.: Fractionation and dose rate in radiotherapy. Thesis, University of Göteborg, 1978.
19. Turesson, I., and Notter, G.: Experimental determination of equivalent radiation doses with continuous low dose-rate and fractionated high dose-rate irradiation on normal tissue, and the potential risk for late effects with high dose per fraction. In *Proceedings Fourth Congress of the European Radiological Society* (Hamburg, September, 1979), pp. 4–8.
20. Turesson, I., and Notter, G.: Early and late effects of multiple daily and conventional fractionation in normal and malignant tissues. Communication at E.O.R.T.C. meeting (Paris, November 1979), pp. 15–16.
21. Wambersie, A., Dutreix, J., Gueulette, J., and Lellouch, J.: Early recovery for Intestinal stem cells, as a function of dose per fraction, evaluated by survival rate after fractionated irradiation of the abdomen of mice. *Radiat Res* **58**:498–515, 1974.

CHAPTER 30

Nonstandard Fractionation: Clinical Observations

L.R. Holsti, M.D.[a]
M. Salmo, M.D.[b]
M.M. Elkind, B.M.E., M.M.E., M.S., Ph.D.[c]

Recent advances in radiobiology have stimulated the development of fractionation regimens based on scientific considerations. Today, nonstandard fractionation schemes are one of the subjects most explored.

What Is Nonstandard Fractionation?

Broadly speaking, all fractionation schemes which differ from daily fractionation with equal daily doses are nonstandard fractionations. These include:

1. *Hypofractionation*–radiotherapy with a reduced number of fractions based on equal individual doses and equal intervals; this type of fractionation has recently been discussed by Cox et al.[5] and Wiernick et al.[17]
2. *Superfractionation*–multiple daily fractionation, recently discussed by Arcangeli et al.;[2] fractionation with multiple daily doses is dealt with in this volume separately.
3. *Split-course fractionation*–two conventionally fractionated parts separated by an interval of rest, or of two differently fractionated parts separated by a rest interval, discussed by Holsti.[11-13]
4. *Unequal or unconventional fractionation*–radiotherapy based on unequal individual doses and unequal intervals[14] or unequal doses and equal intervals.[1]

This chapter will confine itself to the last-mentioned nonstandard fractionation method.

Biological Bases of Unconventional Fractionation

When daily fractions with equal doses and equal intervals are used, sufficient time is obviously not allowed for reoxygenation to exert a significant effect in radiotherapy. According to Elkind,[7-9] a reasonably large degree of cell killing may be required before cell lysis and attendant reoxygenation set in to a significant extent. This suggests that reasonably large initial doses may be the method of choice, and that these perhaps ought to be separated by intervals of 3 to 4 or possibly more cell-cycle times. Once tumor shrinkage and reoxygenation have started, optimal treatment might imply smaller dose fractions and shorter intervals, the latter to ensure that contributions from repopulations remain ineffective.

UFS/1

Based on the ideas on Elkind,[7-9] an un-

[a,b]Department of Radiotherapy and Oncology, University Central Hospital, Helsinki, Finland
[c]The Division of Biological and Medical Research, Argonne National Laboratory, Argonne, Ill.
The Department of Radiology, University of Chicago, Chicago, Ill.

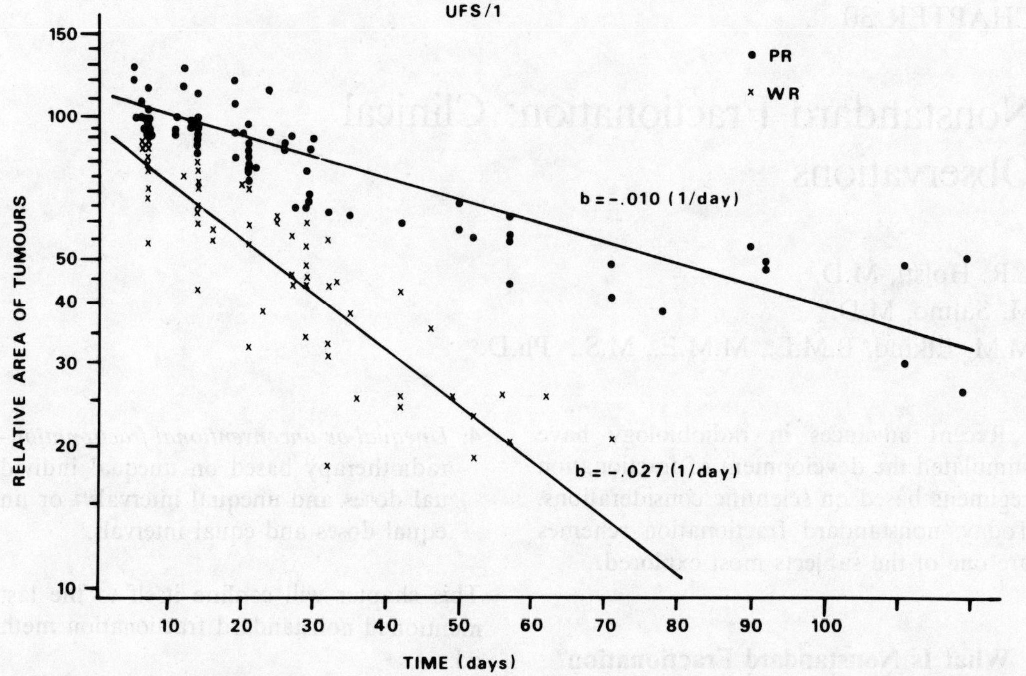

Figure 1. The tumors of the UFS/1 group divided into two subgroups: (x) well-reacting group with shrinking factor b = -0.0268 and (·) poorly reacting group with shrinking factor b = -0.0095.

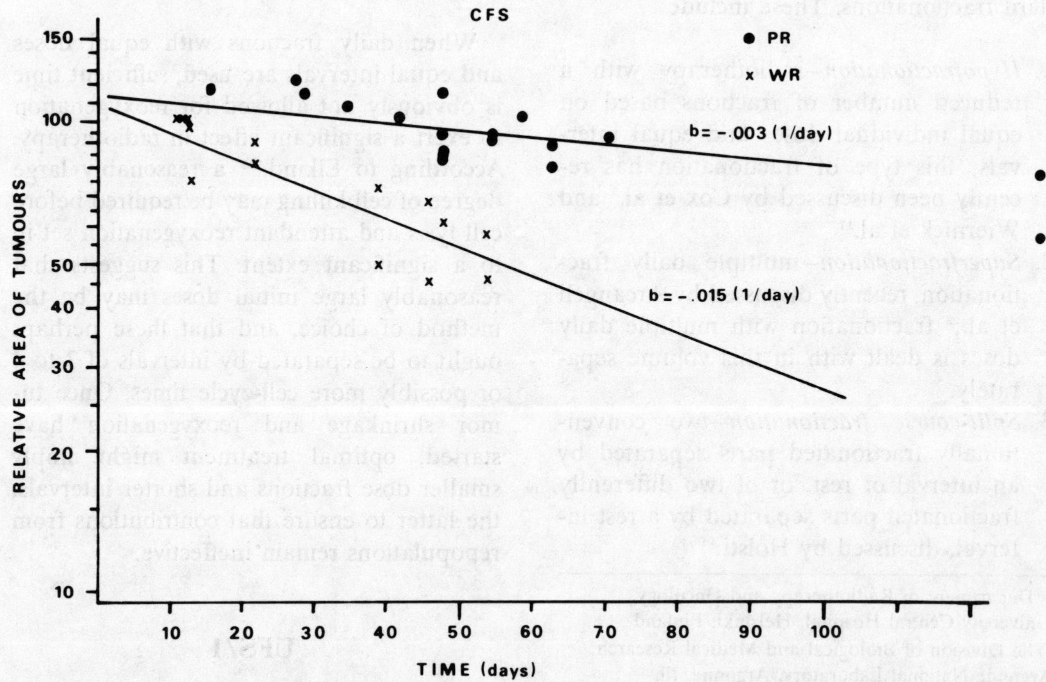

Figure 2. The tumors of the CFS group divided into two subgroups: (x) poorly reacting group with b = 0.0032 and (·) well-reacting group with b = -0.0147.

TABLE 1. The Unconventional Fractionation Scheme 1 (UFS/1)

Week	Mon.	Tues.	Wed.	Thurs.	Fri.
1	1000				
2	700				500
3	300		300		300
4	300		300		300
6	200	200	200	200	200

conventional fractionation scheme with decreasing individual tumor doses, UFS/1 (see Table 1), was tested in a clinical series consisting of primary lung carcinomas and lung metastases from different primaries. The shrinkage rate was calculated by the method of least squares. The results obtained gave two curves whose slopes clearly differ from each other.[14] One curve represents well-responding or rapidly shrinking cases, the other poorly responding or slowly shrinking cases (see Fig. 1). In a conventionally fractionated control group (CFS) the tumors also fell into two subgroups by way of their response (see Fig. 2). It is notable that in the well-responding CFS group the slope is approximately the same as in the poorly responding UFS/1 group.

Individual shrinkage curves show that even very big tumors disappear totally with the UFS/1 regimen (see Fig. 3). The frequency and the degree of lung fibrosis was somewhat higher in the UFS/1 group than in the CFS group.

It is possible that the tumors in the well-responding group respond more favorable because their reoxygenation is sufficient. On the other hand, it could be argued that the improved tumor response reflects a significant improvement in tumor shrinkage rate, due only to increased cell killing resulting from the use of fewer fractionations. The lung fibrosis observed seems to support this interpretation. This is, however, not the only explanation in view of the two subgroups.

A rough estimate suggests that in UFS/1 the total dose could be decreased by 600 to 1000 rad if reduced sublethal damage repair

TABLE 2. The Unconventional Fractionation Scheme 2 (UFS/2)

Week	Mon.	Tues.	Wed.	Thurs.	Fri.
1	800				
2	600				400
3	300		300		250
4	250		250		250
5	200	200	200	200	200

TABLE 3. The Unconventional Fractionation Scheme 3 (UFS/3)

Week	Mon.	Tues.	Wed.	Thurs.	Fri.
1	800				
2			700		
3	300		600		
4	500			500	
5	300		300		300
6	200	200	200	200	200

is the only reason for its greater effectiveness. We, therefore, tried a modified UFS/2 regimen (see Table 2) which starts with 800 rad and in which the total dose is 4400 rad in 5 weeks. If improved reoxygenation plays a role, UFS/2 may be expected to give less normal tissue damage with comparable tumor regression. In order to reduce the degree of fibrosis, we decided to try the unconventional scheme, UFS/3, seen in Table 3.

UFS/2 and UFS/3

The UFS/2 and UFS/3 groups were studied by shrinkage in the same way as UFS/1. In both the UFS/2 and UFS/3 schemes two subgroups of regression patterns were observed; in UFS/3 even a third intermediate group could be identified. The UFS/3 is quite close to UFS/1 in regression behavior (see Fig. 4), whereas the UFS/2 behaves very much like the control group (see Fig. 5).

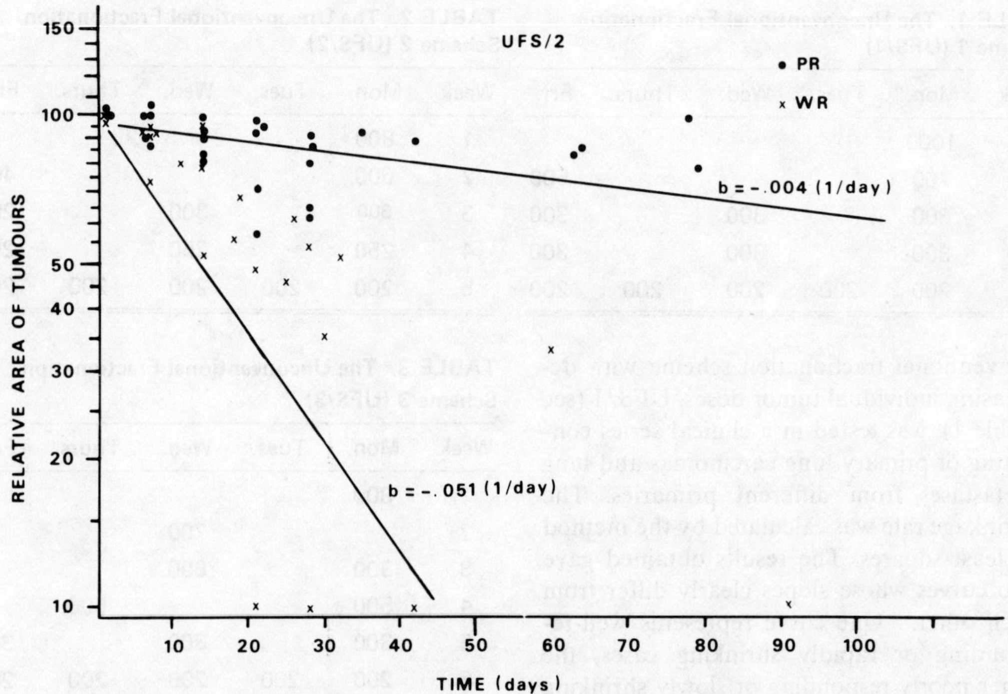

Figure 3. The tumors of the UFS/2 group divided into two subgroups: (x) well-reacting group with shrinking factor $b = -0.051$ and (·) poorly reacting group $b = -0.004$.

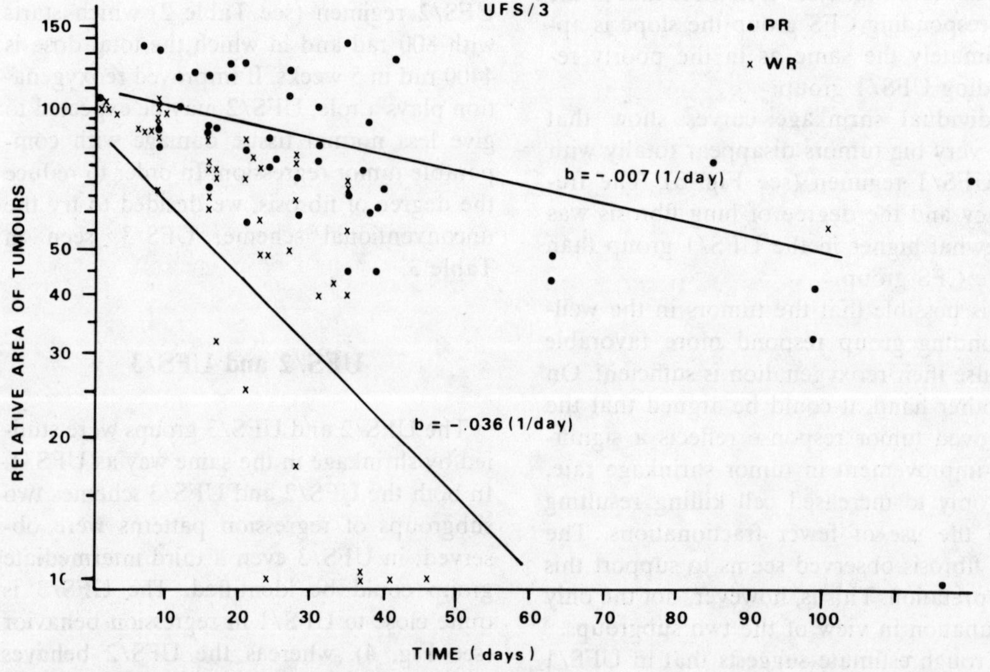

Figure 4. The tumors of the UFS/3 group divided into two subgroups: (x) well-reacting group with shrinking factor $b = -0.036$ and (·) poorly reacting group with $b = -0.007$.

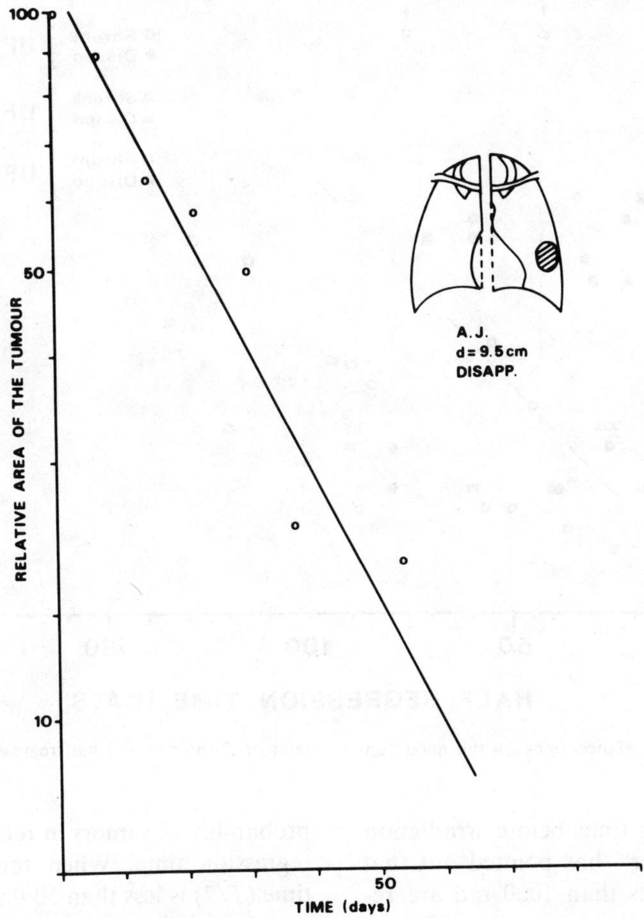

Figure 5. Disappearance of a big epidermoid carcinoma of the lung treated with the UFS/1 scheme.

Tumor Regression

The half-regression time was calculated by the method of least squares taking into account all observations from the weekly chest x-rays. As a criterion of tumor regression we used a 5 mm decrease in diameter within 7 days, irrespective of tumor size. In this way a borderline value for the half-regression time is obtained, by the aid of which tumor shrinkage can be assessed (see Fig. 6).

Our observations indicate that the half-regression time does not correlate with the doubling time of the tumors (see Fig. 7). This observation differs from those reported in fractionated radiotherapy of lung metastases with total doses of 2000 to 5000 rad[4] and single-dose treatment with 1000 rad.[16] Both the authors in question stressed that growth rate is one of the most important parameters in determining radiosensitivity with regard to volume reduction.

According to Malaise et al.,[15] the half-regression time for different types of lung metastases after a single dose of 1000 rad is of the order of 14 days. The interval before the minimum volume was reached was longer

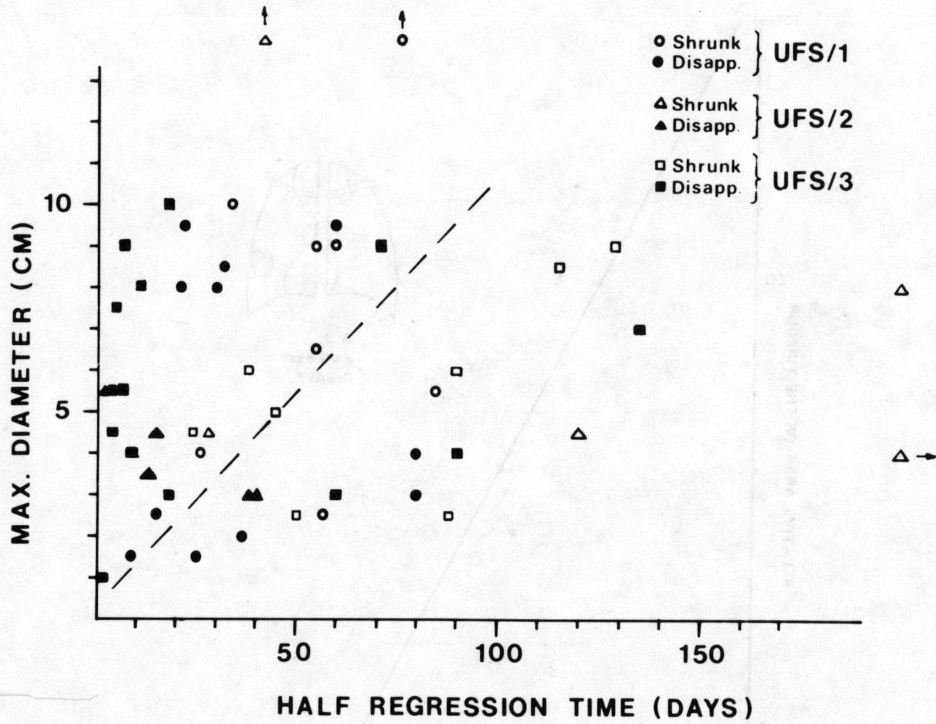

Figure 6. Correlation between the maximum diameter of the tumor and half-regression time.

when the doubling time before irradiation was larger. Fletcher[10] has pointed out that higher weekly doses than 1000 rad are required to initiate the regression of fast-growing masses.

The half-regression time correlates to some degree with tumor size (Fig. 6), though not very strongly. When the diameter is less than 10 cm there is a correlation, but in the few tumors with a diameter exceeding 10 cm there is no correlation. Dutreix, et al.[6] used a concentrated split-course modification consisting of 2 × 850 rad at an interval of 48 hours, a rest interval of 3 weeks, and a second series of 3000 rad in 3 weeks. Tumor regression was faster with concentrated irradiation than with fractionated irradiation.

Local Control

It is useful to consider the disappearance probability of tumors in relation to the half-regression time. When the half-regression time ($T/2$) is less than 50 days, the probability of disappearance of the tumor is great, 83%. On the contrary, when $T/2$ exceeds 50 days, the probability of disappearance is small, only 30% (see Fig. 8).

When the disappearance probability is analyzed by our initial regression criterion–a 5-mm reduction in diameter–the correlation becomes even more pronounced (see Fig. 9). When the half-regression time is less than 36 days, the disappearance probability is 85%, while it is only 25% with a $T/2$ of more than 36 days.

Generally speaking, the probability of disappearance is greater for small tumors less than 10 cm in diameter than for big tumors with a diameter exceeding 10 cm (see Fig. 10). However, this is not a consistent trend. Some big tumors (8–10 cm in diameter) disappeared completely, whereas tumors with diameters of 5–7 cm showed a

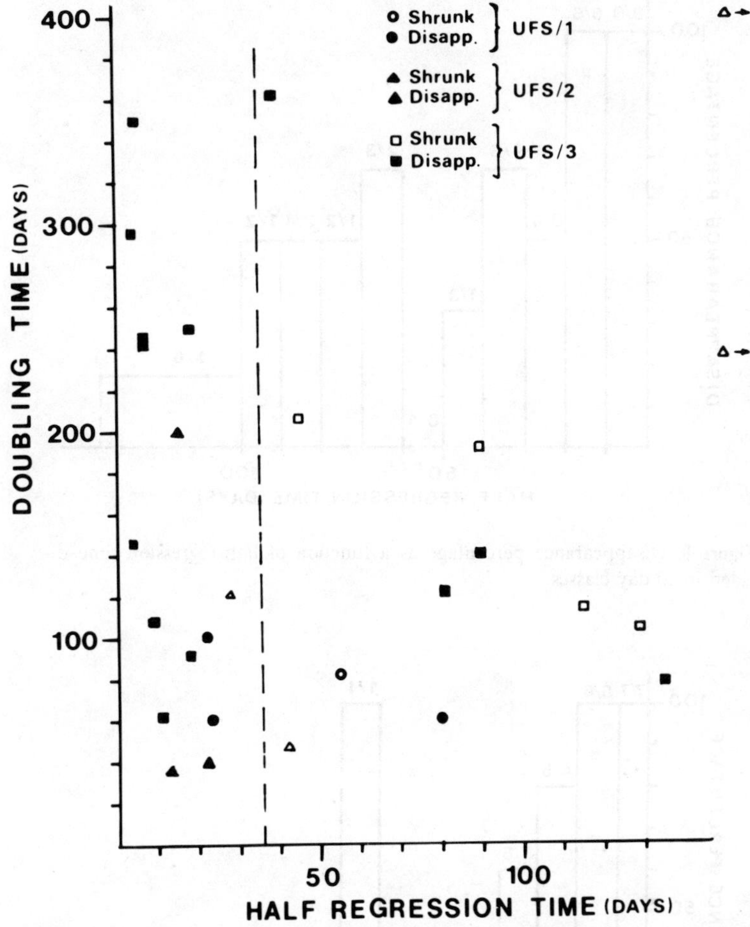

Figure 7. Lack of correlation between doubling time of tumor and half-regression time.

low disappearance frequency. Histology may play a role in tumor disappearance.

No tumors in the group treated with conventional fractionation disappeared.

Normal Tissue Reaction

Observation of the lung fibrosis in the various treatment groups showed that fibrosis develops mainly in cases where the tumor disappears. In these cases there is no great difference between the different schemes with regard to the frequency of fibrosis. The UFS/2 scheme is somewhat better than the other two in this respect, but the probability of tumor disappearance with this regimen is smaller than with UFS/1 and UFS/3. It seems as if the smaller initial dose and the longer time lapse between the first and second fractions reduced the percentage of fibrosis (see Table 4).

When the tumor shrinks very slowly, no heavy fibrosis occurs; there is only fibrosis of slight and medium degree (see Fig. 11). If the half-regression time of the tumor is short, fibrosis will develop early and will be severe in degree (see Fig. 12 and Table 4). This supports our earlier view of the impor-

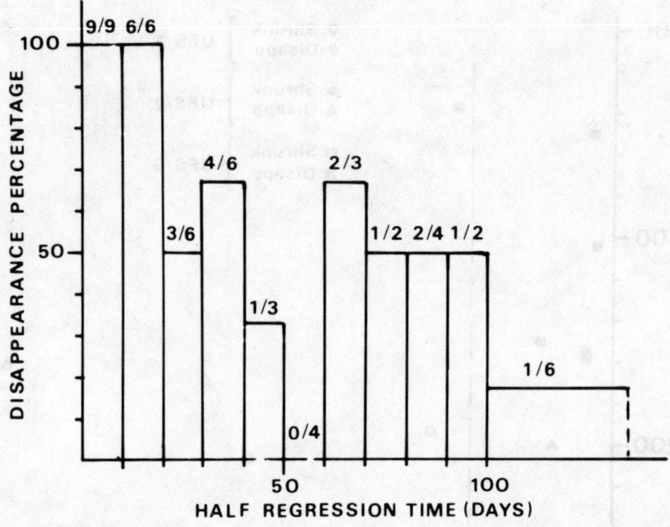

Figure 8. Disappearance percentage as a function of half-regression time divided in 10-day classes.

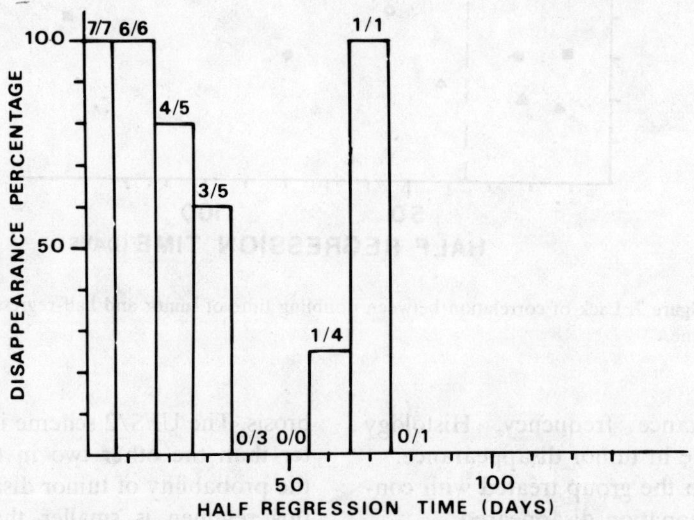

Figure 9. Disappearance percentage as a function of half-regression time divided in closer by using the criterion of tumor regression (5 mm during the first week).

tance of reducing the field size for rapidly shrinking tumors during treatment.

Identification of Radioresistant Tumors

Broadly speaking, the responses to the UFS schemes fall into two classes: tumors that do not start shrinking during the first week are *radioresistant*, while those that do are *radiosensitive*. A shoulder can be seen in the shrinkage curve for poorly responding, resistant tumors. The shoulder is lacking in the shrinkage curve for sensitive tumors. If

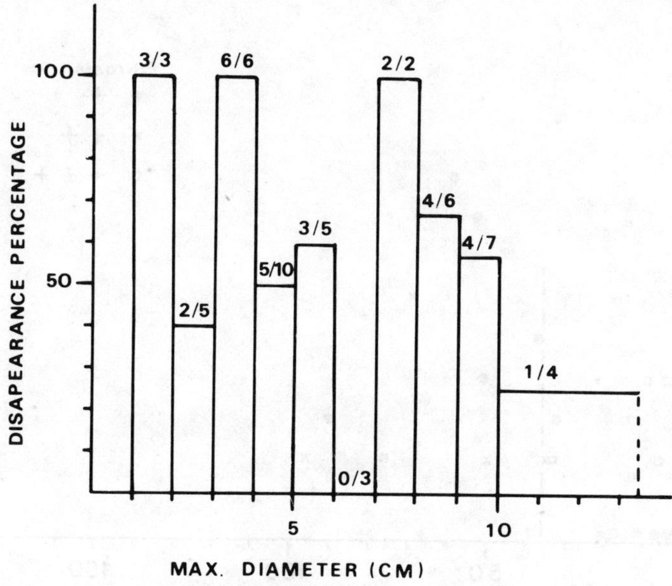

Figure 10. Disappearance percentage as a function of maximum diameter of tumor.

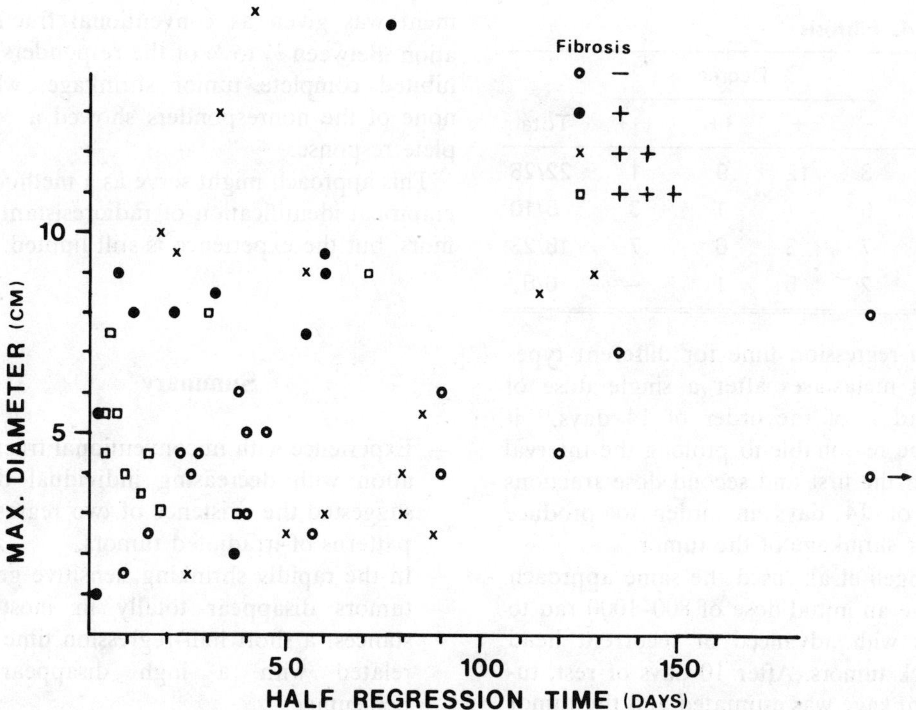

Figure 11. Degree of fibrosis as a function of maximum diameter and half-regression time.

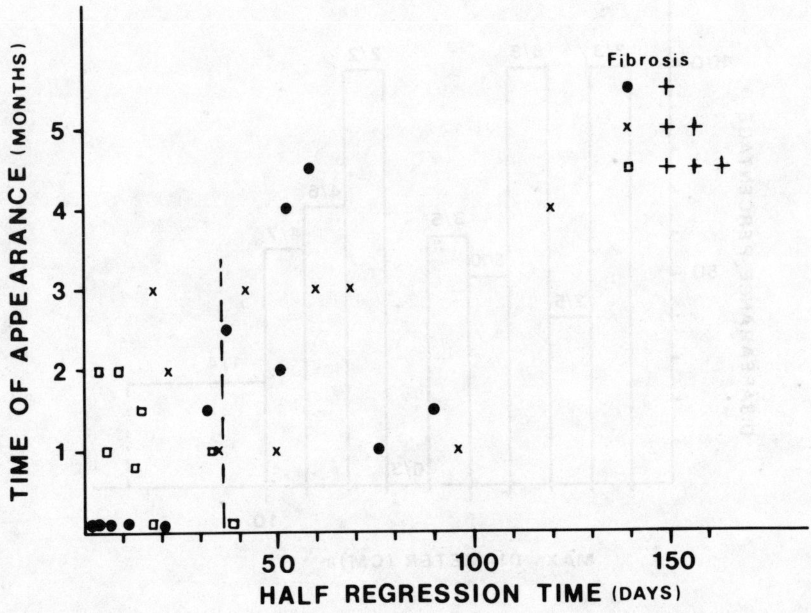

Figure 12. Degree of fibrosis as a function of time of its appearance and the half-regression time.

TABLE 4. Fibrosis

	Degree				
	–	+	++	+++	Total
UFS/1	3	12	9	1	22/25
UFS/2	5	1	1	3	5/10
UFS/3	7	3	6	7	16/23
CFS	2	5	1	–	6/8

the half-regression time for different types of lung metastases after a single dose of 1000 rad is of the order of 14 days,[15] it might be reasonable to prolong the interval between the first and second dose fractions to 10 or 14 days in order to produce stronger shrinkage of the tumor.

Arcangeli et al.[2] used the same approach and gave an initial dose of 800–1000 rad to patients with advanced or recurrent head and neck tumors. After 10 days of rest, tumor shrinkage was estimated and the tumor was classified as a responder or a nonresponder. The remaining part of the treatment was given as conventional fractionation. Between ⅔ to ¾ of the responders exhibited complete tumor shrinkage, while none of the nonresponders showed a complete response.

This approach might serve as a method of empirical identification of radioresistant tumors, but the experience is still limited.

Summary

- Experience with unconventional fractionation with decreasing individual doses suggested the existence of two regression patterns of irradiated tumors.
- In the rapidly shrinking, sensitive group, tumors disappear totally in most instances; a short half-regression time correlated with a high disappearance percentage.
- The half-regression time does not correlate with the doubling time of the tumor,

but it correlates to some degree with tumor size.

- Rapidly shrinking, radiosensitive and slowly shrinking, radioresistant tumors can be identified within a week after an initial large dose fraction.
- Lung fibrosis following unconventional fractionation correlates with the half-regression time; the more rapidly the tumor disappears, the higher the degree of fibrosis.

REFERENCES

1. Abe, M., Yabumoto, E., Nishidai, T., and Takahashi, M.: Trials of new forms of radiotherapy for locally advanced bronchogenic carcinoma. Irradiation under 95% O_2 plus 5% CO_2 inhalation, uneven fractionation and intraoperative irradiation. *Strahlentherapie* **153**:149–158, 1977.
2. Arcangeli, G., Mauro, F., Morelli, D., and Nervi, C.: Multiple daily fractionation in radiotherapy: Biological rationale and preliminary clinical experiences. *Eur J Cancer* **15**:1077–1083, 1979.
3. Arcangeli, G., Mauro, F., Nervi, C., and Starace, G.: A critical appraisal of the usefulness of some biological parameters in predicting tumor radiation response of human head and neck (H & N) cancer. *Br J Cancer* **41**:(IV):39, 1980.
4. Breur, K.: Effectiveness of radiation in relation to growth characteristics of tumors and normal tissues. In *Biological and Clinical Basis of Radiosensitivity,* M. Friedman, ed. Springfield, Ill.: Charles C. Thomas, 1974, pp. 502–527.
5. Cox, J.D., Byhardt, R.W., Komaki, R., and Greenberg, M.: Reduced fractionation and the potential of hypoxic cell sensitizers in irradiation of malignant epithelial tumors. *Int J Radiat Oncol Biol Phys* **6**:37–40, 1980.
6. Dutreix, J., Schlienger, M., Chauvel, C., and Daguin, R.: Concentrated irradiation. Concentrated palliative radiotherapy for tumours affecting the oesophagus, brain, bones and mediastinum. *Ann Clin Res* **3**:9–15, 1971.
7. Elkind, M.M.: Reoxygenation and its potential role in radiotherapy. In *Time and Dose Relationships in Radiation Biology as Applied to Radiotherapy* Carmel Conference Report and Brookhaven National Laboratory Report 50203, 1970, pp. 318–333.
8. Elkind, M.M.: Recovery, reoxygenation and a strategy to improve radiotherapy. In *Biological and Clinical Basis of Radiosensitivity,* M. Friedman, ed. Springfield, Ill.: Charles C. Thomas, 1974, pp. 343–372.
9. Elkind, M.M., Withers, H.R., and Belli, J.A.: Intracellular repair and the oxygen effect in radiobiology and radiotherapy. *Front Radiat Ther Oncol* **3**:55–87, 1968.
10. Fletcher, G.H.: Clinical dose-response curves of human malignant epithelial tumours. *Br J Radiol* **46**:1–12, 1973.
11. Holsti, L.R.: Split-course techniques. In *Time and Dose Relationships in Radiation Biology as Applied to Radiotherapy* Carmel Conference Report and Brookhaven National Laboratory Report 50203, 1970, pp. 292–300.
12. Holsti, L.R.: Alternative approaches to radiotherapy alone and radiotherapy as part of combined therapeutic approach for lung cancer. III. *Cancer Chemother Rep* **4**:165–169, 1973.
13. Holsti, L.R., and Mattson, K.: A randomized study of split-course radiotherapy of lung cancer: long term results. *Int J Radiat Oncol Biol Phys* **6**:977–981, 1980.
14. Holsti, L.R., Salmo, M., and Elkind, M.M.: Unconventional fractionation in clinical radiotherapy. *Br J Cancer* **37**:Suppl. III, 307–310, 1978.
15. Malaise, E.P., Charbit, A., Chavaudra, N., Combes, P.F., Douchez, J., and Tubiana, M.: Change in volume of irradiated human metastases. Investigation of repair of sublethal damage and tumour repopulation. *Br J Cancer* **26**:43–52, 1972.
16. van Peperzeel, H.A.: Effects of single doses of radiation on lung metastases in man and experimental animals. *Eur J Cancer* **8**:665–675, 1972.
17. Wiernick, G., Bleehan, N.M., Brindle, J., Bullimore, J., Churchill-Davidson, I.F.J., Davidson, J., Fowler, J.F., Francis, P., Hadden, R.C.M., Haybittle, J.L., Howard, N., Lanseley, I.F., Lindup, R., Phillips, D.L., and Skeggs, D.: Sixth Interim Progress report of the British Institute of Radiology fractionation study of 3F/week versus 5F/week in radiotherapy of the laryngo-pharynx. *Br J Radiol* **51**:241–250, 1978.

CHAPTER 31

Multiple Daily Fractionation (MDF) Radiotherapy: Clinical Results

Giorgio Arcangeli, M.D.[a]
Francesco Mauro, D.Sc.[b]

The recent fashion of altering a conventional course of radiotherapy by employing different schemes of dose fractionation in the treatment of a large variety of tumors is to be ascribed to both a better understanding of the radiobiological phenomena involved in determining the differential radiation response of normal and tumor tissues and the necessity of enhancing the therapeutic ratio and the final outcome of cancer.

In general, the procedures most commonly employed in altering a conventional radiotherapy course are those allowing a compression of radiation treatment (see Fig. 1):

- Fewer of higher radiation fractions with a fractionation interval longer than 24 hours.
- Hyperfractionation, employing six to eight daily fractions of 0.8–1 Gy with a fractionation interval of 1 hour, thus approaching the "low dose rate" treatment.
- Multiple daily fractionation (MDF), employing three daily fractions of 1.5–1.8 Gy with a fractionation interval of about 4 hours.

In Figure 2, these fractionation schemes are illustrated as a function of the approximate dose and interval scale, according to the specific radiobiological phenomena relevant in determining the radiation response at the dose employed for each particular fractionation course.

Fewer fractions of higher doses of radiation with an interval between fractions longer than 24 hours will surely cause an increased cell killing, possibly larger in normal oxygenated than in neoplastic hypoxic cells because of the marked oxygen effect at these doses. However, intervals longer than 24 hours may allow the hypoxic tumor cells to be fully oxygenated. Therefore, this kind of schedule would be more useful in the treatment of (1) slowly growing tumors in which repopulation and recruitment are considerably less than in normal renewing tissues, (2) tumors in which reoxygenation is a relevant phenomenon, or (3) tumors characterized by a large shoulder in the survival curve (e.g., melanoma).

The other two schemes of "compressed" fractionation (hyperfractionation and MDF) are very similar: no remarkable oxygen effect and repopulation are expected to occur, and all cell killing, at these low doses of radiation, would predominantly be due to irreparable "single-hit" injury rather than to accumulation of sublethal lesions.[7] Furthermore, in both schemes, the response to repeated small dose fractions can be modified to varying extents in different tissues by redistribution (or reassortment) of cells through the cycle.[19] However, in the case of hyperfractionation, the response of both normal and tumor tissues to radiation can be affected by the incomplete repair of sub-

[a]Head, Division of Radiation Therapy, Istituto Medico e di Ricerca Scientifica, Rome, Italy
[b]Senior Scientist, Laboratorio di Dosimetria e Biofisica, Comitato Nazionale per l'Energia Nucleare, Rome, Italy

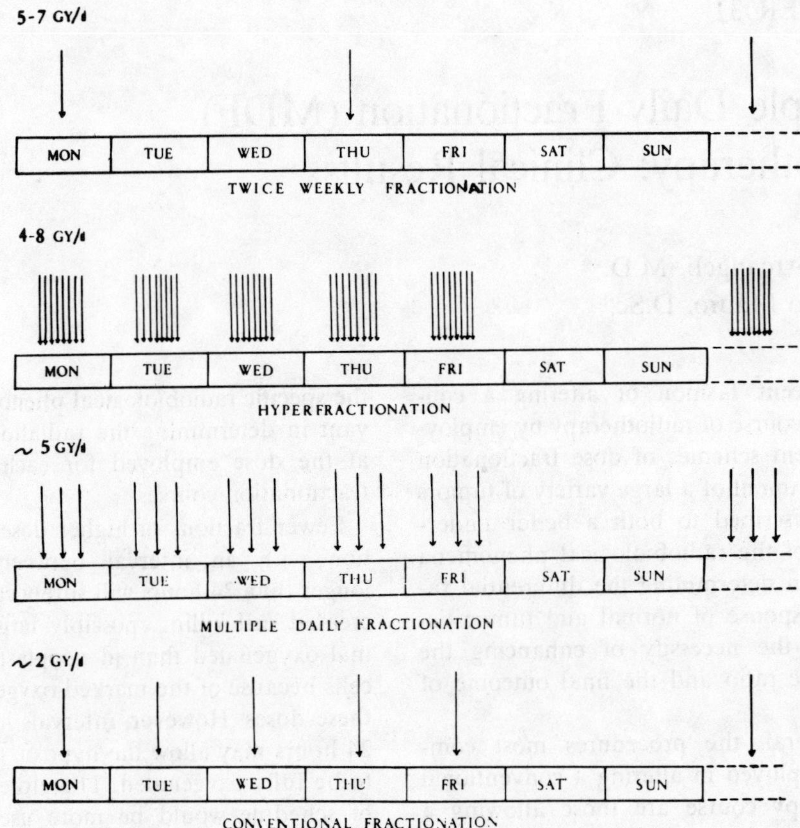

Figure 1. Fractionation modalities in radiotherapy.

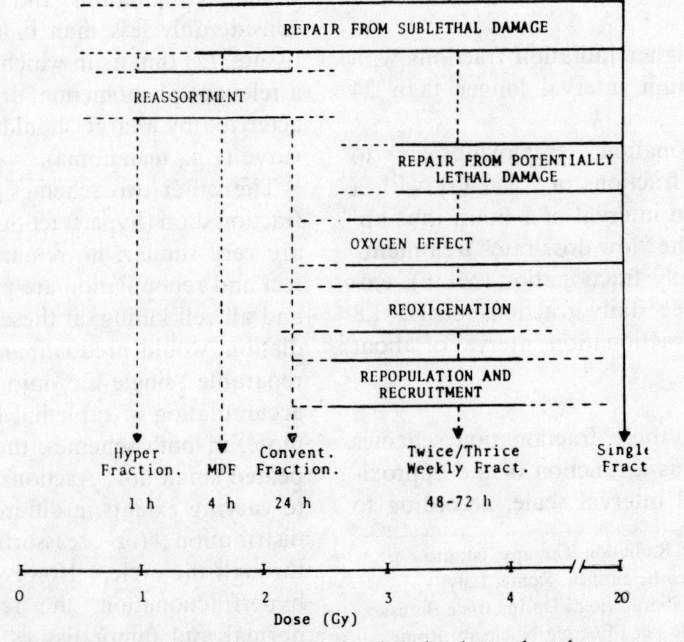

Figure 2. Approximate-dose and fractionation-interval scale as a function of the radiobiological phenomena relevant in determining the radiation response.

lethal injury during the short fractionation interval (1 hour), while the sublethal damage should be completely repaired in normal tissues during the fractionation intervals of 3 to 4 hours of the MDF scheme. In this situation, there is also the possibility that in tumors repair processes are slower than in normal renewing tissues.[5,8] On the other hand, it is likely that, when a small dose is further fractionated, no additional sparing of normal tissue would be obtained.[17] It is clear that this treatment scheme should be useful mainly in the treatment of tumors which grow at least at the same rate as normal renewing tissues. However, it could still be of value in the treatment of hypoxic, slowly growing tumors, in consideration of the fact that the differential oxygen effect and the repair from potentially lethal damage are not likely to occur in these tumors, at these low doses and short fractionation intervals.[9,12]

Effect of MDF on Normal Tissues

The average mucosal reactions from the clinical data available in the current literature is shown in Figure 3. When the weekly dose approximates the conventional fractionation scheme (i.e., two daily fractions of 1.2 Gy each, 5 days per week, for 6–7 weeks), the mucosal reaction tends to be similar to that typically obtainable after a conventional irradiation.[10,14] When more compressed radiotherapy courses are employed (i.e., an MDF of three daily fractions of 1.6–1.8 Gy, 5 days per week, for 11–12 days, optionally followed, after 3–4 weeks of rest, by a 3–5 day boost), the average mucosal reaction tends to develop and subside earlier than that generally observed after noncompressed fractionation schemes.[16]

Skin reactions are difficult to assess from the data available in the current literature. In general, unless some bolus were used, acute skin reactions have rarely been scored as more than intensive erythema, probably because of the skin-sparing effect of the high-energy photon beams currently used in routine radiotherapy.

Using a modification of the Withers technique,[18] we attempted to measure the response of human epithelial cells *in situ* to two different regimens of MDF on two patients by counting repopulating colonies which appeared on the skin after moist desquamation had occurred.[3] Figure 4 shows the survival curve obtained in patient A treated with three daily fractions of 2.5 + 1.5 + 1.5 Gy, at 4-hour intervals between fractions, 5 days per week. The caculated D_o value for this curve is 4.9 ± 1.5 Gy, reflecting the slope of an exponential curve passing from an origin at zero dose through a single-dose survival point intermediate between those of 1.5 and 2.5 Gy. Naturally, no extrapolation number or D_q could be estimated, the initial number of clonogenic cells per unit area being unknown.[18] No moist desquamation was obtained after similar total doses in patient B treated with four daily fractions of 1.5 Gy each, at 3.5-hour intervals between fractions, 5 days per week.

Let us consider the daily treatment in the two patients to be composed of two parts:

Patient A: (1 × 2.5 Gy) + (2 × 1.5 Gy)
Patient B: (2 × 1.5 Gy) + (2 × 1.5 Gy)

Since the second part of the treatment is the same (2 × 1.5 Gy), the experiments on patients A and B compare the relative effectiveness of 1 × 2.5 Gy and 2 × 1.5 Gy. As no moist desquamation occurred in patient B, the effect of 3 Gy in two fractions was less than that from one fraction of 2.5 Gy—that is, that more than 3 Gy must be given in two fractions to achieve equal effects. This strongly suggests that, for skin epithelium, the value of d_f (that is, the range of dose over which the survival curve bends detectably from its exponential slope)[17] is between 1.5 and 2.5 Gy. This means that, with MDF, dose fractions lower than 2.5 Gy should be employed to increase skin tolerance, and that with dose fractions lower

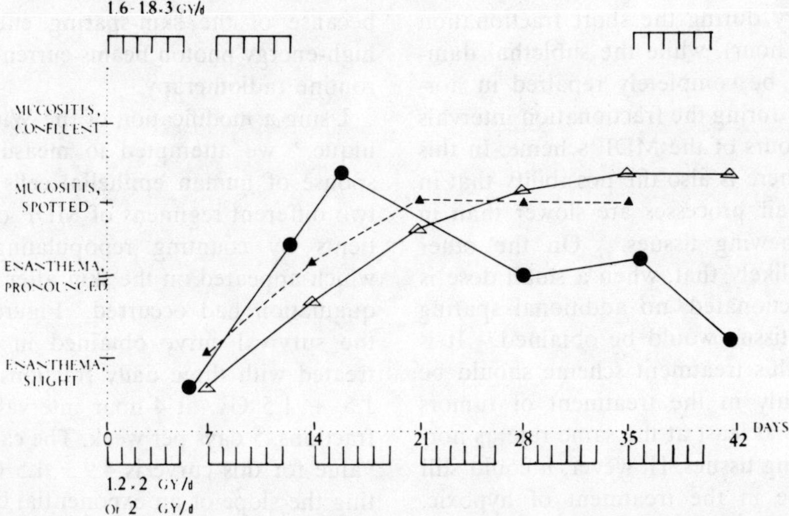

Figure 3. Average mucosal reactions observed with different fractionation schemes: ● = three daily fractions (1.6 to 1.8 Gy/F) (23 cases from van den Bogaert, 1980, and 8 cases from unpublished data of our group); Δ = two daily fractions (1.2 Gy/F) (48 cases from Shukowsky et al., 1976 and Jampolis, et al., 1977); ▲ = conventional fractionation (2 Gy/F) (Schukowsky et al., 1976).

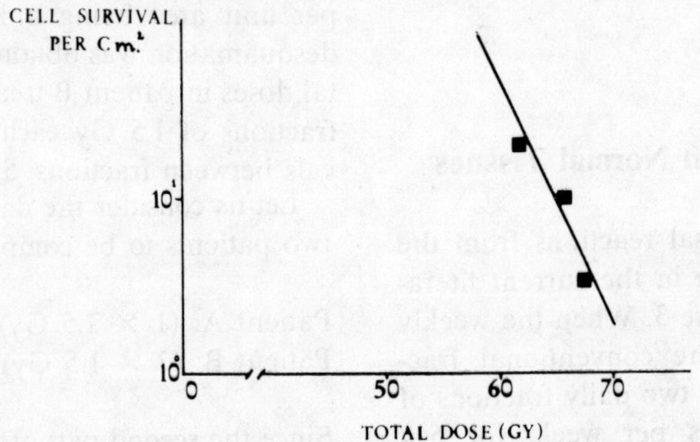

Figure 4. Multifraction dose-survival curve for epithelial cells of human skin treated with a MDF course (2.5 + 1.5 + 1.5 Gy per day). The curve has been fitted by the least squares method and has a D_0 value of 4.9 ± 1.5 Gy (Arcangeli et al., 1980).

than 1.5 Gy no additional sparing of skin would be obtained.

The late effects of MDF on the connective tissue and vascular system underlying the skin are more difficult to evaluate in quantitative terms. Furthermore, the data available in the literature are expressed in a too general way and are lacking in detailed descriptions of the particular damage in each patient. However, we tried to plot together some data, obtained by Svoboda[15] and by our own group, following the irradiation of the chest wall with three daily fractions. The following arbitrary score scale has been used:

0 = No late damage
1 = Pigmentation or questionable fibrosis
2 = Skin atrophy with or without telangiectasis or mild fibrosis
3 = Frank fibrosis and lethering with skin fixation
4 = The above and/or deep muscle fibrosis

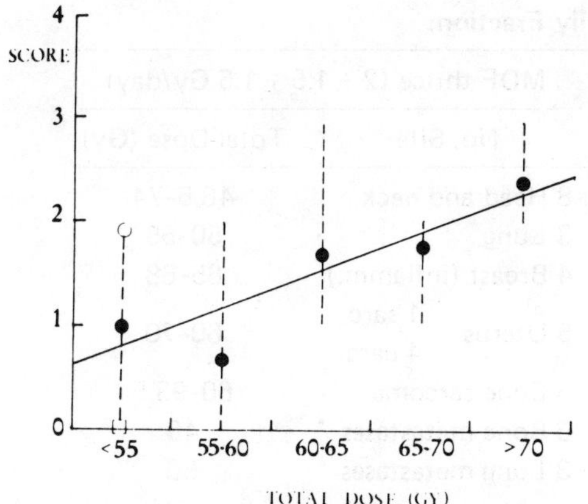

Figure 5. Average late damages after thrice daily fractionation radiotherapy (total dose ranges are indicated on the abscissa): ● = 24 cases treated with daily doses (i.e., sum of three daily fractions) of 5 to 7 Gy (unpublished data); O = 11 cases treated with daily doses >7 Gy (from Svoboda, 1978); □ = 2 cases treated with daily doses < 5 Gy (from Svoboda, 1978); dashed lines represent ranges of score (for the score scale, see text).

In Figure 5, the degree of average late damage is plotted against the total dose ranges. In spite of the small number of cases, the straight line of Figure 5 describes an increased severity of injury and incidence of damage as the total dose bcomes larger, although no damage more than score 3 has ever been recorded. The data plotted along the line refer only to those cases treated with daily doses between 5 and 7 Gy (sum of three dose fractions). Two single points are available in Figure 5 for daily doses higher or lower than such dose range, thus indicating that, in agreement with previous clinical findings[1,4] for the same total doses, the greater the dose per fraction the more severe the late injury. Because of this, and according to our data on skin epithelium, dose fractions of 1.6 Gy are presently employed in our MDF protocols.

Effect of MDF on Tumors

Our main experience in employing MDF in clinical radiotherapy is based on the irradiation of a miscellaneous pilot series of selected patients with advanced and/or generalized radioresistant tumors. The patients have been treated with two or three daily fractions. Table 1 shows the list of patients allotted to the specific treatment group. Preliminary results of this study have already been published elsewhere.[2] In this chapter, the analysis is extended to the results observed after a period of 18 months. The analysis has been discontinued beyond that period in consideration of the fact that the numerous deaths make the evaluation of further observations difficult.

Table 2 shows the results obtained with two (2 + 2 Gy, 8-hour interval) or three (2 + 1.5 + 1.5 Gy, 4-hour interval) daily fractions, 5 days per week, compared with our historical series of patients with the same type of tumors treated with conventional fractionation. In these results, the crude 18-month survival seems to be unaffected by the type of treatment. Nevertheless, the local control rate, either crude or actuarial, appears to be much higher in patients treated with MDF than in those treated with conventional fractionation. The difference is highly significant ($p < 0.01$) at 18 months for patients treated with MDF (two or three daily fractions) as compared with those treated with conventional fractionation. When the percent of successes in surviving patients only are plotted against the period of observation (see Fig. 6), the local control rate seems to be quite similar for the two groups of patients treated with MDF (upper full lines) but still appreciably higher than the rate obtained with conventional fractionation (lower full line). However, when tumors with relatively fast clinical doubling time only (i.e., less than 30 days) are considered, the local control rate (dashed lines) appears to be higher in tumors treated with three than in those treated with two daily fractions. Because of the numerous deaths, the number of patients does not allow, for the moment, a statistically significant difference, although the trend suggests a sharp diverging of the two lines as the period of observation increases.

TABLE 1. Patients Treated with Multiple Daily Fractions

MDF twice (2 + 2 Gy/day)		MDF thrice (2 + 1.5 + 1.5 Gy/day)	
No. Site	Total Dose (Gy)	No. Site	Total Dose (Gy)
6 Head and neck	60–74	8 Head and neck	46.5–74
4 Glioblastoma	58.7–66.5	3 Lung	50–55
2 Ovary	40	4 Breast (inflamm.)	65–68
4 Uterus Sarc. 1 Carc. 3	60–70	5 Uterus 1 sarc. 4 carc.	60–70
4 Prostate	70	3 Bone sarcoma	60–93.5
3 Bone sarcoma	63–80	6 Bone metastases	40
10 Bone metastases	40	3 Lung metastases	50
8 Brain metastases	40–46		
3 Lung metastases	50–54		

TABLE 2. Results of Treatments[a]

Treatment	C.R.[b] at End of Irradiation	C.R.[b] at 18 months	Crude C.R.[b] at 18 months	Crude Survival at 18 months
MDF (twice)	11/46 (0.24)	15/22 (0.68)	15/46 (0.33)	22/46 (0.48)
MDF (thrice)	8/26 (0.31)	9/13 (0.69)	9/26 (0.35)	13/26 (0.50)
Conventional irradiation	38/166 (0.23)	22/80 (0.28)	22/166 (0.13)	80/166 (0.48)

[a] Statistical significance at 18 months for groups 1 and 2 vs. 3: $p < 0.01$.
[b] C.R. = complete response.

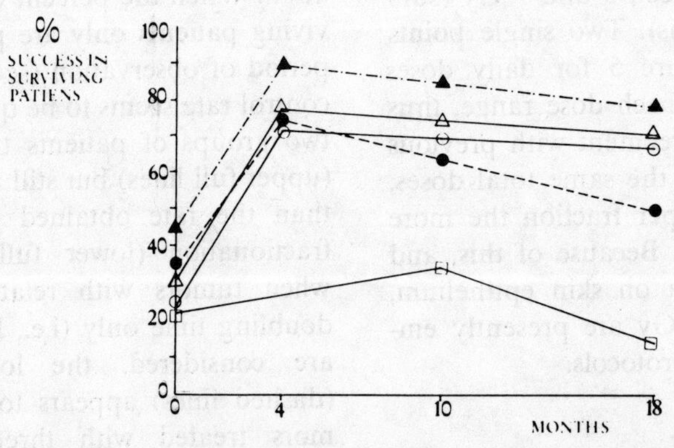

Figure 6. Percent of tumors locally controlled in patients surviving at the time of observation (from Arcangeli et al., 1979 and unpublished data). Twice-daily fractionation (2 + 2 Gy): O = total cases; ● = rapidly growing tumors only. Thrice-daily fractionation (2 + 1.5 + 1.5 Gy): Δ = total cases; ▲ = rapidly growing tumors only. Conventional fractionation: □ = total cases.

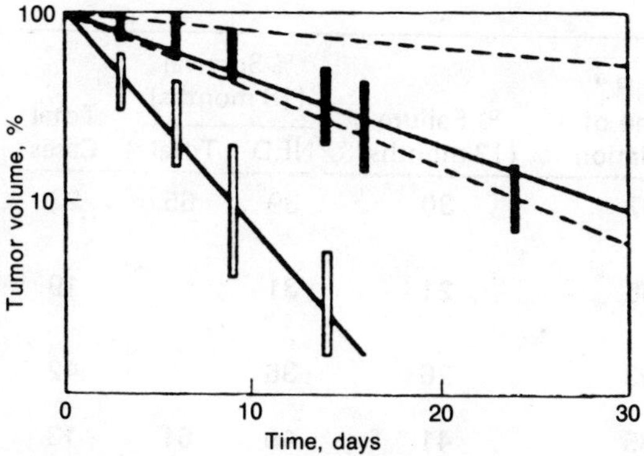

Figure 7. Results for multiple lung metastases from four patients. Lower continuous line represents well-reacting group with fast clinical doubling times (less than 30 days). Higher continuous line represents poorly reacting group with slow clinical doubling times. These results have been obtained with 2 + 1.5 + 1.5 Gy per day, at 5-hour intervals between fractions, 5 days per week, for a total of 50 Gy. The results are compared with similar groups (dashed lines) treated with conventional fractionation (2 Gy per day, 5 days per week) (from Arcangeli et al., 1979).

Also, the regression rate appears to be much faster in rapidly than in slowly growing tumors treated with three daily fractions, as shown in Figure 7, for a group of four patients with multiple lung nodular metastases treated with MDF or conventional fractionation. The response of nodules with a slow clinical doubling time (i.e., more than 30 days) to MDF radiotherapy is similar to that of rapidly growing nodules treated with conventional fractionation.

At present, several studies are merging in the current literature dealing with MDF or hyperfractionation. It is difficult to pool together these results as they are often obtained using very different fractionation schemes and dosages, expressed in widely different ways such as failure, success, or survival, and observed during different periods after the end of treatment. Nevertheless, Table 3 reports some results obtained with MDF in the irradiation of H & N (head and neck) cancer.

In the first two studies[10,14] performed with two daily fractions of 1.2 Gy, the cumulative local failure was 26% at 12 months. The second group includes preliminary results obtained with three daily fractions of 1.6 to 2.3 Gy in some European centers. Following this preliminary approach, a pilot cooperative study was started in Amsterdam, Dijon, Leuven, Porthsmouth, and Rome within the E.O.R.T.C. framework to assess the feasibility of a randomized trial comparing MDF (three daily fractions of 1.6 to 1.8 Gy) with MDF plus misonidazole and with conventional fractionation in advanced H & N cancers. The results after 12 months obtained with MDF only in the first series of 42 patients, all with T_3 - T_4N_3 cancer, are presented in Table 4. Local failure occurred in 14 patients (33%), and 21 (50%) are still alive after 12 months.[16]

In Table 5, the results for other tumors of various sites are reported. These are not randomized trials but in all cases the authors reported some comparison with conventional fractionation.[6,11,13,14] The results indicate that the effectiveness of MDF can be appreciated not only in terms of immediate local response (an important parameter in the case of clinically radioresistant tumors such as glioblastoma multiforme and inflammatory carcinoma of the breast), but also in terms of crude survival rate.

Conclusion

The results reported above indicate that MDF is an effective irradiation scheme for several types of cancer. Our data suggest that three daily fractions are more effective than two daily fractions in the treatment of rapidly growing tumors. Furthermore, high cumulative doses appear to be well tolerated in terms of both acute and late tolerance providing the dose per day is less than 5 Gy. The compression of the overall treatment time, in some MDF schemes, allows the concomitant and/or sequential combination with hyperthermia, hypoxic-cell sensitizers, or cytotoxic drugs. The good local control ob-

TABLE 3. Results of MDF on H & N Cancer

Reference	Dose per Fraction	Total Dose	% C.R.[a] at End of Irradiation	% Failure (12 months)	% Survival (18 months) NED	% Survival (18 months) Total	Total Cases
Jampolis et al., 1977	1.2 X 2	72	87	30	39	65	23
Shukowsky et al., 1976	1.2 X 2	60–75	95	21	31		19
Total	twice a day	60–75	93	26	36		42
Svoboda, 1978	1.6–2.3 X 3	52-55	85	41	46	61	13
Arcangeli, 1980	1.6–1.8 X 3	48 + B[b]	63	50	(50)[c]	(75)[c]	8
van den Bogaert, 1980	1.6–1.8 X 3	48 + B[b]	90	33		(70)[c]	24
Total	thrice a day	48–70	82	40		62	45

[a] C.R. = complete response. [c] Less than 18 months.
[b] B = boost.

TABLE 4. Multifraction—Head & Neck: Follow-Up at 12 Months (42 patients)[a]

NED	10	
Local failure	14	(7 +)
Metastases	5	(4 +)
Dead	21	
Metastases	3	
Local failure and Metastases	1	
Local failure	7	
Intercurrent complications	10	
Insufficient follow-up	4	(All NED at 7,8,9, and 11 months

[a] van den Bogaert, 1980.

tained in several centers with the MDF treatment of advanced or generalized tumors also warrants the use of these schemes on patients with earlier diseases in which the final outcome is more dependent on local control than on distant metastases.

The final demonstration of the higher effectiveness of MDF in respect to conventional fractionation can be obtained only by rigorous clinical trials, some of which are presently underway within the E.O.R.T.C. framework.

Summary

Multiple daily fractionation (MDF) radiotherapy is a treatment scheme based on the exploitation of several biological phenomena. No remarkable oxygen effect and repopulation are expected to occur, and at these low radiation doses, cell killing should be predominantly due to nonrepairable "single-hit" injuries rather than to an accumulation of sublethal lesions. Furthermore, the response to repeated small dose fractions can be modified to varying extents in different tissues by cell redistribution through the cycle. Following this scheme the average mucosal reaction in humans tends to develop and subside earlier than that generally observed after conventional fractionation. The response of human epithelial

TABLE 5. Results of MDF on Various Tumors

Site and Reference	Dose Fraction (Gy)	Total Dose (Gy)	% C.R.[a] at End of Irradiation	% Survival (18 months)	Total Cases
Glioblastoma Multiforme (Douglas, 1977)	1.0 X 3	45		44	31
	conventional	?		13	H[b]
Bladder (Littbrand, 1976)	1.0 X 3	84	64	(58)[c]	36
	conventional	64	44	(41)[c]	41
Breast (inflammatory) (Schukowsky et al., 1976)	1.3 X 2	51–54 + B[d]	100		11
	conventional	?	62		H
Burkitt's Lymphoma (Norin and Onyango, 1977)	0.75–1.85 X 3	16–41	74		34
	conventional	19–51	11		9

[a]C.R. = complete response.
[b]H = historical series.
[c]Between 6 and 40 months.
[d]B = boost.

cells *in situ* to MDF showed a D_o value of 4.9 ± 1.5 Gy and a d_f value between 1.5 and 2.5 Gy. The severity and incidence of late injury, following a MDF scheme, has been found to increase as the local dose becomes larger and, for the same total dose, as the dose per fraction is greater. Our results on different types of advanced tumors indicate that the local control rate is much higher in patients treated with MDF than in those treated with conventional fractionation. The results from several other centers indicate that the effectiveness of MDF can be appreciated not only in terms of immediate local response, but also in terms of crude survival rate.

Acknowledgments

We thank Drs. W. van den Bogaert, D.G. Gonzalez, E. van der Schueren, and V.H.J. Svoboda for the availability of their data and cooperation within the E.O.R.T.C. framework. We are also indebted to Dr. H.R. Withers for the unvaluable critical comments and suggestions. Financial support for this research came from the G. & L. Shenker Research Foundation.

REFERENCES

1. Arcangeli, G., Friedman, M., and Paoluzi, R.: A quantitative study of late radiation effect on normal skin and subcutaneous tissues in human beings. *Br J Radiol* **47**:44–50, 1974.
2. Arcangeli, G., Mauro, F., Morelli, D., and Nervi, C.: Multiple daily fractionation in radiotherapy; Biological rationale and preliminary clinical experiences. *Eur J Cancer* **15**:1077–1083, 1979.
3. Arcangeli, G., Mauro, F., Nervi, C., and Withers, H.R.: Dose-survival relationship for epithelial cells in human skin after multifraction irradiation: Evaluation by a quantitative method *in vivo Int J Radiat Oncol Biol Phys* **6**:841–844, 1980.
4. Chu, F.C.H., Glicksman, A.S., and Nickson, J.J.: Late consequences of early skin reactions. *Radiology* **94**:669–672, 1970.
5. Denekamp, J., and Stewart, F.: Evidence for repair capacity in mouse tumors relative to skin. *Int J Radiat Oncol Biol Phys* **5**:2003–2010, 1979.
6. Douglas, B.G.: Preliminary results using superfractionation in treatment of glioblastoma multiforme. *J Can Assoc Radiol* **28**:106–110, 1977.
7. Elkind, M.M.: The initial part of the survival curve: Implication for low-dose, low-dose rate radiation responses. *Radiat Res* **71**:9–23, 1977.
8. Fowler, J.F., Denekamp, J., Sheldon, W., Smith, A.M., Begg, A.C., Harris, S.R., and Page, A.L.: Sparing effect of x-ray fractionation in mammary tumors and skin reactions in mice. In *Cell Survival after Low Doses of Radiation* T. Alper, ed. London: Institute of Physics and J. Wiley, 1975, pp. 288–292.

9. Jakobson, P.A., and Littbrand, B.: Fractionation scheme with low individual tumor dose and high total dose. *Acta Radiol Ther Phys Biol* **12**:337–346, 1973.
10. Jampolis, S., Pipard, G., Horiot, J.C., Bolla, M., and Le Dorze, C.: Preliminary results using twice-a-day fractionation in the radiotherapeutic management of advanced cancers of the head and neck. *AJR* **129**:1091–1093, 1977.
11. Littbrand, B., and Edsmyr, F.: Preliminary results of bladder carcinoma irradiated with low individual doses and a high total dose. *Int J Radiat Oncol Biol Phys* **1**:1059–1062, 1976.
12. Little, J.B., Hahn, G.M., Frindel, E., and Tubiana, M.: Repair of potentially lethal radiation damage *in vitro* and *in vivo*. *Radiology* **106**:689–694, 1973.
13. Norin, T., and Onyango, J.: Radiotherapy in Burkitt's lymphoma. *Int J Radiat Oncol Biol Phys* **2**:399–406, 1977.
14. Schukowsky, L.J., Fletcher, G.H., Montague, E.D., and Withers, H.R.: Experience with twice-a-day fractionation in clinical radiotherapy. *AJR* **126**:155–162, 1976.
15. Svoboda, V.H.J.: Further experience with radiotherapy by multiple daily sessions. *Br J Radiol* **51**:363–369, 1978.
16. van den Bogaert, W.: Report on multiple daily fractionation in advanced head and neck cancer. Pilot study of the E.O.R.T.C. Radiotherapy Group, reported on October 17, 1980, Paris.
17. Withers, H.R.: The dose-survival relationship for irradiation of epithelial cells of mouse skin. *Br J Radiol* **40**:187–194, 1967.
18. Withers, H.R.: Responses of some normal tissues to low doses of radiation. In *Cell Survival after Low Doses of Radiation* T. Alper, ed. London: Institute of Physics and J. Wiley, 1975, pp. 369–375.
19. Withers, H.R.: Responses of tissues to multiple small dose fractions. *Radiat Res* **71**:24–33, 1977.

CHAPTER 32

Contribution of the Keynote Discussant

Ingela Turesson, M.D.[a]
Gustav Notter, M.D.[a]

Does fractionation change the outcome of local tumor control in radiotherapy and solve the problem of tumor radioresistance?

Unconventional fractionation might be one way to improve the therapeutic ratio and would also be necessary for optimal combination of radiotherapy with hyperbaric oxygen, radiosensitizers, and chemotherapy. In addition to the biological factors, the socioeconomic advantages of some unconventional regimens must also be considered in certain situations.

First we want to make some reflections about the evaluation of the efficiency of unconventional fractionation schedules and then give a short review of the clinical results thus far and the trials which are going on at present.

Evaluation of the Efficiency of Unconventional Fractionation Schedules

There is an obvious need for stringency in clinical research in order to draw valid conclusions. In clinical practice, however, it is extremely difficult to meet all requirements for ethical, practical, and economic reasons. An example from our own clinic illustrates some of the problems.

We have performed a retrospective study of 165 patients irradiated during the period 1963–1977 for glottic cancer T_1 and T_2 (according to UICC, 1978). The patients were irradiated with ^{60}Co x-rays or 5 MV x-rays with two-angled wedge-filter fields.

[a]Department of Radiotherapy, University of Göteborg, Sahlgrenska Hospital, Göteborg, Sweden

Figure 1(*a*) plots the recurrence-free rate at 5 years versus the total tumor dose. It is evident that there is no correlation between local control and tumor dose over a wide dose range. The reason for this is the different fractionation schedules used during the period. Besides different total doses, the dose per fraction and the overall treatment time have varied. Only four to five fractions per week have been used. However, as Figure 1(*b*) shows, there is a good correlation (significant p = 0.013) between 5-year local control and CRE or NSD. CRE (Cu-

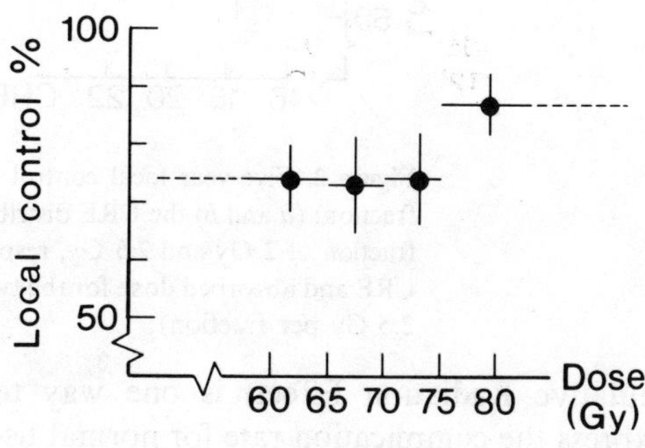

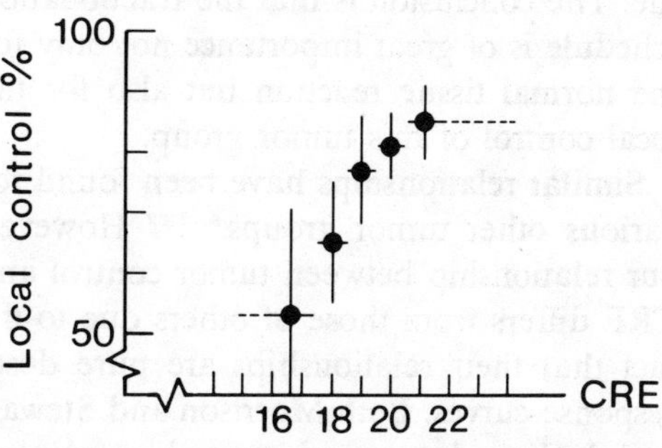

Figure 1. Five-year local control for glottic cancer T1 and T2 as a function of (*a*) the absorbed dose and (*b*) CRE.

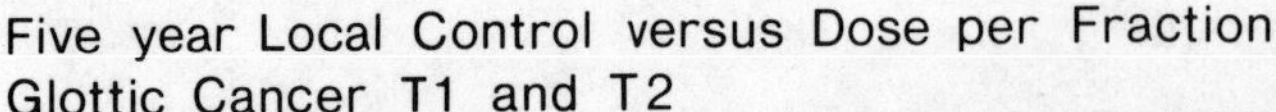

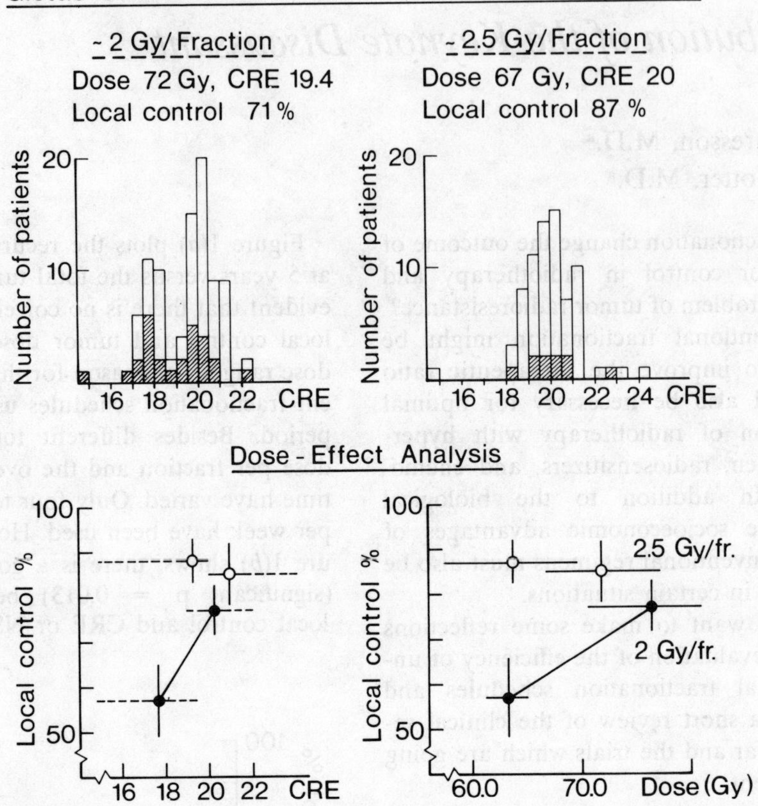

Figure 2. Five-year local control for glottic cancer TI and T2 versus dose per fraction: (*a* and *b*) the CRE distribution for two subgroups with mean doses per fraction of 2 Gy and 2.5 Gy, respectively; (*c* and *d*) 5-year local control versus CRE and absorbed dose for the two subgroups (● = 2 Gy per fraction and ○ = 2.5 Gy per fraction).

mulative Radiation Effect) is one way to express the complication rate for normal tissue. The conclusion is that the fractionation schedule is of great importance not only for the normal tissue reaction but also for the local control of this tumor group.

Similar relationships have been found for various other tumor groups.[9,12,13] However, our relationship between tumor control and CRE differs from those of others due to the fact that their relationships are pure dose-response curves. Both Morrison and Stewart and Jackson have used a fixed number of fractions and a fixed overall treatment time, and Shukovsky's analysis was only based on daily fractionation to 10 Gy per week.

Knowledge of these dose-response curves for conventional fractionation is extremely valuable when one is planning to change to an unconventional fractionation schedule. This is illustrated by a further analysis of our glottic cancer treatments.

The whole group of patients could be divided into two subgroups: one for which the dose per fraction was about 2 Gy and one for which the dose per fraction was about 2.5 Gy. The mean values of dose and CRE for each subgroup are given in Figure 2. The local control was significantly better with the higher dose per fraction ($p < 0.01$). However, keeping the steepness of the relationship between local control and CRE in mind, we have to look at the distribution of CRE within each subgroup, as shown in Figure 2(*a* and *b*). When we performed a dose-effect analysis of each subgroup, which is shown in Figure 2 (*c* and *d*), we got a steep response for 2 Gy per fraction and a flat response for 2.5 Gy per fraction with increasing CRE or dose. It is now possible to evaluate the importance of fraction size at the same and over a narrower CRE range and dose range, respectively.

Statistical analysis demonstrated that the risk for local recurrence decreases with increasing dose per fraction, for fixed CRE and fixed treatment time ($p = 0.07$). For a given dose there is a very pronounced difference in local control between 2 Gy per fraction and 2.5 Gy per fraction ($p < 0.01$), especially in the lower dose range. But the same dose means a higher complication rate with 2.5 Gy per fraction. The effect of the treatment time was analyzed for fixed dose per fraction and fixed CRE. There was no correlation between local control and treatment time.

Thus, there is a clear trend toward a higher local control rate for glottic cancer with a dose per fraction slightly higher than the conventional fraction size of 2 Gy. In view of these results, the discussion should be focused on fraction size. We must point out, however, that in order to evaluate a therapeutic gain for an unconventional fractionation regimen, it is very important to establish that we are comparing the tumor effects at the same complication rates.

The Importance of Fraction Size for Tumor Control

Interest in this session has been focused upon multiple daily fractionation which mainly involves two fractionation principles:

1. Splitting the conventional fraction size of 2 Gy into smaller dose fractions for repeated irradiation two or more times a day.
2. Giving dose fractions of about 2 Gy two or three times a day.

There is also some clinical experience of multiple large dose fractions per day and single large dose fractions repeated once or twice a week.

A crucial point is to establish dose schedules which are equivalent to the conventional schedule with respect to the normal tissue reactions. From our clinical experience of MDF (multiple daily fractionation),[15] we concluded that the CRE formula is relevant for late reactions in human skin provided one takes into account the irregular distributions of fractions in these regimens. The permutation role proved by Kirk *et al.*[7] was used, and an example of the method of calculation has been presented earlier.[16]

The formula also agrees very well with clinical experience of the reactions on other normal tissue end points, as is evident from the review below.

For the purposes of this discussion, I will arbitrarily divide the range of fraction size into (1) small dose fractions, about 1 Gy; (2) conventional dose fractions, about 2 Gy; and (3) large dose fractions.

Small Dose Fractions

Thrice, daily irradiation with dose fractions of 1 Gy has been tried in Burkitt's lymphoma,[10] bladder carcinoma,[8] and glioblastoma[3] with promising preliminary results. In contrast to these results, our own experience of irradiation with 1.0 Gy per fraction 3 times a day in breast carcinoma indicates poorer results compared with conventional fractionation.

Table 1 shows three comparisons of multiple small daily fractions, of about 1 Gy, versus conventional fractionation (the treatment time being the same).

The first is a randomized trial in

TABLE 1. Multiple Small Daily Fractions (about 1 Gy) versus Conventional Fractionation

Squamous Cell Carcinoma (oropharynx) EORTC-22791	Twice a day, versus once a day 5 X 2.0 Gy/week, TD=70 Gy, CRE=19.6 10 X 1.15 Gy/week, TD=80.5 Gy, CRE=19.6 Therapeutic gain: ?
Adenocarcinoma (Breast) Göteborg	Thrice a day, versus once a day 4 X 2.4 Gy/week, TD=76.8 Gy, CRE=21 12 X 1.0 Gy/week, TD=96.6 Gy, CRE=21 Therapeutic gain: negative
Uroepithelial Carcinoma (Bladder) Littbrand, 1976	Thrice a day, versus once a day 5 X 2.0 Gy/week, TD=64 Gy, CRE=18 15 X 1.0 Gy/week, TD=84 Gy, CRE=20 Therapeutic gain: none

squamous cell carcinoma of the oropharynx, within the EORTC, comparing twice-a-day irradiation with 1.15 Gy and once-a-day irradiation with 2 Gy. The CRE formula was applied to these fractionation regimens. It is evident that the CRE formula fits very well with the total doses established by clinical experience for mucosal reactions, even for multiple daily fractionation. This trial has just started, so nothing is yet known about the therapeutic gain.

The second is our own study of adenocarcinoma of the breast in which we compared thrice-a-day irradiation with 1 Gy and once-a-day irradiation with 2.4 Gy. From clinical studies on skin, we know that these fractionation schedules result in equal late effects on normal tissue, as was also verified in this study. Concerning the therapeutic gain, we found that 3 × 1.0 Gy per day was inferior to 2.4 Gy once a day. It seems, therefore, that a dose per fraction of 1 Gy is too low for adenocarcinoma in the breast.

Finally, Table 1 shows a randomized study of uroepithelial carcinoma of the bladder by Littbrand et al.[8] comparing thrice-a-day irradiation with 1 Gy and once-a-day irradiation with 2 Gy. The CRE levels differ by 10%. The results show no therapeutic gain. (Initially there was a higher tumor control rate for 3 × 1.0 Gy, but at 3 years there was no significant difference in local control and the complication rate was somewhat higher after 3 × 1.0 Gy).

For Burkitt's lymphoma, 3 × 1.0 Gy per day is an effective treatment regimen.[10] However, for this tumor group, the total dose level required is at subtolerance level, and the complication rate is therefore low and constitutes a minor problem.

Our conclusions from a review of the literature and ongoing pilot studies of multiple small daily fractions are:

1. No therapeutic gain for uroepithelial carcinoma
2. A negative therapeutic gain for adenocarcinoma
3. A therapeutic gain for lymphoma
4. Inconclusive results for astrocytoma and squamous cell carcinoma

An important question in this context is: Could there be a minimum effective fraction size dependent on histology and tumor site?

Conventional Dose Fractions

Interest has recently been focused on regimens with dose fractions of about 2 Gy repeated two or three times a day. This regimen may drastically reduce the overall treatment time. In spite of this, only a minor reduction in the total dose is required for maintenance of the generally accepted complication rate. This regimen also makes it possible to give high daily doses and still avoid large single dose fractions.

TABLE 2. Multiple Daily Fractions of about 2 Gy

Schedule		Equivalent Total Doses for Normal Tissue		
5 × 2.0 Gy/week		50 Gy	60 Gy	70 Gy
2 × 3.8 Gy/week		38 Gy	45 Gy	53 Gy
10 × 1.8 Gy/week		45 Gy	54 Gy	63 Gy
Arcangeli's schedules		**Equivalent Total Doses for Normal Tissue**		
2.0	Gy/day	50 Gy	60 Gy	70 Gy
2.0 + 2.0	Gy/day	43 Gy	50 Gy	66 Gy[a]
2.0 + 1.5 + 1.5	Gy/day	43 Gy	50 Gy	66 Gy[a]
(4 hour intervals)				

[a] A gap of 3 weeks after 2-weeks treatment.

NORMAL TISSUE

Table 2 shows equivalent total doses concerning late effects on normal tissue. The upper part of the table demonstrates that changing from 2 Gy to 3.8 Gy per fraction means a dose reduction of about 30%. Changing from 2 Gy once a day to 1.8 Gy twice a day means a dose reduction of 10%. The lower part of the table shows the schedules used by Arcangeli (see Chapter 4). The dose should be reduced to be equivalent to the conventional fractionation.

In connection with MDF with dose fractions about 2 Gy, it is pertinent to discuss the importance of treatment time; the problem is illustrated in Figure 3 by three of our own studies on skin according to the method described above.

Figure 3 (*a*) demonstrates the acute erythema after 5 weeks' irradiation with five and two fractions per week.

Figure 3 (*b*) shows that it is possible to give high curative doses without pronounced acute reactions, if we include an interval in the course of treatment. In this case we also avoid irradiation during pronounced skin reactions.

Figure 3(*c*) demonstrates that it is possible to halve the treatment time (here from 5 to 2.5 weeks) without affecting the acute reaction. The maximum acute reaction was the same for both schedules. This is probably explained by an increased sensitivity with single daily fractions as the irradiation is continued, during pronounced reactions with disturbance of the cell kinetics. However, we expect a measurable difference in late reactions.

Only scanty reports about late normal tissue reactions have thus far been published for MDF with a fraction size of about 2 Gy (reviewed by Arcangeli in Chapter 18).

TUMOR EFFECTS

Arcangeli has reported in this session on his extensive experience of twice- and thrice-daily fractionation. An interval of 3 to 4 weeks was allowed after 2 weeks of treatment, which means an overall treatment time of 5 to 6 weeks. The total doses required for these schedules to give the same incidence of late effects as single daily fractions of 2 Gy are given in Table 2. The results are difficult to interpret as data were pooled for different tumor types and a wide dose range was used. Also, the follow-up was rather short. The total doses applied in the historical controls were about the same as for MDF. The acute reactions with MDF were reported to be well and even better tolerated than with the conventional schedule. However, it could be dangerous to rely on the acute reactions, as discussed above and in Chapter 18.

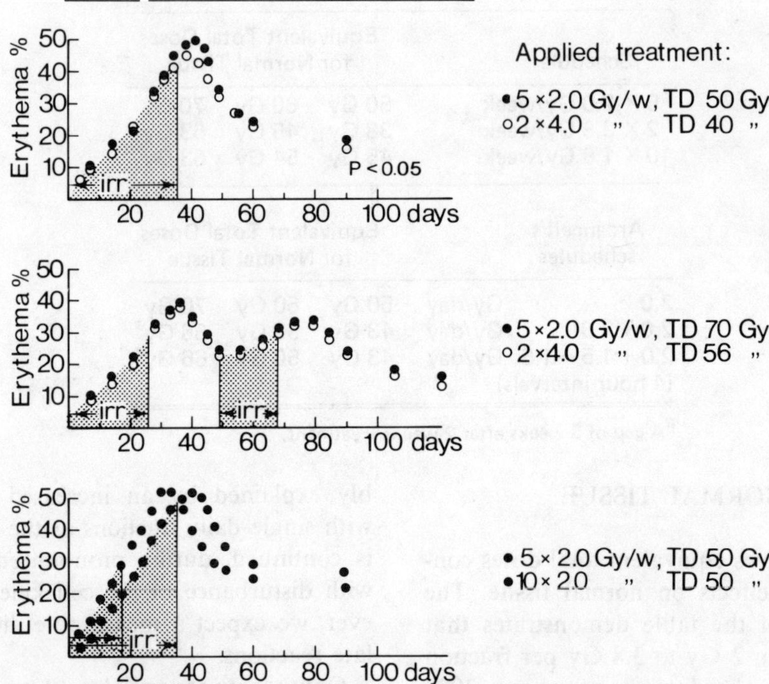

Figure 3. Human skin erythema measured spectrophotometrically after different fractionation schedules. The dashed areas mark the treatment periods. (The skin doses are 90% of the given absorbed doses.)

Results of curative radiotherapy with three and four fractions of 1.6 to 3.2 Gy and an overall treatment time of only 5 to 13 days have been reported by Svoboda[14] for different tumor groups. It is evident that this rapid fractionation regimen is feasible and well tolerated, but no final conclusions about its efficacy can be drawn at the moment.

Pilot studies of MDF (three times a day) with fraction sizes of 1.6 and 2 Gy for squamous cell carcinoma in the head and neck region and for glioblastoma multiforme are being conducted within the EORTC. Both schedules included an interval of 3 weeks after 1 and 2 weeks treatment for gliobastomas and head and neck tumors, respectively. The overall treatment time is 4 weeks for glioblastomas and about 6 weeks for head and neck tumors.

In conclusion, multiple daily fractionation with conventional fraction size makes it possible to give high daily doses and avoid large single dose fractions. Only a moderate reduction in total dose is required compared with the conventional fractionation. This regimen might be effective in the combination with hypoxic radiosensitizers. It also drastically reduces the *effective* treatment time, but the *overall* treatment time can be modified by an interval.

In connection with this regimen the question of the optimal overall treatment time arises.

– Should the course of radiotherapy be given *with* or *without* an interval?
– When is the optimal time for an interval in the treatment?
– What is the optimal length for the interval?

Large Dose Fractions

The many reports of pronounced late re-

• Tumor Effect

	10 fract.	30 fract.
Complete regression	61	58
Recurrence	25	23
Actuarial two-year local control	35.4 %	32.9 %

98 patients in each group

• Normal Tissue Effects

Acute:

	10 fract.	30 fract.
Skin		more severe
Mucosa	more severe	

Late: No difference for
Bone cartilage
Skin
Mucosa

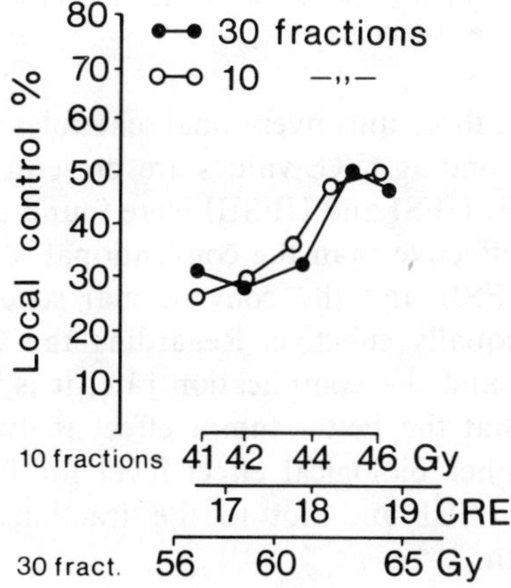

Figure 4. The results of a randomized trial on head and neck carcinomas comparing 10 fractions in 22 days and 30 fractions in 42 days, with 98 patients in each group. Data from Henk and James, 1978.

actions when large dose fractions are used have led to intensive discussion. Evidently, many people have grave doubts about this mode of treatment. However, the complication rate is a question of total dose. Increasing the dose per fraction requires a significant reduction in total dose.

The important question is whether fractionation regimens with large dose fractions are effective after the necessary reduction in total dose. The general opinion is that large dose fractions are less effective.

A randomized trial on squamous cell carcinoma in the head and neck region has been published by Henk and James.[4] They compared 10 fractions in 22 days with 30 fractions in 42 days, keeping the CRE or NSD equal. The doses per fraction were about 4.3 Gy and 2 Gy, respectively. The results, summarized in Figure 4, demonstrate equal tumor effects and late normal tissue reactions.

These results contradict those of Byhardt et al.[2] on squamous cell carcinoma of the oral cavity and oropharynx. However, their study was not randomized. Also, the BIR trial demonstrates a tendency toward poorer tumor control with increasing dose per fraction for squamous cell carcinoma of the larynx. In the BIR trial the mean dose per fraction compared were between 2.0 to 3.9 Gy (five fractions per week). On the contrary, our own results with this tumor group demonstrate a clear trend toward a higher local control rate for fraction sizes of about 2.5 Gy compared with 2 Gy, as presented above.

Malignant melanoma is a tumor for

The Importance of Dose per Fraction for Malignant Melanoma

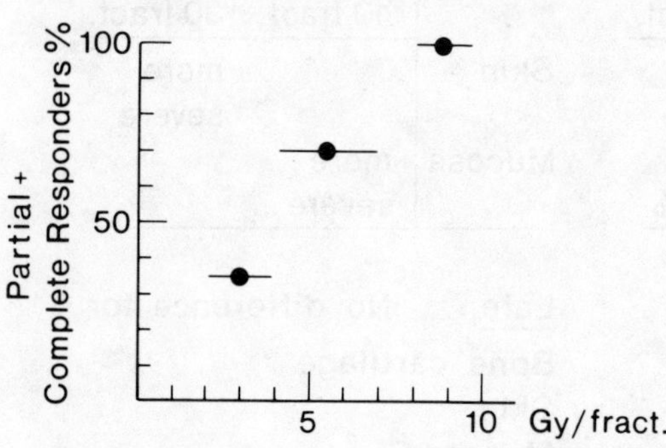

The best schedules:

4 × 8.0 Gy in 28 days, CRE 16 CRE_{corr} 18

3 × 9.0 Gy in 8 days, CRE 16,5 CRE_{corr} 19

Figure 5. Partial and complete responders (%) versus dose per fraction for malignant melanoma. Data from Overgaard, 1980.

which *in vitro* and *in vivo* experiments indicate a pronounced shoulder on the survival curve. Large dose fractions might therefore be favorable for this tumor. This was also established in a clinical study by Overgaard[11] who found schedules with three or four fractions of about 8 to 9 Gy to be superior to those with dose fractions below 4 Gy (see Fig. 5). This result is supported by the findings of others.[6]

Another way to apply large dose fractions has been presented by Holsti in Chapter 30. The total doses given in the conventional and the three unconventional schedules with corresponding CRE values are presented in Table 3. UFSI and UFSIII were found to be more effective than the conventional schedule. UFSII and the conventional schedule were equally effective. Regarding the CRE values and the complication rate, it is possible that the better tumor effect is due to the higher biological effect level for UFSI and UFSIII and not to the fractionation regimen.

TABLE 3. Large-Dose Fractions[a]

Holsti's Schedules		CRE	CRE_{corr}
UFS I:	50 Gy/5 week	19	21
UFS II:	44 Gy/5 week	17	18
UFS III:	50 Gy/6 week	19	20
CFS:	50 Gy/5 week	16	16
	55 Gy/8 week		

[a] UFS I and UFS III feature more rapid tumor regression but more fibrosis than CFS. UFS II and CFS show equal results.

In Table 4 a review of results for large dose fractions are summarized. The conclusion is that large doses per fraction are not generally detrimental. In this context two questions arise:

1. Which tumor types need a higher dose per fraction for better tumor control?
2. How much should the dose per fraction be increased above 2 Gy for these tumors?

TABLE 4. Large Dose Fractions versus Conventional Fractionation

Histology	Dose/Fraction	Therapeutic Gain
Squamous cell carcinoma:		
Henk (1978); random trial	~2 → 4.3 Gy	none
Denmark: random trial	2.0 → 4.1 Gy	not evaluated
BIR: random trial	~2.9 → 4.3 Gy	negative
Wisconsin: no trial	2.0 → 3.0 Gy	negative
Göteborg: no trial	~2 → 2.5 Gy	yes
Astrocytoma, grade III-IV:		
Scand.: random trial	2.0 → 4.0 Gy	not evaluated
Malignant melanoma:		
Overgaard (1980): no trial	2 → ≥8 Gy	yes

REFERENCES

1. Arcangeli, G.: Multiple daily fractionation (MDF) radiotherapy: Clinical results. In *Biological Bases and Clinical Implications of Tumor Radioresistance*, G.H. Fletcher and C. Nervi, eds. New York: Masson, 1982, Chap. 31.
2. Byhardt, R.W., Greenberg, M., and Cox, J.D.: Local control of squamous carcinoma of oral cavity and oropharynx with 3 vs. 5 treatment fractions per week. *Int J Radiat Oncol Biol Phys* **2**:415–420, 1977.
3. Douglas, B.G.: Preliminary results using superfractionation in the treatment of glioblastoma multiforme. *J Can Assoc Radiol* **28**:106–110, 1977.
4. Henk, J.M., and James, K.W.: Comparative trial of large and small fractions in the radiotherapy of head and neck cancer. *Clin Radiol* **29**:611–616, 1978.
5. Holsti, L.: Nonstandard fractionation: Clinical observations. In *Biological Bases and Clinical Implications of Tumor Radioresistance,* G.H. Fletcher and C. Nervi, eds. New York: Masson, 1982, Chap. 30.
6. Hornsey, S.: The relationship between total dose, number of fractions and fraction size in the response of malignant melanoma in patients. *Br J Radiol* **51**:905–909, 1978.
7. Kirk, J., Gray, W.M., and Watson, E.R.: Cumulative radiation effect. I. Fractionated treatment regimes. *Clin Radiol* **22**:145–155, 1971.
8. Littbrand, B., Edsmyr, F.: Preliminary results of bladder carcinoma irradiated with low individual doses and a high total dose. *Int J Radiat Oncol Biol Phys* **1**:1059–1062, 1976.
9. Morrisson, R.: The results of treatment of cancer of the bladder–a clinical contribution to radiobiology. *Clin Radiol* **26**:67–75, 1975.
10. Norin, T., and Onyango, J.: Radiotherapy in Burkitt's lymphoma, Conventional or superfractionated regime–early results. *Int J Radiat Oncol Biol Phys* **2**:399, 1977.
11. Overgaard, J.: Radiation treatment of malignant melanoma. *Int J Radiat Oncol Biol Phys* **6**:41–44, 1980.
12. Shukovsky, L.J.: Dose, time, volume relationships in squamous cell carcinoma of the supraglottic larynx. *AJR* **108**:27–29, 1970.
13. Stewart, J.G., and Jackson, A.W.: The steepness of the dose response curve both for tumour cure and normal tissue injury. *Laryngoscope* **85**:1107–1111, 1975.
14. Svoboda, H.J.: Further experience with radiotherapy by multiple daily sessions. *Br J Radiol* **51**:363–369, 1978.
15. Turesson, I.: Fractionation and dose rate in radiotherapy. An experimental and clinical study of cumulative radiation effect. Thesis, University of Göteborg, 1978.
16. Turesson, I., and Notter, G.: Control dose administered once a week and three times a day according to schedules calculated by the CRE formula, using skin reaction as a biological parameter. *Radiology* **120**:399–401, 1976.
17. Wiernik, G., Bleehan, N.M., Brindle, J., Bullimore, J., Churchill-Davidson, I.F.J., Davidson, J., Fowler, J.F., Francis, P., Hadden, R.C.M., Haybittle, J.L., Howard, N., Lansley, I.F., Lindup, R., Phillips, D.L., and Skeggs, C.: Sixth Interim Progress Report of the British Institute of Radiology fractionation study of 3F/week versus 5F/week in radiotherapy of the laryngo-pharynx. *Br J Radiol* **51**:241–250, 1978.

CHAPTER 33

Keynote Address: Impact of Local–Regional Control on Survival

Simon Kramer, M.D.[a]
David Moylan, M.D.[b]

It is estimated that in 1980 in the United States there will be 785,000 new cancer cases and 405,000 deaths. If one is to extrapolate data provided by Suit,[25] later modified by Powers (personal correspondence) (see Table 1), it is reasonable to suppose that almost one-third of the total cancer deaths will be in patients treated primarily by local-regional intervention in whom such intervention has failed. Most of the remainder will die as the result of disseminated cancer with and without local failure. An appreciable proportion, however, will die of intercurrent disease often related to the neoplasm, and a small proportion will die from truly unrelated disease.

In recent years attention has been directed largely to the problem of disseminated cancer and its treatment by systemic management, with the justification that treatment of local-regional disease had reached a plateau and that in any case it was relatively unimportant to the major problem of survival from cancer. Neither statement can be supported by facts. And indeed, the control of the local-regional disease becomes even more important if ever distant micrometastases can be controlled by systemic therapy. Thus, we believe it is timely to examine the impact of control of local-regional cancer on survival and to try to assess the overall cost benefit ratio of improved local-regional control.

To this end, we will review the facts in cancer in four sites—two where the local-regional disease is primarily responsible for failure and death, namely, cancer of the cervix and cancer of the head and neck; and at two other sites where it has been thought that death is due primarily to distant metastases, namely, in cancer of the lung and cancer of the breast.

Carcinoma of the Uterine Cervix

It has long been considered that patients with carcinoma of the cervix uteri die primarily from local-regional disease. In the preantibiotic era over 80% died as a result

TABLE 1. Potential Candidates for Radiation Therapy and Estimated Proportion of Local Failures[a]

	Deaths 1977	Local Failure
Head, neck, and brain	20,600	12,890
Gastrointestinal	78,000	32,910
Gynecological	21,700	12,940
Genitourinary	29,900	17,030
Lung	89,000	7,960
Skin, bone, and soft tissue	5,100	2,300
Lymphoma	21,900	2,650
Breast	34,000	4,725
	300,200	93,405

[a](Modified from Suit, 1970.)[25] Later modified by Powers, W.E. Personal Correspondence.

[a]Professor and Chairman, Department of Radiation Therapy and Nuclear Medicine, Thomas Jefferson University Hospital, Philadelphia, Penn.
[b]Department of Radiation Therapy and Nuclear Medicine, Thomas Jefferson University Hospital, Philadelphia, Penn.

TABLE 2. Analysis of Cause of Death in 278 Autopsied Cases of Cervical Carcinoma[a]

Primary Cause of Death	Percentage
Uremia	30.0
Sepsis	10.4
Respiratory failure	10.0
Cardiac failure	4.7
Liver failure	2.5
Hemorrhage	2.5
CNS death	2.2
Other primary cancer	7.5
Other causes	30.2

[a](Modified from Badib *et al.*, 1968.[3])

of local sepsis or hemorrhage, almost invariably due to local–regional extension of the tumor.[2] In more recent reports,[3] it has been shown that about one-third died as a result of renal failure (see Table 2). It is interesting to note in Badib's series of 278 autopsied cases that distant metastases were present in 59% of those patients treated by radiation therapy at autopsy; but in four-fifths of these, there was also local pelvic persistence or recurrence (see Table 3).

Homesley et al.[12] reported the relationship of lesion size to local control and survival in patients with stage IB disease treated by radiation therapy alone (see Table 4). In lesions under 4 cm in size, there was one pelvic recurrence in 22 patients and a 95% five-year actuarial survival, while in lesions over 4 cm in size there were 8 out of 23 recurrences with an actuarial five-year survival of 67%, this difference being significant at the 0.05 level.

Bush et al.[5] reported on the effect of hemoglobin levels on the results of the radiotherapeutic management of cervical cancer. Retrospectively, they grouped stage IIB and III patients according to hemoglobin levels and showed that there is a significant increase in survival in patients with hemoglobins greater than 12 g who were treated with definitive radiation therapy (see Fig. 1). Their study indicates that the relative anemia does not impact on distant metastases and that the difference in survival of 10% at 10 years, which is significant with a p value of 0.006, correlates anemia with a failure to control pelvic disease within the irradiated volume, which in turn correlates with survival (See Fig. 2).

Furthermore, the prospective study carried out by these investigators confirms that those anemic patients who were transfused and maintain a hemoglobin level between 12.5 and 13.5 g showed a statistically significant lower pelvic recurrence rate than the untransfused patients. Similarly, survival for stage IIB and III patients were improved although the study was not carried on long enough to reach statistical significance on survival. Similar conclusions can be reached in reviewing the British Medical Research Council Trials[26] of hyperbaric oxygen and radiation therapy in cancer of the cervix. The greatest number of patients occurred with stage III, and here the actuarial local recurrence-free rate is 71% in oxygen versus 44% in air, while the actuarial 5-year survival rate shows a difference of 37% in oxygen to 25% in air (see Table 5).

We are beginning to see a phenomenon here that will repeat itself at other sites. When one compares local–regional control with survival even in a primarily local–regional disease like carcinoma of the cervix, it becomes obvious that a very large advantage in local–regional control is converted into a somewhat less marked advantage in survival. This dilution is due to other causes of death that might befall the locally controlled cancer patient.

Cancer of the Head and Neck

Cancer of the upper aero-digestive passages represent a large group of neoplastic diseases with different biologic and clinical parameters. Here, as in carcinoma of the cervix, a dictum has long existed that the disease kills primarily through extension above the clavicles and that distant metastases are uncommon. We now know this to be untrue, particularly in patients with high-grade carcinomas and those with relatively

TABLE 3. Method of Treatment and Incidence of Persistent or Recurrent Cancer in 278 Autopsied Cases of Cervical Cancer[a]

	Radiation	Surgery	Surgery and Radiation	Other
Stage I	40	17	13	2
Stage II	65	19	13	3
Stage III	62	4	4	4
Stage IV	15	3	2	8
Total	183[b]	44[b]	34[b]	17[b]
Pelvic persistence or recurrence at autopsy	105	31	17	13
Distant metastases	108 (59%)	28 (63%)	18 (53%)	9 (53%)
Local control rate	42%	30%	50%	24%
Mean survival (months)	50.0	26.6	35.7	15.0

[a] (Modified from Badib et. al., 1968.[3]) [b] Four cases apparently unstaged.

TABLE 4. Relation of Size of Tumor in Stage IB Cervical Cancer Treated by Radiation Therapy Alone[a]

	Lesion Size <4 cm	Lesion Size ⩾4 cm	
Number of patients	22	23	
Follow-up:			
pelvic recurrence	1	8	
lost to follow-up	1	1	
dead of other causes	3	2	
5 year actuarial survival	95%	67%	($p < 0.05$)

[a] (Modified from Homesley et. al., 1980.[12])

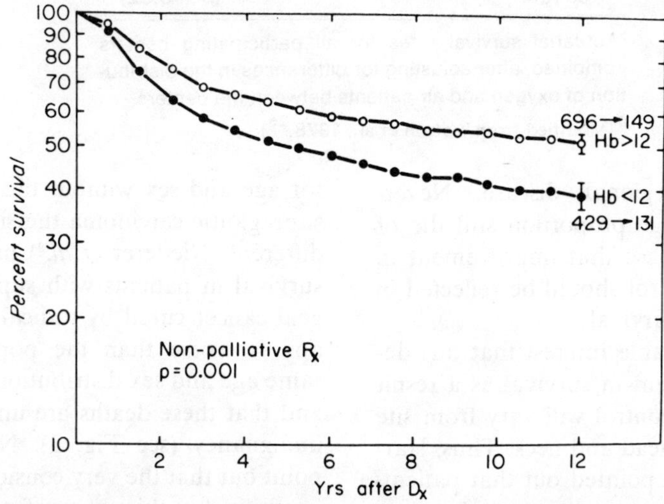

Figure 1. The actuarial survival curves for patients with stages IIB and III carcinoma of the cervix with haemoglobin levels above and below 12 g% during radiation therapy. The number of patients at risk with time is shown by each survival curve. (Data from Bush et. al., 1978.)[5]

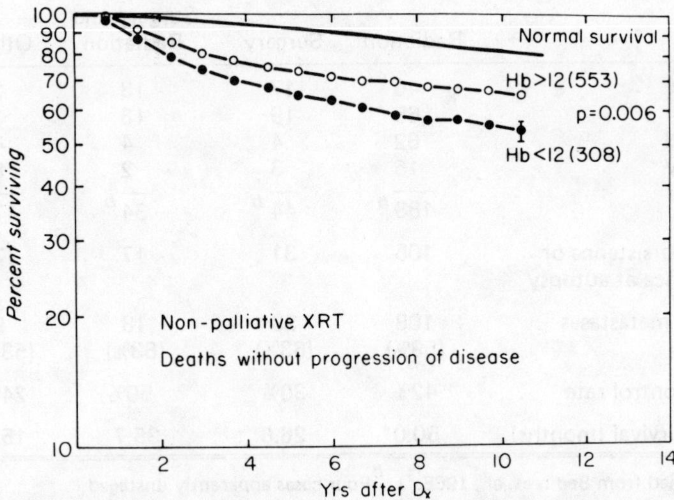

Figure 2. The actuarial survival curve for all the patients represented in Figure 1 except for those who died with evidence of disease only outside the irradiated volume. (Data from Bush *et. al.,* 1978.)[5]

TABLE 5. MRC Hyperbaric Oxygen Trial Stage III Cervical Cancer[a,b]

	Oxygen	Air
Number of patients	119	124
Actuarial 5-year survival	37%	25% ($p = 0.038$)
Actuarial local recurrence-free rate	71%	44% ($p < 0.001$)
Actuarial metastases-free rate	51%	46% ($p = 0.32$)

[a]Actuarial survival rates for all participating centers combined, after adjusting for differences in the distribution of oxygen and air patients between the centers.
[b](Modified from Watson et al., 1978.[26])

advanced local–regional disease. Nevertheless, such a large proportion still die of local–regional disease that improvement in local–regional control should be reflected in better long-term survival.

It is of considerable interest that this degree of improvement in survival as a result of local–regional control will vary from site to site within the head and neck. Thus, Harwood *et al.*[11] have pointed out that patients with early glottic cancer, once they are cured of their disease, have a similar survival to a similar group of patients matched for age and sex without the disease. In the supraglottic carcinoma the situation is quite different. Niederer *et al.*[21] have shown that survival in patients with supraglottic laryngeal cancer cured by radical radiation therapy is worse than the population of the same age and sex distribution without tumor and that these deaths are unrelated to their malignancy (see Fig. 3). Niederer *et al.*[21] point out that the very considerable attrition in survival in this group of patients militates against a major improvement in survival as a result of local–regional manipulation.

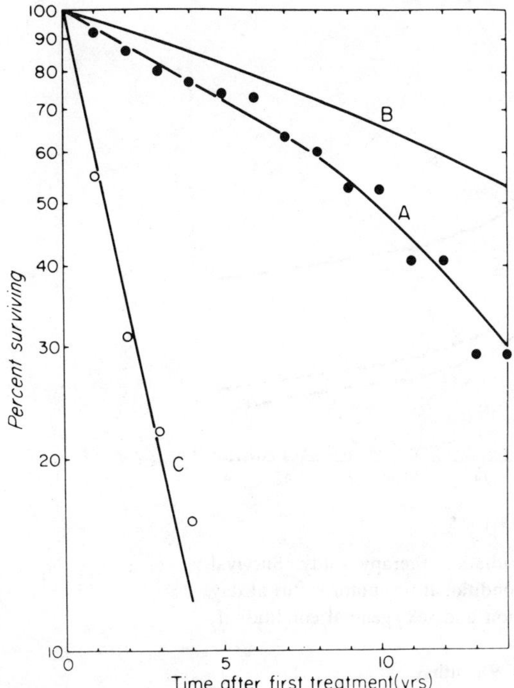

Figure 3. Actuarial survival curves. Curve A: survival curve for patients with supraglottic laryngeal carcinoma first treated by radical radiation therapy in the interval 1958–71, considered to have died of causes unrelated to their malignancy, whether or not evidence of their malignant disease was still present. Curve B: survival curve for a population with the same age and sex distribution, taken from the 1961 Ontario census. Curve C: survival curve for patients who subsequently died of laryngeal cancer. (Data from Niederer *et. al.*, 1977.)[21]

Clearly this is a group of patients with "poor protoplasm" with abuse of alcohol, tobacco, probably malnutrition, who run a considerable risk of dying from other causes.

Our own studies in the Radiation Therapy Oncology Group have lent support, however, to the statement that at least in a proportion of patients, improvement in local–regional control leads to better survival. Thus, in the cooperative study on methotrexate and radiation therapy in advanced head and neck cancer of the oral cavity, oropharynx, supraglottic larynx, and hypopharynx,[15] our results clearly show that the control of the local–regional disease on day 90 (that is, approximately 6 weeks after completion of therapy) is reflected with constancy in survival. Figure 4 shows the results in graphic form for patients with cancer of the supraglottic larynx. Data are similar for the other three sites.

RTOG 73-03 explored the optimal combination of surgery and radiation therapy in a prospective randomized study of advanced cancer of the oral cavity, oropharynx, supraglottic larynx, and hypopharynx (see Fig. 5). The results indicate that local–regional control is statistically significantly better at 2 years when radiation is used postoperatively rather than preoperatively in the supraglottic larynx and in the hypopharynx (p = 0.04).[16] This trend persists when survival is considered, but the difference in survival is not statistically significant (see Table 6 and Fig. 6).

Even more than in cancer of the cervix, it would appear that survival cannot parallel the improvement in local–regional control because of the many factors impinging upon these patients' loss of life.

Carcinoma of the Lung

In cancer of the lung, death due to distant metastases so dominates the picture that the management of the local–regional disease had been deemphasized; yet, uncontrolled local–regional disease remains a major factor in lung cancer.

Loumanen and Watson[17] reported a series of 5000 cases from the Memorial Hospital, New York. They found that one-third of the patients died of complications of the uncontrolled primary tumor. Matthews *et al.*[18] reported another autopsy series of patients who died within 30 days of a "curative" resection of a primary lung cancer. One-third of the patients had persistence of cancer within the thorax, and of these, one-third had no evidence of distant metastases. Considering only patients with squamous cell carcinoma, 44 of 139 patients had persistent intrathoracic tumor, and of these, 50% had no distant metastases. Other autopsy series

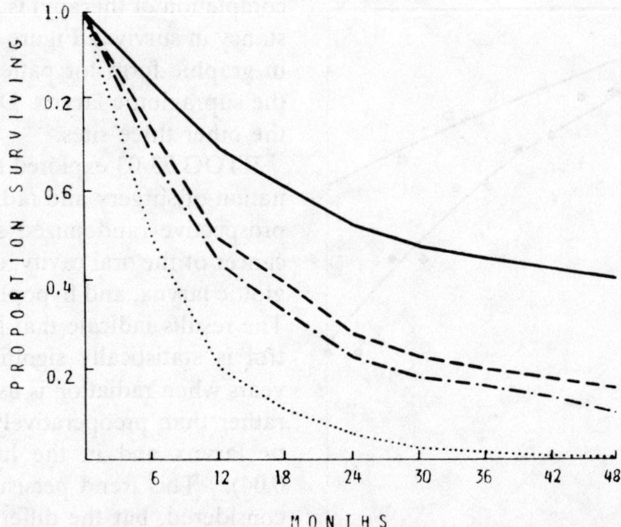

Figure 4. Results of MTX and radiation therapy study. Survival curves for the supraglottic larynx conditional on tumor status at day 90 and adjusted for general condition and sex (general condition 1, male).
primary and node absent (27 cases, 9 deaths);
primary absent, node present (12 cases, 6 deaths);
primary present, node absent (10 cases, 6 deaths);
primary and node present (13 cases, 10 deaths).
(Data from Kramer et. al., 1975.)[15]

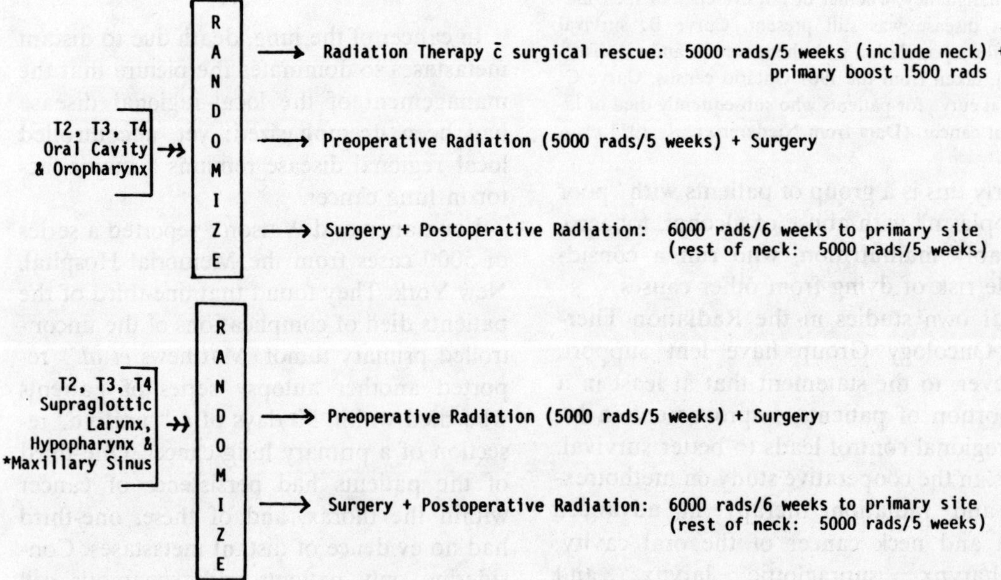

Figure 5. Schema for RTOG study 73-03.

TABLE 6. RTOG 73-03 Case Status, Sites of First Failure, Causes of Death by Treatment and Region[a]

	Supraglottic Larynx		Hypopharynx		Supraglottic Larynx and Hypopharynx	
	PreOp	PostOp	PreOp	PostOP	PreOp	PostOp
Total cases	58	60	35	38	93	98
Alive NED	29%	47%	20%	29%	26%	40%
Alive with Disease	10%	5%	14%	8%	12%	6%
Dead NED	16%	18%	17%	24%	16%	20%
Dead with Disease	45%	30%	49%	39%	46%	34%
Sites of first failure:						
persistent local–regional	10%	3%	11%	8%	11%	5%
recurrent local–regional	24%	15%	26%	16%	25%	15%
distant metastases	16%	15%	23%	16%	18%	15%
local–regional + distant	5%	2%	3%	8%	4%	4%
Causes of death:						
treated primary	14%	10%	20%	16%	16%	12%
new primary cancer	0	3%	6%	3%	2%	3%
cervical nodes	0	0	3%	5%	1%	2%
distant metastases	21%	12%	11%	11%	17%	11%
treatment related	5%	2%	9%	11%	6%	5%
unrelated/unknown	21%	20%	17%	18%	19%	19%

[a] Data from RTOG Group Meeting Minutes, June 1980.

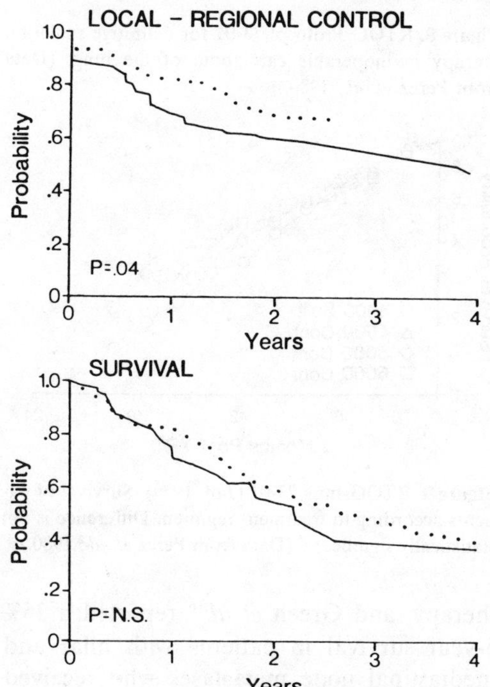

Figure 6. RTOG 73–03 supraglottic larynx and hypopharynx. Treatment: dotted line = postop and solid line = preop. (Data from RTOG Group Meeting Minutes, June, 1980.)

of lung cancer patients (see Table 7) indicate that from 10 to 33% are without distant metastases at the time of death.[1,9,19,20,24] Even where metastases are present the uncontrolled primary tumor contributes to the early demise of the patients in a high proportion of cases, as shown by Petrovich *et al.*[23] in the Veterans Administration Lung Cancer Study Group. The value of improved local–regional control in prolonging survival has been demonstrated in two recent studies. Cox *et al.*[6] reported the experience from the Affiliated Hospitals of the Medical College of Wisconsin. He showed that, where the tumor was controlled locally, median survival was doubled compared to those patients in whom uncontrolled tumor persisted (see Fig. 7).

Our experience in the Radiation Therapy Oncology Group Study 73-01 has been reported by Perez *et al.*[22] Three hundred sixty-five patients with nonresectable nonoat cell carcinoma of the lung were treated by definitive radiation therapy utilizing four treatment regimes. Figure 8 describes the schema.

TABLE 7. Autopsy Series for Lung Cancer Patients

Reference	Number of Patients	% without Distant Metastases
Abadir and Muggia, 1975[1]	48	27
Galluzzi and Payne, 1955[9]	741	30
Moise, 1921[19]	327	10
Neely, 1925[20]	80	33
Rogers, 1932[24]	50	10

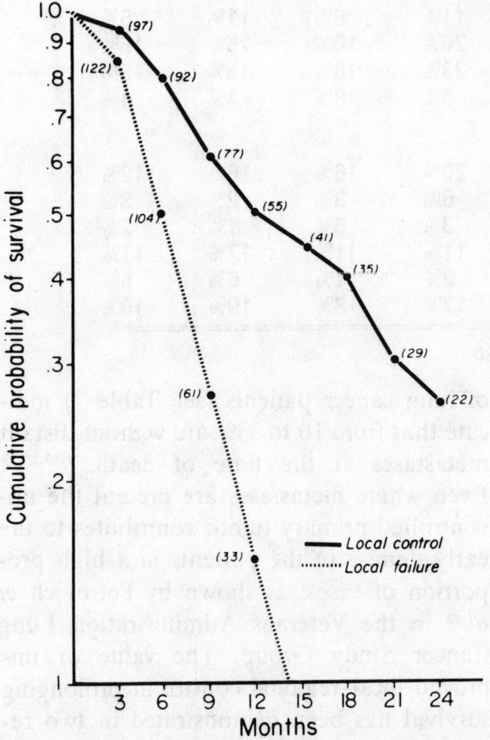

Figure 7. Effect of local tumor control by irradiation on survival in bronchopulmonary cancer. (Data from Cox *et. al.*, 1979.)[6]

Preliminary survival results show a small, but definite, difference related to the dose (see Fig. 9). The dose of radiation correlates with tumor response and tumor response relates with survival, as shown in Figure 10.

The adjuvant use of radiation therapy in operable lung cancer remains controversial, yet a number of reports show very definite advantages. Kirsh *et al.*[14] reported that patients with squamous cell carcinoma and mediastinal node metastases had improved survival following postresection radiation

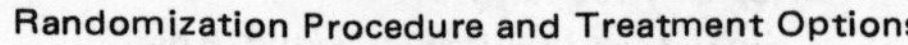

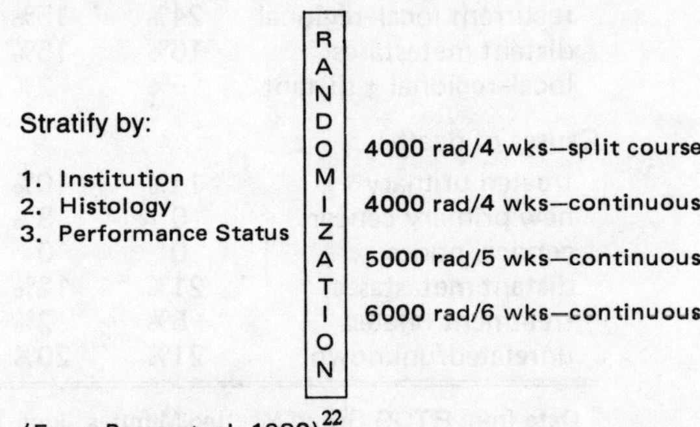

Figure 8. RTOG Protocol 73-01 for definitive radiation therapy in inoperable carcinoma of the lung. (Data from Perez *et. al.*, 1980.)[22]

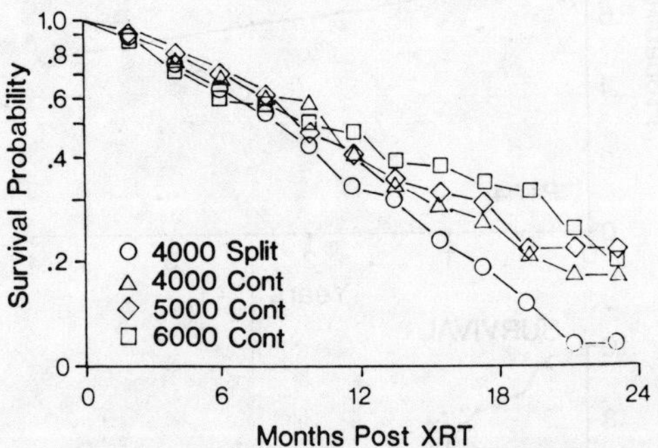

Figure 9. RTOG-lung 73-01 (Jan. 1979). Survival of patients according to treatment regimen. Difference is not statistically significant. (Data from Perez *et. al.*, 1980.)[22]

therapy, and Green *et al.*[10] reported a 35% 5-year survival in patients with hilar and mediastinal node metastases who received post resection radiation compared to 3% of similar patients who had surgery alone. The subgroup of patients where adjuvant radiation therapy is of value has not yet been defined. That may well be small, but the

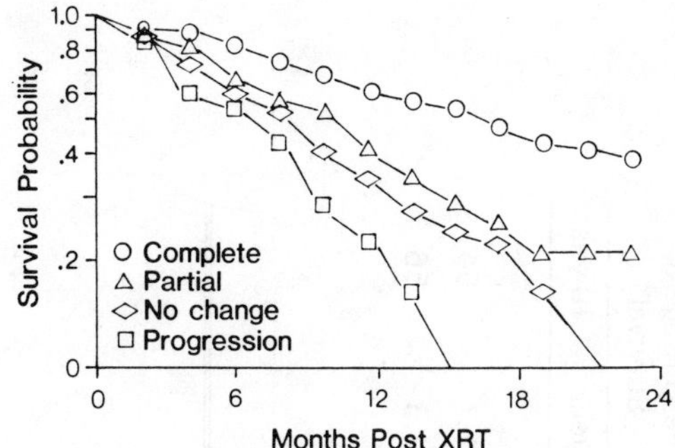

Figure 10. Correlation of survival with degree of local tumor response. (Data from Perez *et. al.*, 1980.)[22]

TABLE 8. Patterns of Recurrence in 423 "Potentially Curable" Breast Cancer Patients[a]

Local recurrence alone	4%
Distant metastases alone	23%
Both types of recurrence	26%
10-year disease-free survival	39%
15-year disease-free survival	35%

[a](Modified from Bruce et al., 1970.[4])

benefit of adjuvant radiation therapy in this group may well be large.

Breast

It is quite proper that the systemic management in patients with breast cancer is attracting a great deal of attention. After all, the great majority of patients die with disseminated disease. Unfortunately, however, it is often overlooked that there is a subset of patients in whom aggressive and successful local–regional treatment eliminates the appearance of metastases and leads to prolongation of life.

How large is the subset? That is difficult to say. Bruce *et al.*[4] (see Table 8), in reviewing the Edinburgh experience, found only 4% with local recurrences alone and as many with both local and distant recurrent disease as with distant metastases alone. There is no way of telling whether, in those patients with both local and distant recurrent disease, these areas are affected synchronously or metachronously, and if so, in what sequence. Still, the existence of the subset cannot be questioned. Fisher[7] reported the NSABP experience comparing patients treated with radical mastectomy and then randomly allocated to receiving or not receiving postoperative irradiation. The incidence of local–regional recurrence and distant metastases shows little difference where the axillary nodes are negative or when there are only one to three positive axillary nodes. However, if there are four or more positive nodes found at surgery, not only would there be a significantly lower incidence of local–regional recurrences, but an improved survival at 5 years with an almost significant p value (0.07) (see Table 9) would also be in order. Fletcher and Montague[8] reported their experience with postoperative radiation therapy in breast cancer (see Table 10). Although not a randomized study, when the group treated by radical mastectomy only is compared with that in which postoperative radiation therapy is given, one sees that the 5- and 10-year survival are essentially the same (although more than five times as many patients in the irradiated series had positive axillary nodes compared to those treated by a radical mastectomy only who should, therefore, have had a markedly worse 10-year survival). Finally, the report of Host and Brennhovd from Norway[13] once again indicates the value of postoperative radiation therapy in a subset of patients with breast cancer. Their series is randomized between postoperative radiation and no radiation. No benefit was seen in stage I patients; but in stage II patients, there was a definite increase in survival, a decrease in local recurrence rate, and a decrease in distant metastases. When those patients who had four or more positive nodes for metastases were reviewed, the difference in survival appears quite marked.

Conclusions

We have seen that in the four tumor systems used in this study, there always appears to be a subset of patients in whom improvement of local–regional control expresses itself as an improved survival. It is also clear that, in the main, we cannot yet identify this subset adequately. The question then arises

TABLE 9. NSABP Study of Disease Status Related to Number of Auxiliary Nodal Metastases[a]

	Negative Nodes			1-3 Positive Nodes			4+ Positive Nodes		
	% NED 5 years	% Local-Regional Recurrence	% Distant Metastases	% NED 5 years	% Local-Regional Recurrence	% Distant Metastases	% NED 5 years	% Local-Regional Recurrence	% Distant Metastases
Postop Irradiation	78.6	8.9	12.5	49.1	5.3	43.9	28.4	10.5	59.7
Thio-Tepa	81.8	0.0	15.9	52.9	17.7	29.4	15.0	27.5	55.0
Placebo	71.2	7.6	21.2	42.4	24.2	33.3	21.9	31.2	46.9
All Controls	76.0	4.2	18.8	47.8	20.9	31.3	18.0	29.1	51.4

[a](Modified from Fisher et al., 1970.[7])

TABLE 10. 5- and 10-year Survival Rates from 1959 through December 1972 (without Adjuvant Chemotherapy)[c]

Treatment Modality	Number of Patients	Patients with Histologically Positive Nodes %	No.	Average Number of Involved Nodes per Patient in the Patients with Involved Nodes	Percentage of Survival[a] 5-year	10-year
Radical mastectomy only	287	11.5	(33/287)	5	71.7	54
Radical mastectomy followed by peripheral lymphatic irradiation (5000 rad in 4 weeks to the supraclavicular area and internal mammary chain with ^{60}Co or ^{137}Cs)[b]	356	65.7	(234/356)	6	71.3	56

[a]Survival rates from Berkson and Gage, not age adjusted.

[b]Presently given in 5 weeks in 25 fractions, 200 rad per fraction.

[c](Data from Fletcher et al., 1978.[8])

whether, given the cost benefit to the subset, all patients with only locally–regionally advanced disease should be submitted to such treatment, rather than only patients in this subset which we cannot yet recognize. In those categories of cancer where the incidence of distant metastases is relatively rare, this question is easy to answer. Where the majority of patients potentially have distant metastases, one must postulate that such treatment is acceptable only when the morbidity is small and, on the whole, nonthreatening to the patients' survival.

Acknowledgments

Research for this chapter has been supported in part by Grant CA 11602 from the Division of Cancer Research, Resources and Centers of the National Cancer Institute, National Institutes of Health.

REFERENCES

1. Abadir, R., and Muggia, F.M.: Irradiated lung cancer: An autopsy analysis of spread pattern. *Radiology* **114**:427–430, 1975.
2. Auster, L.S., and Sala, A.M.: Causes of death in carcinoma of the cervix uteri. *Surg Gynecol Obstet* **71**:231–239, 1940.
3. Badib, A.O., Kurohara, S.S., Webster, J.H., and Pickren, J.W.: Metastasis to organs in carcinoma of the uterine cervix. *Cancer* **21**:434–439, 1968.
4. Bruce, J., Carter, D.C., and Fraser, J.: Patterns of recurrent disease in breast cancer. *Lancet,* 433–435, 1970.
5. Bush, R.S., Jenkin, D.T., Allt, W.E.C., Beale, F.A., et. al.: Definitive evidence for hypoxic cells influencing cure in cancer therapy. *Br J Cancer* **37**: Suppl. III, 302–306, 1978.
6. Cox, J.D., Eisert, D.R., Komaki, R., Mietlowsky, W., and Petrovich, Z.: Patterns of failure following treatment of apparently localized carcinoma of the lung. In *Lung Cancer: Progress in Therapeutic Research* Vol. II, F.M. Muggia and M. Rozencweig, eds. New York: Raven Press, 1979, pp. 279–288.
7. Fisher, B., Slack, N.H., Cavanaugh, P.J., et. al.: Postoperative radiotherapy in the treatment of breast cancer: Results of the NSABP clinical trial. *Ann Surg* **172**:711–730, 1970.
8. Fletcher, G.H., and Montague, E.D.: Does adequate irradiation of the internal mammary chain and supraclavicular nodes improve survival rates? *Int J Radiat Oncol Biol Phys* **4**:481–492, 1978.
9. Galluzzi, S., and Payne, P.M.: Bronchogenic carcinoma: Statistical study of 741 necropsies with special reference to distribution of blood-borne metastases. *Br J Cancer* **9**:511–527, 1955.
10. Green, N., Kurohara, S.S., George, F.W., and Crews, Q.E.: Postresection irradiation for primary lung cancer. *Radiology* **116**:405–407, 1975.
11. Harwood, A.R., Hawkins, N., Rider, W.D., Bryce, D.P.: Radiotherapy of early glottic cancer–I. *Int J Radiat Oncol Biol Phys* **5**:473–476, 1979.
12. Homesley, H.D., Raben, M., Blake, D., et. al.: Relationship of lesion size to survival in patients with stage IB squamous cell carcinoma of the cervix uteri treated by radiation therapy. *Surg Gynecol Obstet* **150**:529–531, 1980.
13. Host, H., and Brennhovd, I.O.: The effect of postoperative radiotherapy in breast cancer. *Int J Radiat Oncol Biol Phys* **2**:1061–1067, 1977.
14. Kirsh, M.M., Prior, M., Gayo, O., et. al.: The effect of histological cell type on the prognosis of patients with bronchogenic carcinoma. *Ann Thorac Surg* **13**:303–310, 1972.
15. Kramer, S.: Methotrexate and radiation therapy in the treatment of advanced squamous carcinoma of the oral cavity, oropharynx, supraglottic larynx, and hypopharynx. *Can J Otolaryngol* **4**:213–218, 1975.
16. Kramer, S., Snow, J., Marcial, V.: Optimal combined use of surgery and radiation therapy in advanced head and neck cancer. A study of the Radiation Therapy Oncology Group (abstract). *Int J Radiat Oncol Biol Phys* **6(1)**:22, 1980.
17. Loumanen, R.K.J., and Watson, W.L.: Autopsy findings. In *Lung Cancer–A Study of Five Thousand Memorial Hospital Cases,* St. Louis: C.V. Mosby, 1968, pp. 504–510.
18. Matthews, M.J., Kanhouwa, S., Pickren, J., and Robinette, D.: Frequency of residual and metastatic tumor in patients undergoing curative surgical resection for lung cancer. *Cancer Chemother Rep* **4**:63–67, 1973.
19. Moise, T.S.: Primary carcinoma of the lung. *Arch Intern Med* **28**:733–772, 1921.
20. Neely, J.M.: Primary carcinoma of the lung: A pathological and clinical study based on eighty cases. *Neb Med J* **20**:693, 1925.
21. Niederer, J., Hawkins, N., Rider, W.D., Till, J.E.: Failure analysis of radical radiation therapy of the supraglottic laryngeal carcinoma. *Int J Radiat Oncol Biol Phys* **2**:621–629, 1977.
22. Perez, C.A., Stanley, K., Rubin, P., et. al.: A prospective randomized study of various irradiation doses and fractionation schedules in the treatment of inoperable non-oat cell carcinoma of the lung. A

preliminary report by the Radiation Therapy Oncology Group. *Cancer* **45**:2744–2753, 1980.

23. Petrovich, Z., Mietlowsky, W., Ohanian, M., and Cox, J.: Clinical report on the treatment of locally advanced lung cancer. *Cancer* **40**: 72–77, 1977.
24. Rogers, W.L.: Primary cancer of the lung: Clinical and pathologic survey of 50 cases. *Arch Intern Med* **49**:1058–1077, 1932.
25. Suit, H.: Introduction: Statement of the problem pertaining to the effect of dose fractionation and total treatment time on response of tissue to x-irradiation. In *Time and Dose Relationships in Radiation Biology as Applied to Radiotherapy* (NCI-AEC Conference, Carmel, California, 1969), Dept. of Commerce, 1970.
26. Watson, E.R., Halnan, K.E., Dische, S., Saunders, M.I., et. al.: Hyperbaric oxygen and radiotherapy: A Medical Research Council trial in carcinoma of the cervix. *Br J Radiol* **51**:879–887, 1978.

CHAPTER 34

Contribution of the Keynote Discussant: Impact of Improved Local–Regional Control on Survival Rates

Norah duV. Tapley, M.D.*[a]

An analysis will be made using data from various groups of patients who have different incidences of control of local–regional disease to ascertain whether the survival rates in these groups are different. An effort will be made to define, based on the initial staging of the disease, which groups of patients may or may not survive. The data analyzed is not based on randomized series, but utilizes the results of patient series treated by current treatment methods.

Head and Neck

In carcinoma of the upper respiratory and digestive passages, the probability of distant metastases is related significantly more to the existence of lymph-node involvement in the neck than to the size and extent of the primary lesion. In two M. D. Anderson Hospital series of patients with squamous cell carcinoma of the pharynx, a relationship has been sought between the incidence of distant metastases and the initial staging of the disease. In a series of patients with nasopharynx or oropharynx carcinoma, the incidence of distant metastases increased as the degree of nodal involvement increased, from 14% for NO and N1 disease to 44% for patients with N2 and N3 nodal involvement, whereas with increasing T stage, the distant metastasis rate was relatively constant.[3] In a series of patients with carcinoma of the pyriform sinus, the incidence of distant metastasis correlated strongly with the extent of neck node disease and not with the stage of the primary lesion.[6] It has also been shown that patients who later develop neck disease after the initial treatment have a higher incidence of distant metastases than those patients who remain free of nodal disease.[13,16]

Combined treatment with surgery and irradiation decreases local–regional recurrence and affects the survival rates. In patients with stage IV carcinoma of the supraglottic larynx, the incidence of local–regional recurrences is decreased if postoperative irradiation is given.[10] The 2-year and 5-year survival rates for patients who receive postoperative irradiation are significantly increased.[8] A statistically significant decrease in the number of recurrences above the clavicles has been shown in the number of patients with squamous cell carcinoma of the pyriform sinus receiving postoperative irradiation compared with patients treated by surgery alone (see Fig. 1).[6] Figure 2 shows that the 5-year survival rate in the patients receiving postoperative irradiation is 38% versus 25% in the group treated by surgery alone. This superiority of results occurs despite a higher incidence of N2 and N3 nodal involvement and T4 primary lesions in the postoperative irradiation

[a]Radiotherapist and Professor of Radiotherapy, Department of Radiotherapy, The University of Texas System Cancer Center, M. D. Anderson Hospital and Tumor Institute, Houston, Texas

*deceased

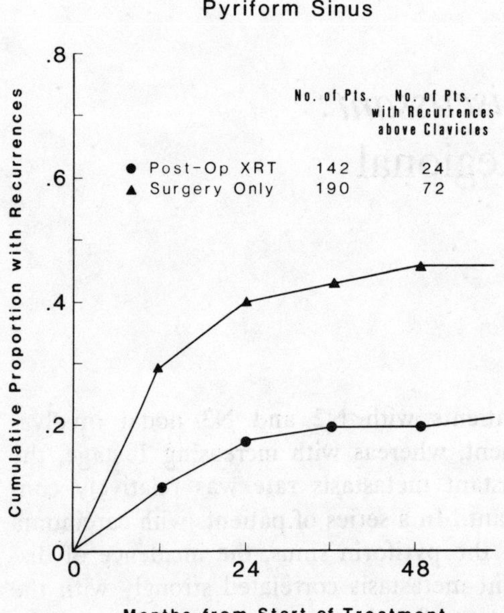

Figure 1. Recurrence rates above the clavicles in patients treated with postoperative irradiation and surgery and with surgery only. The overall comparison between the two curves has a p value of 0.000007.

The Berkson-Gage life-table method (1950) estimates the cumulative proportion of recurrence over time while adjusting for varying periods of follow-up among patients. The raw relative frequency of recurrence in any group at the end of a study does not make this adjustment, and hence, in general, it is not equal to the life-table estimate of recurrence made at the end of the study. (Data from El Badawi, et al., 1982.)[6]

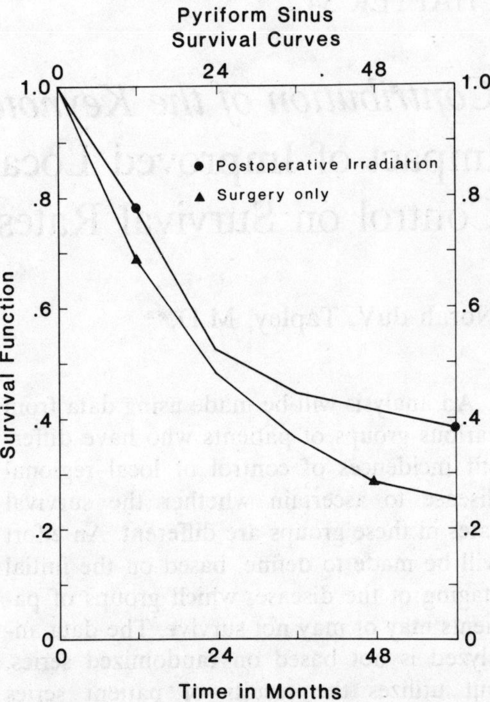

Figure 2. Survival curves according to the Berkson-Gage method for patients receiving postoperative irradiation and those receiving surgery only. At 5 years the survival rates are 38% for the postoperative irradiation group versus 25% for the surgery-only group. The survival rate has a p value of 0.0062, and the overall comparison of the curves has a p value of 0.03. (Data from El Badawi, et al., 1982.)[6]

group than in the group treated by surgery alone. Although the number of patients free of disease above the clavicles is almost double in the irradiated group compared with the surgery-alone group, the 5-year survival rate does not reflect the same degree of improvement because of deaths between 2 and 5 years due to distant metastases or intercurrent disease and, uncommonly, from uncontrolled local–regional disease, since almost all recurrences above the clavicles have appeared by 2 years.

Breast

Table 1 shows that elective irradiation of the supraclavicular and internal mammary chain nodes reduces next to zero the later appearance of manifestation of the disease in these lymphatics. The 10-year survival rate in the patients with no elective postoperative irradiation (12% histologically positive axillary nodes) is 55% as compared with 57% in the patients with elective postoperative irradiation (63.6% histologically positive nodes) (see Table 2). In the group of patients with 63.6% incidence of axillary involvement, the survival rate should be lower than in the group of patients with 12% incidence of involvement since, in patients with breast cancer, survival rates relate to the extent of axillary disease. Furthermore, Table 2 shows the 5- and 10-year survival rates in patients with various degrees of axillary node involvement (not treated with elective chemotherapy) compared with the expected survival rates for individuals of the same

TABLE 1. Effectiveness of Local–Regional Irradiation in Breast Cancer[d]

	Axilla Positive in Surgical Specimen	
	No Irradiation[a]	4500–5000 rad/5 weeks to peripheral lymphatics[b]
Supraclavicular	20–26%	1.5%
	Axilla Positive in Surgical Specimen, Central or Inner Quadrant	
	No Irradiation[c]	4500–5000 rad/5 weeks to peripheral lymphatics (MDAH)
Parasternal	9% (25/264)	0% (0/204)

[a]From Paterson and Russell, 1959.[17]
[b]From Fletcher, 1973.[7]
[c]From Urban, 1952.[21]
[d]Data from Fletcher and Montague, 1978.[9]

race, age, and sex. In the patients with histologically positive nodes who received postoperative irradiation to the peripheral lymphatics, the 10-year survival rate of 47%' must be related to an expected survival rate of 68% and not to 100%.

At M. D. Anderson Hospital, because the patients treated with irradiation alone for stages III and IV disease (inflammatory carcinoma excluded) had too many complications, the indications for simple mastectomy followed by irradiation now include marginally resectable tumors, both in the breast and axilla, and even patients with positive supraclavicular nodes. The mastectomy also includes dissection of the lateral axilla. The concept that all patients with advanced local–regional disease will eventually die of breast cancer is refuted by the comparison given in Table 3 and three series of patients approximately comparable in regard to the extent of disease. The Columbia-Presbyterian series shows the results of irradiation in patients with breast cancer unsuitable for radical mastectomy according to Haagensen's criteria[11] which are essentially American Joint Committee stages III and IV. The radiation doses were low, resulting in a local failure rate of 87% and a 5-year survival rate of 10.7%. In an M. D. Anderson Hospital series of patients treated with high-dose protracted irradiation using ^{60}Co, the local–regional failure rate is reduced to 27.8% and the 5- and 10-year survival rates to 27.7% and 19.3%, respectively. Further improvement is seen in another M. D. Anderson Hospital series in which treatment by simple mastectomy is followed by irradiation, with a local–regional failure rate of 16.1% and 5- and 10-year survival rates of 43.3% and 33.8% respectively. A 34% 10-year disease-free survival rate, which is close to a cure rate, achieved without adjuvant chemotherapy, is substantial in patients with stage III and stage IV disease, and disputes the concept that all patients with advanced local–regional disease have distant metastases and therefore the survival rates cannot be improved by local–regional control.

Pelvic Tumors

UTERUS

Cervix

The effect of regional nodal disease on survival rates in cervix cancer is evident in

TABLE 2. Nondisseminated Breast Cancer. Ratios of Observed 5- and 10 - Year Survival Rates to Normal Expected Survival Rates (Age, Race, and Sex Adjusted; No Elective Chemotherapy) 1959–1972 (analysis May 1978)[e]

Treatment Modality	All Patients Survival Rates 5 years	All Patients Survival Rates 10 years	Histologically Negative Axillary Nodes Survival Rates 5 years	Histologically Negative Axillary Nodes Survival Rates 10 years	Histologically Positive Axillary Nodes: Total + Nodes Survival Rates 5 years	Total + Nodes 10 years	1–3 + Nodes Survival Rates 5 years	1–3 + Nodes 10 years	⩾4 + Nodes Survival Rates 5 years	⩾4 + Nodes 10 years
Radical mastectomy alone	73% A[a]	55% A	76% A	58% A	48% A	33% A	64% A	42% A	31% A	0%
(essentially outer quadrants);	82% E[b]	62% E	82% E	62% E	82% E	62% E	81% E	64% E	83% E	0%
301 patients—12% with histologically positive nodes.	88% R[c]	89% R	92% R	94% R	59% R	53% R	78% R	66% R	38% R	0%
Radical mastectomy followed	74% A	57% A	87% [d]A	76% [d]A	67% A	47% A	77% A	54% A	52% A	36% A
by peripheral lymphatic irradiation;	86% E	68% E	86% E	67% E	87% E	68% E	85% E	65% E	90% E	74% E
368 patients—63.6% with histologically positive nodes.	86% R	86% R	102% R	113% R	77% R	68% R	91% R	83% R	58% R	48% R

[a] A = Actual observed survival rates.

[b] E = Expected survival rates for the group given their age, race, and sex. The general mortality tables used are those from the vital statistics of the United States, 1970.

[c] R = A/E, which is the ratio of observed survival rate to the expected survival rate. This is not a survival rate itself, but an indication of how close to the norm a survival rate is (100% = normal survival expectancy).

[d] Patients with essentially central or inner quadrant lesions.

[e] Adapted from Fletcher, 1980.[8]

TABLE 3. Carcinoma of the Breast—Stages III and IV.[a] Local-Regional Failures vs. Survival Rates (No Adjuvant Chemotherapy)

Treatment	Local Failures	5-year Survival Rate	10-year Disease-Free Survival Rate
Columbia-Presbyterian 1950-1960[b]			
Irradiation only (4000 rad/4 weeks/250 Kv; 5000 rad/4 weeks/22 MeV)	87.2% (34/39)	10.7%	not given
M. D. Anderson Hospital			
Protracted irradiation with ^{60}Co[c]	27.8% (44/158)	27.7%[e]	19.3%[e]
Simple mastectomy and irradiation[d]	16.1% (65/404)	43.3%[e]	33.8%[e]

[a]American Joint Committee Staging System, inflammatory carcinomas excluded.

[b]Unsuitable for radical mastectomy according to Haagensen's criteria (20 patients could have had a simple mastectomy and 19 patients were unsuitable). (Data from Atkins, 1961.)

[c]Spanos et al., 1980.[20]

[d]Montague et al., 1982.[15]

[e]Disease-free 5- and 10-year survival. (Data from Berkson and Gage, 1950,[4] not age adjusted.)

TABLE 4. Preirradiation Therapy Selective Lymphadenectomy. Results According to Nodal Findings July 1971 Thru 1974 (analysis July 1975)[c]

Status of Nodes	Number of Patients	NED[a]	Alive with Cancer	Dead: Cancer	Dead: Complication
Negative	56	34	1	15	6
Positive pelvic only	40	8	3[b]	23	6
Positive common iliac and aortic	24	3	1	12	8
Total	120	45	5	50	20

[a]NED = no evidence of disease.

[b]One patient with metastatic adenocarcinoma of the breast (second primary).

[c]Data from Wharton et al., 1977.[22]

Table 4 which shows the results in a series of 120 patients with squamous cell carcinoma who had a selective lymphadenectomy prior to irradiation. The comparative disease-free survival rates are 60.7% for patients with negative lymph nodes, 20% for those with positive pelvic nodes, and 12.5% for those whose common iliac and aortic nodes were involved. Of 36 patients with positive lymph nodes followed closely at M.D. Anderson Hospital, 25 patients died from distant metastases without clinical manifestation of pelvic or lymphatic disease.

Endometrium

In patients with carcinoma of the endometrium treated with preoperative irradia-

TABLE 5. Pelvic Failures vs. Survival Rates in Bladder and Prostate Carcinoma

	% Pelvic Failure	5-year Survival Rate
Bladder (B_2 + C)[a]		
Irradiation alone (7000 rad)	41%	12%[c]
Preop irradiation (5000 rad) + cystectomy	13%	50.7%[c]
Prostate (C_2 fixed to pelvic wall)[b]		
6500 rad	38.5% (5/13)	30.8%[d] (4/13)
7000 rad	20.6% (7/34)	56.0%[d] (19/34)

[a] Miller and Johnson, 1973.[14]
[b] Hussey, 1980.[12]
[c] $p < 0.02$.
[d] $p = 0.11$.

tion, the pelvic recurrence rate, including central and nodal disease, is on the order of 7%.[19]

BLADDER

The 5-year survival rates in a series of patients with invasive bladder cancer (stages B1, B2, and C) treated by surgery alone or by irradiation alone have been on the order of 20%.[5,23] In patients with B2 and C disease treated by cystectomy alone or by 5000-rad preoperative irradiation to the pelvis followed by cystectomy, the pelvic failure rates are, respectively, 41% and 13%, and the 5-year survival rates are 12% and 50.7%, respectively (see Table 5).[14]

PROSTATE

In a series of patients with carcinoma of the prostate treated with irradiation and followed for a limited time (1 to 50 months), there was an 86.5% free-of-disease survival when the pelvic nodes were negative, 71.4% with positive pelvic nodes, and 30% when both pelvic and periaortic nodes were positive.[2]

In the M. D. Anderson Hospital series of patients with carcinoma of the prostate, local control rates and survival rates were the same for patients with stage B and C1 disease treated with either 6500 or 7000 rad. In patients with stage C2 disease, however, when the dose increased from 6500 to 7000 rad, the incidence of pelvic failure decreased from 38.5 to 20.6% and the 5-year survival rate increased from 30.8 to 56% (Table 5).[12]

Summary

When treatment is optimal for local–regional disease, frequently combining surgery and irradiation, local–regional control can be achieved in a high percentage of patients. Control of local–regional disease improves survival rates in the patients who do not have occult distant metastases on admission. In head and neck and bladder cancer patients, who generally are old, disease-free survival figures, which may be quite good at 2 years, are frequently seriously diminished at 5 years due to death from causes unrelated to cancer or its treatment. In breast cancer patients, 10-year disease-free survival rates, which can be equated with cure rates, must be compared with the survival rates of a general population with the same vital statistics parameters.

Acknowledgments

This work was supported in part by Grants CA06294 and CA05654 from the National Cancer Institute, Department of Health and Human Services, U.S.A.

REFERENCES

1. Atkins, H.L.: Treatment of locally advanced carcinoma of the breast with roentgen therapy and simple mastectomy. *AJR* **85**:860–864, 1961.
2. Bagshaw, M.A., Pistenma, D.A., Ray, G.R., Freiha, F.S., and Kempson, R.L.: Evaluation of extended field radiotherapy for prostatic neoplasms: 1976 progress report. *Cancer Treat Rep* **61**:297–306, 1977.
3. Berger, D.S., and Fletcher, G.H.: Distant metastases following local control of squamous cell carcinoma of the nasopharynx, tonsillar fossa, and base of the tongue. *Radiology* **100**:141–143, 1971.
4. Berkson, J., and Gage, R.: Calculation of survival rates for cancer. *Proc Mayo Clin* **25**:270, 1950.
5. Crigler, C.M., Miller, L.S., Guinn, G.A., and Schillaci, H.G.: Radiotherapy for carcinoma of the bladder. *J Urol* **96**:55–61, 1966.
6. El Badawi, S.A., Goepfert, H., Fletcher, G.H., Herson, J., and Oswald, M.J.: Squamous cell carcinoma of the pyriform sinus. *Laryngoscope* **92**:357–364, 1982.
7. Fletcher, G.H.: *Textbook of Radiotherapy*, 2nd ed. Philadelphia: Lea & Febiger, 1973, pp. 457–493.
8. Fletcher, G.H.: *Textbook of Radiotherapy*, 3rd ed. Philadelphia: Lea & Febiger, 1980, 180–219, 330–363, 527–579.
9. Fletcher, G.H., and Montague, E.D.: Does adequate irradiation of the internal mammary chain and supraclavicular nodes improve survival rate. *Int J Radiat Oncol Biol Phys* **4**:481–492, 1978.
10. Goepfert, H., Jesse, R.H., Fletcher, G.H., and Hamberger, A.: Optimal treatment for the technically resectable squamous cell carcinoma of the supraglottic larynx. *Laryngoscope* **85**:14–32, 1975.
11. Haagensen, C.D., and Stout, A.P.: Carcinoma of the breast. II. Criteria of operability. *Am Surg* **118**:859, 1943.
12. Hussey, D.H.: Carcinoma of the prostate. In *Textbook of Radiotherapy*, 3rd ed., G.H. Fletcher, ed. Philadelphia: Lea & Febiger, 1980, pp. 894–914.
13. Jesse, R.H., Barkley, H.T., Jr., Lindberg, R.D., and Fletcher, G.H.: Cancer of the oral cavity. Is elective neck dissection beneficial? *Am J Surg* **120**:505–508, 1970.
14. Miller, L.S., and Johnson, D.E.: Megavoltage irradiation for bladder cancer: Alone, postoperative, or preoperative. In *Proceedings of the Seventh National Cancer Conference* Philadelphia: J. B. Lippincott, 1973, 771–791.
15. Montague, E.D., Spanos, W.J., Jr., and Fletcher, G.H.: Die Entwicklung der Behandlungsmethoden bei der Primärtherapie des nichtmetastasierten Mammakarzinoms. In *Die Erkankungen der weiblichen Brustdrüse.* Herausgegeben von H.J. Frischbier (ed), New York: George Thieme Verlag Stuttgart, 1982, 201–207.
16. Northrop, M., Fletcher, G.H., Jesse, R.H., Jr., and Lindberg, R.D.: Evolution of neck disease in patients with primary squamous cell carcinomas of the oral tongue, floor of mouth, and palatine arch and clinically positive neck nodes neither fixed nor bilateral. *Cancer* **29**:23–30, 1972.
17. Paterson, R., and Russell, M.H.: Clinical trials in malignant disease. III. Breast cancer: Evaluation of postoperative radiotherapy. *J Fac Radiol* (Lond) **10**:175–180, 1959.
18. Robbins, G.F., Lucas, J.C., Jr., Fracchia, A.A., et. al.: An evaluation of postoperative prophylactic radiation therapy in breast cancer. *Surg Gynecol Obstet* **122**:979–982, 1966.
19. Spanos, W.J., Fletcher, G.H., Wharton, J.T., and Gallager, H.S.: Patterns of pelvic recurrence in endometrial carcinoma. *Gynecol Oncol* **6**:495–502, 1978.
20. Spanos, W.J., Montague, E., and Fletcher, G.H.: Late complications of radiation only for advanced breast cancer. *Int J Radiat Oncol Biol Phys* **6**:1473–1476, 1980.
21. Urban, J.A.: Radical mastectomy in continuity with en bloc resection of internal mammary lymph node chain: New procedure for primary operable cancer of the breast. *Cancer* **5**:992–1008, 1952.
22. Wharton, J.T., Jones, H.W., III, Day, T.G., Rutledge, F.N., and Fletcher, G.H.: Preirradiation celiotomy and extended field irradiation for invasive carcinoma of the cervix. *Obstet Gynecol* **49**:333–338, 1977.
23. Whitmore, W.F., Jr., and Marshall, V.F.: Radical total cystectomy for cancer of the bladder: 230 consecutive cases five years later. *J Urol* **87**:853–868, 1962.

CHAPTER 35

Radiation Boost or Added Limited Surgery as a Means of Improving Local–Regional Control

Gilbert H. Fletcher, M.D.[a]

Historical Background

Baclesse developed the shrinking-field technique based on the concept that peripheral cancer cells are more radiosensitive than those at the center of a mass. It is one of the most important treatment planning schemes in radiotherapy today.

Present Concept of the Relationship of Histology to Radiosensitivity

Present clinical data show that all squamous cell carcinomas, adenocarcinomas of the breast and uterus, mucoepidermoid, malignant mixed, and adenoid cystic carcinomas of the salivary glands, and possibly soft tissue sarcomas have approximately the same radiosensitivity, other factors being equal. The volume of cancer is the predominant parameter because, for a given tumor type, the larger the volume, the greater the number of malignant clonogens and percentage of hypoxic ones. Furthermore, in larger tumors reoxygenation may not be complete before the end of irradiation.

[a]Professor of Radiotherapy, The University of Texas System Cancer Center,
M.D. Anderson Hospital and Tumor Institute, Houston, Texas

Radiocurability of Subclinical Disease

Subclinical disease includes not only microscopic disease, but also macroscopic aggregates of cancer cells that cannot be palpated, even though they are in accessible areas.

Subclinical disease in undisturbed lymphatics of the neck contains relatively few malignant cells which are normally oxygenated. Larger subclinical aggregates of cancer (e.g., 1 mm in diameter, approximately 10^6 cells) may contain hypoxic cells initially, but these should reoxygenate early in an irradiation scheme lasting 5 weeks. A treatment of 5000 rad in 5 weeks has been shown to eradicate close to 100% of subclinical deposits of squamous cell carcinomas of the upper respiratory and digestive tracts and adenocarcinomas of the breast; with smaller doses, lower control rates are obtained.[6,7]

Radiocurability of Gross Cancer

Table 1 shows clinical data from various analyses relating dose and volume in the control of primary lesions and metastatic nodes in adenocarcinomas of the breast and squamous cell carcinomas of the upper respiratory and digestive tracts.[10] In patients with squamous cell carcinoma of the mucous membrane of the upper respiratory and digestive tracts, 50% of clinically positive neck nodes 2 – 3 cm in diameter are controlled with 5000 rad in 5 weeks and

TABLE 1. Probability of Control Correlated with Irradiation Dose and Volume of Cancer.[c]

Dose	Squamous Cell Carcinoma of the Upper Respiratory and Digestive Tracts	Adenocarcinoma of the Breast
5000 rad[a]	>90% subclinical 50% T1 lesions of nasopharynx ≅50% 2–3 cm neck nodes	>90% subclinical
6000 rad[a]	80–90% T1 lesions of pharynx and larynx ≅50% T3 + T4 lesions of tonsillar fossa	
7000 rad[a]	≅90% 1–3 cm neck nodes ≅70% 3–5 cm neck nodes 80–90% T2 lesions of tonsillar fossa and supraglottic larynx ≅80% T3 + T4 lesions of tonsillar fossa	90% clinically positive axillary nodes 2.5–3 cm[b]
7000–8000 rad (8–9 weeks)		65% 2–3 cm primary 30% >5 cm primary
8000–9000 rad (8–10 weeks)		56% >5 cm primary
8000–10,000 rad (10–12 weeks)		75% >5–15 cm primary

[a] 1000 rad/5 fractions/1 week.

[b] The control rate is corrected for the percentage of nodes that would be positive histologically had a dissection of the axilla been performed.

[c] Data from Fletcher and Schukovsky, 1975.[10]

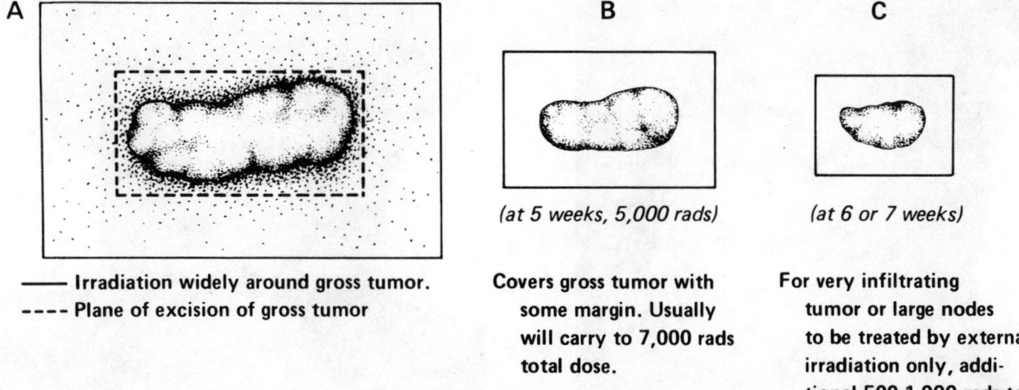
A
B
C
(at 5 weeks, 5,000 rads)
(at 6 or 7 weeks)
—— Irradiation widely around gross tumor.
---- Plane of excision of gross tumor
Covers gross tumor with some margin. Usually will carry to 7,000 rads total dose.
For very infiltrating tumor or large nodes to be treated by external irradiation only, additional 500-1,000 rads to 7,500-8,000 rads total dose.

Figure 1. Diagram illustrating the shrinking-field technique and simple removal of gross tumor. (From Fletcher, 1980.)[8]

90% are controlled with 7000 rad in 7 weeks; approximately 70% of nodes 3 – 5 cm in diameter are sterilized by 7000 rad in 7 weeks.

Treatment Planning

Practically speaking, there are several ways to achieve the effect of a boost:

1. *Simple surgical excision* of easily removable masses at the primary site and/or in the peripheral lymphatics (see Fig. 1). When this is feasible, it may be preferable to a radiation boost.
2. *Interstitial implants.*
3. *Shrinking-field technique.* Initially large portals are used around the main mass or masses to eradicate surrounding microscopic disease, but the added doses to gross disease are given through reduced portals (Fig. 1). The dependence of complications on the volume irradiated is part of the rationale behind the shrinking-field technique. Not only is the size of the portals decreased, but also the depth of irradiated volume may be diminished. For example, in head and neck cancers a laterally located mass may be irradiated with an electron beam alone or combined with the photon beam.

PARAMETERS OF THE BOOST DOSE

The boost dose is considered part of the total dose and is determined by the initial size of the mass(es) and their clinical variety, not the histology.

If gross tumor has clinically disappeared by the third or fourth week, the cancer cells should from there on be euoxic, making the boost dose given in the fourth to seventh week more effective than it would be if induration persisted. However, a fast regression rate must not be the overriding factor in determining the total dose. The probability of control of homogeneous tumors with increasing doses is described by a sigmoid curve. The slope of the curve may vary with the clinical variety and stage of the tumor. For some tumors a portion of the curve can be very steep, so that a relatively small dose increment increases the probability of control from 25% to 75%.[20]

Malignant clonogens respond with accelerated repopulation to the challenge produced by depletion of the tumor population.[21] These kinetic changes can be induced by irradiation or surgical procedure. Repopulation of tumor cells during the rest period may exceed the benefit of potential reoyxgenation; therefore, even if there is clinically residual disease at the end

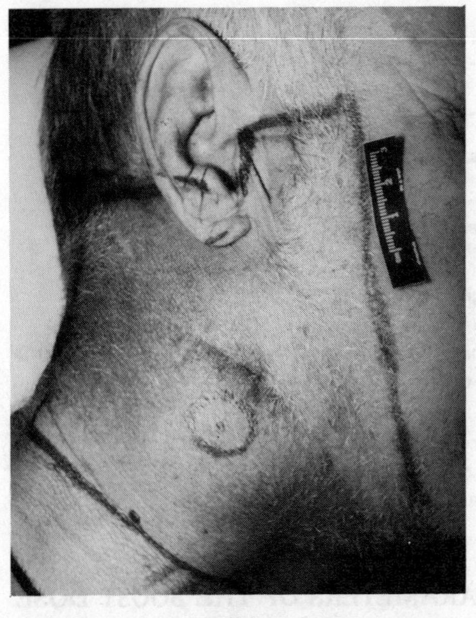

(*a*)

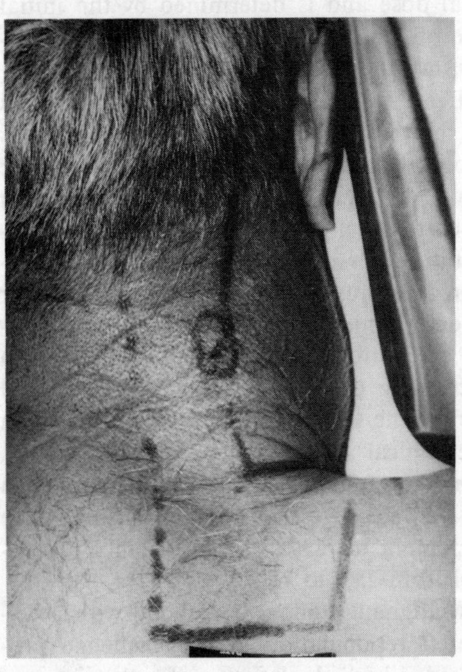

(*b*)

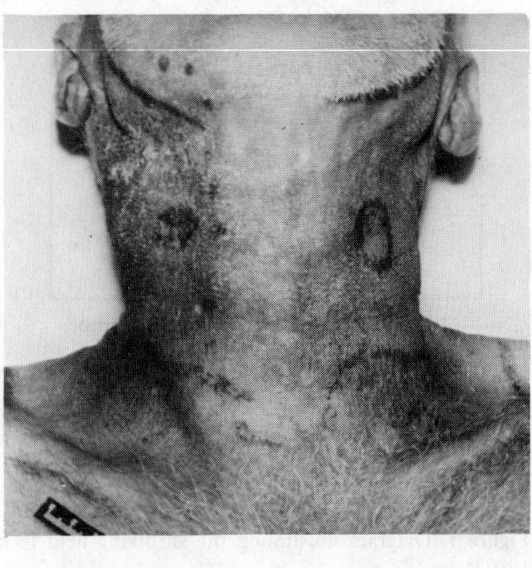

(*c*)

Figure 2. A 57-year-old man, who approximately 2 months prior to admission had noted a swelling in the right side of the neck which at first grew slowly and then increased rapidly in size. When the patient was seen at M.D. Anderson Hospital on December 6, 1979, no diagnosis of primary tumor had been made. On examination, a small exophytic lesion in the right mid-pyriform sinus was found and biopsied. In the right side of the neck there was a large 10 × 10 cm mass in the subdigastric and midjugular area. Biopsies of the primary lesion and node were read as undifferentiated squamous carcinoma.

Through parallel opposed portals (*a*) to the upper neck, 6500 rad was given in 8 weeks at 900 rad per week to the primary lesion, and 5000 rad dose was given through an anterior appositional portal to the lower neck. Three hours after treatment through lateral ports to the primary and neck node, 120 rad was given to the node through alternately anterior and posterior portals so that the node received 1500 rad per week to a total dose of 8500 rad. The dotted line represents the margin of the posterior portal (*b*). Toward the end of treatment, the patient developed only a brisk erythema with patches of moist desquamation in the area glanced by the anterior and posterior portals (*c*). Two months after the completion of therapy, a modified neck dissection was performed. There was no healing delay of the wound of the neck dissection.

The histological description of the surgical specimen is as follows: "No viable-appearing tumor is present. The larger nodule may represent total tumor replacement of a lymph node, with extensive calcification and necrosis. Many scattered, separate small nests of degenerated cells are present in connective tissue and skeletal muscle which are extensively calcified and which have elicited a marked tissue/foreign body reaction. Degenerated cells of squamous carcinoma are identifiable within some of these."

On May 30, 1980, the patient was found to have bilateral lung metastases, NED above the clavicles.

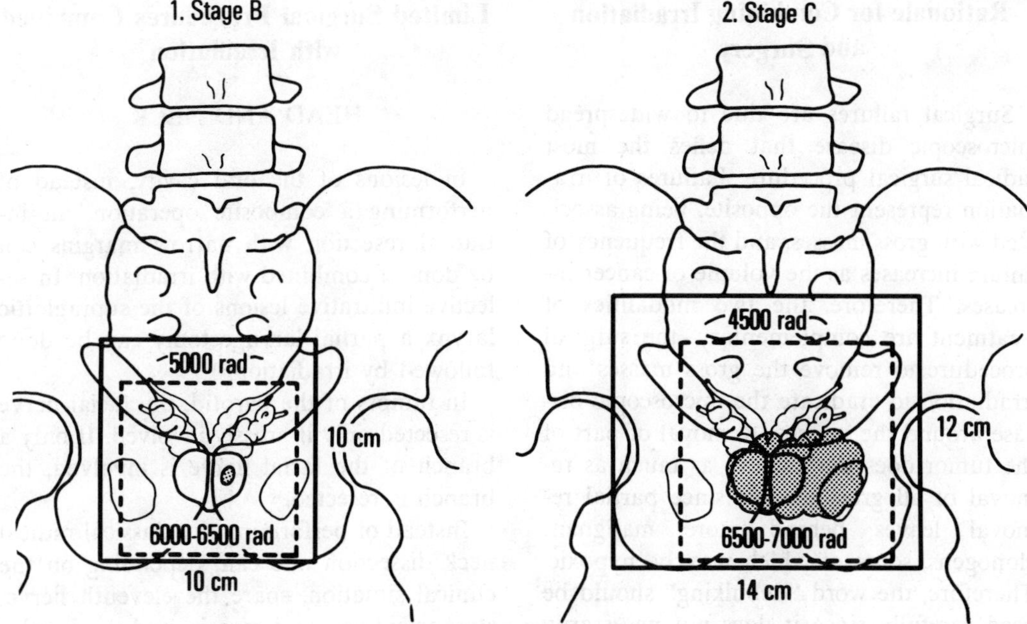

Figure 3. Treatment policy for carcinoma of the prostate with a negative lymphangiogram. Stage B: A dose of 5000 rad in 5 weeks is delivered through the initial portals which measure 10 × 10 cm anteriorly and posteriorly and 10 × 8 cm laterally; the prostate is boosted with 8 × 8 cm portals to a total dose of 6000 to 6500 rad, depending on the size of the tumor. Stage C: A dose of 4500 rad in 4½ to 5 weeks is delivered to the primary tumor and the obturator, hypogastric, and external iliac nodes through 12 × 14 cm anterior and posterior portals and 12 × 8 cm lateral portals; the primary tumor receives 6500 to 7000 rad, depending on the initial bulk of the tumor and the size of the reduced field. (From Fletcher and Hussey, 1980.)[9]

given without waiting for further regression. In fast-growing tumors, a weekly dose of 900–1000 rad does not keep up with tumor cell repopulation. In this situation the boost is given concomitantly.

Although the volume irradiated can be drastically reduced in the treatment of neck nodes, in tumors of the oropharynx it is still quite sizeable. Therefore, the dose per fraction should be kept to a maximum of 200 rad per fraction to minimize late damage, such as fibrosis. Furthermore, at or below 200 rad there is a predominance of single lethal events with a favorable OER.

Figure 2 illustrates a boost given in a patient with a small squamous cell carcinoma of the pyriform sinus and a very large neck node which had grown rapidly. The boost dose was given concomitantly during the basic treatment, through anterior and posterior portals, 3 hours after the irradiation through lateral portals to deliver a 1500-rad weekly tumor dose. During this 3-hour interval, normal tissues have repaired most or all the accumulated sublethal damage of the first irradiation (substantiated by the moderate acute skin reaction and no healing delay of the neck dissection wound), while the hypoxic tumor cells, because of their slower rate of repair, might still have an amount of unrepaired damage.

In treating cancer of the prostate, the pelvis is initially covered to irradiate the obturator and hypogastric nodes which are most commonly involved; then smaller portals are used to irradiate the primary tumor to a dose of 6000 rad for stage B, 6500 rad for stage C1 (tumor not fixed to the pelvic walls), and 7000 rad for stage C2 (tumor fixed to the pelvic walls) (see Fig. 3). With these doses the local control rates are respectively 100%, 94%, and 79.5% for stage B, stage C, and Stage C2 tumors.[17]

Rationale for Combining Irradiation and Surgery

Surgical failures are due to widespread microscopic disease that defies the most radical surgical procedure. Failures of irradiation represent the opposite, being associated with gross masses, and the frequency of failure increases as the volume of cancer increases. Therefore, the two modalities of treatment are complementary–the surgical procedure to remove the gross masses and irradiation to eradicate the microscopic disease around the masses. Removal of part of the tumor does not achieve as much as removal of all gross disease since partial removal leaves behind more malignant clonogens, some of which may be hypoxic. Therefore, the word "debulking" should be used carefully since it does not necessarily imply removal of all gross cancer.

Extent of the Surgical Procedure

The surgical procedure optimally should be limited to the removal of the gross masses (Fig. 1) for the following reasons:

1. With diminished surgical manipulation, there is less opportunity of releasing tumor cells into the blood stream.
2. There is less scar tissue and therefore less possibility of hypoxia for the tumor cells left behind.
3. If postoperative irradiation has been chosen it should be given 3 – 4 weeks following surgery. When surgery is very radical, often using pedicles for reconstruction, it may be months before irradiation can be started. During that time, there is repopulation of the tumor cells, and a gross recurrence is not uncommon when the patient is ready for postoperative irradiation.
4. Conservative surgery leads to a better quality of life.

Limited Surgical Procedures Combined with Irradiation

HEAD AND NECK

In lesions of the oral cavity, instead of performing a composite operation, an intraoral resection with narrow margins can be done if combined with irradiation. In selective infiltrative lesions of the supraglottic larynx a partial laryngectomy can be done followed by irradiation.[11]

In tumors of the parotid, the facial nerve is resected only if grossly involved. If only a branch of the facial nerve is involved, the branch is resected.[19]

Instead of performing the classical radical neck dissection one can, depending on the clinical situation, spare the eleventh nerve, sternocleidomastoid muscle, and the jugular vein with equally good results.[13]

BREAST

With ^{60}Co, using a modified Baclesse fractionation of approximately 70 days, significant control rates can be achieved in patients with very advanced breast cancer treated with external irradiation only (see Table 1). Figure 4 illustrates the considerable fibrosis that can develop later. Because of the direct skin involvement and/or peau d'orange, high doses must be given to the skin which an interstitial implant would not provide.

Because of too many severe complications, the indications for simple mastectomy followed by irradiation were expanded to include even marginally resectable tumors, both at the primary site and in the axilla. Even patients with positive supraclavicular nodes have been treated with this combination if the supraclavicular nodes were small (1 – 2 cm) since the major tumor bulk is in the breast and axilla (See Fig. 5). Initially palpable axillary nodes were not removed,

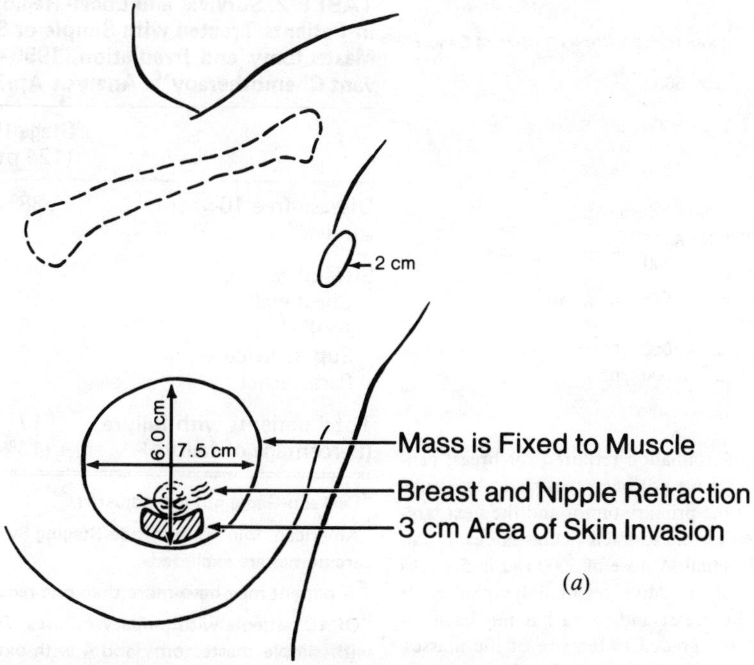

(*a*)

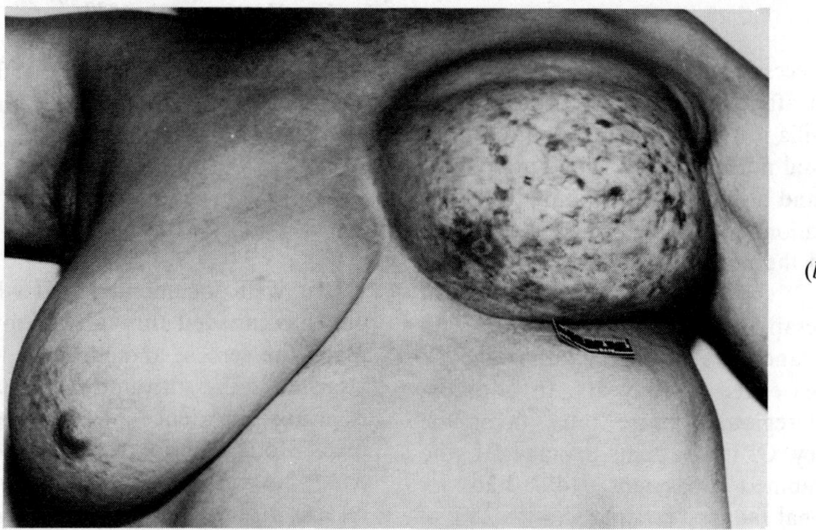

(*b*)

Figure 4. Patient, age 49, presented in July 1960 with a 2-month history of a 7.5 × 6 cm mass in the central portion of the breast, skin involvement, and a clinically positive axillary node (*a*). Aspiration biopsy was positive for tumor.

^{60}Co irradiation began on August 2, 1960 and was completed on October 7, 1960. A tumor dose of 6000 rad was delivered in 8 weeks with five fractions per week with alternating tangential portals. Bolus was used for 20 treatments. The mass in the breast then received 2500 rad tumor dose in 9 fractions and supraclavicular areas received 5000 rad tumor dose in 5 weeks plus 1500 rad through an appositional field to the axilla for the clinically positive axillary node.

The patient remains free of disease in December 1979, but has considerable fibrosis (*b*) and has had repeated episodes of necrosis and infection.

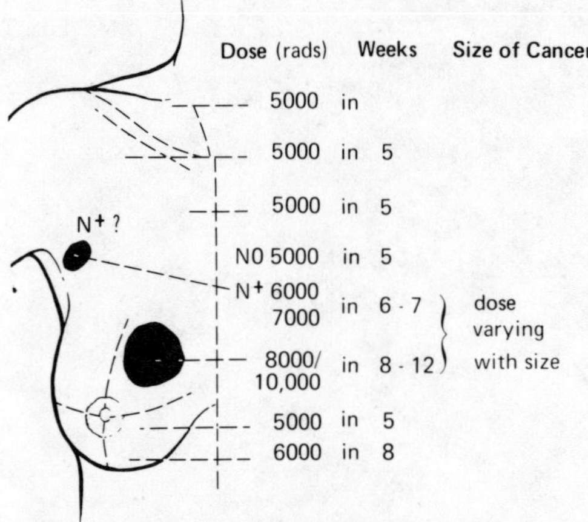

Figure 5. Doses of irradiation required for breast cancer if gross masses have not been removed. As a rule, the largest mass is the primary tumor and the next largest are axillary nodes; the supraclavicular nodes, if palpable, are usually small. A dose of 5000 rad in 5 weeks is given to clinically negative regional lymphatics. If gross cancer in the breast and axilla has not been removed, added doses, graded to the size of the masses, must be given. (Adapted from Calle, Fletcher, and Pierquin, 1973.)[2]

TABLE 2. Survival and Local–Regional Failure Rates in Patients Treated with Simple or Simple Extended Mastectomy and Irradiation, 1955–1975 (No Adjuvant Chemotherapy)[e] Analysis April 1980

	Stage III[b] (124 pts.)	Stage IV[b] (280 pts.)
Disease-free 10-year survival[a]	38%	30%
Sites of failure[c]		
Chest wall	15	34
Axilla[d]	5	13
Supraclavicular	6	11
Parasternal	—	—
Total patients with failure (Percentage of failure)	17 (14%)	48 (17%)

[a] Berkson-Gage, not age adjusted.
[b] American Joint Committee Staging System; inflammatory carcinomas are excluded.
[c] A patient may have more than one recurrence.
[d] Of 18 patients with axillary failures, 14 had been treated with simple mastectomy and 4 with extended simple mastectomy.
[e] Data from Montague et al., 1982.[16]

thereby necessitating an additional boost to the axilla after 5000 rad, but presently the lateral axilla is dissected. The patient of Figure 4 would not be treated with simple mastectomy and dissection of the axilla followed by irradiation, even though there were grave signs and the nodes were large.

Table 2 shows that, without adjuvant chemotherapy, 38% of the patients with stage III and 30% of those with stage IV were disease-free at 10 years. In addition, the local–regional failure rates favor the new policy. Of the patients in stage III who had combined treatment, 14% had local–regional failures, compared with 28% of those treated with protracted irradiation alone; 17% of patients with stage IV disease treated with combined therapy had failures compared to 28% of those treated only with protracted irradiation. Of the 18 patients who had an axillary failure, 14 of 193 had had only a simple mastectomy, whereas only 4 of 211 patients experienced axillary failure following a lateral axillary dissection.

In addition to achieving a better local–regional control, a dose of 5000 rad following a simple mastectomy produces no significant fibrosis.

LARGE BOWEL

It is well documented that when the tumor has invaded through the muscularis to reach the serosa, and more so when it has attached to the surrounding structures, there is a high incidence of local–regional failures.[4] Both anterior resection with end-to-end anastomosis and abdominoperitoneal resection remove only gross cancer without resecting widely around the tumor. Several well-documented series of patients who have received postoperative irradiation show a clear diminution of pelvic and/or peritoneal recurrences.[12,22]

SOFT TISSUE SARCOMAS

The surgical procedures are varied, including simple excision, wide excision,

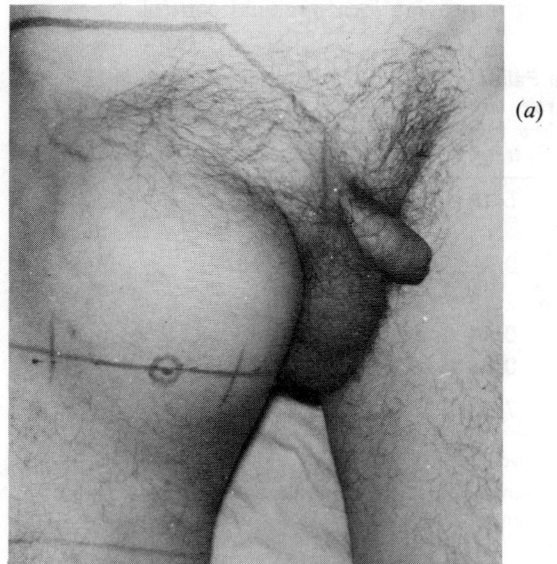

(*a*)

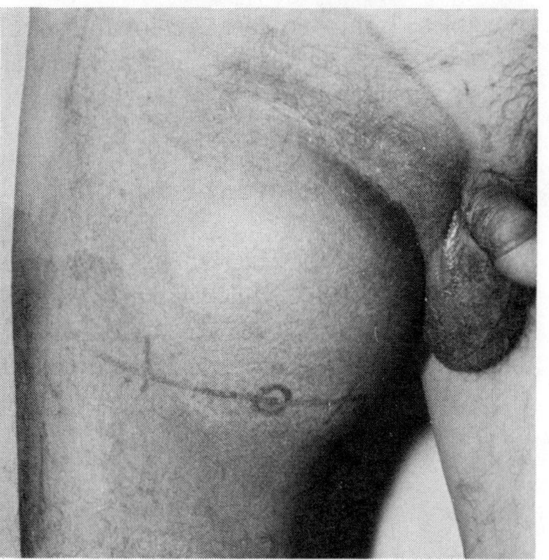

(*b*)

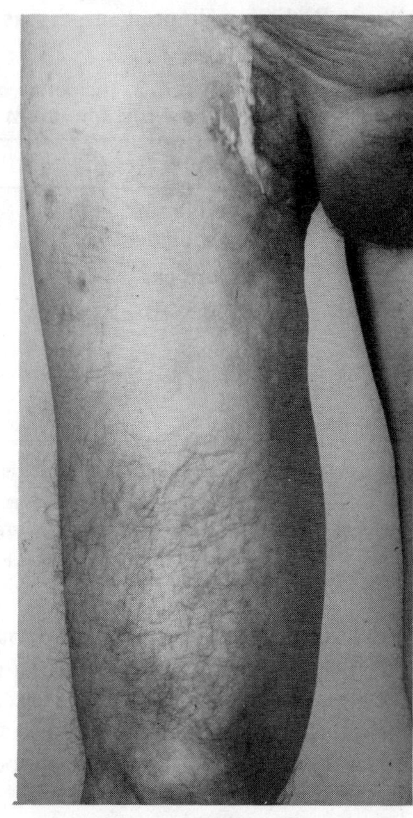

(*c*)

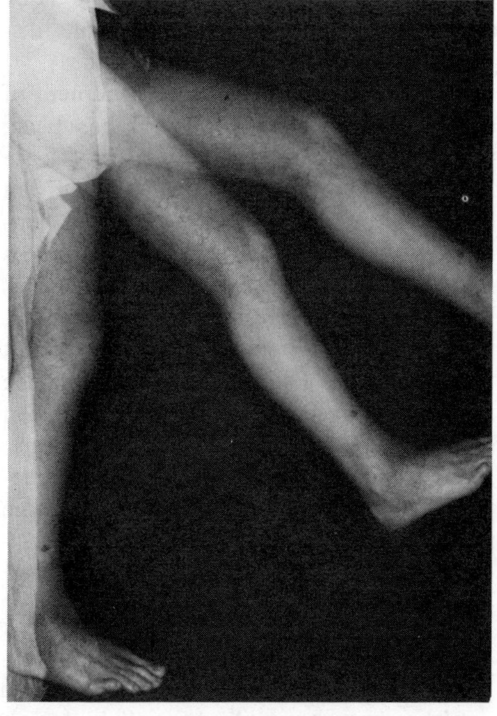

(*d*)

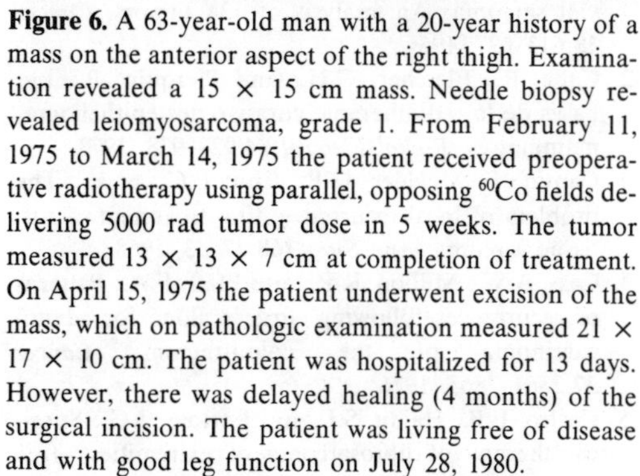

Figure 6. A 63-year-old man with a 20-year history of a mass on the anterior aspect of the right thigh. Examination revealed a 15 × 15 cm mass. Needle biopsy revealed leiomyosarcoma, grade 1. From February 11, 1975 to March 14, 1975 the patient received preoperative radiotherapy using parallel, opposing ^{60}Co fields delivering 5000 rad tumor dose in 5 weeks. The tumor measured 13 × 13 × 7 cm at completion of treatment. On April 15, 1975 the patient underwent excision of the mass, which on pathologic examination measured 21 × 17 × 10 cm. The patient was hospitalized for 13 days. However, there was delayed healing (4 months) of the surgical incision. The patient was living free of disease and with good leg function on July 28, 1980.

(*a*) Tumor mass at the beginning of radiotherapy. (*b*) Tumor mass at completion of 5000 rad tumor dose in 5 weeks. (*c*) View of anterior thigh at 2 years. (*d*) Hip function at 2 years. (From Lindberg, 1980.)[14]

TABLE 3. Incidence of Local Failures, 1963–1973 (Unlimited Follow-up: Minimum 2 Years)[c]

Trunk[a]		Upper Extremity		Lower Extremity	
Axilla and shoulder	1/6 (1)[b]	Arm	5/15 (1)	Thigh	6/30 (1)
Buttocks	2/14	Elbow	0/3	Knee	3/16 (3)
Other sites	4/8 (1)	Forearm	2/13	Leg	6/13 (3)
		Wrist	0/4	Ankle	1/3
		Hand	0/8	Foot	1/3
Total	7/28 (2)		7/43 (1)		17/65 (7)

[a] Intraabdominal primaries are excluded.
[b] Number in parentheses indicates number of geographical misses—i.e., recurrence outside the irradiated volume.
[c] Data from Lindberg et al., 1977.[15]

muscle compartment resection, amputation, and disarticulation. Simple excision of cyst-like tumors has resulted in a recurrence rate of approximately 90% because there is not a true capsule but a pseudocapsule around the mass.[1,5,18]

Even with radical excision, the recurrence rate is 39%.[3] Failures, even after wide excision, are due to the tendency of soft tissue sarcomas to spread for considerable distances along fascial and muscle planes.

For more than 10 years, the treatment of soft tissue sarcomas at MDAH has been, whenever possible, excision of gross disease followed by postoperative irradiation. From the data available, one can state that conservative removal followed by irradiation is highly successful (see Table 3) and preserves limb function. The results are, in the main, independent from the histologic type of soft tissue sarcoma. Failures, essentially in the fleshy parts, result from the wide diffusion of disease along fascial and muscle planes. In large inoperable lesions, 5000 rad, sometimes 6000 rad, followed by resection of the mass, can be very effective (see Fig. 6).

Summary

The addition of a radiation boost or limited surgery for gross masses of cancer has a rationale based on basic radiobiological principles. Improved local-regional control has been shown in various disease areas, as well as considerable increase in the quality of life.

Acknowledgments

Research for this chapter was supported in part by Grants CA06294 and CA05654 from the National Cancer Institute, Department of Health, Education and Welfare, U.S.A.

REFERENCES

1. Cadman, N.L., Soule, E.H., and Kelly, P.J.: Synovial sarcoma: An analysis of 134 tumors. *Cancer* **18**:613–627, 1965.
2. Calle, R., Fletcher, G.H., and Pierquin, B.: Les bases de la radiotherapie curative des epitheliomas mammaires. *Radiol Electrol* **54**:929–938, 1973.
3. Cantin, J., McNeer, G.P., Chu, F.C., et al.: The problem of local recurrence after treatment of soft tissue sarcoma. *Ann Surg* **168**:47–53, 1968.
4. Cass, A.W., Million, R.R., and Pfaff, F.A.: Patterns of recurrences following surgery alone for adenocarcinoma of the colon-rectum. *Cancer* **37**:2861–2865, 1976.
5. Castro, E.B., Hajdu, S.I., and Fortner, J.G.: Surgical therapy of fibrosarcoma of extremities. *Arch Surg* **107**:284–286, 1973.
6. Fletcher, G.H.: Clinical dose-response curves of human malignant epithelial tumors. *Br J Radiol* **46**:1–12, 1973.

7. Fletcher, G.H.: Dose response curve of subclinical aggregates of epithelial tumor cells and its practical application in the management of human cancers. In *Biological and Clinical Basis of Radiosensitivity* M. Friedman, ed. Springfield, Illinois: Charles C. Thomas, 1974, pp. 485–501.
8. Fletcher, G.H.: *Textbook of Radiotherapy*, 3rd ed., Philadelphia: Lea & Febiger, 1980.
9. Fletcher, G.H., and Hussey, D.H.: The role of radiation therapy in the management of regional lymph node metastases in epithelial tumors. *J Eur Radiother* **1**:3–26, 1980.
10. Fletcher, G.H., and Shukovsky, L.J.: The interplay of radiocurability and tolerance in the irradiation of human cancers. *Radiol Electrol* **56**:383–400, 1975.
11. Goepfert, H., Zaren, H., Jesse R., and Lindberg, R.: Treatment of laryngeal carcinoma with conservation surgery and postoperative radiation therapy. *Arch Otolaryngol* **104**:576–578, 1978.
12. Gunderson, L.L.: Radiation therapy of colorectal carcinoma. In *Proceedings of XII International Cancer Congress* (Buenos Aires, Argentina). Oxford: Pergamon Press, in press.
13. Jesse, R.H., Ballantyne, A.J., and Larson, D.: Radical or modified neck dissection. A therapeutic dilemma. *Am J Surg* **136**:516–519, 1978.
14. Lindberg, R.D.: Soft tissue sarcomas. In *Textbook of Radiotherapy* 3rd ed., G.H. Fletcher, ed. Philadelphia: Lea & Febiger, 1980.
15. Lindberg, R.D., Martin, R.G., Romsdahl, M.M., and McMurtrey, M.J.: Conservative surgery and radiation therapy for soft tissue sarcomas. In *The Management of Primary Bone and Soft Tissue Tumors* Chicago: Year Book Medical Publishers, 1977, pp. 289–298.
16. Montague, E.D., Spanos, W.J., Jr., and Fletcher, G.H.: Die Entwicklung der Behandlungsmethoden bei der Primärtherapie des nichtmetastasierten Mammakarzinoms. In *Die Erkankungen der weiblichen Brustdrüse.* Herausgegeben von H.J. Frischbier (ed), New York: George Thieme Verlag Stuttgart, 1982, 201–207.
17. Neglia, W.J., Hussey, D.H., and Johnson, D.E.: Megavoltage radiation therapy for carcinoma of the prostate. *Int J Radiat Oncol Biol Phys* **2**:873–882, 1977.
18. Shieber, W., and Graham, P.: An experience with sarcoma of the soft tissue in adults. *Surgery* **52**:295–298, 1962.
19. Tapley, N. duV.: Irradiation treatment of malignant tumors of the salivary gland. *Ear Nose Throat J* **56**:39–43, 1977.
20. Thames, H.D., Jr., Peters, L.J., Spanos, W.J., and Fletcher, G.H.: Dose response curves for squamous cell carcinomas of the upper respiratory and digestive tracts. *Br J Cancer* **41**:35–38, 1980.
21. Withers, H.R., and Peters, L.J.: Biologic aspects of radiation therapy. In *Textbook of Radiotherapy* 3rd ed. G.H. Fletcher, ed. Philadelphia: Lea & Febiger, 1980, pp. 103–180.
22. Withers, H.R., and Romsdahl, M.M.: Postoperative radiotherapy for adenocarcinoma of the rectum and rectosigmoid. *Int J Radiat Oncol Biol Phys* **2**:1069–1074, 1977.

CHAPTER 36

Results of Conventional Radiation Therapy

Norah duV. Tapley, M.D.[a]*

Conventional radiation therapy is recognized to be either the delivery of total doses of 5000 to 7000 rad in a relatively prolonged course of irradiation, using equal daily fractions of 180–225 rad, 5 days a week, or continuous, low-dosage-rate gamma-ray irradiation. Interstitial and intracavitary gamma-ray therapy may be used to deliver the total dose of irradiation or may precede or follow external beam therapy.

This essay reviews the results, in some of the common cancers, of irradiation of the primary lesion alone or as an adjuvant to a surgical procedure, and of elective treatment to the regional lymphatics.

Treatment of the Primary Disease

HEAD AND NECK

Skin and Lip

Treatment of skin and lip cancers may be by surgical excision, irradiation, or by a combination of both. The determining factors in selection of therapy are cosmetic result, speed of treatment, and ultimate control. In the majority of sites surgery provides the most rapid solution. Lesions involving the eyelids, nose, and ears, where appearance and function may be seriously impaired by surgery, are often best handled by irradiation. When irradiation is used to preserve cosmesis and function, the prolonged fractionation of conventional radiation therapy yields the best results, including a decreased probability of fibrosis and atrophy leading to telangiectasis. The control rate of the majority of irradiated lesions should exceed 90%.[32]

Oral Cavity, Oropharynx, and Larynx

Irradiation alone produces a high local control rate in the treatment of T_1 and T_2 lesions of all sites in the oral cavity, oropharynx, and larynx (see Table 1). In the few failures that occur, surgical salvage is frequently achieved. At the initiation of therapy these lesions of limited size have caused relatively little destruction of normal tissues and minimal functional interference. With the dose-time fractionation of conventional radiation therapy, as the malignant cells are destroyed healing occurs partially or relatively completely reconstituting the involved structure. When only limited volume requires the high dose, late sequelae of fibrosis or necrosis are infrequent and function remains excellent.

For these early lesions the treatment schedule provides 6000 rad in 6 weeks for T_1 lesions and 6500 rad in 6½ weeks for T_2 lesions. For lateralized lesions, the combination of high-energy electrons and photons,

[a]Radiotherapist and Professor of Radiotherapy,
Department of Radiotherapy,
The University of Texas System Cancer Center,
M.D. Anderson Hospital and Tumor Institute,
Houston, Texas
*deceased

TABLE 1. Percentages of Tumor Control Following Irradiation and Rescue Surgery for T_1 and T_2 Lesions of the Upper Respiratory and Digestive Tracts[a,b]

Site	T_1	T_2
Anterior 2/3 of tongue and floor of mouth	96 (98)	85 (91)
Faucial arch	85 (96)	82 (89)
Soft palate	100 (100)	100 (100)
Tonsillar fossa	100 (100)	97 (97)
Base of tongue	93 (100)	75 (81)
Pharyngeal walls	86 (100)	82 (82)
Vocal cords	88 (99)	75 (91)
Supraglottic larynx	90 (95)	80 (90)
Pyriform sinus, nasal cavity, and ethmoids	Good control rates. Too few patients treated with irradiation alone to determine percentage.	

[a] Number in parentheses indicates percentage of ultimate successes after surgical salvage.

[b] Adapted from Lindberg and Fletcher, 1978.[18]

TABLE 2. Comparison of Local-Regional Failure Rates in Patients with Stages I and II Breast Cancer Following Tumorectomy and Irradiation vs. Radical Mastectomy and No Postoperative Irradiation,[a,f] Analysis April 1980

	Outside Excision 1960–1978		MDAH Excision 1960–1978		Radical or Modified Radical Mastectomy at MDAH 1960–1974			
T Stage	T_x[b]		T_1 & T_2		T_1 & T_2 outer quadrants			
N Stage	Clinical N_0 N_1		Clinical N_0 N_1		Histologic N_0			
Number of Patients	117		94		254			
Sites of Recurrences[c]	Breast	Axilla	Breast	Axilla	Chest Wall	Axilla	Supra-clav.	Para-sternal
	10	—	2	1	11	1	3	3
	10/117[d]	(8.6%)	3/94[e]	(3.1%)	18/254		(7.1%)	

[a] American Joint Commission Staging System.

[b] Stage of primary is unknown.

[c] Eleven recurrences occurred within 2 years of follow-up, one at 3 years, and one at 4 years. Eight of 12 breast recurrences occurred in the same quadrant as the original tumor.

[d] Two patients refused further treatment, eight had modified radical mastectomy, four are NED, four have distant metastases.

[e] Three patients have had modified radical mastectomy, two are NED, one has distant metastases.

[f] Data from Montague et al., 1982.[20]

TABLE 3. Squamous Cell Carcinoma of the Cervix—5-year Survival Rate [a] (924 Patients [b]), January 1964 to December 1969, Analysis August 1974[f].

Stage I_B[c]	91%
Stage II_A	82%
Stage II_B	65%
Stage III_A[d]	54%
Stage III_B[e]	40%

[a]Berkson-Gage

[b]Excluding seven analyzable patients with Stages IV_A and IV_B disease.

[c]Includes eight Stage I_B patients treated surgically.

[d]One pelvic wall or lower one-third of the vagina involved.

[e]Two pelvic walls or one pelvic wall and lower third of the vagina involved.

[f]Adapted from Jampolis et al., 1975.[16]

usually in a 1:1 or 2:1 ratio of given doses, has provided an ideal dose distribution. Limiting the high dose to the involved side significantly decreases the dose to the deeper structures. For anterior tongue and floor-of-mouth lesions, 2000 to 3000 rad is added with interstitial therapy after 5000 rad in 5 weeks with external beam irradiation has been given.

BREAST

Small-volume cancer of the breast, classically treated by radical mastectomy, has been shown in several series to be successfully treated by conservation surgery and irradiation.[19,25] When the lesion is of limited extent, permitting simple excision or wedge resection leading to little breast deformity, the delivery of a moderate dose of irradiation to the entire breast has resulted in low local and regional failure rates as shown in Table 2. Unless the surgical removal of breast tissue has been excessive, the cosmetic results are excellent, leaving soft, pliable skin and breast tissue.[20]

The technique of treatment includes irradiation of the entire breast and chest wall through tangential portals and of the adjacent lymphatic areas to a dose of 5000 rad in 5 weeks, five fractions per week. If there is a question of close margins, the site of the primary lesion may receive an additional 1000 rad through a sharply reduced field.

FEMALE GENITAL TRACT

Cervix

Table 3 shows the 5-year survival rates of patients with stage I_B through III_B carcinoma of the cervix who have completed definitive radiation therapy. The survival rates are excellent for patients with stages I and II_A disease. The survival rates of patients with stage II_B (extensive parametrial disease but not fixed to the pelvic wall(s)), stage III_A, and stage III_B disease are still very substantial. From Table 4, which shows the sites of failures, one sees that relatively few patients died from uncontrolled pelvic disease only. The patients who died with pelvic disease and distant metastases would not have been cured even if the pelvic disease had been controlled.

GENITOURINARY TRACT

Bladder

In 112 patients with invasive carcinoma of the bladder, stages B_1, B_2, and C, treated at M. D. Anderson Hospital (MDAH) with 5000 rad preoperative irradiation followed by radical cystectomy without lymphadenectomy, the failure rate has been only 10% (see Table 5). Batata et al.,[2] reporting on a series from Memorial Sloan-Kettering Cancer Center, identified patterns of recurrence in patients with bladder cancer, all stages, treated by cystectomy alone or cystectomy preceded by irradiation. Local recurrence alone occurred in 28% of 137 patients treated by cystectomy alone and in 19% of 119 patients receiving planned irradiation of 4000 rad in 4 weeks prior to cystectomy.

TABLE 4. Squamous Cell Carcinoma of Cervix Treated by Irradiation—Site of Failure, (916 Patients[a]), January 1964 to December 1969, Analysis August 1974[g]

		Known Failures (Patients Dead or Living)			Patients Dead	
Stage	Number of Patients	Pelvis Only	Pelvis + DM[b]	DM Only	Uncertain[c]	LFU[d]
I_B	316	3	13	15	4	5
II_A	178	5	6	23	3	1
II_B	204	9	18	42	9	0
III_A[e]	160	19	14	30	19	0
III_B[f]	58	10	5	9	10	1

[a] Excluding seven analyzable patients with Stage IV_A and IV_B disease and eight Stage I_B patients treated surgically.
[b] DM = distant metastases.
[c] Clinical information is not adequate to determine if the patients died from cancer.
[d] LFU = lost to follow-up.
[e] One pelvic wall involved or lower third of vagina.
[f] Both pelvic walls involved.
[g] Adapted from Jampolis et al., 1975.[16]

TABLE 5. Carcinoma of the Bladder Stages B_1, B_2, and C Treated with 5000 Rad Preoperative Irradiation Followed by Radical Cystectomy Without Lymphadenectomy—January 1969 through December 1977 (Minimum 2-Year Follow-Up)[b]

		Alive			Dead		
Stage	Number of Patients	NED	Pelvic Rec	DM	NED	Pelvic Rec	DM
B_1	29	16	0	1	4	2	6
B_2	38	17	0	3	6	4	8
C	45	21	1	4	3	4	12
Total	112	54	1[a]	8	13	10[a]	26

[a] Failure rate = 10%.
[b] Adapted from Boileau, 1980.

Prostate

Carcinoma of the prostate, even if it has spread beyond the gland, can be controlled by irradiation, using external beam alone or external beam plus interstitial gamma-ray therapy. In the series from MDAH (see Table 6), a high control rate is shown for stages B and C. The doses are 6500 rad in 6½ weeks or 7000 rad in 7 weeks. A substantial improvement, both in local control and in survival, is seen in the massive C_2 tumors when treated with 7000 rad rather than 6500 rad. The price for this improved control rate is a significant increase in the incidence of severe complications which developed in 11% of the patients treated with 7000 rad.

Treatment of Lymphatics

Table 7 correlates the percent of control of expected occult lymphatic infestation

TABLE 6. Carcinoma of the Prostate—Local Control, Survival, and Complications, Rates by Tumor Dose[a] (July 1966 to April 1974 Minimum 4-Year Follow-Up)[e]

	Local Control		Survival[b]		Complications	
Stage	∿ 6500 rad	∿ 7000 rad	∿ 6500 rad	∿ 7000 rad	∿ 6500 rad	∿ 7000 rad
B	100% (3/3)	100% (2/2)	100% (3/3)	100% (2/2)	0% (0/3)	0% (0/2)
C_1[c]	94.1% (16/17)	91.9% (68/74)	64.5% (11/17)	63.5% (47/74)	5.9%[d] (1/17)	10.8% (8/74)
C_2[c]	61.5% (8/13)	79.4% (27/34)	30.8% (4/13)	55.9% (19/34)	0% (0/13)	11.8% (4/34)

[a]Excluding 27 patients diagnosed >6 months before radiotherapy.
[b]Survival rates were computed at the time of analysis (mean follow-up = 6 years, 9 months).
[c]C_1 not fixed to pelvic wall(s); C_2 fixed to pelvic wall(s).
[d]The only complication in the group receiving 6500 rad was in a patient treated with large fields using a rotation technique with ^{60}Co.
[e]Data from Hussey, 1980.[15]

TABLE 7. Percentage of Eradication of Expected Occult Infestation in the Lymphatics of the Neck as Function of Dose[a,b]

Adenocarcinoma of Breast			Squamous Cell Carcinoma of Upper Respiratory and Digestive Tracts		
Number of Patients	Dose (rad)	Control	Number of Patients	Dose (rad)	Control
89	3000–3500	60–70%	50	3000–4000	60–70%
121	4000	80–90%			
273	5000	>90%	356	5000	>90%

[a]1000 rad/week, 5 days a week.
[b]Adapted from Fletcher, 1974.[8]

with the dose given in elective irradiation of regional lymphatics in patients with squamous cell carcinomas of the head and neck and adenocarcinoma of the breast. Close to 100% of occult metastases in peripheral lymphatics are eradicated by 4500 to 5000 rad given in 25 fractions in 5 weeks. Lower doses have less effect. The efficacy of elective irradiation in eliminating occult deposits is similar for all the epithelial tumors, i.e., squamous cell carcinomas, adenocarcinomas of the breast, prostate, uterus, and colon, and malignant salivary gland tumors. With modest doses of irradiation, sequelae are nonexistent or minimal, producing no functional interference.

The alternative to elective irradiation is radical dissection of the draining lymphatic areas performed on all patients in whom the risk of occult infestation is significant. For carcinomas of the upper respiratory and digestive passages, a radical neck dissection would be performed. When midline structures such as the anterior floor of the mouth or base of the tongue are involved, bilateral dissection of the neck would be required. For carcinoma of the breast in a patient with positive axillary nodes and/or the primary lesion located centrally or in the inner quadrants, dissection of the internal mammary node chain would be considered, as opposed to a radical or modified radical mastectomy. For pelvic tumors, therapeutic lymphadenectomies are fraught with complications, including lymphocysts, edema of the extremities, and various degrees, even if often temporary, of hydroureter and hydronephrosis.

HEAD AND NECK

Table 8, adapted from Strong,[30] shows an increasing incidence of nodal involvement with increasing size of the primary in the oral tongue; after radical neck dissection, more than 60% of the patients die of uncontrolled neck disease. Similar data have been obtained for other head-and-neck sites.

Elective irradiation of clinically uninvolved lymphatic areas has been shown in a number of studies to prevent occurrence of nodal disease in initially uninvolved sites, including both ipsilateral and contralateral sides of the neck and in the next relay when the first relay is clinically involved.[3,22]

TABLE 8. Squamous Cell Carcinoma of Oral Tongue Stages T_1, T_2 and T_3 and Neck N_0—Incidence of Patients Later Developing Neck Disease[b]

Stage	Incidence
T_1	29.5%[a] (28/95)
T_2	42.9%[a] (33/77)
T_3	77.0%[a] (10/13)

[a]More than 60% of the patients died of uncontrolled neck disease after radical neck dissection.
[b]Adapted from Strong, 1979.[30]

Table 9 shows examples of the results of elective treatment of the neck lymphatics in MDAH patients with squamous cell carcinoma in selected sites of the upper respiratory and digestive passages. After irradiation of the whole neck to 5000 rad in 5 weeks and control of the primary lesion, there was one nodal failure in 137 patients. Parsons et al.[23] reported 100% control in 266 initially uninvolved carcinoma necks electively irradiated in patients with squamous carcinoma of the upper respiratory and digestive tracts.

BREAST

In carcinoma of the breast, a direct route of spread is to the internal mammary chain nodes as well as to the axillary nodes. The frequency of internal mammary chain involvement is directly associated with the location of the primary lesion in the breast and involvement of the axillary nodes. The incidence of involvement, proven by biopsy, of the internal mammary nodes exceeds 50% for inner quadrant or central lesions when the axillary nodes are histologically positive; even when the axilla is negative, and the primary lesion is in the central or inner quadrants, the probability of internal mammary chain node involvement is high.[12] Elective irradiation is indicated in these clinical situations.

Table 10, compiled from several series, shows the difference of the effectiveness of elective irradiation to the peripheral lym-

TABLE 9. Squamous Cell Carcinoma in Selected Sites of the Upper Respiratory and Digestive Tracts—Results of Elective Irradiation with 5000 rad in 5 weeks (Primary Controlled) Analysis July 1976[b]

Selected Sites—Irradiation of Whole Neck in Initially N_0 Neck, 1970–1973	Supraglottic Larynx—Irradiation of subdigastric and Midjugular Nodes in Initially N_0 Neck, 1948–1973
1/60[a]	0/77[a]

[a]Number of failures/number of patients treated.
[b]Adapted from Fletcher and Hussey, 1980.[11]

TABLE 10. Effectiveness of Peripheral Lymphatics Irradiation in Patients with Histologically Positive Axillary Nodes[a]

	Axilla Positive in the Surgical Specimen	
Incidence of Later Appearance in Supraclavicular Nodes	No Irradiation[a]	4500–5000 rad/5 weeks to Peripheral Lymphatics[b]
	20–26%	1.5%
	Axilla Positive in the Surgical Specimen, Tumor Located Centrally or in the Inner Quadrants	
Incidence of Later Appearance in Parasternal Nodules	No Irradiation[c]	4500–5000 rad/5 weeks to Peripheral Lymphatics[d]
	9% (25/264)	0% (0/204)

[a]From Paterson and Russell, 1959;[24] Robbins et al., 1966.[28]
[b]From Fletcher, 1971.[7]
[c]From Urban, 1952.[31]
[d]From M. D. Anderson Hospital Study.
[e]Data from Fletcher, 1978.[9]

phatics in patients with histologically positive axillary nodes. When these initially clinically uninvolved areas are irradiated with doses of 4500 or 5000 rad in 5 weeks, the incidence of later appearance of disease in supraclavicular nodes is 1.5%, and of parasternal nodules, indicative of internal mammary node involvement, 0%.

The question has remained whether elective irradiation of the internal mammary nodes has affected survival in patients with breast cancer. Recently published results of a randomized series have shown that the 5-year survival rate is significantly higher for patients with positive axillary nodes who receive 5000 rad postoperative radiation therapy to the peripheral lymph nodes than it is for those who do not receive irradiation (see Fig. 1).[14]

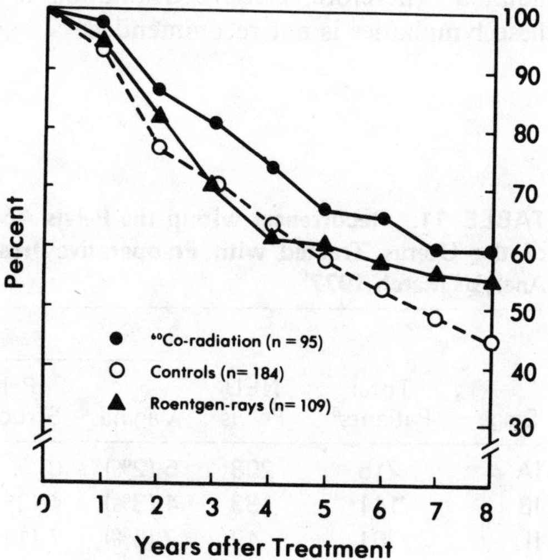

Figure 1. For patients treated with ^{60}Co, the fields covered the internal mammary node chain, the supraclavicular region, and the apex of the axilla nodes. The dose at depth of 3 cm was about 5000 rad over 4 weeks in 20 fractions. The portal is identical to the one used in the MDAH technique. Patients treated by roentgen x-ray had a lesser dose and uncertain coverage of the internal mammary node chain. The proportion of stage II patients treated with ^{60}Co remaining free of disease is higher than that of control patients at every interval. When the curves are analyzed over their entirety by the log rank test, they reveal a significant statistical advantage for the irradiated patients. (From Høst and Brennhovd, 1977.)[14]

FEMALE GENITAL TRACT

Cervix

The incidence of clinical manifestations of pelvic-wall node involvement, such as sciatic pain, hydronephrosis, and edema of the extremities, was 5% in 698 patients with stage I or II disease.[16] In the literature on lymphadenectomy series, the incidence of positive nodes in the surgical specimen ranges from 10 to 25% in stage I patients and from 20 to 40% in stage II patients. This implies that a high percentage of nodes involved by small aggregates of cancer cells have been sterilized by irradiation.

The combined dose of external irradiation and intracavitary gamma-ray therapy is of the order of 5000 to 5500 rad to the external iliac nodes, and somewhat higher to the obturator and hypogastric nodes.

Irradiation of the common iliac and/or paraaortic nodes is fraught with complications.[6,26] The volume of tissue irradiated with the extended field technique to L_4 to cover the common iliac nodes or to T_{12} to cover the paraaortic nodes, is much greater than when only the pelvic wall nodes are irradiated. Therefore, elective irradiation of these lymphatics is not recommended.

Endometrium

Several reviews of lymphadenectomy series in patients with stage I adenocarcinoma of the endometrium who have not had preoperative irradiation have shown an incidence of metastases to the pelvic lymph nodes of close to 11%.[5,17] At MDAH, in 356 patients with stage I disease who had received preoperative irradiation followed by conservative extrafascial hysterectomy without lymphadenectomy, the incidence of clinical manifestations of pelvic-wall node disease is less than 1.0% (Table 11).[29] The preoperative irradiation consists either of two applications of intrauterine and vaginal radium or 4000 rad with external irradiation followed by one radium application. The dose to the pelvic-wall nodes is approximately 4000 rad from two intracavitary radium insertions, or approximately 5500 rad from whole-pelvis irradiation followed by one radium application.

TABLE 11. Recurrences within the Pelvis According to Stage in Patients with Adenocarcinoma of the Uterus Treated with Preoperative Irradiation and Hysterectomy (1947 through 1974) Analysis March 1977[e]

			Recurrences			
Stage	Total Patients[a]	NED Pelvis	Vagina	Pelvic Structures	Possible[b] and Probable[c] Pelvic Wall Nodes	Recurrences percent
IA	215	208	5 (2%)	0	2 (<1%)	3%
IB	141	133	4 (3%)	4 (3%)[d]	0	5.6%
II	61	49	3 (5%)	7 (11.5%)[d]	2 (3%)	19.6%
III	14	11	1 (7%)	2 (14%)[d]	0	21.4%
Total	431	401 (93%)	13 (3%)	13 (3%)	4 (1%)	7%

[a]Excluding patients expiring 2 years due to unknown cause, intercurrent disease, or distant metastases.

[b]Three patients with recurrences localized to one or both pelvic walls but without lower extremity edema or pain.

[c]One patient (stage II) with right pelvic wall recurrence, right lower extremity paraplegia, pain, edema, and right hydronephrosis.

[d]$p < 0.01$.

[e]Data from Spanos et al., 1978.[29]

GENITOURINARY TRACT

Bladder

In stages B_1, B_2, and C bladder cancer, an incidence of involvement of the pelvic lymph nodes has been shown in approximately 30% of surgical specimens of lymph node dissections.[27,34] Whitmore et al.,[33] in their series of patients receiving preoperative irradiation of 4000 rad in 4 weeks to the true pelvis, reported a 13% incidence of nodal disease.

At MDAH, 112 patients with B_1, B_2, and C lesions and negative lymphangiograms have received 5000 rad in 5 weeks in 25 fractions with the box technique prior to radical cystectomy without lymphadenectomy. Only 10% of the patients have developed recurrent pelvic disease (Table 5).[4] This low incidence implies that a significant percentage of nodal involvement has been sterilized. With a width of 12 cm for the AP and PA portals, the dose to the pelvic-wall nodes is approximately 5000 rad in men with a narrow pelvis, while in women it approaches 4000 rad.

Prostate

Pelvic-wall nodal involvement in carcinoma of the prostate has been reported to be 7 – 32% for patients with stage B disease and 28 – 69% for those with stage C.[1,15] In order of frequency of involvement, disease spreads to the obturator, external iliac, and hypogastric lymph nodes.[13]

In the MDAH series, only 3% of the patients whose primary disease was controlled developed clinical evidence of regional metastases (Table 6).[21] Utilizing the box technique to treat patients with stages B and C disease with relatively small treatment portals (AP and PA 10 × 12 cm), approximately 4000 rad is delivered to the obturator and hypogastric nodes.

Summary

In early squamous cell carcinomas of all anatomical sites of the upper respiratory and digestive tracts and squamous cell carcinomas of the uterine cervix, external irradiation alone or combined with interstitial or intracavitary gamma-ray therapy provides high control rates. In carcinoma of the prostate, 6500 rad in 6½ weeks or 7000 rad in 7 weeks results in very high local control, in the range of 80 – 90% in lesions that have spread beyond the prostate. In carcinoma of the urinary bladder, 5000 rad given preoperatively followed by radical cystectomy without lymphadenectomy has resulted in very few pelvic failures.

Elective irradiation with doses in the range of 5000 rad in 5 weeks to lymphatic areas at risk of infestation results in the infrequent, almost near-zero appearance of clinical manifestations of the disease. This relatively low dose is effective for subclinical or microscopic disease because there are fewer malignant clonogenic cells with no hypoxic compartment. With this dose schedule, the sequelae are minimal.

Acknowledgments

Research for this chapter was supported in part by Grants CA06294 and CA05654 from the National Cancer Institute, Department of Health, Education and Welfare, U.S.A.

REFERENCES

1. Bagshaw, M.A., Pistenma, D.A., Ray, G.R., et al.: Evaluation of extended field radiotherapy for prostatic neoplasms: 1976 progress report. *Cancer Treat Rep* **61**:297–307, 1977.
2. Batata, M.A., Whitmore, W.F., Chu, F.C.H., et al.: Patterns of recurrence in bladder cancer treated by irradiation and/or cystectomy. *Int J Radiat Oncol Biol Phys* **6**:155–159, 1980.
3. Berger, D.S., Fletcher, G.H., Lindberg, R.D., and Jesse, R.H., Jr.: Elective irradiation of the neck lymphatics for squamous cell carcinomas of the

nasopharynx and oropharynx. *AJR* **111**:66–72, 1971.

4. Boileau, M.A., Gonzales, M.O., Johnson, D.E., and Chan, R.C.: Bladder carcinoma. Results with preoperative radiation therapy and radical cystectomy without lymphadenectomy. *Urology*, **16**:569–576, 1980.
5. Creasman, W.T., Boronow, R.C., Morrow, C.A., et al.: Adenocarcinoma of the endometrium: Its metastatic lymph node potential. *Gynecol Oncol* **4**:239–243, 1979.
6. El Senoussi, M.A., Fletcher, G.H., and Borlase, B.C.: Correlation of radiation and surgical parameters in complications in the extended field technique for carcinoma of the cervix. *Int J Radiat Oncol Biol Phys* **5**:927–934, 1979.
7. Fletcher, G.H.: Control by irradiation of peripheral lymphatic disease in breast cancer. *AJR* **111**:115–118, 1971.
8. Fletcher, G.H.: Clinical dose response curve of subclinical aggregates of epithelial cells and its practical application in the management of human cancer. In *Biological and Clinical Basis of Radiosensitivity*, M. Friedman, ed., Springfield, Ill.: Charles C Thomas, 1974, pp. 485–501.
9. Fletcher, G.H.: The evolution of the basic concepts underlying the practice of radiotherapy from 1949 to 1977: Erskine Memorial Lecture, 1977. *Radiology* **127**:3–19, 1978.
10. Fletcher, G.H.: *Textbook of Radiotherapy*, 3rd ed. Philadelphia, Lea & Febiger, 1980.
11. Fletcher, G.H., and Hussey, D.H.: The role of radiation therapy in the management of regional lymph node metastases in epithelial tumors. *J Eur Radiother* **1**:3–26, 1980.
12. Handley, R.S.: A surgeon's view of the spread of breast cancer. *Cancer* **24**:1231–1234, 1969.
13. Hilaris, B.S., Whitmore, W.F., Batata, M., et al.: Behavioral patterns of prostatic adenocarcinoma following[125]Implant and pelvic node dissection. *Int J Radiat Oncol Biol Phys* **2**:631–637, 1977.
14. Høst, H., and Brennhovd, I.O.: The effect of postoperative radiotherapy in breast cancer. *Int J Radiat Oncol Biol Phys* **2**:1061–1067, 1977.
15. Hussey, D.H.: Carcinoma of the prostate. In *Textbook of Radiotherapy*, 3rd ed., G.H. Fletcher, ed. Philadelphia: Lea & Febiger, 1980, pp. 894–914.
16. Jampolis, S., Andras, E.J., and Fletcher, G.H.: Analysis of sites and causes of failures of irradiation in invasive squamous cell carcinoma of the intact uterine cervix. *Radiology* **115**:681–685, 1975.
17. Lewis, B.V., Stallworthy, J.A., and Cowdell, R.: Adenocarcinoma of the body of the uterus. *Obstet Gynecol Br Common* **77**:343–348, 1970.
18. Lindberg, R.D., and Fletcher, G.H.: The role of irradiation in the management of head and neck cancer. Analysis of results and causes of failure. *Tumori* **64**:313–325, 1978.
19. Montague, E.D., Gutierrez, A.E., Barker, J.L., et al.: Conservation surgery and irradiation for the treatment of favorable breast cancer. *Cancer* **43**:1058–1061, 1979.
20. Montague, E.D., Spanos, W.J., Jr., and Fletcher, G.H.: Die Entwicklung der Behandlungsmethoden bei der Primärtherapie des nichtmetastasierten Mammakarzinoms. In *Die Erkankungen der weiblichen Brustdrüse.* Herausgegeben von H,-J. Frischbie (ed), New York: George Thieme Verlag Stuttgart, 1982, 201–207.
21. Neglia, W.J., Hussey, D.H., and Johnson, D.E.: Megavoltage radiation therapy for carcinoma of the prostate. *Int J Radiat Oncol Biol Phys* **2**:873–882, 1977.
22. Northrop, M., Fletcher, G.H., Jesse, R.H., Jr., et al.: Evolution of the neck disease in patients with primary squamous cell carcinomas of the oral tongue, floor of mouth, and palatine arch and clinically positive neck nodes neither fixed nor bilateral. *Cancer* **29**:23–30, 1972.
23. Parsons, J.T., Bova, F.J., and Million, R.R.: A reevaluation of split course irradiation for squamous cell carcinomas of the head and neck. *Int J Radiat Oncol Biol Phys* **6**:1645–1652, 1980.
24. Paterson, R., and Russell, M.H.: Clinical trials in malignant disease. III. Breast cancer. Evaluation of postoperative radiotherapy. *J Fac Radiol (Lond)* **10**:175–180, 1959.
25. Peters, M.V.: Wedge resection with or without radiation in early breast cancer. *Int J Radiat Oncol Biol Phys* **2**:1151–1156, 1977.
26. Piver, M.S., Vongtama, V., and Barlow, J.J.: Paraaortic lymph node irradiation for carcinoma of the uterine cervix using split course technique. *Gynecol Oncol* **3**:168–176, 1975.
27. Pomerance, A.: Pathology and prognosis following total cystectomy for carcinoma of the bladder. *Br J Urol* **44**:451–458, 1972.
28. Robbins, G.C., Lucas, J.C., Fracchia, A.A., et al.: An evaluation of postoperative prophylactic radiation therapy in breast cancer. *Surg Gynecol Obstet* **122**:979–982, 1966.
29. Spanos, W.J., Jr., Fletcher, G.H., Wharton, J.T., et al.: Patterns of pelvic recurrence in endometrial carcinoma. *Gynecol Oncol* **6**:494–502, 1978.
30. Strong, E.W.: Carcinoma of the tongue. *Otolaryngol Clin North Am* **12**:107–114, 1979.
31. Urban, J.A.: Radical mastectomy in continuity with en bloc resection of internal mammary lymph node chain: New procedure for primary operable cancer of the breast. *Cancer* **5**:992–1008, 1952.
32. Von Essen, C.F.: Skin and lip: In *Textbook of Radiotherapy* 3rd ed., G.H. Fletcher, ed. Philadelphia: Lea & Febiger, 1980, pp. 271–286.
33. Whitmore, W.F., Jr., Batata, M.A., Hilaris, B.S., et al.: A comparative study for two preoperative radiation regimens with cystectomy for bladder cancer. *Cancer* **40**:1077–1086, 1977.
34. Whitmore, W.F., Jr., and Marshall, V.F.: Radical surgery for carcinoma of the urinary bladder. *Cancer* **9**:596–608, 1956.

CHAPTER 37

Keynote Address: Modifiers of Radiation Response in Tumor Therapy: Strategies and Expectations

Mortimer M. Elkind, Ph.D.,[a]* B.M.E., M.M.E., M.S.

The objective of introducing modifiers of radiation response into tumor radiotherapy is to widen the differential between damage to normal and tumor tissues and thus to effect improved treatment. It is evident that this can be done (1) by increasing tumor damage for the same degree of normal tissue damage, (2) by decreasing normal tissue damage for the same degree of tumor tissue damage, and (3) increasing tumor damage while decreasing normal tissue damage. In the statements above the terms "normal tissue" and "tumor tissue" must be broadly understood if tumor therapy is to be realistically addressed. Thus, the limiting "normal tissue" might not be only what is incidentally irradiated if the modifier significantly affects some other normal tissue(s), and "tumor tissue" has to be understood to include secondary in addition to primary disease.

Using the foregoing as a guide, in this analysis I will discuss, from the viewpoint of a cell biologist, what would appear to be the primary issues in effectively applying one or more agents along with ionizing radiation in the treatment of cancer. I will proceed from the specific to the general. That is, I will first review the cell properties *in vitro* of a particular chemical that has been used in therapy when this chemical is applied by itself or along with radiation. Then I will discuss some of the results obtained when this chemical and radiation are applied to experimental normal and tumor tissue systems, as well as in clinical trials. The preceding will serve as a specific example of the progression from the culture dish to the patient, or from the laboratory to the clinic. Based on this example, I will develop some more general ideas that are applicable to combined-mode chemical-radiation therapy. Lastly, I will comment on how much improvement in differential response is required to effect noticeable improvements in the sterilization of primary tumors.

S-Phase Chemical Cytotoxicity

The antineoplastic agent hydroxyurea (HU) is a simple chemical ($H_2NCONHOH$) but an effective inhibitor of DNA synthesis.[34] Sinclair[25,26] showed that HU in millimolar concentrations is cytotoxic to S-phase Chinese hamster cells and inhibits cell cycle progression at the G_1/S border. Cytotoxicity in S-phase has also been demonstrated in other rodent cells as well as in cultured human cells, and similar cytotoxic effects have been inferred in tumor and in normal rodent cells.[3] Data indicative of a G_1/S-phase progression block have also been obtained *in vivo*.[2,33]

[a]Senior Biophysicist, Division of Biological and Medical Research, Argonne National Laboratory, Professor, Department of Radiology, The University of Chicago, Chicago, Ill.

*Current address: Department of Radiology and Radiation Biology, Colorado State University, Fort Collins, Colorado

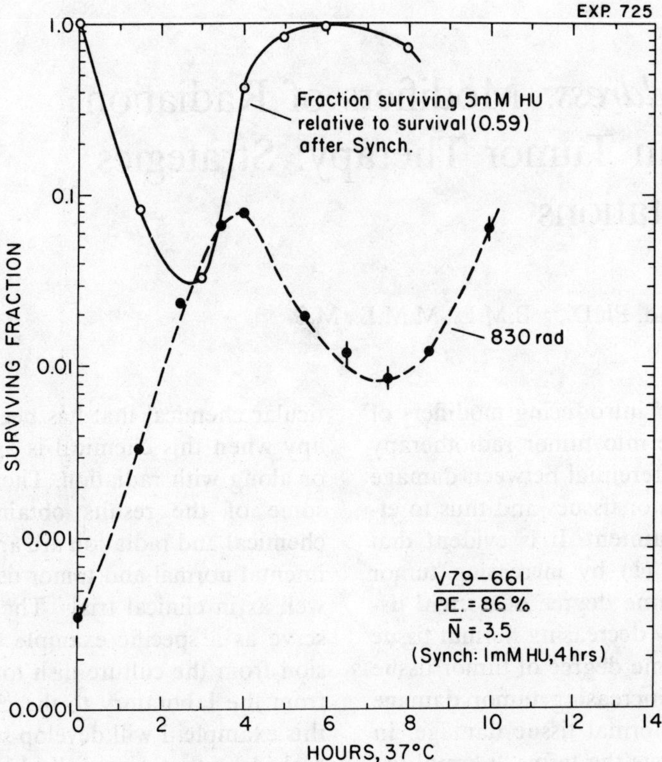

Figure 1. Synchronization and S-phase toxicity of Chinese hamster cells exposed to hydroxyurea (HU) *in vitro*. Asychronous cells were incubated in medium containing 1 mM HU for 4 hours and then exposed to a second treatment with HU1 mM, 5 to 6 hours) at the starting times indicated by the points (upper curve). The consequent minimum in survival results from the cells that were blocked at the G_1/S border cells progressing through the ensuing S phase followed by G_2, M, and then by G_1 of the next cycle (see Fig. 2). The lower curve traces the variation in x-ray survival as G_1/S cells progress through the phases S, G_2, M, and G_1 and S of the next cycle. X-rays: 50 kV, 20 ma, 722 rad/min. *P.E.* = plating efficiency, $\overline{N}$ = average multiplicity. (From Elkind et al., 1968.)

The effects of HU on S-cell viability, as well as the G_1/S block to cell progression, are illustrated with cultured Chinese hamster cells in Figure 1. As schematized in Figure 2, with time HU gathers a cohort of viable cells, held up at the G_1/S border, from an asynchronous population whose initial distribution with cell age is shown in the left panel. That those cells initially in the S phase are killed during the synchronizing exposure to HU may be inferred from the results in Figure 1. Zero time on the abscissa corresponds to the termination of the initial hydroxyurea treatment (which was a 4-hour exposure to 1 mM HU). At the times indicated, cells were either irradiated with a single dose of x-rays, 830 rad, or were exposed to a second HU challenge. The x-ray data indicate the development of a maximum in radioresistance typical of S-phase Chinese hamster cells,[30] while the results of the second HU challenge indicate additional, time-dependent cell killing as cells initially at the G_1/S border progress into and then out of the ensuing S phase. The results in Figure 3 indicate that, at least with cultured Chinese hamster cells, the initial synchronization effected by an HU treat-

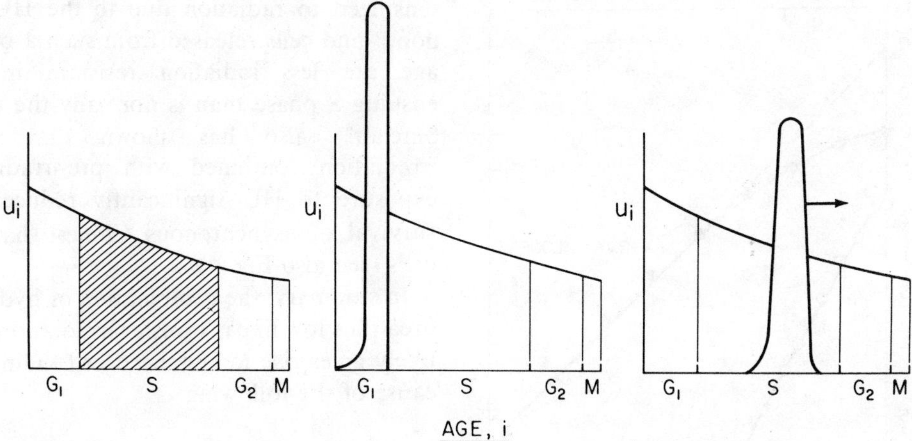

Figure 2. Schematic representation of the synchronization of mammalian cells by hydroxyurea (HU). The left panel shows the cell age-density distribution (U_i) of asynchronously growing cells. Millimolar concentrations of HU kill those cells in the S phase at the time of addition of the HU and allow the remainder of the population to progress to the G_1/S border where they are held up (middle panel). Incubation in the absence of HU permits the latter cohort of cells to progress through the S phase (right panel), making them susceptible to HU cytotoxicity as in the upper part of Figure 1.

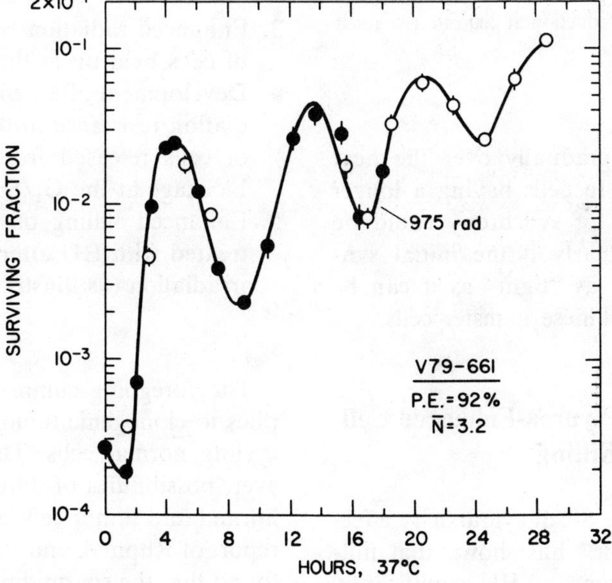

Figure 3. An example of the gradual loss of synchronization of initially asynchronous Chinese hamster cells synchronized *in vitro* with hydroxyurea (HU). Cells were synchronized, as sketched in Figure 2, by exposures to 1.0 mM HU for 4 hours. Following this, they were allowed to progress through several cycles, by incubation in HU-free medium, and exposed to 975 rad as a function of time. Two separate experiments are shown (solid and open circles). Other details as for Figure 1. (From Elkind, Kano, and Kamper, unpublished data.)

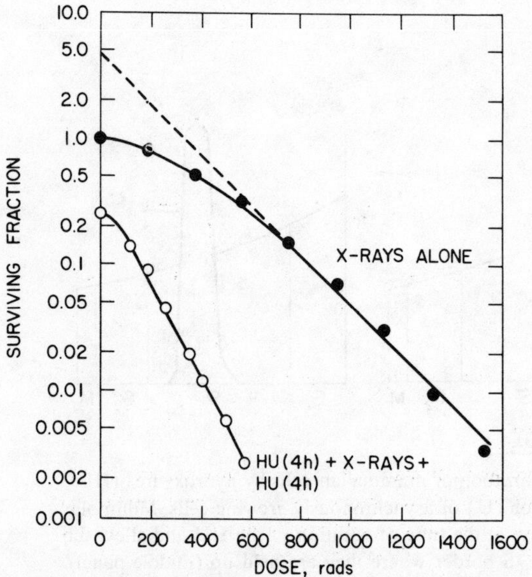

Figure 4. The sensitization by hydroxyurea (HU) of V79 Chinese hamster cells to x-rays. Asynchronous cells were exposed to HU for 4 hours, 1 mM, before and after single x-ray doses as shown. S-phase cytotoxicity plus enhanced radiation cell killing result in more than a 10-fold survival reduction at 200 rad. (Adapted from Sinclair, 1980.[28])

ment is lost only gradually over the next several cell cycles. In cells having a longer G_1 phase, the loss of synchrony could be more rapid particularly if the initial synchronization is not as "tight" as it can be made to be with Chinese hamster cells.

Radiation-Hydroxyurea-Enhanced Cell Killing

In addition to the S-cell cytotoxicity effected by HU, Sinclair[27] has shown that millimolar concentrations of HU significantly enhance x-ray cell killing. Preirradiation incubation of Chinese hamster cells enhances the killing of asynchronous cells at least because of the combined effects of S-phase cytotoxicity plus the accumulation of cells at the G_1/S-phase border—a radiation-sensitive age in the cell-age cycle. In addition, cells blocked at the G_1/S border may be sensitized to radiation due to the HU action,[27] and cells released from such a blockage are less radiation resistant in the ensuing S phase than is normally the case.[7] Sinclair[27] also has shown that post-irradiation combined with pre-irradiation exposure to HU significantly reduces the survival of asynchronous Chinese hamster cells (see also Fig. 4).

In summary, the combination of hydroxyurea plus low linear transfer irradiation very likely gives rise to enhanced cell killing because of the following:

1. S-phase cytotoxicity (presumably because of the inhibition of the reduction of primarily cytidylic acid)
2. Increasing accumulation of cells with time at normally radiation-sensitive ages of the cell cycle, i.e., G_1 and at the G_1/S border
3. Enhanced radiation response due to HU of cells held up at the G_1/S border
4. Development of a deficient pattern of radiation resistance in the ensuing S-phase of cells released from an HU imposed blockage at the G_1/S border
5. Enhanced killing of asynchronous cells treated with HU after, as well as before, irradiation (as illustrated in Fig. 4).

The foregoing summary presumably applies to clonogenic tumor cells as well as to cycling normal cells. There may be, however, possibilities of differentiating between normal and tumor cells as illustrated by the report of Rupniak and Paul.[24] These authors found that the spermidine analogue methylglyoxal bis(guanylhydrazone) (reversibly) arrests normal cells in G_1 while allowing transformed cells to continue to proliferate. Hence, with appropriate timing, cycling normal cells at least could be spared the full impact of the cytotoxic effects of HU by itself if these cells could be arrested in G_1 during HU administration.

TABLE 1. Clinical Trials with Hydroxyurea and Radiation Combined[a]

Site	Reference	Number of Patients	Results
Head and neck	Lerner et al., 1967. Lerner, 1977.	100	Encouraging
	Richards and Chambers, 1969.	40	Encouraging
	Rominger, 1971.	26	Encouraging
	Stefani et al., 1971.	59	Inconclusive to discouraging
	Hussey and Samuels, 1971.	19	Encouraging to inconclusive
	Hussey and Abrams, 1975.	32	Pilot—encouraging
		40	Random—no improvement
Lung	Le Par et al., 1976.	50	Inconclusive
	Landgren et al., 1974.	53	No benefit
Astrocytoma	Lerner et al., 1970.	6	Encouraging
Cervix	Hreshchyshyn, 1967.	15	Pilot-encouraging
	Hreshchyshyn et al., 1979	104	Random—definite improvement with HU
	Piver et al., 1974, 1977.	130	Encouraging
Vulva	Papavasiliou, 1978.		Not stated in abstract

[a]Adapted from Sinclair, 1980.[28]

Animal Studies and Clinical Results of Radiation Plus Hydroxyurea

In the years following the early *in vitro* work, studies were started using experimental rodent systems and a number of clinical trials were also initiated. From the review by Dethlefsen et al.,[2] one may conclude that although in the mouse a number of the consequences predictable from the *in vitro* results are observed, insufficient kinetic data are available upon which to base a design to widen differential response. Further, although experiments with mice impose only limited constraints on the range of doses of HU employed, minimal information is available on the time-dependent concentration of HU in the various normal and tumor tissues of interest and how these depend upon route of administration. As for the clinical data, Sinclair[28,29] has reviewed some 17 studies involving 700 patients. His summary of those clinical results is shown in Table 1; the terms in the last column epitomizing the outcome of the studies are those of Sinclair.[29] Some of these clinical studies attempted to use a timing sequence suggested by *in vitro* studies; for example, see the reports from the Houston group in Table 1.

Of the various results listed in Table 1, those of Hreshchyshyn et al.[10] on the treatment of cervical squamous cell carcinoma with radiation plus HU warrant further comment. Figure 5, reproduced from their report, outlines the protocol for the oral ad-

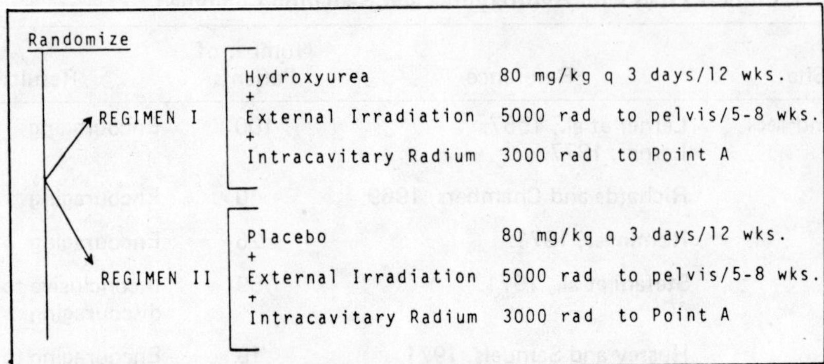

Figure 5. Protocols used in clinical trials of hydroxyurea plus radiation against stages IIIB and IVA cervical squamous cell carcinoma. (From Hreshchyshyn et al., 1979.[10])

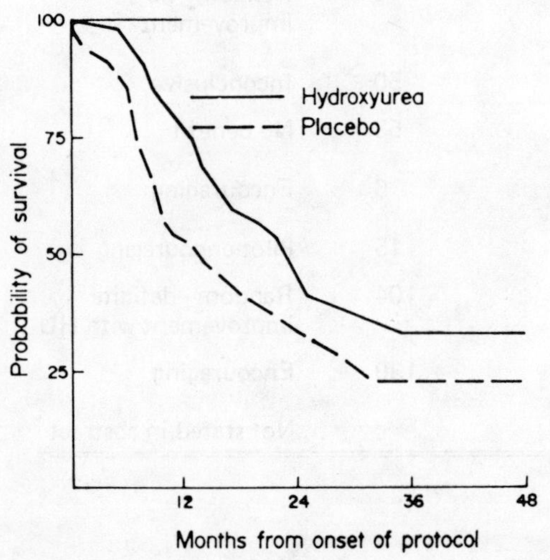

Figure 6. Patient survival, percent, for women having stage IIIB squamous cell cervical carcinoma treated according to the protocols in Figure 5, 42 patients by each regimen. (From Hreshchyshyn et al., 1979.[10])

ministration of HU (or placebo) in respect to the radiation treatments—the HU therapy "starting on the first day of irradiation" and continuing for 12 weeks. Figure 6 from the same report shows that for stage IIIB cervical carcinoma, HU plus radiation was superior (at the 5% level) to placebo plus radiation. (The results for stages IIIB and IV combined, are almost as good.) HU and radiation therapy were more or less contemporaneously administered, but the two modalities were integrated only in a fairly arbitrary sense, as illustrated by the following: (1) external radiation was given daily while HU therapy was given every 3 days;† (2) even on those days when the two agents were both given, their time relationship was not specified and therefore may not have been regulated; (3) if brachytherapy was not to follow external beam therapy, HU treatment was nevertheless spread over 12 weeks, whereas the external beam would have been completed in 6–8 weeks; and (4) when brachytherapy was to follow external beam therapy with a 2-week, radiation-free interval intervening, HU therapy apparently was continued during the interval.

I will comment further on the preceding examples of apparent unrelatedness between drug and radiation therapy. These examples are noted, here, however, because they serve to characterize a principal difference between laboratory and clinical studies. As noted by Sinclair,[29] the gap between the laboratory and clinic has been narrowed in the last 10–15 years; still, it is considerable and significant. Although mindful of the practical problems involved, Sinclair indicates that the gap may be characterized by inadequate kinetic data for human normal and tumor tissues, and inadequate information on the time depen-

†Lerner *et al.* (16) reported that after the oral administration of 80 mg/kg the dose of HU used by Hreschshyshyn *et al.*[10] the maximum serum concentration was reached in 2 hours and the drug was no longer detectable in serum at 24 hours.

dence of drug concentration in the relevant tissues. In view of the time relationships for enhanced interaction indicated by the *in vitro* data summarized in Figures 1–4, and the importance of timing in the widening of differential responses as indicated by the results with mice,[2] it is perhaps not surprising that only a limited number of the studies in which HU is combined with radiation (Table 1) have led to positive results.[29]

General Ideas for Combined-Mode Therapy

The historical and conceptual development just outlined of the combined use of hydroxyurea and radiation for the treatment of cancer, while a specific example, nevertheless illustrates several general points of interest. The first is that laboratory studies can be effectively used to identify combinations of potential usefulness in the clinic. The second is that the ability of the investigator to demonstrate the putative cardinal features of a proposed new combined modality becomes more difficult, for practical reasons at least, as he or she progresses from the dish to the animal to the patient. And the third is that even when a new combination is applied ostensibly to take advantage of the positive features of combined action–i.e., at the least, the two treatment modes are administered more or less contemporaneously–the treatment scheme applied in the clinic may bear little resemblance to one that would maximize combined-mode effectiveness. One must presume that this last point reflects toxic systemic effects of, for example, the chemical agent in a drug-radiation combination. But as illustrated by the timing in the study by Hreshchyshyn et al.,[10] this explanation does not appear to be entirely applicable. The untoward systemic effects observed included those associated with gastrointestinal and hemopoietic damage. Why then, one wonders, was the HU continued either after the completion of radiotherapy or between the external beam therapy treatment course and the beginning of brachytherapy 2 weeks later? If HU is not evident in the serum 24 hours after administration,[16] why was it administered every third day instead of daily? Daily administration of HU probably would have required a reduction of the HU dose, but at least drug-radiation interaction would have been possible for each radiation exposure. And last, one wonders if the HU plus radiation timing was controlled to maximize their combined effect when both agents were given on the same day. Presumably, systemic effects would have been largely independent of this timing whereas the effects on the tumor could have been enhanced.

The foregoing questions are posed in respect to the study of Hreschyshyn et al.[10] because it would appear that their already positive results could have been improved upon even without the desirable, but difficult to obtain, cell kinetic and drug concentration information to which Sinclair referred.[29] Hence, with the HU-radiation experience as a guide, I now undertake to derive some general principles that could be of use in combined-mode therapy.

AGE-RESPONSE PATTERNS

It is well known, particularly from radiation studies, that the response of cells depends upon their position, or age, in their growth cycle at the time that they are are exposed to an agent, all other factors being equal. Taking the curve labeled X in Figure 7 to represent a radiation age-reponse pattern–i.e., the variation of cell survival following a fixed acute dose of, say, x- or γ-rays–we can imagine that a chemical, physical, or biological agent might have patterns such as Y_a, Y_b, etc. While in general an age-response pattern of any shape is possible, Y_a and Y_b typify two particular possibilities. Y_a has approximately the same shape as X, whereas Y_b is intended to complement X. Consequently, for Y_a, G_1, and $(G_2 + M)$-

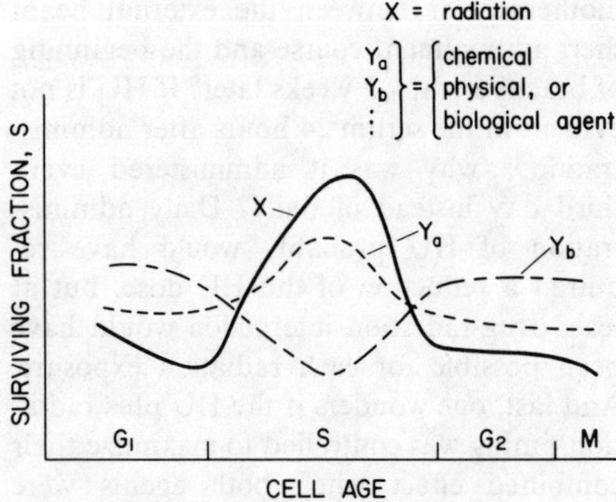

Figure 7. Characteristic age-response patterns for x-rays or γ-rays (X) and other cytotoxic agents (Ya, Yb, , , ,). Surviving fraction following a fixed treatment is sketched as a function of the age of a cell in its growth cycle.

phase cells have qualitatively the same relative sensitivites as for X, whereas for Y_b, the reverse is intended in that G_1- and (G_2 + M)-phase cells are resistant compared to S-phase cells. In general, age-response patterns whose features are combinations of Y_a and Y_b relative to X are possible. I return to a further consideration of Figure 7 presently.

AGENT INTERACTION

In considering optimal strategies for the administration of two (or more) cytotoxic agents, it is useful to distinguish among three possibilities. These possibilities are intended to identify, in operational rather than mechanistic terms, combined effects that represent *sparing* action, *independent* action, or *enhancing* action as sketched in Figure 8. Thus, if dose y_1 of agent Y leads to net survivals greater than, equal to, or less than the product of the survivals expected separately from agents X and Y, we conclude that Y "spares" the killing effectiveness of X, is independent of X, or enhances the effectiveness of X, respectively. (Note that the more conventional terms like *protective, additive,* and *synergistic* action are not used to avoid confusion with the mechanistic meanings that the latter designations have.)

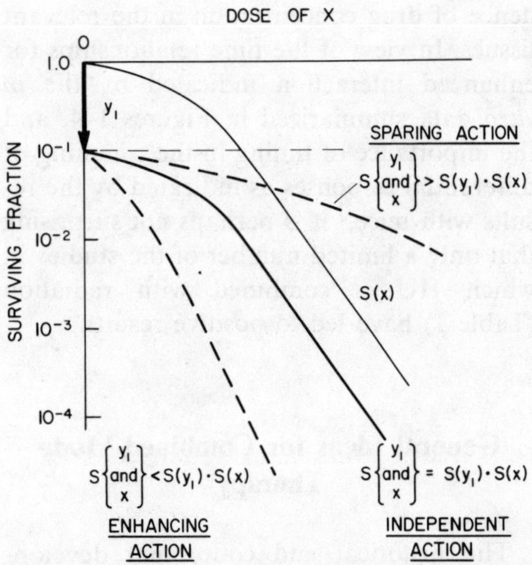

Figure 8. Examples of the net effect on survival of treating a population of cells (normal or tumor cells) with dose y_1, of agent Y followed at some particular time later by graded doses of radiation X. These curves are intended to show the net effect of all processes that may influence combined action.

PROTOCOLS

Based on the types of age-response patterns in Figure 7 and the important additional possibility that agents X and Y may produce enhanced effects because of additive damage and/or the interference with the repair of damage, two basic protocols may be distinguished as shown in Figure 9(a). To begin with, these share the assumption that fractionated treatments will be used because systemic effects have to be kept within tolerable limits and/or compensatory repopulation of normal tissue elements has to take place during the treatment course.

Protocol I is essentially the simultaneous administration of X and Y with the qualification that if it takes some hours for the potential for combined effectiveness of Y to maximize (e.g., time for a drug concentration to maximize in the target tissue), then Y would be administered before X by this interval. Age-response patterns that complement—e.g., X and Y_b in Figure 7—would result in enhanced action (Fig. 8), even if no damage additivity or repair inhibition occurs; enhanced action results if cells resistant to X are sensitive to Y_b and *vice versa*. In contrast, the combination X plus Y_a would result in sparing action if "simultaneous" administration is used and the agents act independently.

Protocol II represents a phase shift, by the interval Δt, in the administration of X and Y to permit age-response complementation. For example, if Δt is long enough to allow the S-phase cells that surgive an x-ray dose to progress to parts of the cycle that are sensitive to Y_a, the latter cohort will be more effectively killed by Y_a and a net enhanced effect may result even if X and Y_a act independently. Similarly, the combined effect of X and Y_b could result in sparing if, in Protocol II, Δt allows S-phase survivors to progress to an age resistant to Y_b.[4,6]

In both Protocols I and II, it is implied in the repetition of the combined-treatment sequence that the effectiveness at each fraction will be the same because the tumor and normal tissue populations return to their starting states of responsiveness by the time of the second, third, etc., treatment sequences. For both kinds of tissue, this assumption is probably not correct, but for different reasons. Tumors are heterogeneous, at least because of a spectrum of metabolic states reflecting active proliferation at one extreme, P cells, and metabolically quiescent cells, Q cells, at the other. Quiescent cells may include or be included in the nutritionally deprived and hypoxic fraction of a tumor—a portion of the population that is added to from cells in active growth and decreased by cell death and cell lysis, at least before the onset of therapy. In addition to the foregoing metabolic heterogeneity, there also may be genetic variants in the tumor cell population due to genomic lability even if the tumor originated from a single transformed cell. As for the cells in normal tissue, proliferation is generally more rapid than for tumor cells, at least in cell-renewal systems, and homeostatic controls and compensatory repopulation may cause cells initially not in cycle, G_0 cells, to start proliferating and/or cells already dividing to be accelerated. In addition, systemic compensatory mechanisms may give rise to altered patterns of differentiation. $G_0 \longrightarrow P$ cell transitions, changes in cell cycle times, and altered patterns of differentiation all may contribute to altered responses to agents X and/or Y during fractionated treatment sequences. (The cell and radiobiological changes that accompany these transitions are largely unknown.)

While generalizations are probably not justified, the large range of cell cycle times that are initially to be expected in a tumor, at least for reasons of metabolic heterogeneity, and the alterations in this distribution that are likely as therapy progresses and tumors shrink, is assumed to be biologically of greater importance than the altered growth and/or differentiation properties of normal tissues. Consequently, Protocols III and IV in Figure 9(*b*) represent two additional schemes of repetitive treatment. In Protocol III, it is assumed that each combined treatment sequence consists of a dose of X plus two or more doses of Y. The separation of repetitive doses of Y would probably depend upon: (1) the nature of the interaction of Y with X (e.g., if Y suppresses the repair of radiation damage, how rapidly the latter damage fades); (2) the persistence of Y at an effective concentration in the relevant tissues; and (3) the possibility that systemic toxicity might require that multiple doses of Y be used in order to avoid exceeding a tolerable level from any given dose of Y while still maintaining a level effective for combination therapy over a long enough interval following a single radiation dose fraction. Similarly, in Protocol IV it is envisaged that the effectiveness of combination therapy is increased if each treatment sequence consists of two or more doses of X per dose

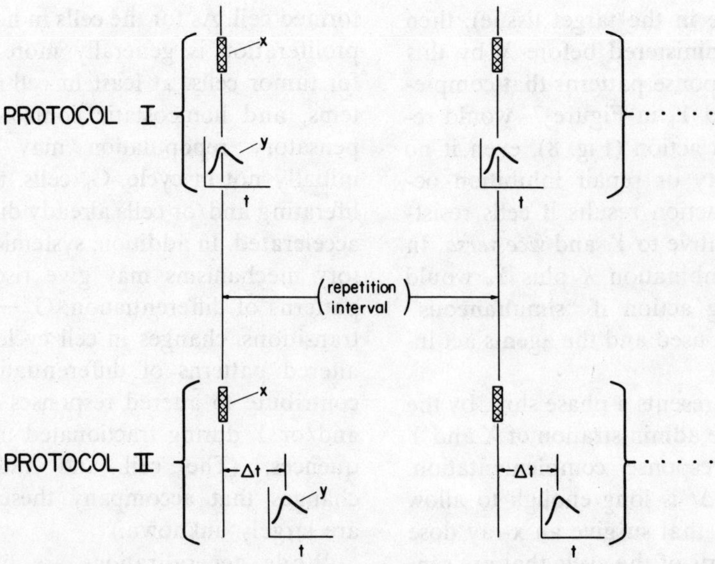

Figure 9. (*a*) Schematic representation of two protocols based on a single radiation dose and a single drug dose per treatment sequence. In Protocol I, it is assumed that the drug is administered sufficiently before the radiation dose x is given so that the drug concentration y reaches a maximum in the site of interest. The bars represent acute radiation doses and the curves the variation of drug concentration with time in the site of interest.

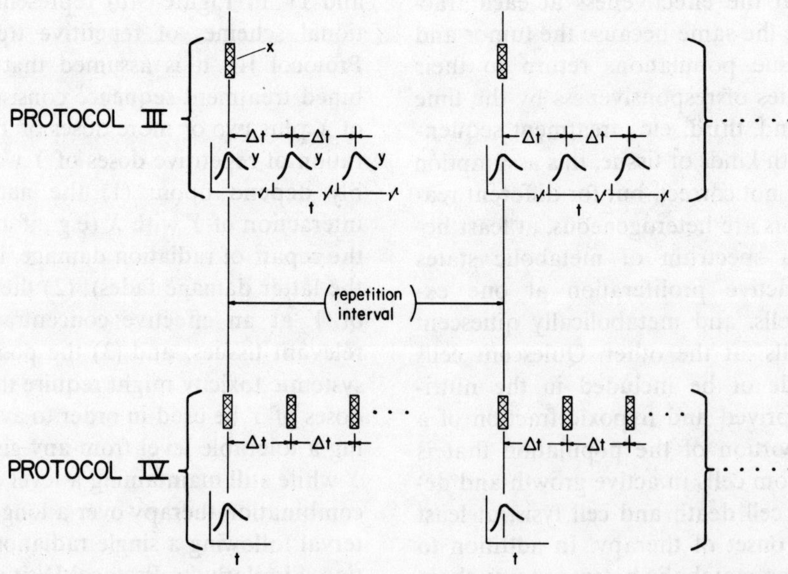

Figure 9. (*b*) Protocols III and IV are similar to I and II except that per treatment sequence two or more drug doses (III) or two or more radiation doses (IV) are given.

of *Y*. Situations in which Protocols III and IV would be more effective than I or II are discussed presently.

INDEPENDENT AND INTERDEPENDENT ACTION

To this point, little distinction was made between independent and interdependent action between *X* and *Y*. The possibilities that age-response complementation might exist (e.g., $Y + Y_b$), or that an enhanced response could be effected by proper timing (e.g., $X + \Delta t + Y_a$), were already discussed in reference to Figure 9(*a*). I now consider more specifically the consequences, or lack thereof, of interactive effects between *X* and *Y* that reflect more than just questions of age-response complementation.

Independent Action

Figure 10(*a*) reiterates in symbolic terms the points made in the earlier discussion of Protocols I and II. If *X* and *Y* are independent in their action, then for age-response patterns that have largely similar shapes, Protocol I is less effective than II, and the reverse is the case when the age-response patterns are largely complementary. Figure 10(*b*) deals with interdependent action, i.e., action which, because of intra- or extracellular factors, results in enhanced responses as in Figure 8. Some examples will make clear the kinds of mechanistic or operational considerations that I am subsuming under interdependent action.

An important case of combined action concerns chemicals that either sensitize (presumably) hypoxic tumor cells or protect (presumably) euoxic normal tissue cells. Possibilities (a) and (b) in Figure 10(*b*) would require that *X* and *Y* be essentially simultaneous, and hence Protocol I is to be favored over II. Further, if cytotoxicity is associated with an hypoxic-cell radiation sensitizer, Protocol I should be used to take full advantage of (a) through (d). Thus, the foregoing is, in part, an example of interdependent action because of chemical modification of radiation-induced molecular damage.

Possibilities (e) through (g) in Figure 10(*b*) illustrate an additional dimension to interdependent action–namely, repair inhibition. If agent *Y* inhibits the repair of radiation damage, then depending on the time course of the repair and the persistence of *Y* in the tumor, multiple doses of *Y* could be useful (i.e., III better than I). Clearly, such action plus hypoxic-cell sensitization would make Protocol III better than either II or I. In principle, it is also possible that radiation may inhibit the repair of damage due to *Y*, in which case Protocol IV would be preferred to I or II.

In addition to molecular interactions, *X* and *Y* may express interdependent action because of time-dependent changes in the microanatomy of a tumor, changes in growth control in the tumor or normal tissue, or both. Possibility (h) concerns shifts in the proportion of proliferating P cells because quiescent Q cells are induced to proliferate. Protocol III would be expected to be superior to I and possibly II if a Q $\longrightarrow$ P transition is due to tumor shrinkage accompanied by reoxygenation, since more than one dose of *Y* might be needed to result in enough cell lysis. Alternatively, repeated doses of *X* per repetition cycle, Protocol IV, could be more effective than a single dose of *X*, Protocols I and possibly II, if the effectiveness of *Y* is restricted to cells undergoing cyclic growth and if the Q $\longrightarrow$ P transition requires a certain minimum level of x-ray cell killing.

The last point alluded to in Figure 10(*b*), $G_0 \longrightarrow$ P transitions, concerns homeostatic controls of proliferation and/or differentiation in normal and tumor tissue. The mechanisms of growth control applicable in such situations are not fully understood, and even less clear is how the cytotoxicity of the cells in question due to *X* or *Y* would depend on one or another protocol. Clearly,

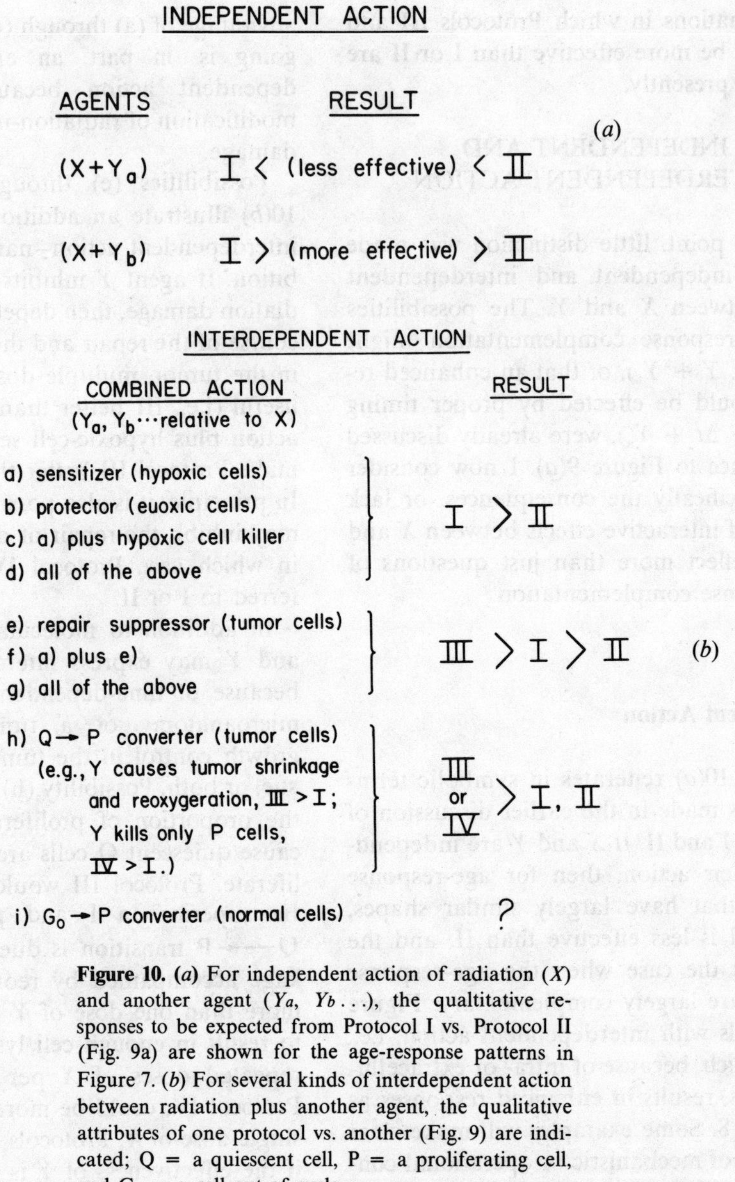

INDEPENDENT ACTION

AGENTS — RESULT

(a)

$(X+Y_a)$ I < (less effective) < II

$(X+Y_b)$ I > (more effective) > II

INTERDEPENDENT ACTION

COMBINED ACTION (Y_a, Y_b···relative to X) — RESULT

a) sensitizer (hypoxic cells)
b) protector (euoxic cells)
c) a) plus hypoxic cell killer
d) all of the above

I > II

e) repair suppressor (tumor cells)
f) a) plus e)
g) all of the above

III > I > II (b)

h) Q → P converter (tumor cells)
(e.g., Y causes tumor shrinkage and reoxygeration, III > I; Y kills only P cells, IV > I.)

III or IV > I, II

i) G_0 → P converter (normal cells) ?

Figure 10. (*a*) For independent action of radiation (*X*) and another agent (*Ya*, *Yb*...), the qualtitative responses to be expected from Protocol I vs. Protocol II (Fig. 9a) are shown for the age-response patterns in Figure 7. (*b*) For several kinds of interdependent action between radiation plus another agent, the qualitative attributes of one protocol vs. another (Fig. 9) are indicated; Q = a quiescent cell, P = a proliferating cell, and G_0 = a cell out of cycle.

the relationship between control of growth and differentiation on one hand and cytotoxicity on the other is a subject in need of sustained research.

Although a cell kinetic characterization of a tumor (or normal tissue) in principle could be important in the scheduling of agents whose age-response patterns have appreciable structure (e.g., as in Figure 7), the possibility of exploiting such information relative to enhanced tumor damage seems unlikely, if only because of the initial kinetic heterogeneity among the cells. To attempt to take advantage of a kinetic approach to widen differentiatial response, two conditions should be sought. The first is to understand the cyclic behavior of normal tissue cells, including the regenerative potential of the tissue, in order to minimize normal tissue damage (e.g., as proposed by Dethlefsen.[1]) The second is either to use for Y a drug whose effectiveness, for example, is minimally dependent upon tumor-cell heterogeneity, or to impose a measure of homogeneity on the tumor. This last possibility brings up again the properties of hydroxyurea and its possible use in a treatment scheme like Protocol III. As noted earlier, HU can synchronize cells at the G_1/S border (e.g., Fig. 3). To do so in a population in which (1) the average cell-cycle time may be several days or more (i.e., many times the one-half persistence time of the drug) and (2) there is a large spread of cell-cycle times, means that multiple doses of HU would be required as in Protocol III. Multiple doses of HU per treatment sequence might enhance systemic toxicity (unless normal cells are protected from HU by being kept out of the S phase;[24] but short of a regimen that accounts for tumor heterogeneity of growth, or one that imposes a pressure toward homogeneity (as well as toward synchronization in the instance of HU) it does not seem likely that tumor cell kinetic data will offer significant opportunities for the improved effectiveness of chemical action, by itself, over the effectiveness of current clinical methods.

Enhanced Effectiveness per Treatment Sequence and Tumor Cure

Thus far, the principles of combined-mode therapy that I have discussed have concerned the features of a single treatment sequence (e.g., Fig. 9) with the implication that the effect of subsequent, equally spaced sequences would be proportionately the same. Particularly for those protocols that are predicated on changes in the micro-anatomy of a tumor (e.g., Protocols III and IV), it is not likely that the assumption of equal effectiveness per sequence will be borne out, if only because of the unpredictable dynamics of growth and shrinkage of a tumor during therapy. Still, the objective of the therapist is to improve the cure rate of at least the primary tumor and, hence, he must shift his sights from the factors pertinent to one or a few repetitions of a particular combined-mode sequence to those which encompass the entire treatment course.

For the purpose of developing the perspective noted above, I now consider the connection between survival decrement per treatment sequence and tumor cure. By treatment sequence, I mean a particular combination of X and Y exposures that are then to be repeated (e.g., as in Fig. 9). And of course tumor cure may not mean patient cure. The management of widespread secondary disease very likely must be via some form of adjunctive therapy.

The bottom part and left ordinate of Figure 11 show a portion of a survival curve for tumor cells. The upper part of the figure is derived from the bottom part as follows. Assume first that a population of tumors, initially all containing 1×10^9 clonogenic cells, is to be treated. If the single-mode therapy, i.e., fractionated radiation alone, cures 10% of the tumors, we inquire how much benefit is needed from combined-mode therapy relative only to the tumor cells to increase the proportion of tumors sterilized to 90% (i.e., to 10% tumor survival, right ordinate). The dose scale of the cell-survival curve is in units of D_o—that is, the "dose" that reduces survival by a factor of $1/e$ ($\simeq 0.37$). (Here "dose" means the net survival reduction of a treatment sequence which, for x-ray fractionation only, includes the effect of sublethal damage repair on cell killing, the sparing effect of hypoxia, the influence of repopulation and reassortment, and so on.) As shown in Figure 11, an additional "dose" of 3.1 D_o's decreases the survival of tumors of size 1×10^9 cells from 0.9 to 0.1.

The required "dose" increment to effect the preceding 80% increase in cure rate may be derived as follows. Let N_o be the initial number of clonogenic tumor cells and let S_c be the cell-surviving fraction. The number

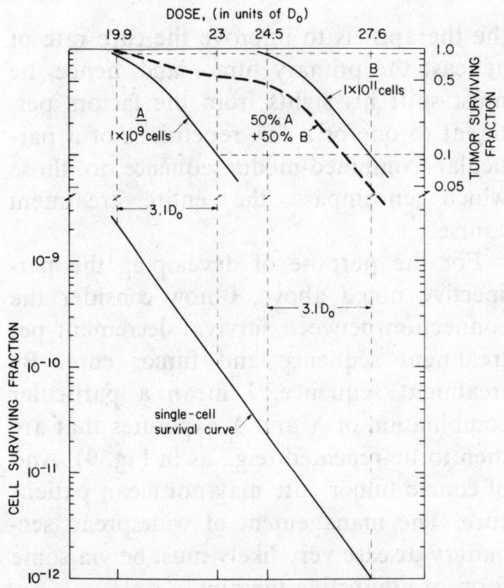

Figure 11. The relationship between cell survival (lower curve) and tumor survival (upper curves) are shown; for details see text. The dashed curve illustrates tumor survival in the instance of a tumor population consisting of an equal mixture of tumors containing 1×10^9 clonogenic cells and 1×10^{11} clonogenic cells (see text). The ordinates are logarithmic and the abscissa, although linear, is in units of the *Do* dose, where *Do* is the "dose" that reduces survival by the fraction 1/e (~0.37) along the exponential part of a dose-response curve. (From Elkind, 1979)[6].

of cells surviving, N_s, a "dose" that produces S_c is

$$N_s = N_o \cdot S_c. \quad (1)$$

When the average number of cells surviving in a tumor is 2.3, from Poisson statistics it may be inferred that tumor survival will be 90% (i.e., 90% of the tumors will contain one or more surviving cells); hence, in equation (1) $S_c = 2.3 \times 10^{-9}$. The "dose" D (in units of D_o) to produce this surviving fraction is

$$D = \ln S_c, \quad (2)$$

which for $S_c = 2.3 \times 10^{-9}$ is 19.9 D_o's. To reach 0.1 tumor-surviving fraction, $S_c = 1.05 \times 10^{-10}$ must be reached, and from equation (2) a total of 23 D_o's is required. Curve A in the upper part of Figure 11 is a plot of tumor surviving fraction versus "dose."

In a similar way, one may derive the survival curve for tumors having 1×10^{11} clonogenic cells per tumor. This is curve B in Figure 11; the dashed curve is the survival curve of an equal-parts mixture of tumors of 1×10^9 and 1×10^{11} cells.

The upper portion of Figure 11 is replotted on linear coordinates in Figure 12. The principal new feature that Figure 12 makes evident is that even for a mixture of tumor sizes—one may easily generalize from an equal-parts mixture to a continuous mixture from 1×10^9 to 1×10^{11} cells—6.6 D_o's [= (26.8 – 20.2) D_o] is required for a tumor population having a 100-fold distribution in clonogenic cell content and presumably, therefore, at least a 100-fold range in size.

For 6.6 D_o's, one may estimate the increase in effectiveness required per treatment sequence as (26.8/20.2 =) 1.33 for the range of tumor sizes noted. Thus, if in practice tumors of a given type at a given site as they are presented in the clinic consist of a population of sizes ranging from 1×10^9 clonogenic cells to 100 times larger, a factor of 1.33 increase in the effectiveness of each treatment sequence will suffice to increase tumor cure from 10 to 90%.

For tumors all of size 1×10^9, the increased effectiveness per sequence that would be required is only (23/19.9 =) 1.16, and for tumors all of size 1×10^{11}, the factor by which each fraction should be increased in effectiveness is (27.6/24.5 =) 1.13. Thus, heterogeneity in tumor size requirs a larger increase in effectiveness per treatment sequence if a given increment in tumor cure is to be effected.

The magnitude of the increased effectiveness factor required varies inversely with the number of clonogenic cells per tumor. For example, for tumors all containing only 1×10^6 cells, the factor is 1.24, and if a 100-fold range of sizes from 1×10^6 to 1×10^8 were to be encountered in the clinic, the factor would increase to 1.52 compared to 1.33 for tumors of size range 1×10^9 to 1×10^{11}.

From these simple calculations, the following points may be extracted.

1. If a given protocol (e.g., radiation therapy only) cures 10% of the tumors, relatively

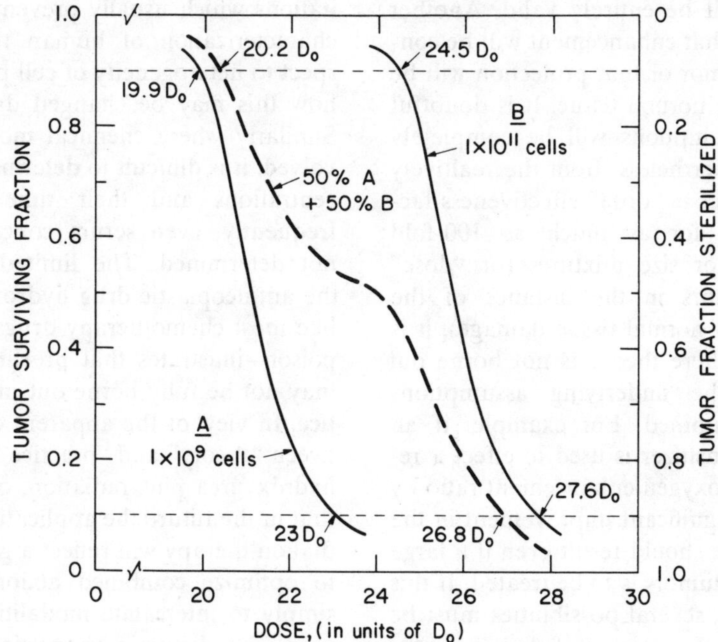

Figure 12. The tumor survival curves (left ordinate) of Figure 11 are replotted on linear coordinates, as well as the corresponding tumor sterilization curves (right ordinate). (From Elkind, 1979.[6])

small increases in the "dose" effectiveness of a combined-mode treatment sequence (e.g., radiation plus a drug) are required to increase substantially the cure rate if the increased effectiveness is confined to the tumor.

2. For a spectrum of tumor sizes from 1 × 10^6 to 1 × 10^8 clonogenic cells (i.e., from ~0.002 cc to ~0.2 cc), a "dose" effectiveness factor of ~1.5 is required to substantially increase tumor cure. This means that the survival decrement per combined-mode treatment sequence must be increased by 40% compared to what it was for radiation alone; for example, if radiation alone reduces survival by a factor of 0.5, each combined-mode sequence would be required to result in a net survival factor of 0.3.

3. For a spectrum of tumor sizes from 1 × 10^9 to 1 × 10^{11} clonogenic cells (i.e., from ~2 cc to 200 cc), a "dose" effectiveness factor of ~1.3 is required. This would require, per combined-mode treatment sequence, a 26% additional reduction in survival compared to radiation alone–e.g., from 0.5 for radiation alone to 0.37 for a combined-mode sequence.

To the foregoing, which focus upon increased killing effectiveness of tumor cells, the following may be added in respect to enhanced protection of normal tissue cells. Reduction of the effective dose to normal cells–e.g., by the use of a radiation protector–in effect permits the dose to the tumor to be increased by the same factor. Thus, in the instance of tumors of clonogenic content from 1 × 10^6 to 1 × 10^8, the ~1.5 tumor "dose" effectiveness factor estimated in point (2) above could be obtained by a combined-mode treatment that effected a one-third reduction in the effective "dose" to the normal tissues.

The foregoing discussion of the changes in "dose" effectiveness required per treatment sequence to effect a large change in tumor cure is based on several assumptions. A principal one is that each treatment sequence has on average an equal effect. As pointed out earlier, it is doubtful that this assumption will be entirely valid. Another assumption is that enhancement will be confined to the tumor or that protection will be confined to the normal tissue. It is doubtful that these assumptions will be completely borne out. Nevertheless, from the realtively modest increases in "dose" effectiveness factors predicted for as much as 100-fold ranges of tumor size mixtures (or "dose" protection factors in the instance of the modification of normal tissue damage), it is evident that where theory is not borne out in practice, the underlying assumptions must be reexamined. For example, if an hypoxic-cell sensitizer is used to effect a reduction in the oxygen enhancement ratio by ~1.3, then a significant improvement in the tumor cure rate should result even if a large range of large tumors is to be treated. If this does not occur, several possibilities must be considered: (1) the number of clonogenic tumor cells that have to be killed is of the order of 1×10^7 and not 1×10^{10}; (2) even though serum levels of the sensitizer may be monitored (see Chapter 40), adequate concentrations may not be present in the regions of hypoxic cells at the time of irradiation; (3) the sensitization of hypoxic tumor cells is not maintained for the entire treatment course; or (4) tumor cells are not hypoxic for the entire course of therapy. Similarly, if neutron therapy is supposed to reduce the oxygen enhancement ratio from ~3.0 to ~1.9–i.e., by a factor of ~1.7–then if a large improvement in cure rate is not effected one must question the assumptions made about normal versus tumor tissue RBE's and/or the persistence of hypoxic tumor cells throughout the treatment course.

Summary

While considerable potential exists for the development of modifiers of radiation response via the use of preclinical cell and animal studies, the fruits of this potential have not been fully realized in the clinic.

To begin with, there are the practical limitations which usually prevent an adequate characterization of human tumors, in respect to heterogeneity of cell properties, and how this may be changed during therapy. Similarly where chemical modifiers are involved, it is difficult to determine tissue concentrations and their time dependence; frequently, even serum concentrations are not determined. The limited success with the antineoplastic drug hydroxyurea–which like most chemotherapy drugs is a systemic poison–illustrates that preclinical potential may not be fully borne out in clinical practice. In view of the apparent differences between "theory" and "practice" in the case of hydroxyurea plus radiation, one must hope that in the future the application of drug-radiation therapy will reflect a greater attempt to optimize combined action rather than simply to intercalate modalities. In this regard, the dynamic properties of a tumor which, to a large degree, are responsible for its heterogeneity, suggest yet another problem since, as treatment progresses, one can expect cell death and cell lysis to add a further measure of time variation to what at the outset is a complex kinetic picture. Consequently, although treatment sequences usually are based on daily and weekly rhythms, such periodicities may not be optimal nor are there compelling biological reasons for maintaining a given periodicity for the entire course of treatment. If a single characteristic time were to be chosen as a fundamental parameter upon which to base variations in lengths of treatment sequences during the course of therapy, I would recommend the average generation time of euoxic tumor cells. The limited data available indicate that few tumors have cycle times as short as 1 day, and that most cycle times are 2 or more days long.[31] The effects of low oxygen tensions and the depletion of other nutrilites in regions of a tumor distant from capillaries would be expected to lengthen cell-cycle times further. Hence, repetition intervals which are at the start of therapy long compared to euoxic-cell transit times, but which are reduced as tumors begin to shrink, would appear to be needed if combined action intended to exploit cyclic variations in cell responses (e.g., Fig. 7) is to be obtained. Alternatively, if systemic toxicity is limiting and if supportive therapy is not adequate, treatment intervals may have to be at least long enough to permit adequate levels of compensatory repopulation in the limiting tissues.

It is evident that combined-mode, and particularly chemical-radiation therapy, has considerable potential. However, "practice" still remains well separated from "theory." When viewed from the vantage point of the laboratory researcher, at present the gap is due to a lack of knowledge of the cyclic properties of tumor and (limiting) normal tissue cells, the progressive effect of therapy on these properties, and the time variations of drug concentrations in both kinds of tissues. Added to the foregoing are the related changes associated with P $\longrightarrow$ Q and $G_o \longrightarrow$ P cell transitions. These processes, whose biology is poorly understood and the radiobiological consequences of which are not clear, are part of the host-related cellular dynamics of both abnormal and normal tissues. Hence, in addition to cell kinetic characterizations of tumor heterogeneity and drug concentration data, progress in combined-mode cancer therapy will probably require a determination of the importance of growth control in tumor sterilization and in normal tissue tolerance. The report of Rupniak and Paul[24] offers hope that characteristic differences in growth control between tumor and normal tissue cells may be exploited further to widen differential responses.

Acknowledgments

This analysis was made possible by support from the United States Department of Energy, Contract No. W-31-109-ENG-38, and from the United States National Cancer Institute, Grant No. CA18081.

REFERENCES

1. Dethlefsen, L.A.: Cellular recovery kinetic studies relevant to combined-modality research and therapy. *Int J Radiat Oncol Biol Phys* **5**:1197–1203, 1979.
2. Dethlefsen, L.A., Ohlsen, J.D., and Roti-Roti, J.C.: Cell synchronization in vivo: Fact or fancy? In *Growth Kinetics and Biochemical Regulation of Normal and Malignant Cells* B. Derwinko and R.M. Humphrey, eds. Baltimore: Williams & Wilkins, 1977, pp. 493–507.
3. Dethlefsen, L.A., Sorensen, S.P., and Riley, B.M.: Effects on double and multiple doses of hydroxyurea or mouse duodenum and mammary tumors. *Cancer Res* **35**:694–699, 1975.
4. Elkind, M.M.: Some principles for a rational, cell-based development of combined radiation-drug therapy. *Front Radiat Ther Oncol* **4**:76–78, 1969.
5. Elkind, M.M.: Introduction to session on drug lethality and sublethal damage: Cytotoxic damage and repair. *Cancer Treat Rep* **60**:1777–1780, 1976.
6. Elkind, M.M.: Fundamental questions in the combined use of radiation and chemicals in the treatment of cancer. *Int J Radiat Oncol Biol Phys* **5**:1711–1720, 1979.
7. Elkind, M.M., and Kano, E.: Radiation-induced age-response changes in Chinese hamster cells: Evidence for a new form of damage and its repair. *Int J Radiat Biol* **19**:547–560, 1971.
8. Elkind, M.M., Sakamoto, K., and Kamper, C.: Age-dependent toxic properties of actinomycin D and x-rays in cultured Chinese hamster cells. *Cell Tissue Kinet* **1**:209–224, 1968.
9. Hreshchyshyn, M.M.: Hydroxyurea (NSC-32065) with irradiation for cervical carconoma–preliminary report. *Cancer Chemother Rep* **52**:601–602, 1968; *Am Surg* **35**:525–534, 1967, 401–402, 1970.
10. Hreshchyshyn, M.M., Aron, B.S., Boronow, R.C., Franklin, E.W., Shingleton, H.M., and Blessing, J.A.: Hydroxyurea or placebo combined with radiation to treat stages IIIB and IV cervical cancer confined to the pelvis. *Int J Radiat Oncol Biol Phys* **5**:317–322, 1979.
11. Hussey, D.H., and Abrams, J.P.: Combined therapy in advanced head and neck cancer: Hydroxyurea and radiotherapy. *Prog Clin Cancer* **6**:79–86, 1975.
12. Hussey, D.H., and Samuels, M.L.: Combined therapy in advanced cancer: Hydroxyurea and radiotherapy. *Cancer Bull* **23**:42–45, 1971.
13. Landgren, R.C., Hussey, D.H., Barkley, H.T., and Samuels, M.L.: Split course irradiation compared to split course irradiation in inoperable bronchogenic carcinoma–a randomized study of 53 patients. *Cancer* **34**:1598–1601, 1974.
14. LePar, E., Faust, D.S., Brady, L.W., and Beckloff, G.L.: Clinical evaluation of the adjunctive use of

hydroxyurea in radiation therapy of carcinoma of the lung. *Radiology* **36**:32–40, 1967.

15. Lerner, H.J.: Concomitant hydroxyurea and irradiation: Clinical experience with advanced head and neck cancer at Pennsylvania Hospital. *Am J Surg* **134**:505–509, 1977.
16. Lerner, H.J., Beckloff, G.L., and Goodwin, M.C.: Hydroxyurea (NSC-32065) intermittent therapy in malignant diseases. *Cancer Chemother Rep* **53**:385–395, 1969.
17. Lerner, H.J., Beckloff, G.L., and Goodwin, M.C.: Treatment of astrocytoma with hydroxyurea and irradiation: Report of six patients with 18-month follow up. *Am Surg* **36**:401–402, 1970.
18. Lerner, H.J., Beckloff, G.L., Lipschutz, H., Campbell, R., and Ritchie, D.: Hydroxyurea in management of head and neck cancer. *Plas Reconstr Surg* **40**:233–239, 1967.
19. Papavasiliou, C.: Combined treatment of carcinoma of the vulva by irradiation and hydroxyurea. In *CROS Conference on Combined Modalities* Hilton Head Island, November 1978.
20. Piver, M.S., Barlow, J.J., Vongtama, V., and Blumenson, L.: Hydroxyurea as a sensitizer in women with carcinoma of the cervix. *Am Obstet Gynecol* **129**:379–383, 1977.
21. Piver, M.S., Barlow, J.J., Vongtama, V., and Webster, J.: Hydroxyurea and radiation therapy in advanced cervical cancer. *Am J Obstet Gynecol* **120**:969–972, 1974.
22. Richards, G.J., and Chambers, R.G.: Hydroxyurea: A radiosensitizer in the treatment of neoplasms of the head and neck. *AJR* **105**:555–564, 1969.
23. Rominger, C.J.: Hydroxyurea and radiation therapy in advanced neoplasms of the head and neck. *AJR* **111**:103–108, 1971.
24. Rupniak, H.T., and Paul, D.: Selective killing of transformed cells by exploitation of their defective cell cycle control by polyamines. *Cancer Res* **40**:293–297, 1980.
25. Sinclair, W.K.: Hydroxyurea; Differential lethal effects on cultured mammalian cells during the cell cycle. *Science* **150**:1729–1731, 1965.
26. Sinclair, W.K.: Hydroxyurea: Effects on Chinese hamster cells grown in culture. *Cancer Res* **27** (Part I);297–308, 1967.
27. Sinclair, W.K.: The combined effect of hydroxyurea and x-rays on Chinese hamster cells *in vitro*. *Cancer RRes* **28**:190–206, 1968.
28. Sinclair, W.K.: Hydroxyurea revisited: A decade of clinical effects studies. *Int J Radiat Oncol Biol Phys* **5**:(suppl 2,) 132–133, 1979.
29. Sinclair, W.K.: Hydroxyurea revisited: A decade of clinical effects studies. *Radiology*, submitted, 1980.
30. Sinclair, W.K., and Morton, R.A.: X-ray sensitivity during the cell generation cycle of cultured Chinese hamster cells. *Radiat Res* **29**:450–474, 1966.
31. Steel, G.G.: In *Growth Kinetics of Tumors* Oxford: Clarendon Press, 1977, pp. 202–203.
32. Stefani, S., Eells, R.W., and Abbate, J.: Hydroxyurea and radiotherapy in head and neck cancer. *Radiology* **101**:391–396, 1971.
33. Tubiana, M., Frindel, E., and Vassant, F.: Critical survey of experimental data on *in vivo* synchronization by hydroxyurea. *Recent Results Cancer Res* **52**:187–205, 1975.
34. Young, C.W., and Hodas, S.: Hydroxyurea: Inhibitory effect on DNA metabolism. *Science* **146**:1172–1174, 1964.

CHAPTER 38

Adriamycin-Resistant Cells Express Multiple Phenotypes

James A. Belli, M.D.[a]
Neil Howell, Ph.D.[a]

Radiation resistance expressed by subpopulations of tumor cells is due, in large part, to physiologic factors. These factors are well known and include changes in cell-cycle age distributions, hypoxia, and as yet undefined interrelationships between tumor and host. The development of hypoxic-cell sensitizers and nonstandard fractionation schemes are directed toward circumventing these physiologic and biological contraints on tumor responses. On the other hand, the presence of tumor cells which are intrinsically radiation resistant, under physiological conditions comparable to most normal tissues, is unlikely to account for the sometimes unsatisfactory local control probabilities for certain tumor types. The degree of inherent radioresistance among tumor cells may not be sufficient to account for radiotherapeutic failure.

Radiotherapeutic success is largely dependent upon normal tissue tolerance; when tumors recur after x-irradiation, these tumors are not less responsive than when initially treated except *within the constraints of normal tissue tolerance.* The latter may limit the amount of radiation that can be safely delivered to recurrent tumor masses. In contrast, failure of chemotherapeutic agents to control human neoplastic disease is often associated with the emergence of drug-resistant tumor cell populations. While initial tumor response may be influenced by tumor physiology, the induction of drug resistance represents a change in the *intrinsic* sensitivity at a cellular level. This change may be genetic and reflected as membrane restriction to the drug and/or differences in intracellular processing. Current therapeutic strategies for these patients include the use of agents to which tumor cells are not likely to be cross-resistant, development of new chemotherapeutic agents, and the use of more effective combinations of drugs. These strategies are designed to circumvent the emergence of tumor cells which have become inherently drug resistant. Under these circumstances, it is important to know whether or not drug-resistant tumor cells are more or less responsive to x-irradiation. Apart from this consideration, it is also important to understand the long-term effects of these chemotherapeutic agents especially as these may relate to mutagenic effects and the risk for second neoplasms.

In this chapter we show that second-step mutants selected from adriamycin-resistant cells derived from Chinese hamster lung fibroblasts (V79) express multiple phenotypic changes with respect to DNA content, chromosome number, x-ray survival response, growth-rate and growth properties, and cellular and colony morphology.

Continuous growth of Chinese hamster fibroblasts in the presence of low levels of adriamycin (0.05 μ/ml) eventually resulted in the emergence of cells resistant to adriamycin. Resistance was found to be stable because growth in drug-free medium was not accompanied by reversion to parental (V79) drug response.[1,2] To select for second-step mutants, stable, resistant cells (77A) were exposed for 1 hour to 25 μg adriamycin/ml growth medium (alpha-MEM with

[a]Department of Radiation Therapy, Joint Center for Radiation Therapy, Harvard Medical School, Boston, Mass.

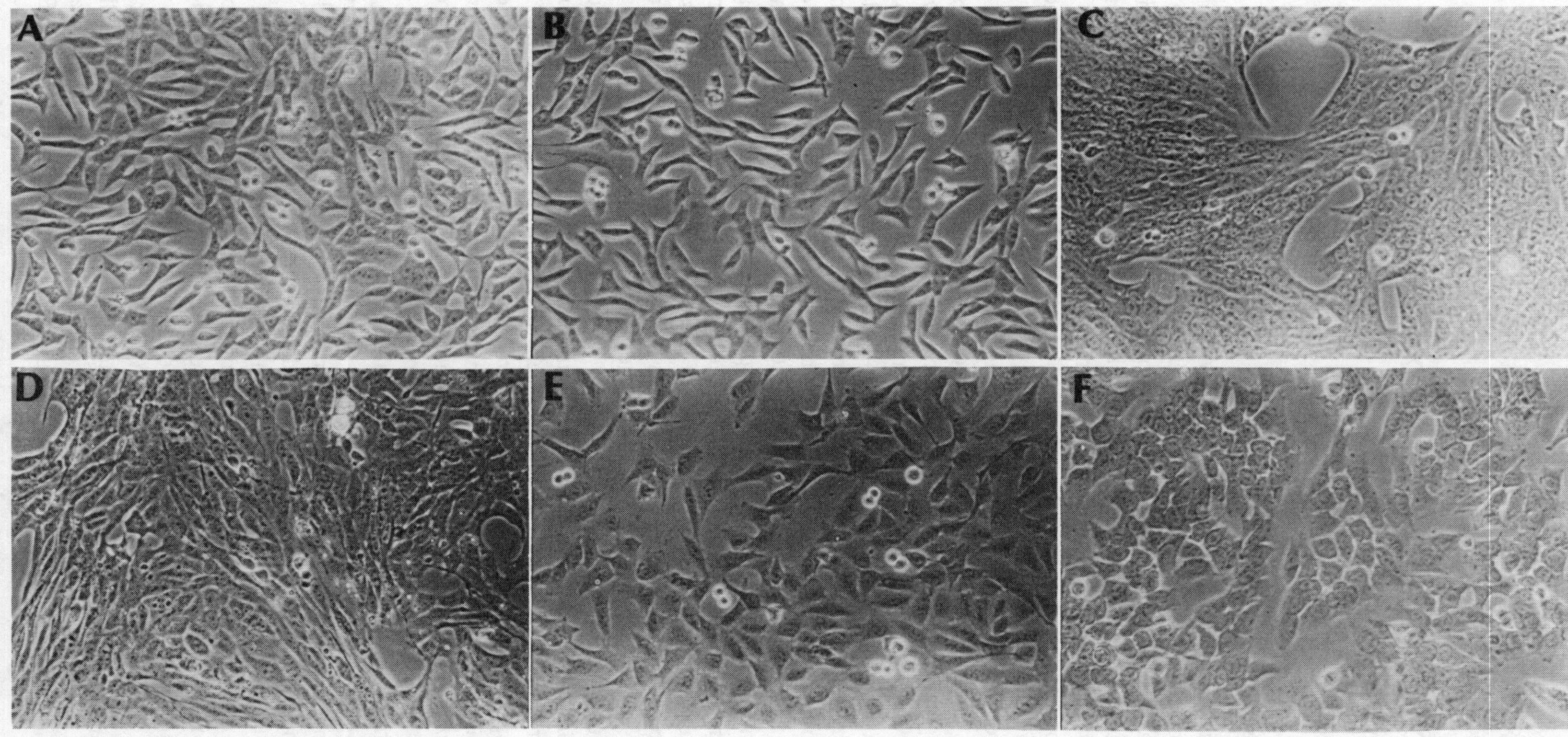

Figure 1. Cellular morphologies of parent and mutant lines isolated from an adriamycin-resistant line: (*a*) V79; (*b*) 77A; (*c*) 77A-1; (*d*) 77A-6; (*e*) 77A-3; (*f*) 77A-51S. 77A-1 and 77A-6 cells show typical fibroblastlike morphology. 77A-3 and 77A-51S cells are more typical of epithelial cells. Modal chromosome numbers are given in Table 1. Phase contrast, 256×.

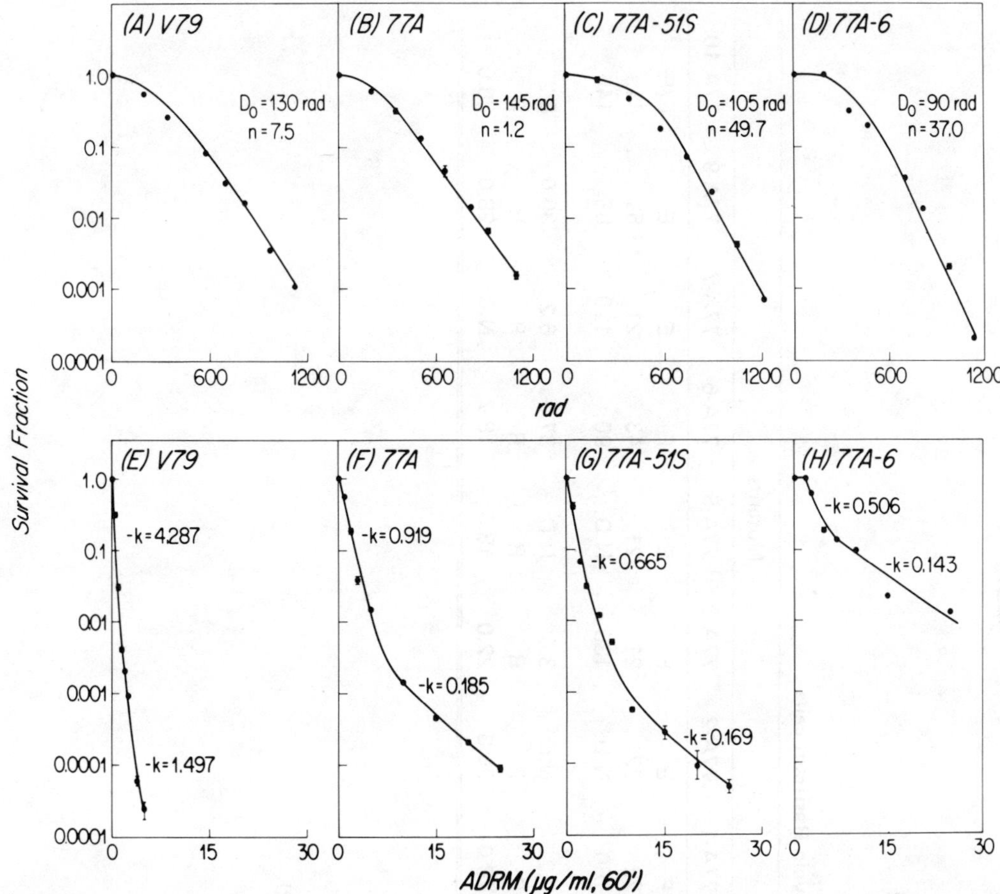

Figure 2. Radiation and adriamycin dose-response curves for selected adriamycin-resistant cells and V79 cells. Survival responses were determined with exponentially growing cells plated at cell concentrations chosen to yield approximately 200 colonies at all survival levels. X-rays were produced in an OEG-60 Machlett beryllium end-window tube operated at 50 kVp and 20 mA. The x-ray survival curves were obtained with single cells. D_o = radiation dose required to reduce survival by e^{-1} on the exponential portion of the curve; n = extrapolation number determined from the intersection of the straight line portion to dose = 0. Adriamycin dose-response curves were determined for microcolonies (average number of cells per colony = 2-3). k = inactivation constant, determined for the sensitive and resistant portions of the curve by regression analysis. k^{-1} = microgram • ml^{-1}. Following adriamycin exposure, cells were rinsed with Puck's saline A and refed with growth medium for colony formation.

10% donor calf serum), rinsed with Puck's saline A, harvested with 0.05% trysin, diluted in growth medium, and plated into 60 mm Falcon plastic petri dishes at cell numbers required to yield, on the average, one surviving cell per dish. This treatment resulted in a survival fraction of approximately 10^{-4}. After 2 weeks, petri dishes were examined for the presence of colonies and those dishes containing only one colony selected for subculture. Table 1 summarizes the characteristics of clones isolated in this manner. Four of the nine lines were found to be aneuploid (77A-51S, 77A-6, 77A-9, 77A-10). Cellular and colony morphology were also found to vary among the second-step mutants isolated. Representative examples of the morphologies observed, compared to V79 and 77A cells, are shown in Figure 1. Colony and cellular morphology were not dependent upon chromosome number.

All second-step mutants studied remained adriamycin-resistant. However, some mutants exhibited significant differences in x-ray survival properties compared to V79 or 77A cells. Figure 2 shows adriamycin and x-

TABLE 1. Phenotype of Second-Step Mutants from Adriamycin-Resistant cells

Phenotype	Parents		Mutants								
	V79	77A	77A-516S	77A-1	77A-2	77A-3	77A-5	77A-6	77A-7	77A-9	77A-10
Morphology (cellular)	F[a]	F	E[b]	F	E	E	E	F	E	E	E/F[c]
Chromosome number (mode)	22	22	36	22	22	21	21	43	21	51	41
Radiation response D_o (rad)[d]	130	145	105	160	N.D.[e]	130	N.D.	90	120	85	145
Extrapolation number[f]	7.5	1.2	49.7	2.2	N.D	3.6	N.D	37.0	6.2	30.0	8.2
Adriamycin response	S[g]	R[h]	R	R	R	R	R	R	R	R	R
Doubling time (hours)	9.0	10.5	21.0	18.0	25.0	22.0	18.5	18.7	N.D	28.0	20.0

[a] Fibroblast.
[b] Epithelial.
[c] Mixed.
[d] D_o = slope^{-1} (see fig. 2).
[e] Not determined.
[f] Extrapolate of exponential part of the curve to zero dose (see fig. 2).
[g] Sensitive.
[h] Resistant.

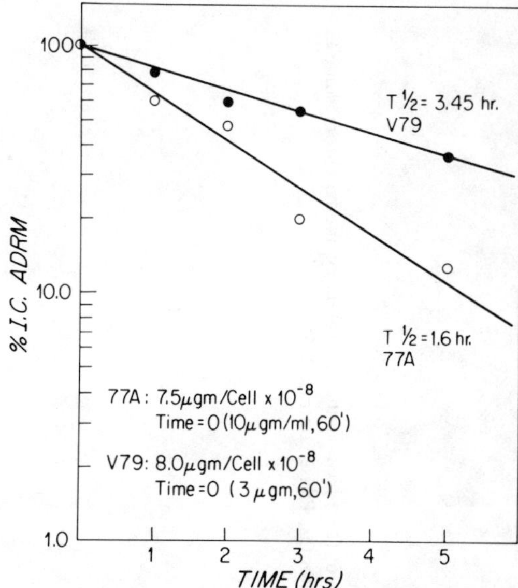

Figure 3. Uptake and efflux of adriamycin in sensitive (V79) and resistant (77A) cells. Drug concentrations were chosen to give comparable intracellular concentrations at time = 0. Adriamycin was measured by flurescence of butanol extract of disrupted cells using excitation and emission wavelengths of 485 nm and 590 nm, respectively. Efflux was more efficient in resistant cells.

ray survival curves for V79 and 77A cells and two aneuploid clones isolated from the latter. Aneuploidy was associated with x-ray survival properties characterized by increased radiation sensitivity as measured by the reciprocal slope (D_o) of the straight line portion of the x-ray survival curve and by an increased capacity to accumulate sublethal radiation injury (Figure 2, [*c*] and [*d*]).

One of the aneuploid mutants (77A-6) also demonstrated increased resistance to adriamycin. This change in resistance may reflect gene amplification resulting in greater levels of the gene product responsible for adriamycin resistance. In addition, the doubling time of this mutant was found to be 18.7 hours compared to 10.5 hours for its resistant parent, 77A. This increase in cell-cycle time, if at the expense of the proportion of cells in DNA synthesis and a prolongation of G_1, may result in an increased proportion of cells in an adriamycin-resistant compartment of the cell cycle (G_1).

Adriamycin resistance is mediated through drug transport across the cell membrane.[3] Resistant cells also appeared to have the capacity for increased efflux of drug. Figure 3 shows the time course of drug release, measured with fluorescence techniques, from 77A and V79 cells for comparable intracellular concentrations at time-zero. 77A cells lost intracellular adriamycin with a $T^{½}$ which is one-half that for V79 cells (1.6 hours versus 3.45 hours).

One of the radiosensitive mutants, 77A-51S, demonstrated spontaneous reversion of cellular morphology after prolonged subculture. These morphological changes are shown in Figure 4 and were accompanied by loss of chromosomes. Currently, this clone has a modal chromosome number of 22, remains adriamycin-resistant, and has x-ray survival properties similar to its parent 77A (n = 2.5 and D_o = 145 rad).

These observations suggest the following conclusions: (1) adriamycin, a widely used chemotherapeutic agent, is an effective mutagen of mammalian cells in culture; (2) some second-step mutants with increased chromosome numbers became radiation sensitive, but with the additional property of increased threshold for radiation damage; and (3) when second-step mutants which were aneuploid were isolated, this property was not necessarily associated with changes in cellular morphology. When changes in cellular morphology were expressed, this phenotype may be unstable because one of the aneuploid mutants with an epithelial cell morphology (77A-51S) reverted to fibroblast morphology as chromosomes were lost. This reversion was also associated with a change in x-ray survival properties. Some second-step mutants isolated from adriamycin-resistant cells following a single large exposure to adriamycin demonstrated changes in x-ray survival responses which were in the direction of increased radiation sensitivity. This finding has important implications relative to the possible x-ray responses of adriamycin-resistant tumor cells in patients who have failed chemotherapeutic combinations containing adriamycin.

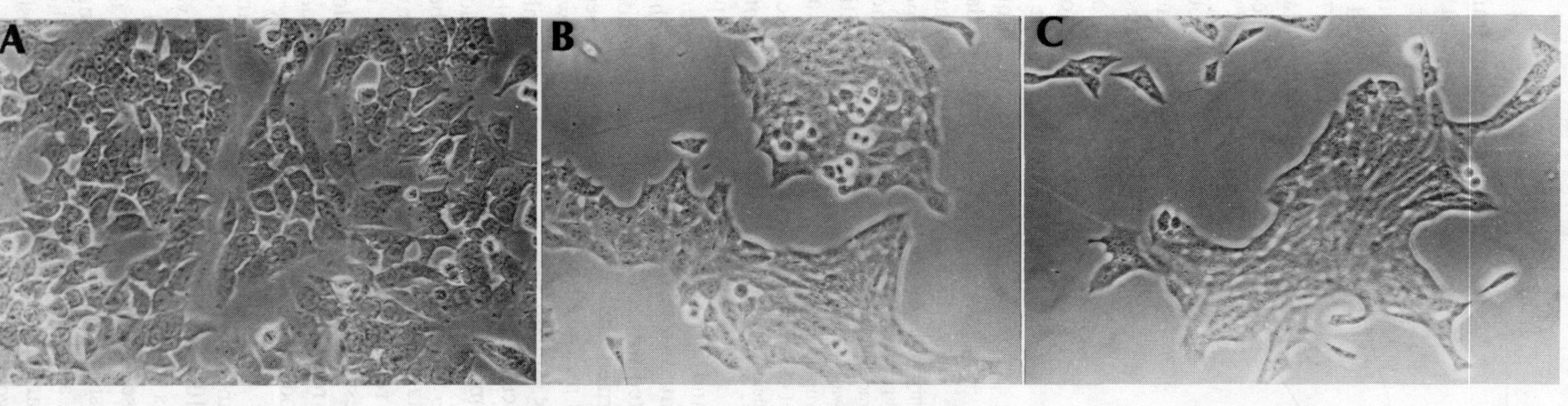

Figure 4. Morphological reversion of 77A-51S: (*a*) epithelial morphology, modal chromosome number = 36; (*b*) mixed cellular morphology, modal chromosome ≅ 30; (*c*) complete reversion to fibroblastlike morphology, modal chromosome number = 22. Time course was 4 months. Phase contrast 256×

Apart from this, the data presented in this paper suggest that adriamycin is a strong mutagen capable of inducing a number of phenotypes within resistant populations suggesting that adriamycin-resistant cells may have increased mutability. Genetic analysis of these phenotypes may provide insight into the genetic control mechanisms of drug transport across cell membranes and the expression of cellular radiation damage.

Summary

Following prolonged exposure to adriamycin, Chinese hamster cells developed resistance to this chemotherapeutic agent. The resistant phenotype was stable for long periods after cells were removed from low levels of drug. Second-step mutants from adriamycin-resistant cells expressed multiple phenotypes, including aneuploidy, change in growth properties, cell and colony morphology, and increased sensitivity to radiation. All mutants isolated remained adriamycin-resistant. Cellular and colony morphology was not dependent upon chromosome number or the presence or absence of other phenotypes. Increased radiation sensitivity was most often associated with aneuploidy. One second-step mutant, which was polyploid, had an epithelial morphology, was radiation sensitive, but reverted to fibroblast morphology and parent-type radiation response with loss of chromosomes during a prolonged culture period.

Acknowledgments

Research for this chapter was supported by USPHS Grants CA25333, CA12662, and CA28608 from the National Cancer Institute, National Institutes of Health.

REFERENCES

1. Belli, J.A.: Radiation response and adriamycin resistance in mammalian cells in culture. *Front Radiat Ther Oncol* **13**:9–20, 1978.
2. Belli, J.A., and Harris, J.R.: Adriamycin resistance and radiation response. *Int J Radiat Oncol Biol Phys* **5**:1231–1234, 1979.
3. Harris, J.R., Timberlake, N., Henson, P., Schimke, P., and Belli, J.A.: Adriamycin uptake in V79 and adriamycin resistant Chinese hamster cells. *Int J Radiat Oncol Biol Phys* **5**:1233–1239, 1979.

CHAPTER 39

Chemical Inhibition of Host Toxicity as a Means of Overcoming Tumor Resistance

John M. Yuhas, Ph.D.[a]
M. Chiara Pardini, D.Sc.[b]

WR-2721 is presently entering initial clinical trials in solid tumor radiotherapy since, in experimental systems, it has been shown to protect normal tissues selectively while leaving the solid tumors studied to suffer the full effects of the exposure. Although this drug would appear to be of general effectiveness, it does not protect the CNS, and its activity in certain tissues could be improved upon. We are presently engaged in studies on the mechanism of action of this drug in the hope that even better agents could be developed. Progress to date has included dissociation of the mechanisms responsible for the lack of CNS and solid tumor protection, demonstration of active drug concentration against a gradient *in vivo* and *in vitro*, with the latter studies including surgically derived human tissues and extension of the potential application of WR-2721 to include alkylating agent therapy, either alone or in combination with radiation. It would appear, therefore, that WR-2721 can play a role in overcoming tumor resistance, and, in those cases where it is ineffective, the information is at hand such that more appropriate agents could be developed.

The proposal that radioprotective drugs might selectively protect normal tissues against radiation injury while leaving solid tumors to suffer the full effects of the radiation exposure is more than 30 years old; yet a definitive evaluation of this proposal is still lacking. Many drugs have been tested and shown to be inappropriate, but the possibility remains that a nontoxic drug which selectively protects normal tissues might still be developed. The search for such a drug began shortly after Patt and colleagues[10] first reported that injection of cysteine protected rats against otherwise lethal doses of x-rays. By 1965, however, the prospects for developing such a drug appeared dismal[6] in that those drugs which did show selective normal tissue protection were relatively weak, and what little protection was afforded required the injection of near toxic drug doses.

Consequently, this approach to overcoming the relative radioresistance of tumors was all but abandoned until 1969, when the first reports began to appear on WR-2721. Building on the observations of Akerfeldt,[2-4] the United States Army Anti-Radiation Drug Development Program synthesized a series of phosphorothioates for potential military application. The most effective of these, in terms of protection of mice against radiation-induced hematopoietic death, proved to be WR-2721 or S-2-(3-aminopropylamino) ethylphosphorothioic acid.[24] In addition to offering selective protection of normal tissues,[25] this drug was effective at relatively small fractions of the maximum tolerated dose,[15] suggesting that this drug overcame the limitations which had hampered this approach for more than 20 years.

Since that time, this drug has been stud-

[a]Department of Radiation Therapy, University of Pennsylvania and Children's Hospital of Philadelphia, Philadelphia, Penn.
[b]On leave from Instituto Medico e di Ricerca Scientifica, Rome, Italy

TABLE 1. Summary of the Radioprotective Effectiveness of WR-2721 in Normal Tissues [b]

Tissues Protected by WR-2721	Tissues Not Protected by WR-2721
Bone marrow	Brain
Skin	Spinal Cord
G.I. epithelium	
Salivary gland	
Oral mucosa	
Immune system	
Wound healing	
Liver	
Kidney	
Esophagus	
Lung	
Vasculature[a]	

[a] From J.F. Utley, personal communication, 1980.
[b] Data from Yuhas, 1980.[20]

ied in a variety of normal tissue and tumor systems of mice, rats, rabbits, guinea pigs, dogs, and monkeys, and Table 1 summarizes our present evaluation of its effectiveness in both normal and malignant tissues. With the exception of the brain[24] and the spinal cord,[16] WR-2721 has been shown to protect all normal tissues studied against radiation injury. The extent of protection against single doses of radiation varies widely, and we will return to this point below. Of the 12 solid tumors studied, none have been significantly radioprotected by WR-2721. In the rare instances where marginal levels of tumor radioprotection were reported,[25] more complete testing, especially tests involving multiple treatments, have failed to confirm this protection.

Therefore, WR-2721 appears able to protect most normal tissues against radiation injury and would appear clinically applicable in those instances in which the CNS is not the radiation dose-limiting tissue. This presupposes that WR-2721 will be well tolerated by man, as it is by all other species studied. The initial clinical studies on WR-2721 are conflicting in this regard, however. The phase I clinical trial being conducted at the University of New Mexico[8] has escalated through single doses as high as 450 mg/m^2 without encountering any significant toxicity.

On the contrary, Sugahara and Tanaka[11] reported a dose-limiting hypotension at drug doses of 100 mg/m^2–i.e., at a dose which is four times lower than that which has been well tolerated in the New Mexico study. Whether this gross difference in toxicity reflects differences in the drug samples or other study variables remains to be determined. Based on these encouraging initial results, including the demonstration of radioprotection in man,[11] a multiple dose phase I/phase II study has been initiated involving the Universities of New Mexico, California, Alberta, and Pennsylvania, the Mallinkrodt Institute, and the National Cancer Institute.

Although WR-2721 would appear to hold promise of eventual clinical appliction, it is not without limitations. First and most clearly, WR-2721 does not protect the central nervous system, and the effectiveness of radiotherapy at many sites could be improved if we could increase the radiation tolerance of the brain and spinal cord. Second, although it is difficult to extrapolate single-dose radiation data in mice to multiple-dose situations in the clinic, it is obvious that the protection which WR-2721

TABLE 2. Potential Mechanisms Which Might Account for the Inability of WR-2721 to Radioprotect Solid Tumors and the CNS.

Level of Organization	Potential Mechanism	
	Solid Tumors	CNS
Tissue	Deficient vascularity	Blood-brain barrier
Cell	Membrane restriction	Membrane restriction
Subcellular	Metabolic handling	Metabolic handling
	Quality of injury	Quality of injury

affords certain tissues (e.g., the lung) could be improved. Lastly, although WR-2721 is relatively nontoxic, it would be highly desirable to develop agents which offered similar levels of protection but at lower fractions of the maximum tolerated dose. In order to address each of these problems logically, it will be necessary to understand the basis of selective normal tissue protection and toxicity.

Mechanism of Selective Normal Tissue Protection

Table 2 lists the three potential mechanisms which might be able to account for the inability of WR-2721 to protect either solid tumors or the CNS. At the grossest level of organization, one could argue that vascular factors restrict absorption of WR-2721 by these two tissues. At a slightly more refined level, it is possible that the cell membranes of the two tissues restrict the absorption of the drug. Lastly, even if the vascularity is sufficient and the drug crosses the cell membrane, these two tissues could metabolize the drug to a nonprotective form, or suffer a type of injury which WR-2721 cannot protect against.

Initial studies demonstrated that these two tissues failed to absorb significant quantities of WR-2721 following injection,[14] suggesting that one or both of the mechanisms which would restrict absorption (Table 2) were involved in selective normal tissue protection, except for the CNS. Since Harris and Phillips[7] had reported that normal and tumor cells alike, when studied *in vitro*, absorbed WR-2721 passively down a concentration gradient, it appeared that deficient vascularity was responsible for the failure of the tumors to absorb the drug. Until recently[1] no further studies have been reported on the basis of limited CNS absorption.

The third potential mechanism, that the tumor cells do not respond to the radioprotective effects of WR-2721, was considered by a number of investigators.[7,13,22] All three groups reached essentially the same conclusion, i.e., that hypoxic cells are not protected as effectively by WR-2721 as are their well-oxygenated counterparts. The reasons for this relatively poor protection of hypoxic cells have never been established unequivocally, but the observation itself suggests that the small amount of WR-2721 which is absorbed would be even less effective if we assume that the critical tumor cells are hypoxic.

Until recently, the foregoing represented our understanding of the mechanism of selective protection. The inconsistency of this interpretation occurred to us when we initiated studies on the combined use of radioprotectors and radiosensitizers.[26] Injection of misonidazole, another passively absorbed drug, produced roughly equal drug levels in normal tissues and tumors alike; yet in the same animals WR-2721 was not absorbed by the tumor. Of all the possibilities which could account for the gross differences in distribution of these two passively absorbed

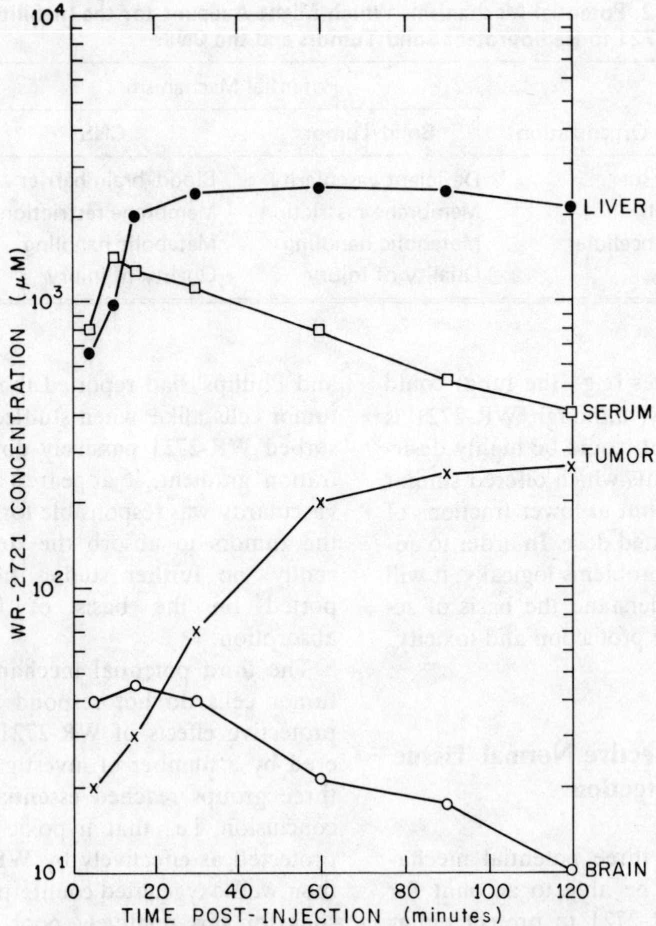

Figure 1. Concentration of WR-2721 in the serum, liver, brain, and 3M2N tumor of Fisher 344 rats as a function of time after injection of 200 mg/kg of WR-2721.

drugs, the simplest one, that WR-2721 was not being passively absorbed by most normal tissues, proved to be the correct one. Figure 1 is a plot of the concentration of WR-2721 in the serum, liver, brain, and 3M2N tumor of rats as a function of time after the I.P. injection of 200 mg/kg of WR-2721.[1,18] As the serum concentration declines with time postinjection, the liver concentration continues to rise, indicating that the liver (and other normal tissues not shown) can actively concentrate WR-2721 against a concentration gradient. Quite the reverse, the concentration of WR-2721 in the tumor gradually approaches equilibrium with the declining serum concentration, suggesting passive absorption kinetics (Fig. 1). A third pattern is seen in the brain (Fig. 1) in which minimal absorption occurs, and what little is absorbed declines in parallel with the serum concentration. This would suggest that the limited amounts which are detected in the brain actually represent a serum contaminant.

To allow more detailed study of these differing patterns of absorption, we developed an *in vitro* assay for WR-2721 absorption.[1,18] Figure 2 summarizes the results of a typical study in which 1 mm cubes of liver, brain, and 3M2N tumor were incubated in 100 μm WR-2721 for up to 4 hours. Within the 4-hour incubation period the concentration of

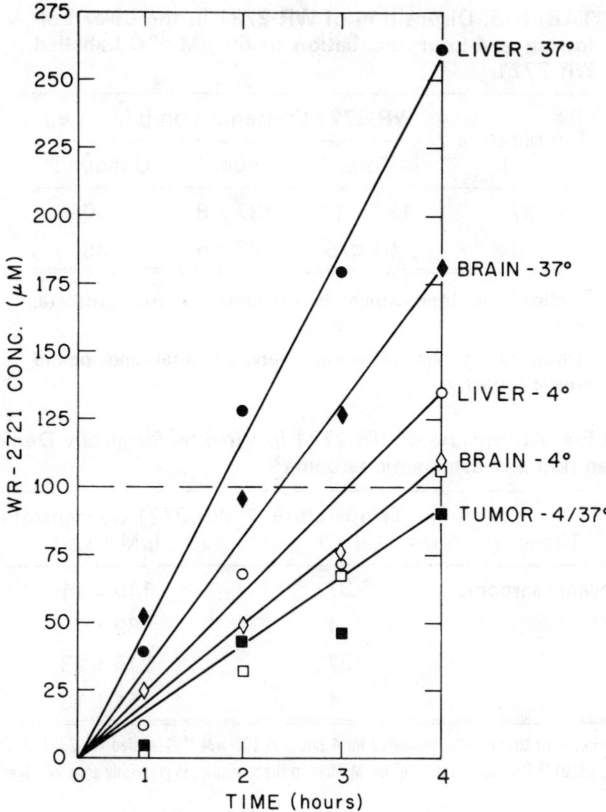

Figure 2. Concentration of WR-2721 in the liver, brain, and 3M2N tumor as a function of time that 1-mm cubes of these tissues were incubated in 100 μM WR-2721 at 37°C or 4°C.

the WR-2721 in the liver rises to 2.7 times greater than that in the surrounding medium, indicating that the active concentration mechanism operates at the cellular level. When the incubations are carried out at 4°C, as opposed to 37°C, the effectiveness of the active concentration mechanism is grossly impaired (Fig. 2).

In these studies, active concentration of WR-2721 was also observed for brain samples, which suggests that the limited absorption of WR-2721 by this tissue *in vivo* (Fig. 1) is a product of the blood-brain barrier (Fig. 2). However, even when the tumor is given free access to WR-2721 in this *in vitro* system, we were unable to demonstrate active concentration (Fig. 2).

Before concluding that the failure of this tumor (and others in our laboratory) to concentrate WR-2721 actively was due to a membrane restriction, we had to discount a potential artifact. At this point, it remained possible that portions of the tumor were actively concentrating WR-2721, but that this process was more than counterbalanced by necrotic areas of the tumor which did not absorb WR-2721 at all. Clearly, this is not the case since grossly necrotic samples of tumor can actively concentrate WR-2721 while grossly viable samples cannot.[18] Further, if we destroy the integrity of the cell membrane by freeze-thaw or by hypotonic shock,[1,18] we can promote active concentration of WR-2721 by grossly viable tumor samples.

Our present understanding of the active concentration mechanism is that it is a facilitated diffusion in which the drug, once inside the cell, is dephosphorylated and bound to endogenous macromolecules,

TABLE 3. Disposition of WR-2721 in the Liver Following a 4-hour incubation in 50 μM ^{14}C-Labelled WR-2721

Temperature (°C)	WR-2721 Concentration (μM ± s.e.)		
	Total	Bound[a]	Unbound[b]
37	187 ± 11	137 ± 8	50
4	61 ± 5	23 ± 5	38

[a] Defined as that which is insoluble in trichloroacetic acid.
[b] Obtained as the difference between total and bound drug absorbed.

TABLE 4. Absorption of WR-2721 *In Vitro* by Surgically Derived Human skin and osteogenic sarcoma[a]

Tissue	Temperature (°C)	WR-2721 Concentration (μM ± s.e.)
Osteogenic sarcoma	37	115 ± 11
	4	89 ± 7
Skin	37	215 ± 23
	4	151 ± 18

[a] 1-mm cubes of tissue were incubated for 4 hours in 100 μM ^{14}C-labeled WR-2721 (from Yuhas, 1980).[18] The participation of Dr. M Khan in these studies is gratefully acknowledged.

thereby allowing the entrance of more drug. A large fraction of the intracellular drug can be shown to be bound (see Table 3) with the unbound forms, being in approximate equilibrium with the surrounding medium. This would account for the failure of Harris and Phillips[7] to detect active concentration of WR-2721 by normal cells since their wet chemical methods could not detect the bound forms of the drug, as they pointed out. Further support for this facilitated diffusion hypothesis comes from the observation that the pH optima for dephosphorylation of WR-2721 and for active concentration of the drug are near identical–6.0 to 6.2 (see Fig. 3). This suggested to us that acid phosphatase is a critical enzyme in this process, and, indeed, one can demonstrate that acid phosphatase can catalyze the binding of WR-2721 to reporter proteins (Table 3).

In addition to providing us with a tool for studying the active concentration mechanism, the development of this *in vitro* assay has allowed us to compare the results obtained with normal tissues and transplanted tumors in animals with the data obtained from surgically derived patient material. An example of such studies with human tissues is given in Table 4, and it is readily apparent that temperature-dependent active concentration of WR-2721 is observed in normal human tissues, but not in the tumors derived from the same patient. Therefore, active concentration of WR-2721, which is the basis of its selective protection, is not an artifact of transplanted experimental tumors, but occurs also in man.

Prospects for Developing Clinically Useful CNS Radioprotectors

The question of whether it will be pos-

TABLE 5. Potential CNS Radioprotectors

Agent	Chemical Formula	Comments[a]
WR-187093[b]	$NH_2(CH_2)_3CH(CH_2)_2SH_2PO_3$	Active p.o.
WR-76842	$NH_2-\overset{NH_2}{\underset{NH}{C}}-CH_2SH$	Active p.o
WR-1607	$CH_3(CH_2)_9NH(CH_2)_2SSO_3H$	CNS protectors in monkeys

[a] Refers to potential basis for expecting CNS radioprotection.
[b] More complete data on these compounds can be found in Sweeney, 1980.[12]

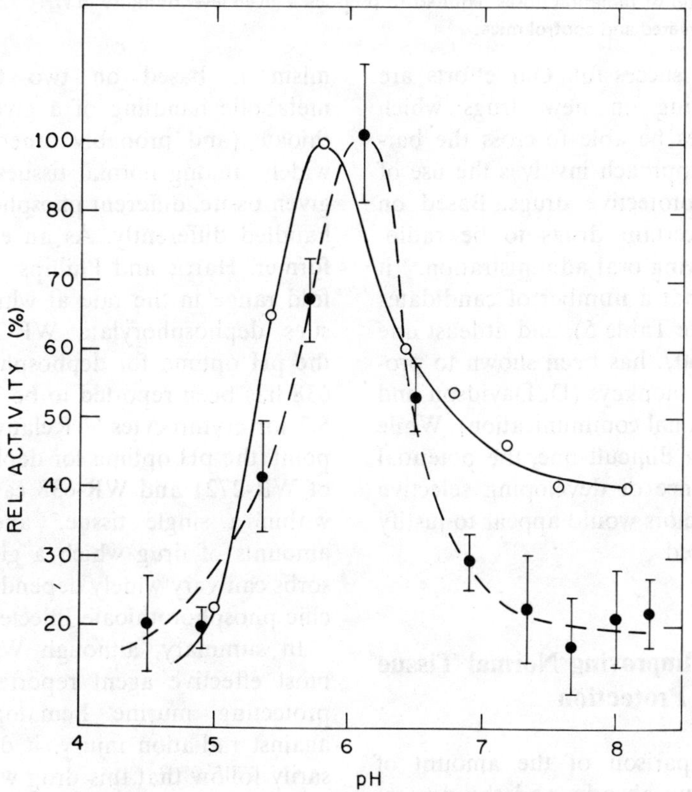

Figure 3. pH dependence for dephosphorylation of WR-2721 (o) and for active concentration of WR-2721 (•). (Data on dephosphorylation taken from Harris and Phillips, 1971.)

sible to develop CNS protectors which would have a role in clinical radiotherapy is actually a series of three sequential questions:

1. Can radioprotective drugs be developed which will cross the blood–brain barrier?
2. Will the brain tolerate the drug levels required for protection?
3. Will a drug which protects the CNS fail to protect solid tumors?

We are presently approaching the first question in two ways, by altering the manner in which WR-2721 is administered and by testing other drugs. Administration of WR-2721 in solvents which might carry it across the blood–brain barrier (e.g., DMSO)

TABLE 6. Dissociation of the Concentration of WR-2721 Observed in a Series of Normal Tissues[a] and the Protection Which This Drug Affords Them Against Radiation Injury.

Tissue	WR-2721 Concentration (μM ± s.e.)	Dose-Reduction Factor[b]
Lung	807 ± 21	1.2
Kidney	1103 ± 38	1.5
Bone marrow	904 ± 51	2.5

[a] Determined at 30 minutes after the injection of 200 mg of WR-2721 per kg of body weight in mice.

[b] Ratio of radiation doses required to produce a given level of injury in WR-2721 pretreated and control mice.

has not proven successful. Our efforts are now concentrating on new drugs which might themselves be able to cross the barrier. One such approach involves the use of lipophilic radioprotective drugs. Based on the ability of certain drugs to be radioprotective following oral administration,[12] it would appear that a number of candidates are available (see Table 5), and at least one of them, WR-1607, has been shown to protect the CNS in monkeys (D. Davidson and M. Heiffer, personal communication). While the problem is a difficult one, the potential clinical importance of developing selective CNS radioprotectors would appear to justify the effort required.

Prospects for Improving Normal Tissue Protection

From a comparison of the amount of WR-2721 a tissue absorbs and the protection afforded, it is readily apparent that protection is not a simple function of drug concentration (see Table 6). Rather, it would appear that more subtle measures of the quality and location of the WR-2721 will be required in order to account for and, in certain cases, rectify the levels of protection observed. Just as is the case for the development of CNS radioprotectors, these studies are only now beginning, but the prospects for rational improvement of normal tissue protection are high. This optimism is based on two facts: (1) the metabolic handling of a given phosphorothioate (and probably other drugs) varies widely among normal tissues, and (2) in a given tissue, different phosphorothioates are handled differently. As an example of the former, Harris and Phillips[7] reported a 15-fold range in the rate at which normal tissues dephosphorylate WR-2721. Further, the pH optima for dephosphorylating WR-638 has been reported to be 7 for brain but 5.7 for erythrocytes.[2,3] Relative to the latter point, the pH optima for dephosphorylation of WR-2721 and WR-638 can differ widely within a single tissue,[7] and the relative amounts of drug which a given organ absorbs can vary widely depending on the specific phosphorothioate injected.[9,14,18]

In summary, although WR-2721 is the most effective agent reported to date for protecting murine hematopoietic tissues against radiation injury, it does not necessarily follow that this drug will be the most efficient radioprotector of other tissues. There would appear to be significant variation in tissue response and drug behavior to merit an attempt to develop specific drugs for specific tissues.

An Expanded Role for WR-2721

Once it was apparent that WR-2721 was being actively concentrated by normal tissues but not by tumors (Fig. 1), we initiated

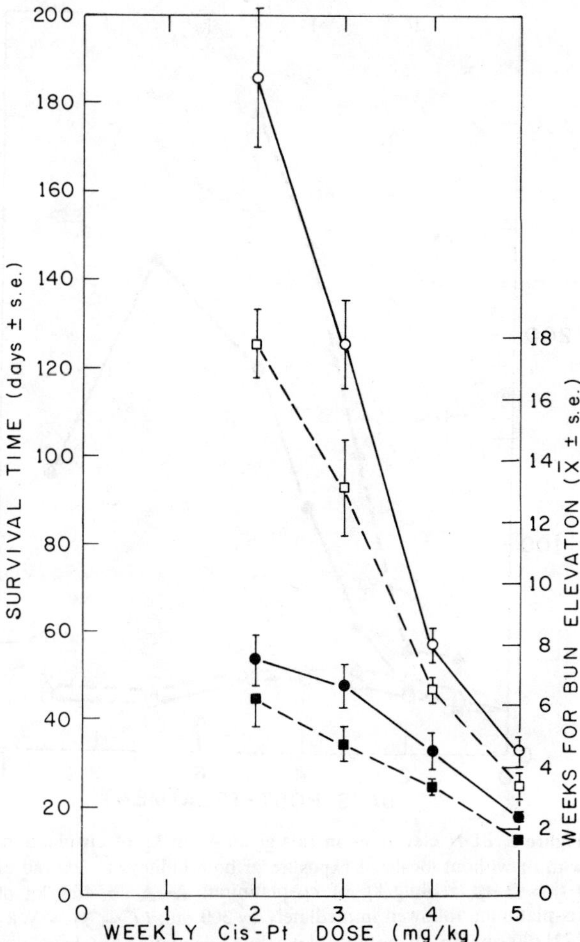

Figure 4. Mean number of weeks before the BUN surpassed 40 mg/ 100 ml and mean survival time for rats receiving weekly doses of 2 – 5 mg/kg of *cis*-platinum. Circles represent mean survival time and squares represent BUN elevation; open symbols are for rats given 200 mg/kg of WR-2721 30 minutes before each *cis*-platinum dose and closed symbols are for rats which received no WR-2721 pretreatment.

studies to determine whether WR-2721 might also offer selective normal tissue protection against alkylating agents. It had been established by others that radioprotective drugs also offered protection against alkylating agents,[5] but we neglected this potential application of WR-2721 due to our misunderstanding of its mechanism. If both WR-2721 and the alkylating agent were passively absorbed, their appeared to be little reason for expecting a differential protection. Given, however, the active concentration of WR-2721 by most normal tissues, the potential of WR-2721 in alkylating agent therapy was obvious. Thus far, we have demonstrated that WR-2721 offers selective protection of normal tissues (bone marrow and kidney) against such agents as nitrogen mustard,[17] *cis*-platinum,[21,23] cyclophosphamide,[18,23] and L-phenylalanine mustard.[18] A typical result is plotted in Figure 4 which shows the average time before the appearance of nephrotoxic injury and the mean survival time in rats being given

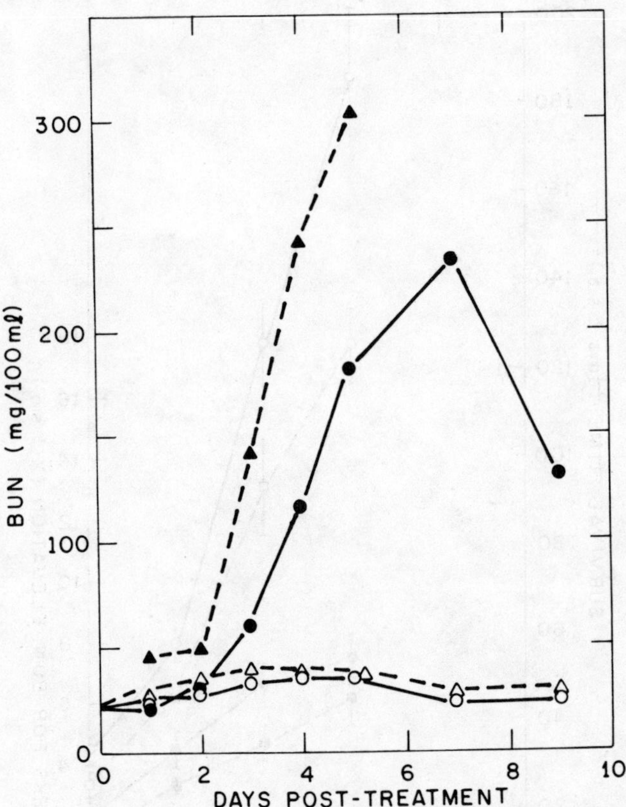

Figure 5. BUN elevations in rats given 4 mg/kg of *cis*-platinum with or without localized exposure of both kidneys to 300 rad of x-rays ●—● ⅔ 4mg/kg of *cis*-platinum; ▲--▲ ⅔ 4mg/kg of cis-platinum, followed immediately by 300 rad; (○—○) = WR-2721 (200 mg/kg), 30 minutes, 4 mg/kg of cis-platinum; (△--△) = WR-2721, 30 minutes, 4 mg/kg of cis-platinum, followed immediately by 300 rad.

weekly doses of 2-5 mg/kg of *cis*-platinum, with or without injection of 200 mg/kg of WR-2721 30 minutes before each treatment. It is quite apparent from these data that WR-2721 is very effective in protecting the rat against the nephrotoxic effects of *cis*-platinum and that under appropriate conditions, the factor increase in resistance can exceed 3.

In none of our studies, however, have we detected protection in five different tumor systems when the animals were given WR-2721 prior to single, five daily, or weekly doses of the agents listed above. The only precaution one must take is that the alkylating agent must be given after protective metabolites have been cleared from the circulation, i.e., 30 minutes later in the mouse.[17]

As might be expected from the fact that WR-2721 protects against ionizing radiation and alkylating agents when they are given singly, it is also effective in selectively protecting normal tissues against the combined effects of these agents.[19] This selective normal tissue protection has been shown in the rat skin versus the 3M2N mammary tumor[19] and in the same tumor considered relative to the kidney (see Fig. 5).

As a last point, one must consider the possibility that WR-2721 might protect micrometastases against alkylating agents and

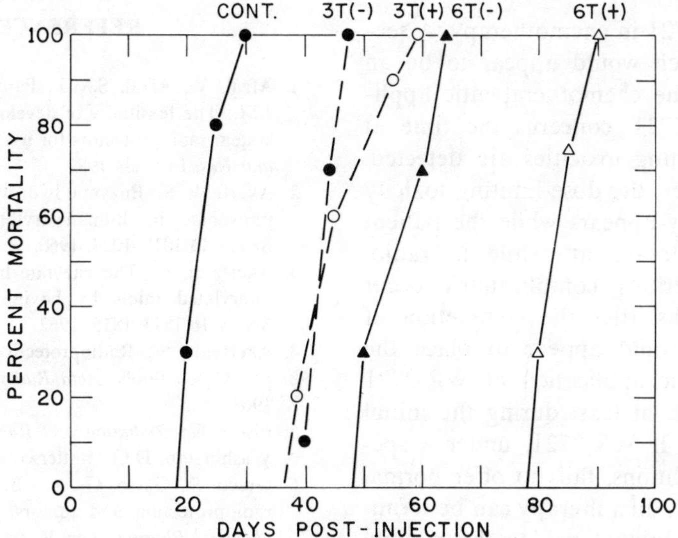

Figure 6. Percent mortality as a function of time after BALB/c mice were given 50,000 line 1 lung carcinoma cells and no further treatment (CONT), 3 weekly i.p. doses of cyclophosphamide starting on day 0, with (3T+) or without an injection of 200 mg/kg of WR-2721 before each CYC dose, or 6 weekly doses of 100 mg/kg of cyclophosphamide starting on day 0, with (6T+) or without (6T–) an injection of 200 mg/kg of WR-2721 before each CYC dose. WR-2721 was given by i.p. injection 30 minutes before cyclophosphamide.

thereby obviate one of the main advantages of combined-modality therapy. This might occur, in spite of the lack of an active concentration process in the micrometastases, simply because they have already access to the circulation and the amount of WR-2721 they absorb passively is sufficient to offer protection. In none of the studies we have performed thus far (e.g., Fig. 6) have we been able to detect protection of artificial micrometastases. We tentatively conclude that this lack of protection results from failure of the micrometastases to absorb protective levels of WR-2721 or that the protective levels they absorb are irrelevant because of the supralethal concentrations of the alkylating agent to which they are exposed.

Prospects for Clinical Application in Radiotherapy and/or Alkylating Agent Chemotherapy

In spite of the relatively large amounts of information which are available on WR-2721, it would be pure speculation to comment on how effective WR-2721 will prove to be in a clinical setting. This will be determined largely by the amount of WR-2721 which can safely be administered in a clinical setting. As pointed out above, the phase I studies being conducted in New Mexico are encouraging in this regard, but we have no idea, as yet, as to how large a dose can be administered or what the chronic toxicity of the drug will be. It should be noted that we have already administered 100 mg/m² weekly for 3 weeks and have observed no detectable toxicity. (M.M. Kligerman and J.M. Yuhas, unpublished observations.)

This raises an interesting point relative to the potential application of WR-2721 in chemotherapy versus radiotherapy. In many instances, chemotherapy is given at weekly to monthly intervals, and even if we find that patients will not tolerate protective levels of WR-2721 on a daily basis, this should not seriously hamper the potential application of WR-2721 in chemotherapy. A second factor, which would appear to be an advantage for the chemotherapeutic application of WR-2721, concerns the time at which dose-limiting toxicities are detected. In most instances, the dose-limiting toxicity in chemotherapy appears while the patient is undergoing treatment, while in radiotherapy the serious complications occur weeks to months after the completion of therapy. This would appear to place the chemotherapeutic application of WR-2721 at an advantage, at least during the initial efficacy testing. If WR-2721, under a specific set of conditions, fails to offer normal tissue protection, then therapy can be terminated at no additional risk to the patient. However, should normal tissue protection be observed, the therapy can be continued beyond the normal period until such time that normal tissue injury appears.

Summary

Largely because we have accumulated so much information on WR-2721 in the past decade, we know that this drug is not a universal panacea which will solve all the problems which confront us. However, in those instances where it would appear applicable, clinical testing would appear appropriate. Thanks largely to the efforts of M.M. Kligerman, these studies have been initiated. In those instances where WR-2721 would appear inappropriate or not of sufficient activity, the information we have already accumulated should point the way to the development of qualitatively and/or quantitatively superior drugs which selectively inhibit host toxicity.

Acknowledgments

Research for this chapter was supported by Grant CA19236 from the National Cancer Institute, National Institute of Health, Department of Health, Education and Welfare.

REFERENCES

1. Afzal, V., Afzal, S.M.J., Pardini, C., and Yuhas, J.M.: The feasibility of developing central nervous system radioprotectors for use in radiotherapy. *Radiat Res*, In press 1982.
2. Akerfeldt, S.: Enzymic hydrolysis of cysteamine-S-phosphate by human erythrocytes. *Acta Chem Scand* **14**:1019–1024, 1960.
3. Akerfeldt, S.: The enzymic hydrolysis of S-phosphorylated thiols by bovine brain. *Acta Chem Scand* **16**:1813–1815, 1962.
4. Akerfeldt, S.: Radioprotective effects of S-phosphorylated thiols. *Acta Radiol* [*Ther*] **L:** 465–470, 1963.
5. Elson, E.: *Radiation and Radiomimetic Chemicals* Washington, D.C.: Butterworth, 1963.
6. Greco, S., Gasso, G., and Billitteri, A.: Chemical radioprotection and tumors. In *Progress in Biochemical Pharmacology* R. Paoletti and R. Vertua, eds. Washington, D.C.: Butterworth, 1965, pp. 277–305.
7. Harris, J.W., and Phillips, T.L.: Radiobiological and biochemical studies of thiophosphate radioprotective compounds related to cysteamine. *Radiat Res* **46**:362–379, 1971.
8. Kligerman, M.M., Shaw, M.T., Slavik, M., and Yuhas, J.M.: Phase I clinical trials with WR-2721. *Cancer Clin Trials* **4**:469–474, 1981.
9. Kollman, G., Martin, D., and Shapiro, B.: The distribution and metabolism of the radiation protective agent aminopentylaminoethylphosphorothioate in mice. *Radiat Res* **48**:542–550, 1971.
10. Patt, H., Tyree, E.B., and Straube, R.: Cysteine protection against x-irradiation. *Science* **110**:213–215, 1949.
11. Sugahara, T., and Tanaka, Y.: Clinical experiences of chemical radiation protection in radiotherapy in Japan. *Cancer Clin Trials*, in press.
12. Sweeney, T.R.: A survey of compounds from the antiradiation drug development program of the U.S. Army Medical Research and Development Command. US. Government Printing Office, Washington, D.C., 1980.
13. Utley, J., Phillips, T.L., and Kane, L.J.: Differential radioprotection of euoxic and hypoxic mouse mammary tumors by a thiophosphate compound. *Radiology* **110**:213–216, 1974.
14. Washburn, L.C., Carlton, J.E., Hayes, R.L., and Yuhas, J.M.: Distribution of WR-2721 in normal and malignant tissues of mice and rats bearing solid tumors: Dependence on tumor type, drug dose and species. *Radiat Res* **59**:475–483, 1974.
15. Yuhas, J.M.: Biological factors affecting the radioprotective effectiveness of WR-2721: $LD_{50(30)}$ doses. *Radiat Res* **44**;621–628, 1970.
16. Yuhas, J.M.: Misonidazole enhancement of acute and late radiation injury to the rat spinal cord. *Br J Cancer* **40**:161–163, 1979.

17. Yuhas, J.M.: Differential protection of normal and malignant tissues against the cytotoxic effects of mechlorethamine. *Cancer Treat Rep* **63**:971–976, 1979.
18. Yuhas, J.M.: Active versus passive absorption kinetics as the basis for selective protection of normal tissues by WR-2721. *Cancer Res,* **40**:1519–1524, 1980.
19. Yuhas, J.M.: A more general role for WR-2721 in cancer therapy. *Br J Cancer* **41**:832–834, 1980.
20. Yuhas, J.M.: On the potential application of WR-2721 in radiotherapy. In *Radiation-Drug Interactions in Cancer Management* G. Sokol, ed. New York: J. Wiley, pp. 113–136, 1980.
21. Yuhas, J.M., and Culo, F.: Selective inhibition of the nephrotoxicity of cis-platinum by WR-2721 without altering its anti-tumor properties. *Cancer Treat Rep,* **64**:57–64, 1980.
22. Yuhas, J.M., Proctor, J.O., and Smith, L.H,: Some pharmacologic effects of WR-2721: Their importance in toxicity and radioprotection. *Radiat Res* **54**:222–223, 1974.
23. Yuhas, J.M., Spellman, and Jordan, S.W.: Multiple treatment studies with the combination of WR-2721 and *cis*-dichlorodiammineplatinum or cyclophosphamide. *Br J Cancer* **42**:574–585, 1980.
24. Yuhas, J.M., and Storer, J.B.: Chemoprotection against three modes of radiation death in the mouse. *Int J Radiat Biol* **15**:233–238, 1969.
25. Yuhas, J.M., and Storer, J.B.: Differential chemoprotection of normal and malignant tissues. *J Natl Cancer Inst* **42**:331–335, 1969.

CHAPTER 40

Hypoxic-Cell Sensitizers

Stanley Dische, M.D., F.R.C.R.[a]

Misonidazole was first given to a patient as an hypoxic-cell sensitizer in November 1974. We now have experience with over 3000 doses, 4 kg of the drug, and 240 patients. Worldwide experience must now extend to several thousands of patients.

The total dose of misonidazole which may be given is unfortunately limited by drug-induced neurotoxicity, and we have observed this complication in 63 of our 240 patients. Peripheral neuropathy occurred in 28% of those given multiple doses of the drug. We have shown evidence that the incidence of peripheral neuropathy is directly related to the area under the curve of plasma concentration.[5,6] A simple method of calculating this area is to multiply the concentration at 3½ to 4 hours after administration by the half-life of the drug, the latter being derived from the concentration at 3½ to 4 hours and that at 24 hours. The relationship with peripheral neuropathy is clearly shown in an analysis of 76 of our patients who were scheduled to receive misonidazole in six doses to a maximum of 12 g per square meter of surface area over a period of 18 days (see Table 1).

How can we employ this limited dose of misonidazole, which under most conditions should not exceed 12 g per square meter of surface area, to achieve the greatest benefit to a patient undergoing a course of radiotherapy?

First, we can give misonidazole with radiotherapy on a limited number of occasions. Theoretically, the combination of the high drug and radiation dose should lead to considerable advantage over a control group given the same radiotherapy without the drug. We have performed a trial in locally advanced carcinoma of the bronchus in which a total of 60 patients were included. No benefit has been shown; however, in these patients we may well have been dealing with a too-advanced situation for an hypoxic-cell sensitizer to give benefit. We must approach a local eradication of tumor before such a method can yield a betterment of result. Professor Sealy in Cape Town has treated advanced tumors in the oral cavity using the same fractionation and dose of radiation with and without misonidazole. In an interim report, he showed that a margin of benefit developed in the early months following treatment, but that this seemed to be lost by the time 18 months had passed. We must wait for his final report.[9]

Second, as a further means of taking advantage of a high dose of sensitizer and radiation, some have treated patients once weekly with the drug, giving radiotherapy on other days without it. Professor Bleehen in glioblastomas grades III and IV has found no benefit.[1] In Vienna, Kogelnik and his colleagues, with similar patients, using large doses of sensitizer and radiation at the beginning and at the end of a prolonged course of radiotherapy, found that the patients given the drug in an interim analysis seemed to be faring better.[8]

Third, in a further extension of the technique of giving a single dose of sensitizer each week, the RTOG in the United States

[a]Marie Curie Research Wing for Oncology, Regional Radiotherapy Centre, Mount Vernon Hospital, Northwood, Middlesex, England

TABLE 1. Mount Vernon Misonidazole Study—Plasma Concentration and Peripheral Neuropathy in 74 Patients Scheduled for 6 Doses on the Basis of 12 g/Square Meter of Surface Area

	Neuropathy		
	Yes—23 Mean and S.D.	No—51 Mean and S.D.	*p*
Total Dose (g)	17.8 (3.0)	17.5 (3.0)	0.7
Plateau Level (μg/ml)	69.8 (5.8)	64.2 (8.5)	0.005
Half-Life (hours)	14.2 (3.2)	12.8 (2.2)	0.04
Exposure (Plateau Level × Half-Life)	58.6 (15.0)	48.1 (10.2)	0.001

and Bataini in Paris, working with head and neck tumors, give radiotherapy twice on the day the sensitizer is given and also again early on the following day when appreciable concentrations may still be present in the tumor. Two further radiation treatments are given later in the same week without the drug. A dose in excess of 12 g per square meter of surface area may be given with safety when a once-a-week administration is extended over a period of 7 or 8 weeks. Bataini has described, in an interim assessment of patients with advanced oral cancer, a margin of benefit in those given the drug (personal communication).

Fourth, multiple treatments can be given when doses of sensitizer are given on more than 1 day of the week. In this way all, or a great part, of the course of radiotherapy can be given with sensitizer. So far, pilot studies and interim reports of trials concerned with head and neck, bladder, and brain tumors in European centers have yielded results which are considered promising.

Finally, sensitizer can be given with every treatment in a conventional course of radiotherapy. This is the form of application most generally under test in the United Kingdom. However, only modest sensitizing concentrations may be achieved in the tumor on each occasion. In our own center, small trials in carcinoma of breast and bladder have so far shown no benefit to misonidazole; but in a pilot study in 10 patients with advanced carcinoma of cervix, all showed complete regression of tumor by the time treatment was concluded—a most promising prognostic sign, as was shown in our previous experience with hyperbaric oxygen.

In order to give a higher dose on each treatment day, some give the drug with every treatment in the first 2 and the last 2 weeks of a course of radiotherapy which is extended over 6 or 7 weeks, and there have been reports of benefit in the early stages of trials in pharyngeal cancer. In other trials the drug is given either in the first few weeks of treatment or in the final weeks.

We have all seen remarkable responses when the drug has been given, but experience tells us how fallacious is an assessment entirely based on such case experience. We must await the results of the randomized controlled studies underway. There is no doubt some disappointment that so far no clear benefit has been shown in any one study. One has the impression that trends toward benefit are most often observed when most of a multifraction course of radiotherapy is given under conditions where the highest concentration of sensitizer is present.

We must consider the extent to which hypoxic tumor cells are being sensitized with misonidazole given in the various ways described. With Professor Adams and other colleagues, we presented a relationship between the concentration of radiosensitizer and enhancement ratio derived from *in vitro* experiments but supported by our work with hypoxic skin in humans.[6] Based on 742

TABLE 2. Plateau Plasma and Levels in Hypoxic Tumor Cells[a]

Fractionation	Dose g/m²	Plateau Plasma Concentration		Probable Levels in Hypoxic Tumor Cells	
		μg/ml	Enhancement	μg/g	Enhancement
6	2.0	80	1.65	40	1.50
10	1.2	50	1.55	25	1.40
20	0.6	24	1.40	12	1.20
24	0.5	20	1.35	10	1.20
30	0.4	16	1.25	8	1.15

[a]Plateau plasma and levels in hypoxic tumor cells if 50% of the plasma concentration is achieved when misonidazole is given in different fractionation regimes using the dose limit of 12 g per square meter of surface area; enhancement ratios for hypoxic cells relating to the concentrations achieved.

observations we have calculated that a dose of 1 g per square meter of surface area will give approximately 40 μg/ml in the plasma at the usual time of treatment, 3½ to 4 hours after administration. With this figure we can relate the curve of radiosensitization and enhancement ratio to the actual plasma concentration (see Table 2).

We know that in the majority of cases, however, tumor concentrations lie between 60 and 100% of the plasma concentrations at the time the sample is taken. The concentration of misonidazole in necrotic tissue is generally low. This may be of academic interest only or it may give us some indication as to the depth to which a drug will penetrate in viable tumor. Whatever the situation, it seems more realistic to consider that the hypoxic tumor cells contain a concentration of approximately 50% of that in the plasma at the time radiotherapy is given. If we look again at the concentration of sensitizer with enhancement ratio of hypoxic cells (Table 2) we can see that under most conditions of delivery of the drug we are at low levels of enhancement of response. It seems quite possible that with the present schemes of radiotherapy with misonidazole we may only show benefit in those situations where, using conventional radiotherapy, radioresistant hypoxic cells are the strongly dominant cause for failure. Such conditions may apply in head and neck tumors and in squamous carcinoma of the cervix, as the experience with hyperbaric oxygen would suggest.[3]

We need to be able to combine the hypoxic cell sensitizer safely with conventional radiotherapy and obtain enhancements toward the upper end of the steep part of the curve relating concentration with enhancement ratio. We would like to achieve enhancement ratios of 1.5 or 1.6 in the hypoxic cells in tumors. To do this we must obtain radiosensitizing levels several times greater than those presently being achieved with misonidazole.

Our colleagues in radiobiology are working hard to produce new drugs which may achieve this. Much attention has been given to the nitroimidazoles which have low lipophilicity and which combine a shorter half-life with a lower uptake in nervous tissue.[2] We have long been interested in desmethylmisonidazole since learning of reports of lower neurotoxicity in dogs some 4 years ago. In January 1980, due to the kind cooperation of Roche Products Ltd., we were able to administer some of this drug to normal volunteers and found that despite predictions to the contrary it was well absorbed, peak concentrations being 80% of those with misonidazole when equal amounts of the two drugs were given. The drug is cleared from the plasma at twice the rate of misonidazole and double the quantity is excreted in the urine in the first 24 hours.[4]

A study of tumor concentration and cerebrospinal fluid concentrations in patients has now been completed.[7] The area under the curve of CSF concentration is approximately one-third of that with misonidazole. The risk of central neurotoxicity should therefore be one-third of that with misonidazole. We do not know whether these levels in CSF give an indication of the uptake in peripheral nerve, but the curve of plasma concentrations in patients give an area under the curve of 55% of that under the area under the curve of misonidazole concentration. Therefore, we should at least be able to double the amount which we can safely give.

We have found that good concentrations of the drug are achieved in tumors. The optimum time for treatment may be at 90 minutes after administration compared with 3½ hours for misonidazole. At 90 minutes there is very little concentration in the CSF, and so there should be no enhancement of radiation response in normal brain cells that may be hypoxic. The ratio of tumor to plasma concentration seen in tumor samples, which histologically show no evidence for necrosis, is 0.83 for desmethylmisonidazole compared with 0.82 for misonidazole. In the presence of gross necrosis in tumor samples there is a tendency for higher concentrations of desmethylmisonidazole to be present. As in laboratory experiments equimolar concentrations of the two drugs are equal in effectiveness as hypoxic-cell radiosensitizers, and as desmethylmisonidazole has a smaller molecule we can expect a 7% advanatage to desmethylmisonidazole when using equal quantities of the two drugs. Taking all factors into consideration, it seems likely we will obtain equal radiosensitization with desmethylmisonidazole compared with misonidazole when a similar dose by weight is given.

There are, therefore, reasonable grounds for optimism that desmethylmisonidazole will take us at least part of the way toward the levels of sensitization of hypoxic cells which we require if in clinical practice such drugs can be expected to make a major contribution. We hope that with newer drugs we will do better. With desmethylmisonidazole the future use depends upon the toxilogical studies now underway in man in which multiple doses of the drug are being given.

No measure other than hypoxic-cell sensitizers, when tested in the whole range of animal tumors, has shown such consistent improvement in response to radiotherapy. We hope that this great promise will be realized in man, for any benefit obtained may be added to all existing techniques of radiotherapy and be employed in every center for treatment throughout the world, regardless of size or affluence.

Summary

There is now 6 years of clinical experience with misonidazole as a hypoxic-cell sensitizer. Neurotoxicity limits the total dose which may be given, and so relatively low concentrations of radiosensitizing drugs are likely to be achieved in hypoxic cells in man as compared with those in animal tumors. It is likely that benefit will only be shown in those situations where radioresistant hypoxic cells strongly dominate as a cause of radiation failure. Many clinical trials are underway, and thus far some show no benefit while in others there is a definite advantage to the patients given the drug. These trials must be continued to their conclusion, but misonidazole must be regarded as the first of a series of radiosensitizers to reach the clinic for trial. There is a promise of more effective drugs becoming available within the next few years. Those showing a lower lipophilicity than misonidazole have been found to have a shorter half-life and a lower uptake in neural tissue in animal studies. One such drug, desmethylmisonidazole, is presently undergoing clinical trial.

REFERENCES

1. Bleehen, N.M.: The Cambridge glioma trial misonidazole and radiation therapy with associated pharmacokinetic studies. *Cancer Clin Trials*, submitted 1980.
2. Brown, J.M., and Workman, P.: Partition co-efficient as a guide to the development of radiosensitizers which are less toxic than misonidazole. *Radiat Res* **82**:171–190, 1980.
3. Dische, S.: Hyperbaric oxygen. The Medical Research Council trials and their clinical significance. *Br J Radiol* **51**:888–894, 1978.
4. Dische, S., Saunders, M.I., Anderson, P., Lee, M., Fowler, J.F., Stratford, M., and Minchinton, A.: A drug for improved radiosensitization in radiotherapy. *Br J Cancer* **42**:153–155, 1980.
5. Dische, S., Saunders, M.I., Flockhart, I.R., Lee, M.E., and Anderson, P.: Misonidazole. A drug for trial in radiotherapy and oncology. *Int J Radiat Oncol Biol Phys* **5**:851–860, 1979.
6. Dische, S., Saunders, M.I., Lee, M.E., Adams, G.E., and Flockhart, I.R.: Clinical testing of the radiosensitizer Ro 07-0582: Experience with multiple doses. *Br J Cancer* **35**:567–579, 1977.
7. Dische, S., Saunders, M.I., Riley, P.J., Hauck, J., Bennett, M.H., Stratford, M.R.L., and Minchinton, A.I.: The concentration of desmethylmisonidazole in human tumours and in cerebro-spinal fluid. *Br J Cancer*, submitted 1980.
8. Kogelnik, H.D.: Clinical experience with misonidazole. High dose fractions versus daily low doses. *Cancer Clin Trials* **3**:179, 1980.
9. Sealy, R., Williams, A., Cridland, S., Stratford, M., Minchinton, A. and Hallet, C.: A report on misonidazole in a randomized trial in locally advanced head and neck cancer. *Int J Radiat Oncol Biol Phys* **8**:339–342, 1982.

CHAPTER 41

Hyperthermic Modification of the Radiation Response in Solid Tumors

Jens Overgaard, M.D.[a]

Among the different aspects of hyperthermic cancer therapy, the potential use of hyperthermia as an adjuvant to radiation therapy has been the most widely studied. The current role of hyperthermia in clinical cancer treatment appears most attractive with such a combined treatment. Naturally, most work on hyperthermia and radiation has been performed in experimental systems, but hyperthermic treatment equipment for clinical use has recently been developed more successfully. Consequently, more attention has been given to clinical phase 1 and 2 studies which have supplied us with early information about the effect of local hyperthermia in malignant and normal tissues in man.

Biological Bases for the Hyperthermic Modification of Radiation Response in Solid Tumors

The interaction between hyperthermia and radiation is complex and involves two principally different mechanisms: (1) a hyperthermic radiosensitization, and (2) a direct hyperthermic cytotoxicity against radioresistant tumor cells (see Table 1). There are several reasons why adjuvant hyperthermic treatment may be used to overcome the radioresistance of solid tumors. The following shortly describes the interaction between heat and radiation.

[a]Senior Research Fellow in Experimental Radiotherapy and Oncology, The Institute of Cancer Research, Radiumstationen, Aarhus, Denmark

HYPERTHERMIC RADIOSENSITIZATION

The interaction between heat and radiation manifests itself in several ways. Among the most important are: (1) direct radiosensitization (a decreased D_o), (2) decreased repair of sublethal and potentially lethal damage, and (3) sensitization of cells in relatively radioresistant phases of the cell cycle (e.g., late S phase).[6,11,36,38,41,52] Furthermore, heat has been reported to sensitize hypoxic cells more than oxygenated cells, thus causing a decreased oxygen enhancement ratio. However, the data supporting such preferentially hypoxic radiosensitization are ambigious.[11,36,38,52]

The magnitude of hyperthermic radiosensitization depends on the time interval between the two modalities. In general, the maximum sensitization occurs after simultaneous treatment.[6,38,41] The hyperthermic radiosensitization further depends on the temperature and the treatment time in that an increase in either produces an increase of the thermal enhancement–the temperature probably being the most critical of these two factors.[38] Experimental studies in animal tumors indicate that if a simultaneous treatment is applied, the thermal enhancement ratio (TER) approximately doubled for each degree of increased treatment temperature (see Fig. 1). Unfortunately, the hyperthermic radiosensitization seems to be of the same magnitude in both tumor and normal tissues (Fig. 1), and if both tumor and critical surrounding tissue is heated to the same temperature an improvement of the therapeutic effect is unlikely to result. This im-

TABLE 1. Phenotype of Second-Step Mutants from Adriamycin-Resistant cells

A. Hyperthermic Radiosensitization (Maximal with Simultaneous Treatment)
   1. direct radiosensitization (decreased D_o)
   2. reduced repair of sublethal damage
   3. increased sensitivity of cells in radioresistant phases of the cell cycle
   4. reduced repair of potential lethal damage
   5. (decreased OER?)

B. Hyperthermic Cytotoxicity (Independent of Sequence and Interval)
   1. nutritional deprivation
   2. chronic hypoxia
   3. acidity (most important)

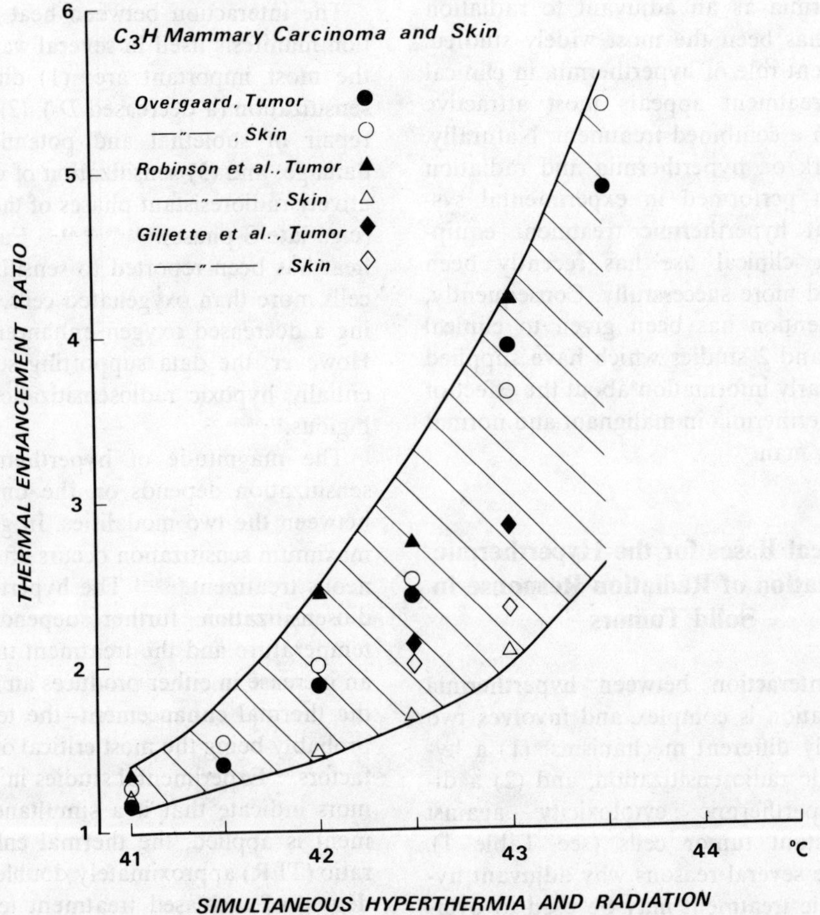

Figure 1. Thermal enhancement ratios for tumors and skin radiated simultaneously with a 1-hour heat treatment. (From Gillette and Ensley,[13] Overgaard[38] Robinson et et al.,[46])

plies that a clinical utilization of the hyperthermic radiosensitization is only suitable if a tumor can be heated to a temperature higher than that of the surrounding tissue, or if radiation is given to the tumor only (e.g., by an implant).[27] Although the current heating technique is far from sufficient in this regard, there are indications that heat treatment itself may cause collapse of the microvascularization especially in central areas of the tumor, whereas it will result in an increased blood flow in the surrounding normal tissue.[8,47] This, in turn, tends to create a temperature difference, the higher temperature being in the tumor center.[51] Under such conditions it is likely that an improved therapeutic effect can be observed as a result of the steep temperature gradient of the hyperthermic radiosensitization.

The fact that both normal tissue and tumors are sensitized to the same degree despite differences in proliferation kinetics and oxygen status makes it reasonable to assume that the direct radiosensitization and the reduced accumulation of sublethal damage carry the main responsibility for the hyperthermic radiosensitization.

CYTOTOXIC EFFECT OF HYPERTHERMIA

Hyperthermia alone is also directly cytotoxic to malignant cells and may with an acceptable degree of normal tissue damage control some experimental tumors.[6,36,44] This cytotoxicity is strongly enhanced under certain environmental conditions. Cells situated in an environment characterized by insufficient nutrition, chronic hypoxia, and increased acidity, which is typically found in large areas in poorly vascularized tumors, are considerably more vulnerable to hyperthermic destruction than are similar cells kept under physiological conditions.[7,11,36,41,44,52] Hyperthermia may, furthermore, enhance these environmental conditions in that it alters the tumor cell metabolism[4,35] and reduces the blood flow.[3,8,47] This implies that a moderate heat treatment almost selectively is able to destroy a large proportion of the clonogenic cells situated in a chronic hypoxic environment.[43,44] The fact that such heat-sensitive hypoxic cells may be the most radioresistant probably indirectly influences the response to the combined heat and radiation treatment. Thus, a smaller radiation dose may be adequate to secure control of the remaining viable cells which are relatively heat resistant but at the same time radiosensitive due to their localization in a well-oxygenated and more physiological environment.[38,41]

This hyperthermic cytotoxicity probably has no well-defined time relationship with the radiation treatment. As the hyperthermic cytotoxicity probably represents the only modality by which a major radioresistant tumor cell population can be destroyed selectively, it may have great potential implications for the problem of overcoming the radioresistance in large solid tumors. This is illustrated in Figure 2, which shows the absolute number of oxygenated clonogenic tumor cells in an experimental tumor following exposure to a 1-hour hyperthermic treatment at different temperatures. The presence of a selective heat-induced destruction of cells in poorly vascularized tumor areas has also become apparent in morphological studies and from experiments in which the tumor environment has been changed due to clamping.[15,44] Although several environmental conditions, including insufficient nutrition, low proliferation, hypoxia, and increased acidity, are known to enhance the hyperthermic cell killing, the latter appears to carry the main responsibility for the increased heat sensitivity, and the other conditions may mainly act indirectly, changing the metabolism to a more acidic type.[41,44,52] Poor vascularization in such areas may tend to increase accumulation of acidic metabolic products as well.

Importance of Sequence and Interval for the Therapeutic Gain Obtained by Combined Radiation and Heat Treatment

Consideration of the two different types of interaction between heat and radiation and their different time relationship makes it natural to ask the question: How should heat and radiation be applied in order to obtain the optimal therapeutic effect?

Recently, several investigators have focused on this problem and they seem to agree on the conclusions unanimously; max-

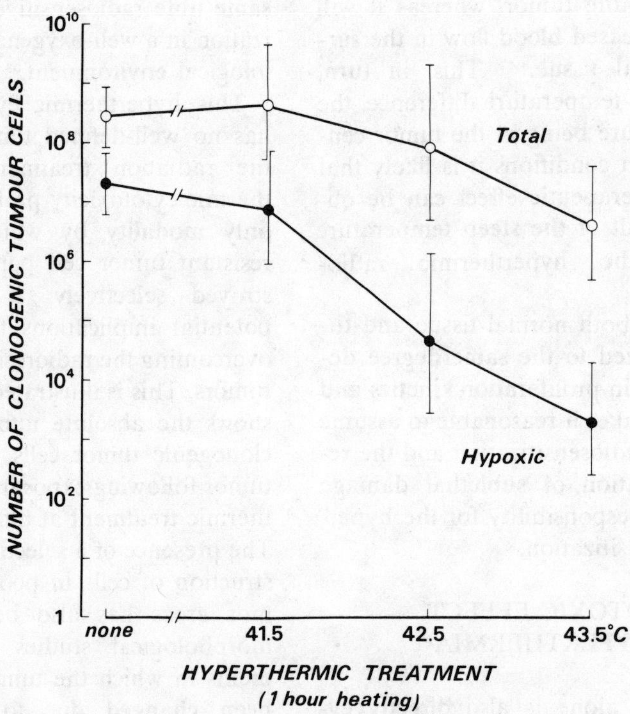

Figure 2. Estimated values of absolute numbers of clonogenic cells in a C3H mammary tumor as a function of different heat treatment. Hyperthermia destroy preferential hypoxic cells, resulting in a reduced hypoxic fraction after heat treatment. (From Overgaard, in press (d).)

imal thermal enhancement ratios are obtained when radiation and hyperthermia is applied simultaneously.[11,13,16,23,38,41,48,49] The enhancement depends both on the heating time and especially on the treatment temperature. Any time interval between the two modalities tends to decrease the thermal enhancement, but the TER values in both tumors and different normal tissues are within the same range if the treatment is given either simultaneously or applied within intervals of a few minutes. Therefore, it is unlikely that simultaneous treatment results in an improvement of the therapeutic gain if both tumor and surrounding normal tissues are heated to the same degree. If a preferential tumor-heating can be achieved an improved therapeutic effect can be expected, and the magnitude will depend on the temperature difference between the tumor and the surrounding tissue.[38,41]

The introduction of an interval between the two modalities decreases the thermal enhancement ratio to a different extent in tumors and normal tissues.

In the tumor the decrease is independent of the sequence between heat and radiation. However, the TER decreases gradually with intervals up to 4 hours after which it reaches a plateau with a constantly enhanced TER value which depends on the temperature and heating time applied (see Fig. 3).[13,16,38,41,49] This plateau level seems to last for at least 24 hours.

The normal tissue response is dependent on the sequence.[11,13,23,31,38,41,48] When hyperthermia is given before radiation the TER values decrease as time intervals are increased; but it appears that a prolonged thermal enhancement results in most normal tissues when heat is given before radiation (see Fig. 4), and the level of this enhancement is within the same range as that observed in tumors given a similar treatment. A therapeutic advantage is therefore not obtained with this sequence. If hy-

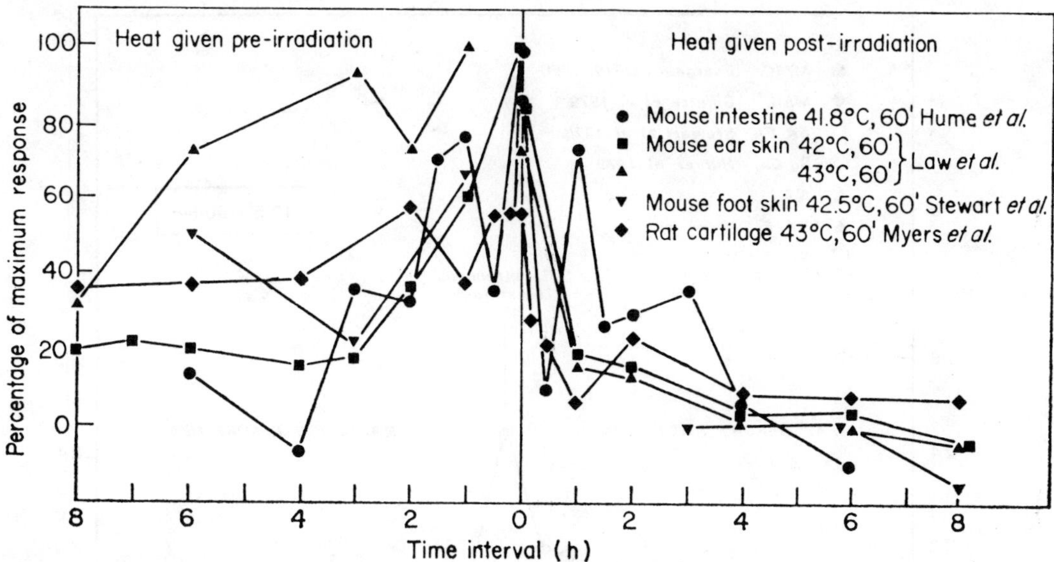

Figure 3. The time course of decay of heat potentiation of radiation damage in different normal tissues for hyperthermia given either before or after irradiation. The TER values have been normalized to the percentage of the maximum response for each curve. Heat preceding radiation causes a longer and higher thermal enhancement than when heat is given after radiation. For this sequence there is no thermal enhancement with split intervals greater than 4 hours. (From Field and Bleehan, 1979.[11])

perthermia is applied *after* radiation, all normal tissue systems show a rapid decrease in the TER, and no thermal enhancement is observed in normal tissues when intervals between the two modalities exceed 3 - 4 hours. This contrasts with the tumor response which after a similar treatment has a persistent increase in TER, thereby affecting the therapeutic effect.[13,16,38,41,50] In an experimental system where tumor and normal tissues are heated to the same degree, the therapeutic gain factor will gradually increase with increasing intervals between radiation and hyperthermia, reaching a maximum plateau level after 3 - 4 hours (see Fig. 5). The magnitude of this therapeutic gain factor is dependent of the hyperthermic treatment[38] and can be explained as a consequence of the hyperthermic cytotoxic destruction of radioresistant tumor cells.

Fractionated Heat and Radiation Treatment

There are only few experimental studies of the effect of fractionated hyperthermia and radiation.[12,22,39,42,50] Despite some variation in the results from different experimental systems, it is likely that fractionated treatment schedules will yield TER values in both tumor and normal tissues similar to those observed after a single treatment (see Fig. 6). However, there are several unsolved problems related to this treatment. Most important is whether the heat-induced temporary resistance to a subsequent hyperthermic treatment (thermal tolerance)[10] influences the interaction between heat and radiation. Although there are indications of such an influence, the magnitude of this may be rather small.[22,24,33] However, it is clearly a subject which deserves further attention in order to outline the optimal fractionation schedules. The fractionation interval is important if heat is given 3 - 4 hours after radiation (sequential treatment). Since the opposite sequence results in normal tissue enhancement, persisting for a long period, it is necessary to use fraction intervals not shorter than about 3 days to avoid enhancement of normal tissue damage (i.e., heat treatment from the previous fraction enhances the radiation effect of the

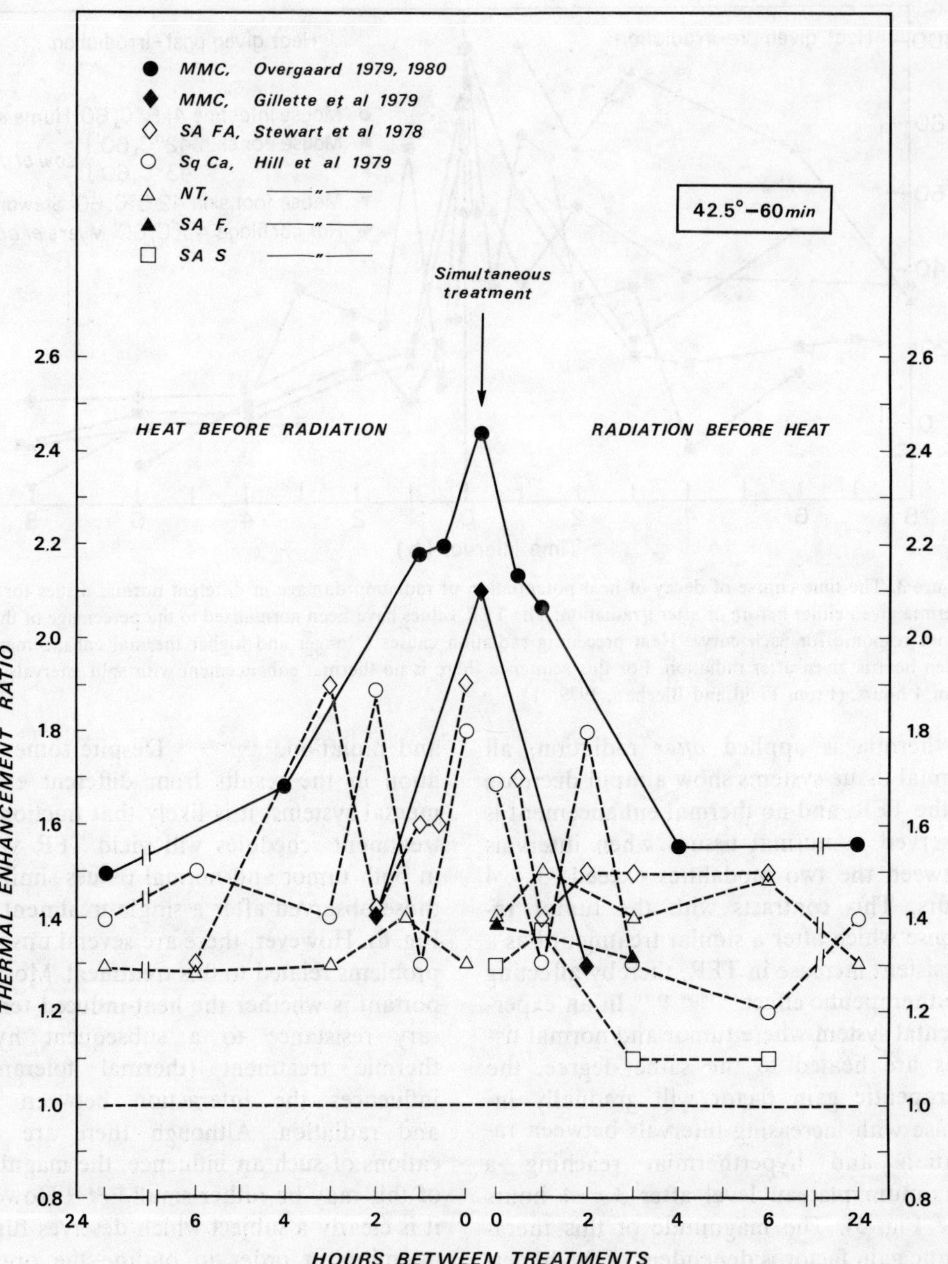

Figure 4. Thermal enhancement ratio as a function of time interval and sequence between hyperthermia (42.5°C for 1 hour) and radiation in different tumors. Maximal TER values are observed with simultaneous or immediate application between the modalities, and the TER is reduced with increasing intervals after about 4 hours. In all tumors but one there was a persistent thermal enhancement for intervals greater than 4 hours with maximal TER values in the range of 1.3 to 1.5, independent of the sequence. True simultaneous treatment (solid lines) apparently causes a higher TER than treatment with close applications between the modalities (dashed lines). (From Field and Ensley, 1979; Hill and Denekamp, 1979;[15] Overgaard, 1980a;[38] Stewart and Denekamp, 1978.[49])

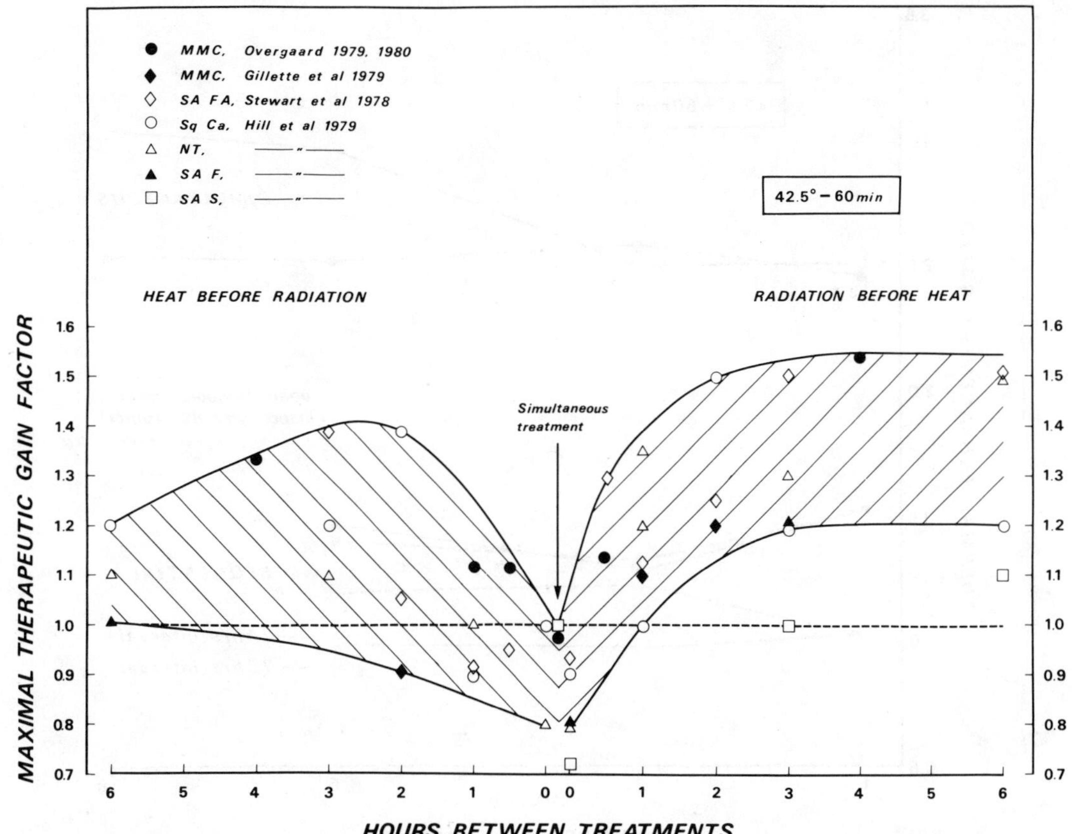

Figure 5. Maximal therapeutic gain factor as a function of time interval between radiation and hyperthermia (42.5°C/min). The figure is a survey of studies where tumor and normal tissues have been compared. Heat treatment given simultaneously or immediately before or after radiation causes no significant increase in therapeutic effect. Increased TGF is obtained with increasing intervals when radiation is given before heat. This effect reaches a plateau with split intervals longer than 3 to 4 hours with TGF values between 1.2 and 1.6. The only exception to this was the slow-growing sarcoma (SA S). (From Field and Ensley, 1979; Hill and Denekamp, 1978;[14] Overgaard, 1980a;[58] Stewart and Denekamp, 1978.[49])

subsequent fraction).[39,40,42] However, experiments suggest that a single large hyperthermic treatment given after multiple radiation fractions may yield the same results as if the heat treatment were given in connection with all radiation fractions.[40,42]

Implications for Clinical Treatment Based on Experimental Observations

The design of schedules for combined heat and radiation treatment is linked to the technical problems of heat application and temperature measurements. At present, the difficulties in applying a well-defined and homogeneous local heating selectively to a tumor area appears to be the greatest hurdle to a useful application of clinical hyperthermia.[18,21,30,37,40,51,53]

However, assuming that such selective tumor heating can be obtained, the optimal therapeutic effect is achieved by way of simultaneous treatment utilizing the direct hyperthermic radiosensitization. Such treatment should be given at the highest possible temperature. Since one of the main effects of heat in this situation is reduced repair of radiation damage, it is important to apply

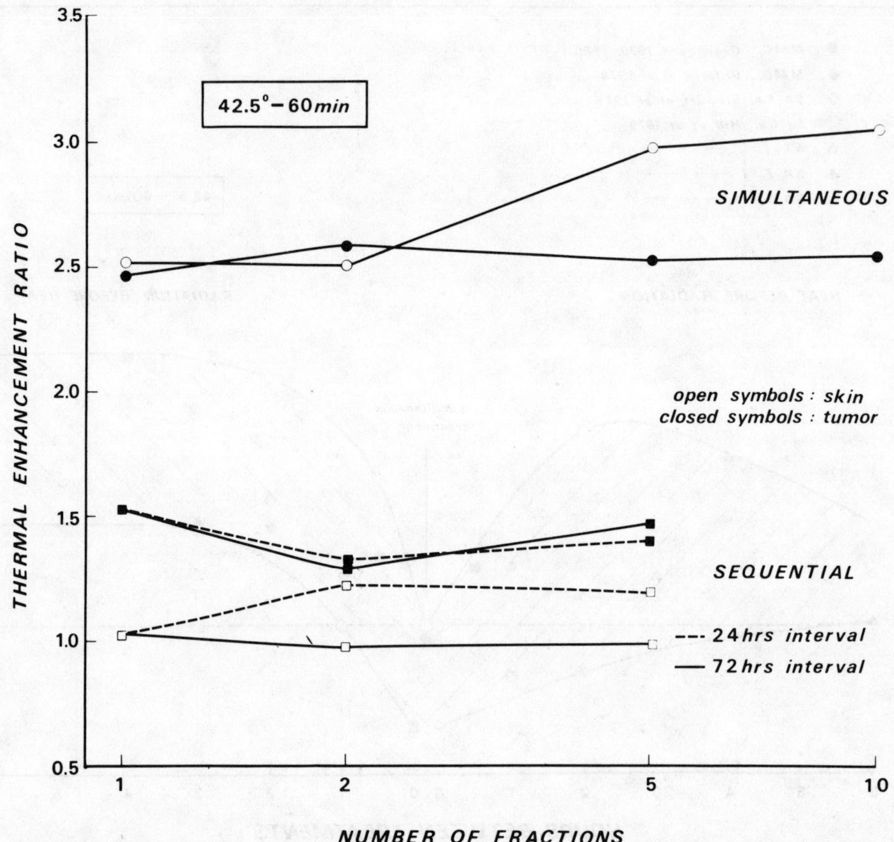

Figure 6. Effect on TER of fractionated hyperthermia and radiation in a C3H mammary carcinoma and its surrounding skin. Heat treatment was given either simultaneously or sequentially (4 hours after radiation) with all radiation fractions. No significant difference in tumor TER was observed as the number of fractions was increased. In the skin the TER slightly increased with increasing number of fractionated simultaneous treatment. With sequential treatment a moderate increase in the skin TER was observed with fractionation intervals of 24 hours. With intervals of 72 hours any thermal enhancement in normal tissue was avoided. (From Overgaard, in press (b) and (c).[40,41])

hyperthermia together with each radiation fraction.[42]

Although it is doubtful whether such treatment is currently feasible, the differential changes in the vascular pattern between tumor and surrounding tissue, which occur during heating of especially large tumors,[47,51] may result in a semiselective tumor-heating. Due to a collapse of the microvasculature and a reduced tumor blood flow,[38,47] more heat may be accumulated in the tumor area, whereas the increased blood flow in the surrounding normal tissue may tend to cool this, thus creating a temperature difference. Unfortunately, it is difficult to predict in which tumors such differential heating changes will occur, and a definitive rationale of such therapy requires further knowledge about the effect of hyperthermia on blood flow.

If a preferential tumor-heating cannot be obtained, the treatment rationale should be based on a sequential application of radiation and heat which utilizes the hyperthermic cytotoxic destruction of the nutritionally deprived, acidic, and chronically hypoxic radioresistant tumor cells. Such treatment should avoid the direct hyperthermic radiosensitization, and therefore it must be given with a sequence in which radiation is applied more than 3 - 4 hours before hyperthermia. With such a schedule, no thermal enhancement of normal tissue is likely to occur, and due to the selective destruction of radioresistant tumor cells, an improved therapeutic gain may result. The magnitude of the heat treatment in such a schedule is limited by the heat tolerance and the involved critical normal tissue; but in most well-vascularized tissues a local heating to about 43°C for 1 hour is normally acceptable. In fractionated schedules it may be applied only in connection with a single or a few radiation fractions. Otherwise it is important to allow a time interval of probably about 3 days between the previous hyperthermic treatment and the subsequent radiation fraction in order to avoid thermal sensitization of the radiation damage in normal tissue.

Clinical Experience

The clinical experience with hyperthermia has accumulated rapidly during the last few years. Thus, during the period 1977–1980 at least 66 studies including more than 3000 patients have been reported (see Table 2). Most studies have applied local hyperthermia given with different techniques, but whole-body hyperthermia and regional limb perfusion have also been used–the latter being an almost-established therapy for malignant melanoma. However, both whole-body and regional heating normally are not applied together with radiotherapy, and therefore this kind of treatment is outside the scope of the present review.

On the contrary, local hyperthermia has most frequently been given in combination with irradiation (Table 2). Most investigations have been phase 1 and 2 studies giving special attention to the technical problems

TABLE 2. Clinical Studies with Hyperthermia, 1977–1980

	Number of Studies	Treatment	Number of Patients
Local Hyperthermia	16	heat alone	605
	15	heat and radiation	717
	1	heat vs. heat and radiation	47
	7	radiation vs. heat and radiation	172
	3	radiation vs. heat and radiation vs heat alone	60
	4	heat with other modalities	87
	46		1688
Regional Hyperthermia	8	heat or heat + chemotherapy	884
Whole-Body Hyperthermia	12	heat or heat + chemotherapy	452
All Studies	66		3024

TABLE 3. Effect of Local Hyperthermia Alone

Reference	Treatment Technique	Number of Patients	Response CR	Response PR	Response NR	Response Rate
Luk, 1980.[26]	2450 mhz 915 mhz	11	1	2	8	27%
Fazekas and Nerlinger, 1980.[9]	2450 mhz	4	1	0	3	25%
Perez et al., 1980.[45]	915 mhz	5	2	0	3	40%
Kim et al., 1977; 1978.[20,21]	27 mhz	19	4	6	9	53%
Marmor et al. 1978; 1979.[28,30]	us	42	5	20	17	60%
U et al., 1980.[53]	915 mhz 2450 mhz	6	0	3	3	50%
Corry et al., 1980.[5]	us	8	1	3	4	50%
Israel and Besenwal, 1980.[19]	13.6 mhz	36	1	13	22	39%
LeVeen et al., 1980.[25]	13.6 mhz	30	2	9	19	37%
Okada et al., 1977.[34]	bladder perfusion	69	15	28	26	62%
Overgaard, 1979; in press (a).[37,40]	bladder perfusion or 27 mhz	11	0	4	7	36%
Hall et al., 1974.[14]	bladder	35	4	19	12	66%
	Total	276	36 (13%)	109 (39%)	133 (48%)	52%

TABLE 4. Effect of Adjuvant Hyperthermia on the Radiation Response in Human Tumors

Study	Number of Patients/Tumors	Frequency of Complete Response: Radiation alone[a]		Radiation[a] + Heat
Arcangeli et al., 1980.[1]	39	47%	→	85%
U et al., 1980.[53]	7	14%	→	85%
Overgaard, in press (a).[40]	22	37%	→	77%
Kim et al., in press.[19]	86	33%	→	80%
Bede et al., 1980.[2]	24	0%	→	9%
Corry et al., 1980.[5]	6	0%	→	40%
Total	186	31%	→	74%

[a] Identical radiation dose in both arms.

of heat delivery and temperature measurements.

Nevertheless, some experience of the tumoricidal effect of hyperthermia alone has been obtained. Table 3 shows that heat alone is able to cause a substantial regression in many tumors which is indicated by an overall response rate of about 50%. However, neither the heating technique nor the given temperature seem to be of any major importance for the response rate. It also appears from the literature that a single treatment may give almost the same response rate as multiple fractions. This certainly has not been investigated sufficiently, but it may suggest that the development of thermal tolerance exists in human tumors as well. The lack of a well-defined time-temperature relationship in the early clinical studies is probably a consequence of a heterogeneous tumor-heating to an often unknown temperature.

The observation that large tumors often respond better than smaller tumors may be of importance.[27] Although this is a preliminary clinical finding, it corresponds to experimental studies[54] and may be due to the fact that larger tumors in great areas have an environment dominated by increased acidity and nutritional deprivation.[3] A further indication to use hyperthermia in the treatment of large solid tumors may be their ability to reach a relatively higher temperature[51] due to a collapse of the microvasculature.Thus, the term "big is beautiful" may apply to hyperthermic treatment.

Despite the relatively high response rate induced by heat alone, a complete tumor control is rare, and this makes it reasonable to conclude that, generally, local hyperthermia alone is not a feasible modality.

Many investigators, therefore, combine hyperthermia with radiation. Unfortunately, most of these studies have not been elaborated in a way that permits comparison between the effect of radiation alone and a combined heat and radiation treatment. Therefore, most experience on combined heat and radiation treatment cannot be utilized to illustrate the potential beneficial effect of adjuvant hyperthermic treatment but only to provide an understanding of the technical applicability of such combined treatment. So far, only a few studies have been able to give significant information about potential hyperthermic radiosensitization.[1,2,18,19,29,37,40,45] In these studies comparable lesions have been treated with either radiation alone or combined heat and radiation. Although the number and size of heat and radiation fractions as well as the sequence and interval between the two modalities differ, a remarkable heat improvement of the radiation response has been achieved (see Table 4). In most of these studies hyperthermia has been given either

TABLE 5. Effect of Hyperthermia (43°C/30 min) Given Simultaneously or Sequentially with Radiation to Malignant Melanoma Metastases[f]

Response	Radiation Alone			Simultaneous Treatment			Sequential Treatment		
	Dose/Fraction[a] (Gy)	TER[d]	TGF[e]	Dose/Fraction[a] (Gy)	TER	TGF	Dose/Fraction[a] (Gy)	TER	TGF
Tumor (cr in 50% of treated tumors)	8.8	—	—	6.1	1.44	1.10	6.7	1.31	1.30
Skin (marked erythema in)	8.5	—		6.5	1.31		8.4	1.01	

[a] Three fractions in 7 days.
[b] Heat immediately after radiation.
[c] Heat 3 to 4 hours after radiation.
[d] TER: Thermal Enhancement Ratio.
[e] TGF: Therapeutic Gain Factor.
[f] Data from Overgaard, 1979; in press (a).[37,40]

immediately before or after radiation, and it is therefore, interesting to note that some investigators describe a very moderate enhancement of the radiation damage to the normal tissue contrary to what would have been expected from animal studies. A likely explanation of this is that the heat has been distributed predominantly to the tumor area while the overlaying skin has been cooled actively during the heating. Therefore, the observation neither presents a biological difference between mice and men, nor gives a proper answer to the question whether or not a close sequence between heat and radiation always enhances normal tissue response. It does indicate, however, that higher tumor temperatures can be achieved in the treatment of superficial tumors. The only study in which sequential and simultaneous heat and radiation have been compared[40] showed that, although a higher TER was observed in the tumor after simultaneous treatment, a similar enhancement occurred in the noncooled overlaying skin as well, which resulted in a small therapeutic gain factor (see Table 5). A sequential heat treatment given 3 – 4 hours after radiation also caused an improved thermal enhancement in the tumor without causing any heat-induced radiation damage to the skin, thus securing a higher therapeutic gain factor. Consequently, this study confirms the observations of experimental systems and indicates that, if heat and radiation were applied with close time intervals, an enhanced radiation response would be likely to occur in the heated normal tissue, an observation which is in accordance with recently published data.[18,29] This is especially important if the radiation dose approximates the tolerance level. More studies are needed to clarify whether a sequential heating schedule should be recommended or if the heating technique and the heat-induced alterations in the microvascularization may allow us to use a simultaneous application due to a preferential tumor-heating. Although the latter certainly is the most attractive and produces the highest thermal enhancement ratios, the present technique and biological knowledge is not sufficiently developed to recommend such treatment.

In conclusion, recent years have provided abundant experimental experience and numerous early clinical studies indicating that adjuvant hyperthermic treatment can be applied to human tumors, significantly improving the radiation response. Further development of heating technique and temperature measurements, as well as improved knowledge of the physiological changes induced by hyperthermia, is needed before heat can be more widely introduced as an adjuvant to radiation therapy.

Summary

There are several reasons why adjuvant hyperthermic treatment may have a great potential in overcoming the radioresistance of solid tumors.

First, heat has a radiosensitizing effect. This is most prominent with a simultaneous application of heat and radiation, but is likely to occur to the same degree in both normal and tumor tissue. Therefore, it is only possible to utilize hyperthermic radiosensitization if the tumor can be heated to a higher temperature than the surrounding normal tissue. In this situation, it will be possible to deliver a higher biological dose of radiation to the tumor when compared to the surrounding normal tissue. The sensitizing efect depends on the treatment temperature and heating time, but a two- to three-fold increase in biological effect is likely to occur after treatment with a moderate heating which itself does not involve any normal tissue damage. Such treatment is, therefore, likely to result in an improved therapeutic effect, but depends on the technical ability to produce a selective local tumor-heating.

Second, moderate heat treatment alone is almost selectively cytotoxic against tumor cells situated in an environment characterized by nutritional deprivation, chronic hypoxia, and increased acidity. Since such cells are the most resistant to radiation therapy, a smaller overall radiation dose is needed to control the remaining more radiosensitive tumor cells. This cytotoxicity can be utilized in a sequential treatment schedule where radiation is given about 4 hours before hyperthermia. With such a treatment, any hyperthermic radiosensitization is avoided, and no selective tumor-heating is required since no enhanced radiation damage will occur in the normal tissue due to its physiological environment.

The early clinical experiences obtained in different institutions are used to illustrate the clinical relevance of these biological principles.

Acknowledgments

Research for this chapter was supported by the Danish Cancer Society, Grant 24/79, and "Ingeborg and Leo Danin's Foundation for Scientific Research."

References

1. Arcangeli, G., Barocas, A., Mauro, F., Nervi, C., Spano, M., and Tabocchini, A.: Mulitple daily fractionation (MDF) radiotherapy in association with hyperthermia and/or misonidazole: Experimental and clinical results. *Cancer* **45**:2707–2711, 1980.
2. Bede, Z., Diven, Z., and Shoexion, W.: The clinical effects of radiofrequency diathermy and radiation in bladder cancer: A preliminary report. Presented at the Third International Symposium: Cancer Therapy by Hyperthermia, Drugs and Radiation, Fort Collins, Colorado, June 22–26, 1980.
3. Bicher, H.I., Hetzel, F.W., Sandhu, T.S., Frinka, S., Vaupel, P., O'Hara, M.D., and O'Brien, T.: Effects of hyperthermia on normal and tumor microenvironment. *Radiology* **137**:523–530, 1980.
4. Cavaliere, R., Ciocatto, E.C., Giovanella, B.C., Beppino, C., Heidelberger, C., Johnson, R.O., Margottini, M., Mondovi, B., Moricca, G., and Rossi-Fanelli, A.: Selective heat sensitivity of cancer cells. Biochemical and clinical studies. *Cancer* **20**:1351–1381, 1967.
5. Corry, P., Barlogie, B., Spanos, W., Armour, E., Barkley, H., and Gonzales, M.: Approaches to clinical application of combinations on nonionizing and ionizing radiations. In *Radiation Biology in Cancer Research* R.E. Meyn and H.R. Withers, eds. New York: Raven Press, 1980, pp. 637–644.
6. Dewey, W.C., Freeman, M.L., Raaphorst, G.P., Clark, E.P., Wong, R.S.L., Highfield, D.P., Spiro, I.J., Tomasovic, S.P., Denman, D.L., and Coss, R.A.: Cell biology of hyperthermia and radiation. In *Radiation Biology in Cancer Research* R.E. Meyn and H.R. Withers, eds. New York: Raven Press, 1980, pp. 589–621.
7. Dewey, W.C., Hopwood, L.E., Sapareto, S.A., Gerweck, L.E.: Cellular responses to combinations of hyperthermia and radiation. *Radiology* **123**:463–474, 1977.
8. Eddy, H.A.: Alterations in tumor microvasculature during hyperthermia. *Radiology* **137**:515–521, 1980.
9. Fazekas, J., and Nerlinger, T.: Clinical hyperthermia pilot studies Thomas Jefferson University Hospital. Results of 42°C adjuvant to irradiation. In *Proceedings from the Symposium on "Clinical Hyperthermia Today"* Henry Ford Hospital, Detroit, 1980, pp. 39–46.
10. Field, S.B., and Anderson, R.L.: Thermotolerance: A review of observations and possible mechanisms. *J Natl Cancer Inst*, in press.
11. Field, S.B., and Bleehan, N.M.: Hyperthermia in the treatment of cancer. *Cancer Treat Rev* **6**:63–94, 1979.
12. Field, S.B., and Law, M.P.: The response of skin to fractionated heat and x-rays. *Br J Radiol* **51**: 221–222, 1978.
13. Gilette, E.L., and Ensley, B.A.: Effect of heating order on radiation response of mouse tumor and skin. *Int J Radiat Oncol Biol Phys* **5**:209–213, 1979.
14. Hall, R.R., Schade, R.O.K., and Swinney, J.: Effects of hyperthermia on bladder cancer. *Br Med J* **2**:593–594, 1974.
15. Hill, S.A., and Denekamp, J.: The effect of vascular occlusion on the thermal sensitization of a mouse tumor. *Br J Radiol* **51**:997–1002, 1978.
16. Hill, S.A., and Denekamp, J.: The response of six mouse tumors to combined heat and x-rays: Implications for therapy. *Br J Radiol* **52**:209–218, 1979.
17. Israel, L., and Besenval, M.: Local hyperthermia with 13.56 MHZ in 46 patients with deep-seated solid tumors. Presented at the Third International Symposium: Cancer Therapy by Hyperthermia, Drugs and Radiation, Fort Collins, Colorado, June 22–26, 1980.
18. Johnson, R.J.R., Sandhu, T.S., Hetzel, F.W., Song, S.Y., Bicher, H.I., Subjeck, J.R., and Kowal, H.S.: A pilot study to investigate skin and tumor thermal enhancement ratios of 41.5–42.0°C hyperthermia with radiation. *Int J Radiat Oncol Biol Phys* **5**:947–953, 1979.
19. Kim, J.H., Hahn, E.W., and Antich, P.P.: Radio-

frequency hyperthermia for clinical cancer therapy. *Natl Cancer Insti*, in press.

20. Kim, J.H., Hahn, E.W., and Toketa, N.: Combination hyperthermia and radiation therapy for cutaneous malignant melanoma. *Cancer* **41**:2143–2148, 1978.
21. Kim, J.H., Hahn, E.W., Tokita, N., and Nisce, L.Z.: Local tumor hyperthermia in combination with radiation therapy. 1. Malignant cutaneous lesions. *Cancer* **40**:161–169, 1977.
22. Law, M.P.: Some effects of fractionation on the response of the mouse to combined heat and x-rays. *Radiat Res* **80**:360–368, 1979.
23. Law, M.P., Ahier, R.G., and Field, S.B.: The response of mouse skin to combined hyperthermia and x-rays. *Int J Radiat Biol* **32**:153–163, 1977.
24. Law, M.P., Ashier, R.G., and Field, S.B.: The effect of prior heat treatment on the thermal enhancement of radiation damage in the mouse ear. *Br J Radiol* **52**:315–321, 1979.
25. LeVeen, H.H., Ashmed, N., Piccone, V.A., Shugaar, S., and Falk, G.: Radiofrequency therapy: Clinical experience. *Ann NY Acad Sci* **335**:362–371, 1980.
26. Luk, K.H.: An updated analysis of microwave hyperthermia at 2450 megahertz and 915 megahertz frequencies. In *Proceedings from the Symposium "Clinical Hyperthermia Today"* Henry Ford Hospital, Detroit, 1980, pp. 71–76.
27. Manning, M.R., Gerner, E.W., and Cetas, T.C.: Interstitial thermoradiotherapy. *Natl Cancer Inst*, in press.
28. Marmor, J.B., and Hahn, G.M.: Ultrasound heating in previously irradiated sites. *Int J Radiat Oncol Biol Phys* **4**:1029–1032, 1978.
29. Marmor, J.B., and Hahn, G.M.: Combined radiation and hyperthermia in superficial human tumors. *Cancer* **46**:1986–1991, 1980.
30. Marmor, J.B., Pounds, D., Postic, T.B., and Hahn, G.M.: Treatment of superficial human neoplasms by local hyperthermia induced by ultrasound. *Cancer* **43**:188–197, 1979.
31. Myers, R., and Field, S.B.: The response of the rat tail to combined heat and x-rays. *Br J Radiol* **50**: 581–586, 1977.
32. Myers, R., and Field, S.B.: Hyperthermia and the oxygen enhancement ratio for damage to baby rat cartilage. *Br J Radiol* **52**:415–416, 1979.
33. Nielsen, O.S., and Overgaard, J.: Hyperthermic radiosensitization of thermotolerant tumor cells in vitro. *Int J Radiat Biol* **35**:171–176, 1979.
34. Okada, K., Kiyotake, S., Kawazoe, K., Sato, Y., Tahara, R., Kinoshita, M., Kumagai, S., Kitazima, K., Onoe, Y., Rakimoto, Y., and Kishimoto, T.: II. Hyperthermic treatment for the bladder tumor. *Jpn J Urol* **68**:128–135, 1977.
35. Overgaard, J.: Effect of hyperthermia on malignant cells in vivo. A review and a hypothesis. *Cancer* **39**:2637–2646, 1977.
36. Overgaard, J.: The effect of local hyperthermia alone and in combination with radiation, on solid tumors. In *Cancer Therapy by Hyperthermia and Radiation*, Baltimore and Munich: Urban and Schwarzenberg, 1978, pp. 49–61.
37. Overgaard, J.: Hyperthermia and radiotherapy. In *Basis for Cancer Therapy 2* Advances in Medical Oncology, Research and Education, vol. 6, M. Moore, ed. Oxford: Pergamon Press, 1979, pp. 235–245.
38. Overgaard, J.: Simultaneous and sequential hyperthermia and radiation treatment of an experimental tumor and its surrounding normal tissue in vivo. *Int J Radiat Oncol Biol Phys* **6**:1507–1517, 1980a.
39. Overgaard, J.: Effect of fractionated hyperthermia and radiation on an experimental tumor and its surrounding skin. In *Hyperthermia in Radiation Oncology*, G. Arcangeli and F. Mauro, eds. Milan: Masson Italia Eglitori, 1980b, pp. 241–246.
40. Overgaaard, J.: Fractionated radiation and hyperthermia. Experimental and clinical studies. *Cancer*, in press (a).
41. Overgaard, J.: Influence of sequence and interval on the biological response to combined hyperthermia and radiation. *Natl Cancer Inst*, in press (b).
42. Overgaard, J.: Fractionated hyperthermia and radiation in vivo. *Natl Cancer Inst,* in press (c).
43. Overgaard, J.: Effect of hyperthermia on the hypoxic fraction in an experimental mammary carcinoma in vivo. *Br J Radiol,* in press (d).
44. Overgaard, J., and Nielsen, O.S.: The role of tissue environmental factors on the kinetics and morphology of tumor cells exposed to hyperthermia. *Ann NY Acad Sci* **335**:254–282, 1980.
45. Perez, C.A., Kopecky, W., Baglan, R., Rao, D.V., Johnson, R.: Local microwave hyperthermia in cancer therapy. Preliminary report. In *Proceedings from the Symposium "Clinical Hyperthermia Today"* Henry Ford Hospital, Detroit, 1980, pp. 23–38.
46. Robinson, J.E., Wizenberg, M.J., and McCready, W.A.: Radiation and hyperthermal response of normal tissue in situ. *Radiology* **113**:195–198, 1974.
47. Song, C.W., Kang, M.S., Rhee, J.G., and Levitt, S.H.: Effect of hyperthermia on vascular function in normal and neoplastic tissues. *Ann NY Acad Sci* **335**:35–47, 1980.
48. Stewart, F.A., and Denekamp, J.: Sensitization of mouse skin to X-irradiation by moderate heating. *Radiology* **123**:195–200, 1977.
49. Stewart, F.A., and Denekamp, J.: The therapeutic advantage of combined heat and x-rays on a mouse fibrosarcoma. *Br J Radiol* **51**:307–316, 1978.
50. Stewart, F.A., and Denekamp, J.: Fractionation studies with combined x-rays and hyperthermia in vivo. *Br J Radiol* **53**:346–356, 1980.

51. Storm, F.K., Harrison, W.H., Elliott, R.S., and Morton, D.L.: Normal tissue and solid tumor effects of hyperthermia in animal models and clinical trials. *Cancer Res* **39**:2245–2251, 1979.
52. Suit, H., and Gerweck, L.E.: Potential for hyperthermia and radiation therapy. *Cancer Res* **39**: 2290–2298, 1979.
53. UR., Noell, T.K., Woodward, K.T., Worde, B.T., Fishburn, R., and Miller, L.S.: Microwave-induced local hyperthermia in combination with radiotherapy of human malignant tumors. *Cancer* **45**:638–646, 1980.
54. Urano, M., Gerweck, L.E., Epstein, R., Cunningham, M., and Suit, H.D.: Response of a spontaneous murine tumor to hyperthermia: Factors which modify the thermal response in vivo. *Radiat Res* **83**:312–322, 1980.

CHAPTER 42

Preliminary Report of Combined Neutron and Photon Irradiation for Advanced Head and Neck Tumors

David H. Hussey, M.D.[a]
Moshe H. Maor, M.D.[a]

In October 1972, The University of Texas System Cancer Center M. D. Anderson Hospital and Tumor Institute (MDAH) initiated a pilot study of fast-neutron therapy using the Texas A & M variable energy cyclotron (TAMVEC). During the first phase of this program, patients with locally advanced head and neck tumors were usually treated with neutrons alone using a twice-weekly fractionation scheule. The pilot study results of this treatment schedule have been reported previously.[8,11]

Since October 1974, the majority of patients with advanced head and neck tumors have been treated with a combination of neutrons and ^{60}Co gamma rays using a mixed-beam fractionation schedule. In the mixed-beam treatment schedule, patients were treated five times weekly—twice weekly with neutrons and three times weekly with photons.

The cyclotron was not available for clinical use between July and December 1975 and between July and December 1976. During these times, patients who were candidates for the neutron therapy pilot study were registered in a "control group" and treated with conventional treatment methods. Although these patients were not prospectively randomized, they would have been treated with mixed-beam irradiation had the cyclotron been available clinically.

[a]Department of Radiotherapy, The University of Texas System Cancer Center, M. D. Anderson Hospital and Tumor Institute, Houston, Texas

A prospective clinical trial for locally advanced head and neck cancer has been underway since January 1977. In this study, patients have been randomized to receive mixed-beam irradiation or conventional treatment with photons or combined surgery and photons.

This is a report of the MDAH-TAMVEC study of mixed-beam irradiation for locally advanced head and neck cancers. The specific objective is to compare the results of mixed-beam therapy with those of conventional treatment with surgery, photons, or a combination of surgery and photons. The preliminary results of the prospective randomized trial are also discussed.

Energy and Dosage Conventions

The neutron treatments were delivered with a neutron beam produced by bombarding a thick beryllium target with 50 MeV deuterons (50 $MeV_{d\rightarrow Be}$). This beam has skin-sparing and depth-dose properties similar to those of x-rays from a 4 MeV linear accelerator.[7] The photon treatments were delivered with ^{60}Co gamma rays, occasionally supplemented with 18-25 MeV x-rays or 6-18 MeV electrons.

The neutron beam doses were determined by measurements with a tissue-equivalent ionization chamber immersed in tissue-equivalent liquid (ρ = 1.07 g/cm^3). The physical doses have been expressed in rad including both the neutron and gamma components ($rad_{n\gamma}$). The gamma dose for the 50 $MeV_{d \rightarrow Be}$ neutron beam is approximately 7% of the total physical dose at a depth of 7 cm.

The mixed-beam doses are reported in terms of: (1) the physical dose, listing the neutron and photon beam doses separately ($rad_{n\gamma}$ + rad), and (2) the total equivalent dose of the combined regimen (rad_{eq}). The equivalent doses (rad_{eq}) were determined by multiplying the physical dose delivered with neutrons by an RBE of 3.1 and adding this to the dose delivered with photons. The RBE of 3.1 was determined clinically by comparing the late effects of neutrons twice weekly with the late effects of photon irradiation delivered in fractions of 200 rad five times weekly.[8]

Materials and Methods

CLINICAL MATERIAL

The clinical material is comprised of 138 patients with locally advanced head and neck cancers treated between October 1974 and January 1979. This includes 73 patients in the prospective randomized trial. There were 64 patients in the mixed-beam group and 74 in the conventional treatment group.

All the patients had locally advanced carcinomas (stages $T_{3-4}N_{0-3}$, $T_{0-2}N_3$ or recurrent tumors following surgical management). With the exception of two patients in the mixed-beam group with a diagnosis of adenoid cystic carcinoma, all patients presented with squamous carcinomas. The tumors were not graded histopathologically.

The patients are listed by tumor site in Table 1. There were more patients with oral cavity tumors, particularly floor of mouth and oral tongue lesions, in the conventional treatment group (33%, 24/74) than in the mixed-beam group (13%, 8/64). On the other hand, more patients presented with recurrent tumors in the mixed-beam group (19%, 12/64) than in the conventional treatment group (5%, 4/74). About half of the patients in each group had oropharyngeal cancers.

The patients are listed by clinical stage in Table 2. On the average, the patients in the mixed-beam group presented with slightly more advanced tumors than those in the conventional treatment group. In the mixed-beam group, 63% (40/64) of patients presented with stage T_4N_{0-3}, $T_{0-3}N_3$, or massive recurrent tumors compared to 54% (40/74) of patients in the conventional treatment group. Although the distribution by N stage was similar for both treatment groups, the distribution by T stage was more advanced in the mixed-beam group.

TREATMENT TECHNIQUES

Mixed-Beam Group

The standard photon treatment policies at M. D. Anderson Hospital were adapted for mixed-beam treatment. In general, the same treatment portals, total equivalent dose, and overall time were employed as would have been used with photon irradiation. The primary tumors in this group were treated entirely with radiotherapy, usually with external-beam irradiation. However, patients with oral tongue and floor of mouth tumors were evaluated after 4500–5000 rad_{eq} for completion of treatment with interstitial radium implants. The neck was treated with radiotherapy, usually as the sole modality. Modified neck dissections were permitted for patients with bulky but technically resectable lymph node metastases. The mixed-beam treatments were given twice weekly with neutrons using a fraction size of 65 $rad_{n\gamma}$ and three times weekly with photons using a fraction size of 200 rad. A neutron fraction of 65 $rad_{n\gamma}$ is equivalent to 200 rad with photons, assuming an RBE of 3.1.

For most tumor sites, the aim was to deliver 6000–6500 rad_{eq} in 6–6½ weeks for

TABLE 1. Distribution of Patients by Tumor Site (October 1974–January 1979)

Site	Mixed-Beam Number		Mixed-Beam %		Conventional Treatment Number		Conventional Treatment %	
Oral cavity	8		13%		24		33%	
floor of mouth		4		6%		9		12%
oral tongue		2		3%		11		15%
hard palate		—		—		2		3%
buccal mucosa		1		2%		1		1%
gingiva		1		2%		1		1%
Oropharynx	36		56%		37		50%	
faucial arch		7		11%		3		4%
tonsillar fossa		6		9%		12		16%
base of tongue		16		25%		15		20%
pharyngeal wall		7		11%		7		9%
Larynx and pyriform sinus	2		3%		6		8%	
Other primary sites	2		3%		1		1%	
Nodal metastases (T_O or T_X)	4		6%		2		3%	
Recurrent tumor	12		19%		4		5%	
at primary site		6		9%		1		1%
in nodes		6		9%		3		4%
Total	64				74			

moderately advanced tumors and 6500–7000 rad_{eq} in 6½–7 weeks for massive cancers. The average tumor dose was 6741 ± 435 rad_{eq} (4174 ± 617 rad with photons and 836 ± 142 $rad_{n\gamma}$ with neutrons) (see Table 3). On the average, 38% of the total equivalent dose to the gross cancer was delivered with neutrons. Four patients completed treatment with interstitial radium implants (2000–3000 rad), and seven had planned modified neck dissections for bulky lymphadenopathy.

The portal arrangements were determined by the site of the primary tumor and the distribution of the regional lymph node metastases. The primary tumor and upper neck nodes were usually treated through parallel-opposing lateral portals. If the main bulk of the cancer was midline—e.g., tumors of the base of tongue—the given doses were equally loaded. If the gross cancer was located laterally—e.g., lesions of the tonsillar fossa—the given doses were weighted 3:2 or 2:1 to the ipsilateral side. Patients with tumors confined to the parotid gland or to nodes on one side of the neck were usually treated with wedged fields.

The spinal cord dose was limited to no more than 4500 rad_{eq} in 4½ weeks using an RBE of 4.1 for spinal cord injury.[9] When there were posterior cervical lymph node metastases or a significant risk of subclinical disease in this area, part of the treatment was given with electrons to limit the dose to the spinal cord.

The regional lymphatics of the lower neck were treated with a single anterior treatment portal. When the lower neck was clinically negative, the treatment to this area was delivered with ^{60}Co gamma rays using a given dose of 4500 rad in 15 fractions in 5 weeks or 5000 rad in 25 fractions in 5 weeks.

Conventional Treatment Group

The treatment for patients in the conventional treatment group was determined by the site and extent of the cancer and the

TABLE 2 Distribution of Patients by Clinical Stage (October 1974–January 1979)

Stage	Mixed-Beam[a] T_0-X	T_1	T_2	T_3	T_4	Total	Conventional Treatment[b] T_0-X	T_1	T_2	T_3	T_4	Total
N_0				13	6	19 (30%)				13	9	22 (30%)
N_1				4	5	9 (14%)				8	1	9 (12%)
N_2				5	2	7 (11%)				12	8	20 (27%)
N_3	4			3	10	17 (26%)	2	1	1	5	10	19 (26%)
Total	4 (6%)			25 (39%)	23 (39%)		2 (3%)	1 (1%)	1 (1%)	38 (51%)	28 (38%)	

[a]Plus 12 patients with recurrent tumors (19%) (2 moderately advanced, 10 massive).
[b]Plus 4 patients with recurrent tumors (5%) (1 moderately advanced, 3 massive).

general condition of the patient. In general, patients with oral cavity tumors were selected for treatment with surgery or combined surgery and irradiation, whereas those with oropharyngeal or hypopharyngeal lesions were treated with radiation therapy alone. The primary tumors were treated with surgery alone in 7 patients, with radiotherapy alone in 39 patients, and with combined surgery and radiotherapy in 28 patients. Of the 28 patients treated with combined surgery and radiotherapy, preoperative radiotherapy was used in 6 patients and postoperative radiotherapy in 22 patients.

The average tumor dose for patients treated with photon irradiation alone (7102 ± 560 rad) was greater than that employed for the mixed-beam group (Table 3). The average preoperative dose was 4650 ± 399 rad, and the average postoperative dose was 5660 ± 522 rad. Three patients in the conventional treatment group completed treatment with interstitial radium implants (2000–3000 rad), and five of those whose primary tumor was treated with radiotherapy alone had planned modified neck dissections for bulky lymphadenopathy. The treatment portals for this treatment group were the same as those described for the mixed-beam group.

Results

TOTAL POPULATION

The data were analyzed in August 1979. The average interval from the start of radiation therapy to the date of analysis was 26.7 months (range: 8–57 months) for the mixed-beam group and 27.1 months (range: 6–48 months) for the conventional treatment group. The preliminary results for the total population are shown in Tables 4 and 5 and Figure 1.

The patients were scored as having their

TABLE 3. Total Population: Treatment Methods and Average Tumor Dose

Treatment Method for Primary Tumor	Number of Patients		Average Tumor Dose ± 1 Standard Deviation
Mixed beams	64[a]		6741 ± 435 rad_{eq}[b] (neutrons: 836 ± 142 $rad_{n\gamma}$ photons: 4174 ± 617 rad)
Conventional treatment	74		
surgery only		7	
radiotherapy only		39[c]	7102 ± 560 rad[d]
preoperative radiotherapy + surgery		6	4650 ± 399 rad
Surgery + postoperative radiotherapy		22	5660 ± 522 rad

[a]7 patients in the mixed-beam group had modified neck dissections.

[b]Includes the dose delivered with radium implants (4 patients in the mixed-beam group).

[c]5 patients in the conventional treatment group whose primary tumor was treated with radiotherapy alone had modified neck dissections.

[d]Includes the dose delivered with radium implants (3 patients in the conventional treatment group).

tumor locally controlled if they were alive with no evidence of disease at the time of analysis or if they had died of distant metastasis or intercurrent disease with no clinical evidence of local cancer. Complications developing in an area of residual recurrent disease were attributed to persistent cancer and were not scored as complications of treatment.

Local Control

About half of the patients were scored as having local control of their disease–53% (34/64) in the mixed-beam group and 49% (36/74) in the conventional treatment group (Table 4). However, the patients in the mixed-beam group presented with slightly more advanced disease, on the average, than those in the conventional treatment group. For moderately advanced cancers (T_3N_{0-2} or recurrent tumors <6 cm in diameter), the local control rate with mixed-beam irradiation (71%, 17/24) was superior to that achieved with conventional treatment (50%, 17/34) (χ^2, p = 0.11). The local control rates for patients with massive tumors (stages T_4N_{0-3} or $T_{0-3}N_3$, or recurrent tumors >6 cm in diameter) were similar for both groups.

Local tumor control is analyzed by tumor site in Table 5. For oropharyngeal neoplasms the local control rate with mixed-beam irradiation (61%, 22/36) was superior to that achieved with conventional treatment (49%, 19/37), although the difference is not statistically significant (χ^2, p = 0.40). For oral cavity tumors the local control rate with conventional treatment was better than that achieved with mixed-beam irradiation, although the number of oral cavity tumors treated in the mixed-beam group is very small.

Complications

Thirteen patients (9%) developed major complications (Table 4). Surgery was at

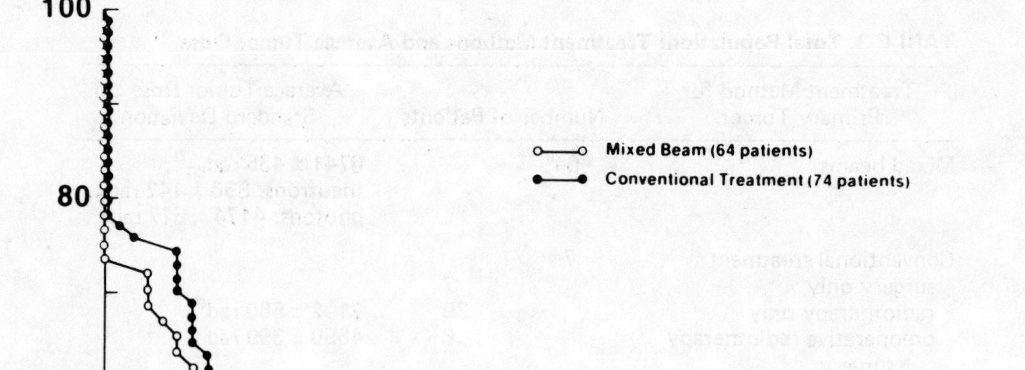

Figure 1. Actuarial local control, complication, and survival curves for the total population. (from Kaplan and Meier, 1958[10]).

least a contributory factor in the majority of these patients, and only two complications developed in patients treated with radiation therapy alone. There were significantly more major complications in the conventional treatment group (14%, 10/74) than in the mixed-beam group (5%, 3/64) (χ^2, $p = 0.08$).

Two patients in the mixed-beam group developed wound-healing complications following a planned modified neck dissection after radiotherapy. The other complication in this group occurred in a patient treated with radiotherapy alone. This patient developed contralateral hypopharyngeal wall necrosis 16 months following treatment for a T_3N_0 squamous carcinoma of the base of tongue. In retrospect, this may have resulted from an overlap of the upper neck neutron portals with the lower neck photon portals.

In the conventional treatment group, three complications developed following treatment by surgery alone, two following treatment by preoperative radiotherapy and surgery, and four following treatment by surgery and postoperative radiotherapy. Only one patient treated with photon irradiation alone developed a major complication. This patient developed oropharyngeal necrosis following 8000 rad in 60 fractions

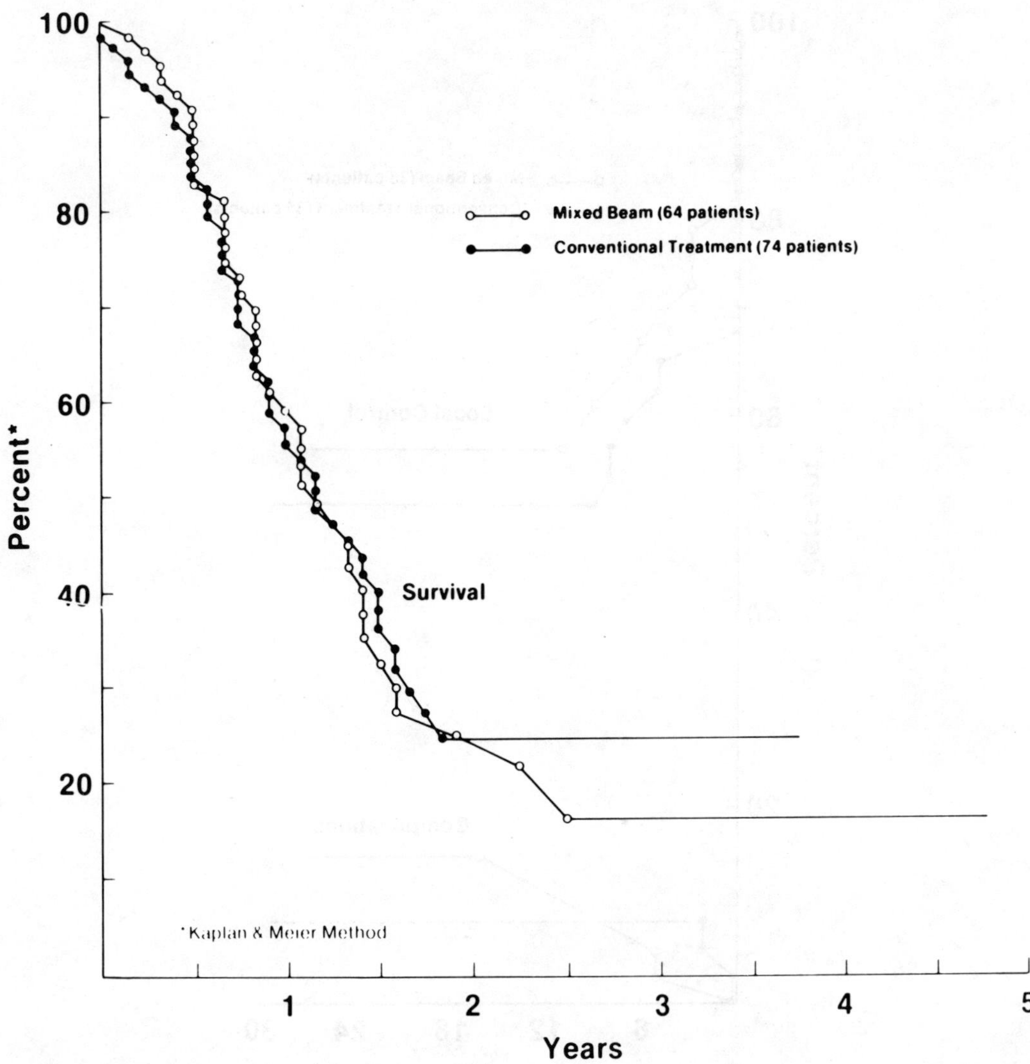

Figure 1 (continued)

over 49 days using twice-daily fractionation for a T_4N_0 squamous carcinoma of the tonsillar fossa.

Survival

The survival rates for the mixed-beam and conventional treatment groups were the same (Table 4). At the time of analysis, 34% (22/64) of the patients in the mixed-beam group were alive, compared to 36% (27/74) of those in the conventional treatment group.

Actuarial Analysis

Actuarial local control, complications, and survival curves[10] are plotted in Figure 1. By this method of analysis, the local control and survival curves were almost identical for the two treatment groups. However, the complication rate for patients in the conventional treatment group was significantly greater than that for patients treated with mixed-beam irradiation (Wilcoxon test, p = 0.07).

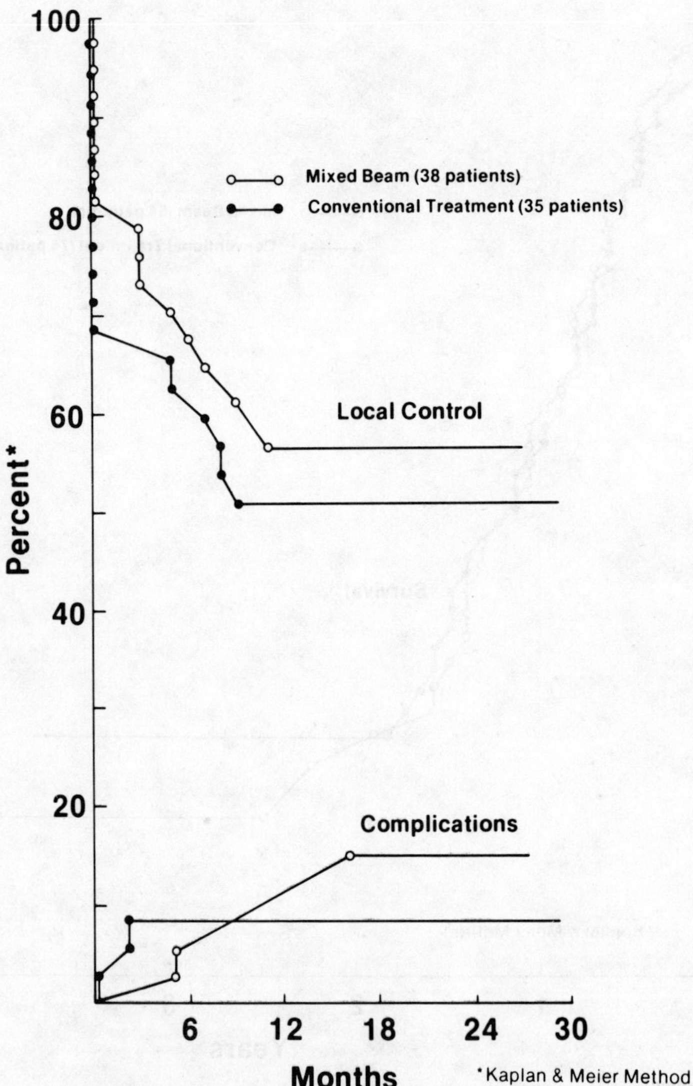

Figure 2. Actuarial local control, complication, and survival curve for patients treated in the randomized trial (from Kaplan and Meier, 1958[10]).

PRELIMINARY RESULTS OF THE RANDOMIZED TRIAL

Between January 1977 and January 1979, 73 patients with locally advanced head and neck cancer were randomized to receive mixed-beam radiotherapy or conventional treatment with photons or combined surgery and photons. There were 38 patients in the mixed-beam group and 35 in the conventional treatment group; 27 of the patients in the conventional treatment group were treated with photons and 8 with combined surgery and photons. The tumor site and stage distributions were similar for the two groups.

The preliminary results are listed in Table 6. In the mixed-beam group, 61% (23/38) of patients had achieved local control of their disease, 8% (3/38) developed major complications, and 45% (17/38) were alive at the time of analysis. In the conventional treat-

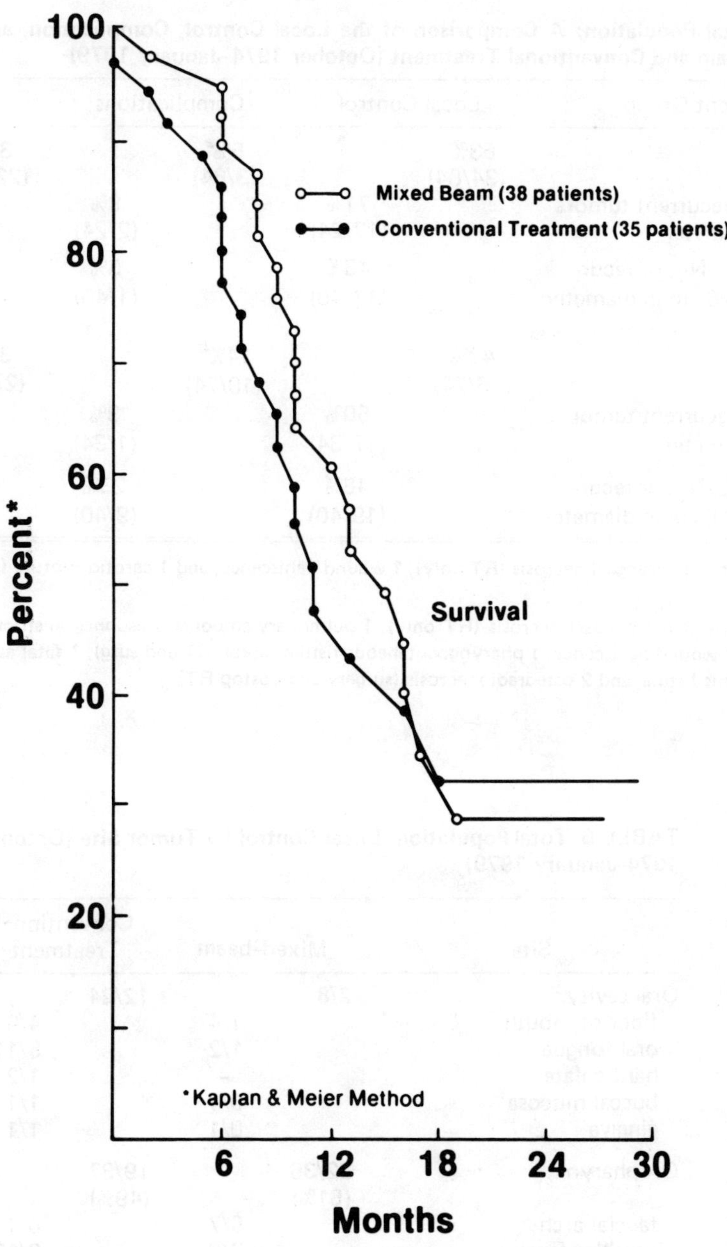

Figure 2 (continued)

ment group, 51% (18/35) were scored as having local tumor control, 9% (3/35) developed major complications, and 43% (15/35) were alive.

Actuarial local control, complication, and survival curves[10] were plotted because of the limited follow-up interval (see Fig. 2). Although the local control and survival curves are superior with mixed-beam irradiation, the differences are not statistically significant (Wilcoxon test: local control, $p = 0.18$; survival, $p = 0.11$).

TABLE 4. Total Population: A Comparison of the Local Control, Complication, and Survival Rates with Mixed-Beam and Conventional Treatment (October 1974–January 1979)

Treatment Group	Local Control	Complications	Survival
Mixed-Beam	53% (34/64)	5%[a] (3/64)	34% (22/64)
T_3N_{0-2}, or recurrent tumors <6 cm in diameter	71% (17/24)	8% (2/24)	54% (13/24)
T_4N_{0-3}, $T_{0-3}N_3$, or recurrent tumor >6 cm in diameter	43% (17/40)	3% (1/40)	23% (9/40)
Conventional	49% (36/74)	14%[b] (10/74)	36% (27/74)
T_3N_{0-2} or recurrent tumor <6 cm in diameter	50% (17/34)	3% (1/34)	50% (17/34)
T_4N_{0-3}, $T_{0-3}N_3$, or recurrent tumor >6 cm in diameter	48% (19/40)	23% (9/40)	25% (10/40)

[a] 3 complications: 1 pharyngeal necrosis (RT only), 1 wound dehiscence, and 1 carotid rupture (RT and neck dissection).

[b] 10 complications: 1 oromucosal necrosis (RT only), 1 pulmonary embolus, 1 esophageal stricture, 1 postop death (surgery only), 1 wound dehiscence, 1 pharyngocutaneous fistula (preop RT and surg), 1 fatal aspiration pneumonitis, 1 orocutaneous fistula, and 2 osteoradionecrosis (surgery and postop RT).

TABLE 5. Total Population: Local Control by Tumor Site (October 1974–January 1979)

Site	Mixed-beam	Conventional Treatment
Oral cavity	**2/8**	12/24
floor of mouth	1/4	4/9
oral tongue	1/2	5/11
hard palate	—	1/2
buccal mucosa	0/1	1/1
gingiva	0/1	1/1
Oropharynx	22/36 (61%)	19/37 (49%)
faucial arch	5/7	0/1
tonsillar fossa	3/6	8/12
base of tongue	9/16	7/15
pharyngeal wall	5/7	4/7
Larynx and pyriform sinus	1/2	3/6
Other primary sites	2/2	0/1
Nodal metastasis (T_0 or T_x)	3/4	2/2
Recurrent tumor	4/12	0/4
Total	34/64 (53%)	36/74 (49%)

TABLE 6. Preliminary Results of the Randomized Trial (January 1977–January 1979)

Treatment Group	Local Control	Complications	Survival
Mixed-Beam	61% (23/38)	8%[a] (3/38)	45% (17/38)
T_3N_{0-3}, or recurrent tumors <6 cm in diameter	86% (12/14)	14% (2/14)	71% (10/14)
T_4N_{0-3}, $T_{0-3}N_3$, or recurrent tumor >6 cm in diameter	46% (11/24)	4% (1/24)	29% (7/24)
Conventional	51% (18/35)	9%[b] (3/35)	43% (15/35)
T_3N_{0-3}, or recurrent tumor <6 cm in diameter	77% (10/13)	0% (0/13)	92% (12/13)
T_4N_{0-3}, $T_{0-3}N_3$, or recurrent tumor >6 cm in diameter	36% (8/22)	13% (3/24)	14% (3/22)

[a] 3 complications: 1 pharyngeal necrosis (RT only), 1 wound dehiscence, and 1 carotid rupture (RT and neck dissection).

[b] 3 complications: 1 pulmonary embolus (surgery only), 1 wound dehiscence, and 1 pharyngocutaneous fistula (preop RT and surgery).

Discussion

Locally advanced cancers of the head and neck are difficult to control with surgery or conventional radiation therapy alone. Surgery fails in a high percentage of cases because the tumor frequently extends beyond the margins of resection, whereas conventional irradiation fails because of the inability to eradicate bulky cancer in the center of the treatment portals. In some situations, local tumor control can be improved by using combinations of surgery and radiation therapy.[3] The rationale for the combined approach is that the surgical procedure can remove gross masses that are too large to be eradicated by moderate doses of irradiation, and radiation therapy eradicates microscopic extensions of tumor that cannot be excised.

It has been postulated that hypoxic tumor cells are often responsible for the failure of radiotherapy to control gross cancers because these cells are inherently more resistant to X- and gamma irradiation than are well-oxygenated cells.[6] If this is so, fast neutrons, because of their decreased dependence on oxygen for their biological effects, should be more effective than photons for local tumor control.

Catterall[2] has reported the results of a clinical trial of 134 patients with stages $T_{2-4}N_{0-3}$ squamous carcinomas of the head and neck randomized for treatment with 16 $MeV_{d\rightarrow Be}$ neutrons or photons. Local control was achieved in 76% (54/71) of the patients in the neutron group, compared to only 19% (12/63) of those in the photon group. However, there was no signiicant difference in survival between the two groups. Because the majority of patients in the photon group were treated at institutions other than Hammersmith, critics have argued that the photon group may not have been treated as precisely, or to as high a biological dose, as those treated with neutrons at Hammersmith. This criticism may have some validity since the patients treated with neutrons had a greater incidence of late normal tissue damage (17%, 12/71) than those treated with photons (3%, 2/63).

The results with neutrons only twice weekly in the MDAH-TAMVEC pilot study are poorer than those reported from Hammersmith Hospital. With neutrons alone at TAMVEC, 44% (30/68) of the patients scored as having local tumor control and 16% (11/68) developed major complications.[11]

The preliminary results with the mixed-beam fractionation schedule in the MDAH-TAMVEC trial are at least as good as those achieved with conventional treatment methods. The local control and survival rates for the mixed-beam group were the same as those achieved in the conventional treatment group, but the patients receiving mixed-beam irradiation presented with slightly more advanced cancers. Furthermore, the incidence of complications was greater for the patients treated conventionally. There is a slight indication of improved local control and survival rates with mixed-beam irradiation in the randomized study, but these results are only preliminary.

The results of the mixed-beam treatment schedule are superior to those previously reported for the neutrons-only treatment schedule at TAMVEC.[11] With neutrons alone, 44% (30/68) of the patients were scored as having local tumor control and 16% (11/68) developed major complications. On the other hand, 53% (34/64) of the patients treated with mixed-beam irradiation achieved local tumor control and only 5% (3/64) developed major complications. This was not a randomized study, however, and the patients treated with neutrons alone may have had more advanced cancers than those treated with mixed-beam irradiation. Furthermore, they were treated in the initial phase of the program when dosage schedules were uncertain.

One should not discount the possibility that the mixed-beam treatment schedule is superior to both the neutrons-only and the photons-only treatment schedules in certain clinical situations. This could occur if neutrons were more effective than photons for the eradication of hypoxic tumor cells, but less effective than photons for the eradication of well-oxygenated tumor cells—for the same degree of normal tissue injury.

In this situation, the relative merits of neutrons-only, photons-only, and mixed-beam treatment schedules would depend on the proportion of hypoxic and well-oxygenated cells present during treatment. This, in turn, would be influenced by the degree of reoxygenation achieved with each treatment schedule. For severely hypoxic tumors, the neutrons-only schedule would be superior to either of the other treatment schedules, whereas for well-oxygenated tumors, the photons-only schedule would be superior. When the proportion of hypoxic and well-oxygenated tumor cells is such that either are likely to persist, the mixed-beam treatment schedule would be superior to treatment with either neutrons or photons alone.

The greater effect of neutrons on hypoxic cells is well established by numerous radiobiology studies and a variety of cell systems. However, other differences in the way neutrons and photons interact with tissues could determine their comparative effectiveness on well-oxygenated cells. With neutron irradiation, there is: (1) greater absorption in fat and other hydrogen-rich tissues,[1] (2) less repair of sublethal and potentially lethal damage,[4] and (3) less variation in radiosensitivity with position in the cell cycle[5] than there is with photon irradiation. Under the right circumstances, any of these factors could result in diminished effectiveness of neutron irradiation (compared to photon irradiation) on well-oxygenated tumor cells for the same degree of normal tissue injury.

Summary

Between October 1974 and January 1979, 64 patients with locally advanced head and neck tumors were treated with a combination of 50 $MeV_{d \rightarrow Be}$ neutrons and photons using a mixed-beam treatment schedule (two neutron and three photon fractions per week). During the same period, 74 patients with similar tumors were treated conventionally with surgery, photons, or combined surgery and photons. As of August 1, 1979, 53% of the patients treated with mixed-beam irradiation had achieved local tumor control, 5% developed complications, and 34% were surviving. By comparison, 49% of the patients treated with conventional treatment methods had achieved local tumor control, 14% had developed complications, and 36% were surviving.

Seventy-three patients were treated in a prospective randomized trial—38 with mixed-beam irradiation and 35 with photons or combined surgery and photons. In the randomized trial, 61% of patients treated with mixed-beam irradiation achieved local tumor control, 8% developed complications, and 45% were surviving. Of those allocated to conventional treatment, 51% achieved local tumor control, 9% developed complications, and 43% were surviving.

ACKNOWLEDGMENTS

Research for this chapter was supported in part by Grants CA12542 and CA06294, awarded by the National Cancer Institute, Department of Health, Education and Welfare.

REFERENCES

1. Bewley, D.K.: Fast neutron beams for therapy. *Curr Top Radiat Res* **:**251–292, 1970.
2. Catterall, M.: Experience with fast neutrons and results of controlled clinical trials. In *Progress in Radio-Oncology* (International Symposium, Baden, Austria), K.H. Karcher, H.D. Kogelnik, and H.J. Meyer, eds. Stuttgart: Georg Thieme Verlag, 1980, pp. 44.
3. Fletcher, G.H.: Combination of irradiation and surgery. *Int Adv Surg Oncol* **2**:55–98, 1979.
4. Gragg, R.L., Humphrey, R.M., and Meyn, R.E.: The response of Chinese hamster ovary cells to fast-neutron radiotherapy beams. II. Sublethal and potentially lethal damage recovery capabilities. *Radiat Res* **71**:461–470, 1977.
5. Gragg, R.L., Humphrey, R.M., Thomas, H.T., and Meyn, R.E.: The response of Chinese hamster ovary cells to fast-neutron radiotherapy beams. III. Variations in RBE with position in the cell cycle. *Radiat Res* **76**:283–291, 1978.
6. Gray, L.H., Conger, A.D., Ebert, M., Hornsey, S., and Scott, O.C.A.: Concentration of oxygen dissolved in tissues at time of irradiation as factor in radiotherapy. *Br J Radiol* **26**:638–648, 1953.
7. Hussey, D.H., and Fletcher, G.H.: Clinical features of 16 and 50 $MeV_{d \rightarrow Be}$ neutrons. *Eur J Cancer* **10**:357–360, 1974.
8. Hussey, D.H., Fletcher, G.H., and Caderao, J.B.: A preliminary report of the MDAH-TAMVEC neutron therapy pilot study. In *Proceedings of the Fifth International Congress of Radiation Research* O.F. Nygaard, H.I. Adler, and W.K. Sinclair, eds. New York: Academic Press, 1975, pp. 1106–1117.
9. Hussey, D.H., Smathers, J.B., and Meyn, R.E.: Neutron Therapy. In *Radiation Therapy Planning* N.M. Bleehan, E. Glatstein, and J. Haybittle, eds. New York: Marcel Dekker, in preparation.
10. Kaplan, E.L., and Meier, P.: Nonparametric estimations from incomplete observation. *Am Statist Assoc J* **53**:457–480, 1958.
11. Peters, L.J., Hussey, D.H., Fletcher, G.H., Baumann, P.A., and Olson, M.H.: Preliminary report of the M. D. Anderson Hospital/Texas A & M variable energy cyclotron fast neutron therapy pilot study. *AJR* **132**:637–642, 1979.

CHAPTER 43

Results of Phases I and II Trials of Pion Radiotherapy

Morton M. Kligerman, M.D.,[a,b,d]
Steven E. Bush, M.D.,[a]
Makoto Kondo, M.D.,[c]
Stephany Wilson, B.A.,[a]
Alfred R. Smith, Ph.D.[a]

Clinical trials have been underway at the Los Alamos Meson Physics Facility (LAMPF) since 1974 and with treatment of large, deep-seated neoplasms since November 1976. The clinical studies are the result of cooperative efforts of the University of New Mexico Cancer Research and Treatment Center and the Los Alamos Scientific Laboratory. Since the original prediction by Fowler and Perkins[1] of the potential therapeutic advantages of negative pi meson radiotherapy, considerable interest has developed in the international radiotherapy community regarding implementation of this modality. Because of formidable technical challenges, the necessity for extensive preclinical studies in beam characterization and radiobiology, and the availability of beam time with adequate current, the initiation of clinical programs has been gradual. The purpose of the phase I and II trials was to implement as rapidly as possible a randomized study comparing pion radiotherapy to conventional radiotherapy with minimum risk to the patients in the study. The results of treatment of 96 patients with 97 tumors receiving pion radiotherapy with curative intent between May 1977 and April 1980 are presented.

[a]Cancer Research and Treatment Center, University of New Mexico, Albuquerque, New Mexico
[b]Los Alamos Scientific Laboratory, Los Alamos, New Mexico
[c]Department of Radiology, School of Medicine, Keio University, Tokyo, Japan
[d]Present address Department of Radiation Therapy, University of Pennsylvania, Philadelphia, Pennsylvania

Methods and Material

LAMPF operates a one-half-mile-long, 800 MeV proton linear accelerator with a beam current of about 550 microamperes and a design potential of 1 milliampere. Negative pi mesons (pions) are produced in quantities necessary for biomedical applications by proton bombardment of a graphite target with collection of particles of appropriate momenta and charge by a series of quadrupole and bending magnets previously described by Paciotti *et al.*[6] The pion channel produces a fixed vertical, slightly divergent beam. Field sizes were variable with diameters between 5 and 20 cm. The dose rate varied with beam tuning (penetration) and spread of the peak from 5 to 20 rads a minute depending on total volume. Penetration may be varied from 0 cm to 28 cm in water-equivalent density. Approximately 10–15% of the total dose is contributed by electron and muon contaminants. Techniques for patient positioning and immobilization have been previously reported by Kligerman *et al.*[3] Computerized treatment planning by use of CT data has been described by Hogstrom *et al.*,[2] and simula-

TABLE 1. Exclusions from Analysis

Total tumors	141[a]
Exclusions	
skin metastases	9
distant metastases	15
low dose, tolerance study	7
low dose, machine malfunction	10
low dose, medical reasons	3
total excluded	44
Total tumors analyzed	97

[a]140 patients, 1 with simultaneous prostate and bladder primaries.

TABLE 2. 97 Tumors Treated with Curative Intent

Pions alone	68[a]
Pions + XRT	19
Pions + surgery	10
Total	97

[a]67 patients, 1 with simultaneous prostate and bladder primaries.

tion and port check techniques have been reported by Tsujii et al.[7]

One hundred forty patients received pion irradiation for biopsy-proven neoplasms between October 1974 and April 1980. The original nine patients were treated for subcutaneous metastases using small volumes and superficially penetrating beams in order to establish a relative biological effectiveness (RBE) for pions as compared to orthovoltage x-rays.[4] One hundred thirty-one patients were treated for large, deep-seated tumors between November 1976 and April 1980. All have been followed for a minimum of 6 months, and none have been lost to follow-up.

Of the total 131 patients, 96 with 97 tumors received treatment with curative intent (one patient had histologically proven separate primaries of the urinary bladder and the prostate). The reasons for exclusion from analysis are shown in Table 1 and include known distant metastases at start of treatment in 15 cases; low dose (less than 2700 π^- rad maximum) due to planned tolerance studies or machine malfunction in 7 and 10 patients, respectively; and 3 patients who had unplanned discontinuation of therapy due to medical causes. All patients were treated as outpatients and began treatment with a minimum Karnofsy status of 60.

Patients included in this analysis received at least 2700 π^- rad maximum, a dose below which complete tumor regression has not been observed,[5] with the exception of five patients who received planned conventional whole-brain irradiation (4500 rad/4½ weeks) with boosting pion irradiation (1250–1650 π^- rad/2 weeks) for malignant gliomata. Other patients received doses of 2700 π^- rad maximum/25 fractions over 5 weeks to 5400 π^- rad maximum/51 fractions over 11 weeks. As shown in Table 2, 68 tumors were treated with pion irradiation alone, while 19 had combined pion and conventional irradiation by external or interstitial techniques, and 10 had subsequent surgical procedures. Ethical considerations have dictated a cautious approach to incrementation of pion doses. Particularly in the early clinical experience, a large safety factor led to expected underdosage in some advanced lesions and resulted in persistent disease necessitating additional treatment with conventional radiations. Occasional patients treated to high dose with pions have had locally persistent or early recurrent disease managed by interstitial implant or surgery.

The majority of patients included in this analysis have been treated for advanced neoplasms of the head and neck (36 patients) and high grade gliomata (23 patients). The former category includes patients with squamous carcinomas of the oral cavity, 6; nasopharynx, 4; oropharynx, 14; hypopharynx, 2; larynx, 4; sinuses, 2. There were 3 patients with minor salivary gland tumors and 1 with anaplastic carcinoma of the nasopharynx. Of 23 patients with primary brain tumors, 8 had Grade III astrocytoma and 15 had glioblastoma multi-

TABLE 3. Survival by Site and Dose

Site	Pion Boost	Dose (π^- Rad Maximum) 2700–3999	4000–4999	>5000	Survival
Head and neck	0/0	6/12	7/18	3/6	16/36 (44%)
Brain	4/5[a]	5/11	4/7	0/0	13/23 (57%)
Prostate	0/0	4/4	10/11	0/0	14/16 (93%)
Pancreas	0/0	0/6	0/5	0/0	0/11 (0%)
Other	0/0	4/6	2/5	0/1	6/12 (50%)

[a]Planned conventional whole-brain irradiation with pion boost.

TABLE 4. Local Control by Site and Dose

Site	Pion Boost	Dose (π^- Rad Maximum) 2700–3999	4000–4999	>5000	Local Control
Head and neck	0/0	6/12	8/18	3/6	17/36 (47%)
Brain	3/5[a]	1/11	2/7	0/0	6/23 (26%)
Prostate	0/0	4/4	11/11	0/0	15/15 (100%)
Pancreas	0/0	0/6	0/5	0/0	0/11 (0%)
Other	0/0	4/6	2/5	0/1	6/12 (50%)

[a]Planned conventional whole-brain irradiation with pion boost.

forme. Other major treatment sites include 15 cases with T3 and T4 adenocarcinoma of the prostate and 11 cases with locally advanced, unresectable adenocarcinoma of the pancreas. Groups of 1–3 patients were treated for primary carcinomas of the esophagus, lung, stomach, skin, uterine cervix, urinary bladder, and rectum. A total of 12 patients are represented in this group. Planned accession of scattered sites occurred in the early phase I and II studies for two reasons: (1) to assess, as rapidly as possible, the tolerance of various normal tissues, and (2) to determine whether any sites exhibited an unexpected therapeutic gain for pions versus experience with conventional treatment.

Results

Tables 3 and 4 present survival and local control data as related to dose range and site of disease for the entire population of 96 patients with 97 tumors. Overall survival and local control, i.e., without evidence of disease in the treatment volume at last follow-up or at death, are 51% and 45%, respectively, with follow-up from 6 to 40 months. The best results for a single site were obtained in treatment of prostatic carcinoma with all 15 patients controlled locally from 6 to 36 months, although one patient expired from hepatic metastases. Sixteen of 36 patients with head and neck tumors survive, although 2 have known local disease. Fourteen survivors are without evidence of disease, and 3 patients died of intercurrent disease or distant metastases without local–regional disease.

Review of all patients treated for primary brain tumors shows survival of 13 of 23 (57%), with follow-up of 6–21 months and a median survival of 14 months in those 13 patients treated more than 12 months ago. Eight of 10 patients treated during the last year survived. Eight of the 23 had lesions of histologic Grade III, while 15 had lesions of

TABLE 5. Local Control, Pions Only, by Site and Dose

Site	Dose (π^- Rad Maximum) 2700–3999	4000–4999	>5000	Local Control
Head and neck	1/4	4/9	0/3	5/16 (31%)
Brain	1/10	2/6	0/0	3/16 (19%)
Prostate	4/10	11/11	0/0	15/15 (100%)
Pancreas	0/5	0/5	0/0	0/10 (0%)
Other	3/6	1/4	0/1	4/11 (36%)

TABLE 6. Acute Reactions to Pion Irradiation Alone

Dose (π^- Rad Maximum)	Severity	Number of Patients	Average Severity
2700–3999	0	2	
	1	9	1.7
	2	13	
	3	4	
4000–4999	0	0	
	1	11	2.0
	2	12	
	3	12	
⩾5000	0	0	
	1	0	2.8
	2	1	
	3	3	

Grade IV. Of those with Grade III lesions, 7 of the 8 survive, with follow-up times of 8 – 21 months. Three of 4 with Grade III lesions treated more than a year ago survive, with a median survival time of 18 months. Among the 15 Grade IV lesions, 6 survive with follow-up times of 6–18 months. Three of 10 with Grade IV lesions treated more than a year ago survive, with a median survival time of 11 months. Using the criteria of neurologic stability, absence of steroid dependence, and absence of contrast enhancement of CT scan, 6 of the 8 Grade III patients and none of the 15 Grade IV patients has locally controlled disease at follow-up times of 6–21 months.

None of the 11 patients with pancreatic carcinoma survive, and all had clinical or autopsy evidence of locally active disease. Six of these patients received between 2700–3999 peak pion rad. Only 5 of the 11 received doses in the current working tolerance dose range (4000–4999 rad). Nine of 11 had evidence of distant metastases at time of death. Six of 12 patients with carcinomas of miscellaneous sites survive, 5 of whom have no evidence of disease. A sixth patient, with carcinoma of the bladder, died of intercurrent gastrointestinal bleeding with autopsy proof of local control and distant metastasis.

Analysis of 67 patients with 68 tumors treated with pion irradiation alone shows similar results to those of the entire group. Survival and local control in the group receiving pions only were 31/68 (46%) and 29/68 (43%), respectively. Table 5 shows local control by site and dose with pion irra-

TABLE 7. Chronic Reactions Related to Pions Alone*

Dose (π^- Rad Maximum)	Severity	Number of Patients	Average Severity
2700–3999	0	9	
	1	10	1.0
	2	9	
	3	0	
4000–4999	0	9	
	1	16	1.1
	2	8	
	3	2	
⩾5000	0	0	
	1	2	1.5
	2	2	
	3	0	

diation alone. Sixteen of 36 head and neck patients received pions alone and 5 of these have local control (31%). Five of 16 patients treated for gliomata with pions alone had local control, and all 15 patients with prostate cancer had local control as determined by physical examination and CT scan. No patients with pancreatic carcinoma, but 4 of 11 with miscellaneous carcinomas, had eradication of local disease by pion irradiation.

Acute reactions to therapy have been generally well tolerated, and only four patients have had interruption of their planned course of irradiation by such reactions. Table 6 shows tabulation of numbers of patients having reactions of varying severity related to dose range. The scoring system is based on a scale from 0, i.e., no detectable reaction, to 4, i.e., acute life-threatening reaction. Grade 1 injury includes cutaneous erythema, mucosal injection, taste alteration, diarrhea without mucus or tenesmus, dysuria, and nocturia less than three times per night. Grade 2 includes such symptoms and signs as dry desquamation, patchy mucositis, mild to moderate xerostomia, diarrhea with mucus, and nocturia occurring more than three but less than six times per night. Grade 3 describes acute reactions such as moist desquamation, confluent mucositis, severe xerostomia, diarrhea with bleeding, and nocturia with frequency greater than six times per night.

Table 6 demonstrates a definite tendency toward increasingly severe acute reactions with escalating dose, particularly for those few patients receiving more than 5000 π^- rad. No patient, however, has sustained life-threatening acute injury. Acute reactions related to pion irradiation have demonstrated a pattern of resolution similar to that following curative doses of conventional irradiation, namely healing over a 2- to 4-week period.

Late reactions related to pion irradiation have been recorded according to the end-results format adopted by the Radiation Therapy Oncology Group (RTOG) and the European Organization for Research on Treatment of Cancer (EORTC) and are analyzed in Table 7 by dose range and severity. Again, the trend toward increasingly severe chronic effects is observed with escalating dose; however, only two patients have sustained severe injury related to pion irradiation alone and none has had life-threatening injury. The 2 patients with severe chronic reactions include one patient with symptomatic pulmonary fibrosis persisting 2 years after 3900 π^- rad maximum for a carcinoma of the left lower lobe and another with laryngeal edema 1 year following 5000 π^- rad maximum for a T4 carcinoma of the larynx. Of 19 patients scored with Grade 2 or moderate chronic injury, 10 had complete alopecia in part or all of the treatment field following irradiation of gliomata and 5 had moderate xerostomia following head and neck irradiation. In none of these cases did the reaction impair the patient's lifestyle.

Discussion

Negative pi mesons have attractive physical and biological properties that suggest theoretical advantages over conventional radiation modalities both in terms of dose distribution and biological effect within the peak region. The first clinical project to explore these possibilities has been underway at LAMPF with treatment of locally advanced neoplasms since 1976. Results of studies intended to elucidate acute and chronic tolerance of normal human tissues and response of various neoplasms to pion irradiation are presented as direction for future clinical research. These studies have necessarily encompassed a wide spectrum of clinical situations, including varying time, dose, and fractionation schedules, tumor sites, treatment volumes, and types of adjunctive therapy. The data presented indicate that pion irradiation can be effectively delivered by currently available technology, that this type of radiation can destroy some locally advanced neoplasms and effect control of such lesions for periods of 3 years, and that this benefit may be obtained with moderately acute toxicity and minimal chronic toxicity.

Review of data concerning acute reactions suggests that doses of 4500 π^- rad maximum delivered in 105–125 π^- rad fractions will produce moderate to severe acute reactions in nearly all patients, although very rarely will they necessitate interruption or abbreviation of the planned treatment. This has led to adoption of 4500 π^- rad maximum in 36 fractions over 50 days as the usual dose for most sites in the pelvis and head and neck, as well as cone-down volumes of the brain. Small volumes, especially in the head and neck, may tolerate boosting doses to the range of 5000–5200 π^- rad maximum. The follow-up in these cases as a group is brief, although 76 were followed more than 12 months. Chronic radiation effects have been, with rare exceptions, mild to moderate in degree. They have not been disproportionately severe as compared to acute reactions, and do not indicate that normal tissue tolerance has been exceeded. As yet, follow-up is too brief and numbers of patients too small to make definitive observations regarding long-term survival or local control; however, preliminary results are encouraging for a variety of disease sites including some lesions of the head and neck, malignant gliomata, and locally advanced prostatic carcinoma. As a result, a Phase III randomized trial has been implemented comparing pion and conventional radiotherapy for stage III and IV squamous carcinoma of the oral cavity and pharynx. Similar trials have been approved for locally recurrent or inoperable adenocarcinoma of the rectum and for T3 and T4 transitional cell carcinoma of the bladder. Gliomata continue to be treated in a nonrandomized fashion pending elucidation of maximum tolerable doses for normal brain. The nonrandomized pilot study of prostatic carcinoma has been closed to provide the long follow-up necessary to assess whether a randomized trial with conventional radiation is warranted, given the relative efficacy of conventional treatment in this site as compared to most others being treated. It is clear that the phase III trials underway will provide methodologically sound answers regarding survival and local control and that further follow-up of previously treated patients will offer additional guidance regarding future clinical trials with pion radiotherapy.

Summary

One hundred forty patients were treated

with pion radiotherapy at the Los Alamos Meson Physics Facility prior to April 1980. Ninety-six patients with 97 tumors receiving definitive therapy with curative intent are analyzed with regard to survival, local control, and acute and chronic reactions. Twenty-nine patients received additional conventional radiation therapy or surgery. Cases analyzed include 36 with neoplasms of the head and neck, 23 with high grade gliomata, 15 with prostatic carcinoma, 11 with pancreatic carcinoma, and 12 with locally advanced carcinomas of various sites, including rectum, bladder, uterine cervix, lung, skin, stomach, and esophagus. Thus, the local control rate, assessed clinically, varied from 0% for pancreatic cancer to 100% for advanced prostatic cancer. Survival rates must be evaluated with caution since only 24 patients received a dose now considered at a working tolerance level, i.e., 4500 π^- rad in 36 fractions over 7 weeks. The local control rate, assessed clinically, varied from 0% for pancreatic carcinoma to 100% for advanced prostatic carcinoma. Acute reactions increased with escalating dose but have rarely resulted in interruption of treatment. Only two cases of severe chronic radiation injury have been ascribed to pion irradiation alone.

ACKNOWLEDGMENTS

Research for this chapter was supported in part by U.S. Public Health Service Grant CA16127 from the National Cancer Institute and by the U.S. Department of Energy.

REFERENCES

1. Fowler, P.H., and Perkins, D.H.: The possibility of therapeutic applications of beams of negative π^- mesons. *Nature* **189**:524–528, 1961.
2. Hogstrom, K.R., Smith, A.R., Kelsey, C.A., Simon, S.L., Somers, J.W., Lane, R.G., Rosen, I.I., von Essen, C.F., Kligerman, M.M., Berardo, P.A., and Zink, S.M.: Static pion beam treatment planning of deep seated tumors using computerized tomographic scans at LAMPF. *Int J Radiat Oncol Biol Phys* **5**:875–886, 1979.
3. Kligerman, M.M., Hogstrom, K.R., Lane, R.G., and Somers, J.: Prior immobilization and positioning for more efficient radiotherapy. *Int J Radiat Oncol Biol Phys* **2**:1141–1144, 1977.
4. Kligerman, M.M., Smith, A., Yuhas, J.M., Wilson, S., Sternhagen, C.J., Helland, J.A., and Sala, J.M.: The relative biological effectiveness of pions in the acture response of human skin. *Int J Radiat Oncol Biol Phys* **3**:335–339, 1977.
5. Kligerman, M., Tsujii, H., Bagshaw, M., Wilson, S., Black, W., Mettler, F., and Hogstrom, K.: Current observations of pion radiation therapy at LAMPF. In *Treatment of Radioresistant Cancers* M. Abe, K. Sakamoto, and T.L. Phillips, eds. Amsterdam: Elsevier/North-Holland Biomedical Press, 1979, pp. 145–157.
6. Paciotti, M., Bradbury, J., Hutson, R., Knapp, E., and Rivera, O.: Tuning the beam shaping section at the LAMPF biomedical channel. *IEEE Trans Nucl Sci* **NS-24**:1059, 1977.
7. Tsujii, H., Bagshaw, M., Smith, A., von Essen, C., Mettler, F., and Kligerman, M.: Localization of structures for pion radiotherapy by computerized tomography and orthodiagraphic projection. *Int J Radiat Oncol Biol Phys* **6**:319–325, 1980.

CHAPTER 44

Contribution of the Discussion Initiator: Combined Modalities–Possibilities and Liabilities

Shirley Hornsey, D.Sc., F.I. Biol.

The motive for using combined modalities of treatment is to enhance the destruction of tumor cells without an equal enhancement of damage to limiting normal tissues. In his review, Elkind suggested that by a study of the characteristics of cell sensitivity to combined modalities, such as hydroxyurea (HU) and radiation, we should be able to propose combined treatments which will give enhanced tumor control. However, he pointed out that the clinical results of combining HU and radiation had all fallen far short of the enhancement that appeared theoretically possible. This may have been because the drug had not been given at optimum times for combined treatment. Perhaps radiobiological theory can effectively and usefully be used in criticizing such clinical protocols.[4] It remains questionable whether theoretical expectation derived from cell studies *in vitro*, where cells progress through the cell cycle at roughly similar rates, can ever be realized in practice. In recent studies on the mouse intestine, Griffin and Hornsey have found that the sensitization and synchrony produced by HU in the ileum was very much less than in the jejunum (Fig. 1), and this can be explained entirely by the small differences in proliferation rates in these two similar tissues. The differences in cycle time seen within a tumor are much greater than those observed between the ileum and jejunum. In a tumor with a heterolegous cell population, therefore, the HU would have to be given over long periods to accumulate a significant proportion of cells at the G_1/S border, or to kill significant numbers of cells in S. It is unlikely that the limiting tissues, intestine and haemopoietic, would tolerate an adequate regime. Indeed, Madoc Jones *et al.*,[10] in a randomized trial of HU with radiation on carcinoma of the cervix using the same drug regimen used by Hreshchyshyn et al.,[7] reported that the drug had to be reduced or discontinued in 26/28 patients because of gastrointestinal or bone marrow toxicity. The satisfactory combination of such chemotherapeutic agents to enhance the radiosensitivity of the primary tumor may in practice be difficult to achieve. Belli[1] drew to our attention the fact that highly toxic chemotherapeutic agents are also highly mutagenic and that the mutants are fre-

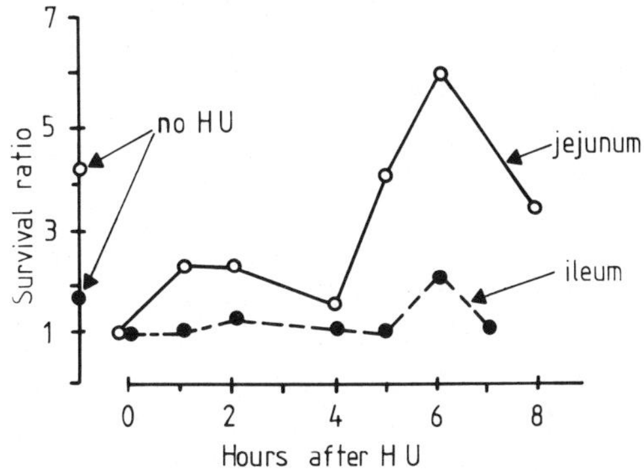

Figure 1. The effect on intestinal crypt counts of 1025 rad x-rays given to mice at various times after HU (1.5 mg/g I.P. followed after 2 hours by a second dose of 0.6 mg/g body weight).

Medical Research Council, Cyclotron Unit, Hammersmith Hospital, London, England

quently drug resistant and some may also be radiation resistant. Inadequate combined treatments may therefore also prejudice retreatment.

The enhancement of tumor sensitivity by hyperthermia or by hypoxic sensitizers may not be so limited by normal tissue sensitivity because for a given heat input tumor temperature rises much more than the normal tissue temperature. Furthermore, with few, if any, hypoxic foci in normal tissues, sensitivity is unchanged by hypoxic sensitizers. The neurotoxicity of some of the less lipophilic sensitizers being developed is significantly less than that observed with misonidazole. There appears to be an optimum for the 2-nitrosureas at a partition coefficient (octanol/water) of 0.04 giving a good uptake into tumor calls but little uptake in nervous tissue.[2]

Fears have been voiced that neutrons could reduce the recovery from photon-produced sublethal damage and that RBE values are therefore difficult to predict for combinations of neutrons and photons.[3] Hussey and Maor,[8] in their report on the mixed-beam trial of neutrons and photons, have shown no enhanced normal tissue effects, thus giving no indication that the RBE values were other than predicted from neutron-only studies. In other trials of mixed-beam treatment, there have been no reports of serious late complications,[9] possibly because of the smaller contribution to damage from neutrons; but in some trials using neutrons only, late damage, particularly to the CNS, had been greater than expected. This was due to insufficient knowledge of RBE for late effects but also in some cases to the use of an RBE of 3 to convert a satisfactory photon schedule to a neutron-limiting dose. RBE is related to the dose/fraction and at a photon dose of 200 rad, the RBE for a 16 MeVd-Be beam, for example, is 4.2 for skin damage and 5.2 for damage to the CNS.[6] The RBE's for higher energy beams will be lower, and it is interesting to note that Hussey and his colleagues have used a value of 4.1 at 200 rad/fraction of neutrons for the CNS for their neutron beam. It is important when converting acceptable photon schedules to neutron dose to use the RBE at the photon dose/fraction used in the conventional arm of the trial.

REFERENCES

1. Belli, J.A.: Adriamycin-resistant cells express multiple phenotypes. In *Biological Bases and Clinical Implications of Tumor Radioresistance* G.H. Fletcher and C. Nervi, eds. New York: Masson, 1982.
2. Brown, M.: Personal communication.
3. Denekamp, J.: Gamma contamination of neutron beams. *Br J Radiol* **53**:819, 1980.
4. Elkind, M.M.: Modifiers of radiation response in tumor therapy: Strategies and expectations. In *Biological Bases and Clinical Implications of Tumor Radioresistance* G.H. Fletcher and C. Nervi, eds. New York: Masson, 1982.
5. Griffin, C., and Hornsey, S., Personal communication.
6. Hornsey, S., Morris, C.C., Myers, R., and White, A.: Relative biological effectiveness for damage to the central nervous system by neutrons. *Int J Radiat Oncol Biol Phys* **7**:185, 1981.
7. Hreshchyshyn, M.M., Aron, B.S., Boronow, R.C., Franklin, E.W., Shingleton, H.M., and Blessing, J.A.: Hydroxyurea or placebo combined with radiation to treat stages III B and IV cervical cancer confined to the pelvis. *Int J Radiat Oncol Biol Phys* **5**:317–322, 1979.
8. Hussey, D.H., and Maor, M.H.: Preliminary report of combined neutron and photon irradiation for locally advanced head and neck tumors. In *Biological Bases and Clinical Implications of Tumor Radioresistance* G.H. Fletcher and C. Nervi, eds. New York: Masson, 1982.
9. Laramore, G.E., Blasko, J.C., Griffin, T.W., Croudine, M.T., and Parker, R.G.: Fast neutron teletherapy for advanced carcinomas of the oropharynx. *Int J Radiat Oncol Biol Phys* **5**:1821–1827, 1979.
10. Madoc-Jones, H., Perez, C.A., Kao, M.S., and Jennings, F.: Hydroxyurea with radiation in the treatment of advanced carcinoma of the cervix: A prospective randomized trial. In *Biological Bases and Clinical Implications of Tumor Radioresistance* G.H. Fletcher and C. Nervi, eds. New York: Masson, 1982.

CHAPTER 45

Keynote Address: Adjuvant Chemotherapy and Cancer Cure

Joseph R. Bertino[a]

The term adjuvant chemotherapy has enjoyed wide popularity in recent years. In order to avoid confusion, we will define it as chemotherapy following definitive primary therapy designed to eradicate all *detectable* malignant disease. This definition is more restrictive than commonly employed but allows less confusion with terms such as combined-modality therapy which may or may not imply this usage. It follows that the need for adjuvant chemotherapy is based on the historical observations that in a given set of patients, despite "eradication" of the primary tumor, tumor cells remain. This recurrence can be local, regional, or metastatic.

Definition of risk of recurrence then becomes the key to optimal use of chemotherapy; the usual clinical and pathologic guidelines used for most circumstances are the size of the primary tumor, degree of regional node involvement, and the degree of differentiation. At the present time, these prognostic determinants are useful, but only approximate; what is more important is that they are useless for helping us with the individual patient.

Table 1 indicates that adjuvant therapy need not be chemotherapy. In some circumstances chemotherapy may be primary therapy and may be successful in eradicating all evidence of disease (clinical complete remission), and surgery or radiation therapy may be employed as adjuvant treatment in an attempt to eradicate clinically undetectable residual foci of disease (e.g., testicular cancer, advanced Hodgkin's disease).

The rationale and enthusiasm for adjuvant chemotherapy derives from experimental considerations, i.e., that chemotherapy (or x-ray therapy) is more effective when the tumor burden is small, and that it has the potential for eradication of micrometastasis.[24,25] However, there is a contrary theoretical argument that suggests that small tumor burdens may require larger amounts of drug for eradication.[16] Clinical support is for the former view, however, and there is reasonable evidence to indicate that curability of several human cancers with chemotherapy is inversely proportional to the tumor burden.[27]

Considerations in the Use of Adjuvant Chemotherapy

The following section will attempt to provide both experimental and clinical evidence to indicate that for successful adjuvant chemotherapy (1) the dose is important, (2) timing of chemotherapy after primary therapy is important (i.e., the earlier the better), and (3) combination therapy may be more effective than single-agent treatment in the adjuvant situation, as it usually is for treatment of advanced disease.

The importance of dose is easily documented by the experimental work by Schabel and co-workers. Tumor eradication requires a maximum dose of chemotherapy in most circumstances.[25] The recent data of Bonnadonna and his colleagues[22] in the clin-

[a]American Cancer Society Professor of Medicine and Pharmacology, Departments of Medicine and Pharmacology, Yale University School of Medicine, New Haven, Conn.

TABLE 1. Surgery, X-Irradiation or Chemotherapy as Adjuvant Therapy

Cancer Type	Primary Therapy	Adjuvant Therapy	Reference
Breast cancer	Surgery	Chemotherapy	Bonnadonna et al., 1978[5]
Hodgkin's disease (IIIA)	Radiation Therapy;	Chemotherapy;	Rosenberg et al., 1979[21]
(IIIB, IV)	Chemotherapy	Radiation Therapy	Prosnitz et al., 1976[20]
Testicular cancer	Chemotherapy	Surgery	Anderson et al., 1979[29]
Acute leukemia	Chemotherapy	Radiation Therapy	Pinkel, 1976[17]

ical situation would also seem to support this concept: postmenopausal women receiving an *adequate* dose of CMF appear to benefit from adjuvant chemotherapy–those given a suboptimal dose do not.

Timing of chemotherapy following definitive treatment also appears to be important but has not been given sufficient attention. It is customary to wait 2–4 weeks following surgery to initiate adjuvant chemotherapy; in one very provocative study, cyclophosphamide administered immediately following surgery was associated with an improvement in survival. In one hospital that delayed this treatment 2–4 weeks after surgery, no survival advantage was seen over patients not receiving chemotherapy.[15] The importance of early initial chemotherapy is also clearly demonstrated with experimental tumor models.[25]

Unless a tumor is unusually sensitive to single-agent therapy (a rare circumstance–choriocarcinoma and Burkitt's lymphoma are examples), even in the adjuvant situation where the residual tumor burden is likely to be small ($< 10^9$ cells), single-agent therapy is not likely to be effective unless the tumor burden is $< 10^5$ cells. This conclusion derives from mutation frequencies that range from 1 in 10^5 - 10^6 cells for drug-resistant cells. It is not surprising, therefore, to find ample experimental evidence to indicate that an effective drug combination is more likely to be successful in adjuvant chemotherapy as compared to single-agent therapy.[24] Clinically, these considerations seem correct, especially in breast cancer where drug combinations such as CMF and CMFVP appear to result in lower relapse rates than L-PAM alone.[10,22]

Problems with Adjuvant Chemotherapy

The dilemma of using adjuvant therapy is that all patients at risk are treated, some of whom are cured by primary therapy. In the situation after the primary has been removed in breast cancer, the relative risk may be defined if the axillary node status is known. The size of the primary and the estrogen receptor (ER) status help further in defining the risk.[1] Nevertheless, these predictions are only approximate, and even in situations of high risk (i.e., four or more nodes positive, ER negative), a substantial number of patients may not relapse. Since the drugs currently employed have short-term as well as long-term toxicities and since adjuvant therapy is associated with increased medical costs and can cause severe emotional stress in patients,[13] it is desirable to be able to define the risk of recurrence for the individual patient. Clearly, as has been emphasized by Ultman,[28] "salvage" therapy as well as the relative risk of recurrence are considerations in the choice of patients to be treated.

For example, patients with stage I and II Hodgkin's disease who relapse after radiation therapy (10–20%) may in a majority of cases be cured by salvage chemotherapy with or without additional small doses of x-ray.[19,20] Since current chemotherapy regimens in this disease, e.g., MOPP, have the potential for causing sterility as well as an increased risk of a second malignancy, especially acute leukemia, it may not make sense to treat stage I and II patients with adjunctive chemotherapy unless less toxic drug regimens than MOPP are developed. Thus, the therapeutic index or gain to be expected

TABLE 2. Strategy for Increasing Cure Rates in Solid Tumors[a]

1. Test new drugs and combinations in advanced disease.
2. Develop optimum chemotherapy regimen for primary treatment of disseminated disease.
3. Integrate optimum chemotherapy regimen into combined-modality approach for primary treatment of local and regional disease.

[a] Data from Carter, 1974.

depends not only on the risk of recurrence versus the toxicity of the drugs employed, but also on the effectiveness of "salvage" therapy.

Strategy of Drug-Combination Development for Adjuvant Chemotherapy—Are Alkylating Agents Necessary?

The strategy for development of effective adjuvant regimens proposed by Carter[7] and commonly practiced is shown in Table 2. An effective drug combination is developed to treat advanced disease (i.e., MOPP in Hodgkin's disease, CMF for breast cancer), and this regimen is then employed in the adjuvant situation. Experimental considerations and evidence argue that an alkylating agent (a noncycle active agent), as a component of these regimens may not be necessary. If this premise is correct, then the significant risks (sterility, secondary malignancies) associated with adjuvant treatment may be avoided, and consequently chemotherapy may be offered even to patients with a relatively low risk of recurrence. In breast cancer, the doubling time of early disease has been estimated to be 25 days, while in advanced disease it is estimated to be over 120 days.[26] These estimates are compatible with "Gompertzian" kinetics, and are similar to tumor-growth kinetics observed in animal tumor models. Thus, when tumors are growing rapidly (i.e., in the adjuvant situation), if effective antimetabolites are available, then these drugs may be effective alone, and alkylating agents may not be necessary for maximum cell kill. An example of this is shown in Table 3. In the early treatment of mice bearing the L1210 leukemia, use of cytosine arabinoside and methotrexate, an

TABLE 3. Antimetabolites vs. Cyclophosphamide and Antimetabolites in the Treatment of Early and Late Stage L1210 Leukemia[a]

Initiated Treatment[b]	Treatment	Survival (days)	WTΔ (day 7)
Day 3	Control	9.3	+3.3
	MTX (12 mg/kg)	13.5	−0.8
	ARA-C (180 mg/kg)	13.0	+1.0
	MTX/ARA-C	24.5	−1.5
	Cy (150 mg/kg)	15.5	−2.2
	Cy/MTX/ARA-C	20.5	−2.9
Day 6	Control	9.0	+3.0
	MTX (12 mg/kg)	10.5	+2.3
	ARA-C (180 mg/kg)	12.0	+3.6
	MTX/ARA-C	12.0	+3.6
	Cy (150 mg/kg)	13.0	+1.0
	Cy/MTX/ARA-C	20.0	−3.1

[a] Unpublished observations by Skeel, Capizzi, Hyrniuk, Skeltorp, and Bertino.

[b] Drug treatment was initiated 3 or 6 days after I.P. inoculation of BDF_1 with 10^6 leukemia cells (n = 8/group). Antimetabolite regimens consisted of methotrexate (MTX) and cytosine arabinoside (ARA-C), alone or in combination in the dose indicated. The alkylating agent, cyclophosphamide (Cy), was tested alone or in combination with both antimetabolites at the doses indicated.

TABLE 4. Toxic Effects of Sequential MTX → 5-FU[a]

Leukopenia[b]	3
Mucositis (grade 1)	2
Nausea and vomiting	1
No side effects	6
—	—
Total patients	12

[a] Dose schedule given in Table 4.

[b] 2400–4000 WBC/mm^3.

effective combination, results in long survival; the addition of cyclophosphamide does not appreciably add to this survival. However, in the treatment of advanced disease, these same two drugs have little effect, and the addition of cyclophosphamide to the regimen is necessary to increase survival, presumably because the cells are now in plateau phase growth and less sensitive to antimetabolites.[12] In addition, with larger tumor burdens, the chance of drug-resistant mutants being present is increased.[3]

During the past several years, based on experimental studies,[4,6,8] we have developed an effective sequential program utilizing methotrexate and fluorouracil that has modest antitumor effects in advanced breast and head and neck cancer.[9,18] Based on concepts discussed above, this regimen should be as effective in the adjuvant situation as CMF. We have offered this therapy to a small number of patients who have refused adjuvant therapy containing cyclophosphamide because of the risks of acute and long-term toxicity associated with this drug. Table 4 indicates that this regimen in the doses employed is extremely well tolerated, and half of the patients reported no toxicity. Table 5 summarizes the clinical data on the subjects treated, and this data has provided encouragement for testing this concept and this particular regimen in larger, controlled trials. The NSABP at the present time is considering this combination for an arm of one of their adjuvant trials.

Future Needs and Prospects

Clearly, a better definition of which pa-

TABLE 5. MTX/FU in Adjuvant Breast[a]

			Stage	Nodes	RAD/RX	ER Status	Clinical Status
Premenopausal	(1)	A.C.	III	?	yes	n.d.	74+ months
	(2)	A.E.	II	1/11	no	n.d.	51+ months
	(3)	L.W.	II	2/11	no	n.d.	52+ months
	(4)	C.G.	III	Palpable	yes	+(6)	41+ months
	(5)	D.D.	II	2/38	no	+	26+ months
	(6)	C.J.	III	9/26	no	+(4)	Relapse at 14 months + (CEA = 83)
	(7)	V.R.	III	?	yes	+(7)	23+ months
	(8)	H.B.	II	12/14	no	+(91)	18+ months
Postmenopausal	(9)	M.A.	II	1/11	no	n.d.	53 + months
	(10)	G.M.	III	7/20	no	n.d.	51+ months
	(11)	M.V.	II	5/13	no	+(25.2)	34+ months
	(12)	A.D.	III	6/6	no	n.d.	18+ months

[a] Methotrexate, 30 mg/m^2, followed by 5-fluorouracil, 600 mg/m^2, 1 hour later were administered intravenously to 9 of the patients above. They were treated weekly for 3 doses each month; duration of treatment was 18 months. In 3 patients, methotrexate, 200 mg/m^2, followed by 5-fluorouracil, 600 mg/m^2, 1 hour later and leucovorin, 10 mg/m^2 q6h × 6, 24 hours later were administered on days 1 and 8 of each month for 18 consecutive months.

tients are in danger of relapse, which sites may be at risk, and the sensitivity of patients' tumor cells to drugs or combinations of drugs are needed. Some developments are encouraging in this regard. For example, the ER status helps predict hormone sensitivity, soft agar systems for cloning human tumor stem cells are being evaluated as *in vitro* predictive tests,[23] and it may be possible eventually to predict the metastatic behavior of tumors, perhaps by analysis of tumor cell membrane glycoproteins.

We also need more sensitive markers to detect small amounts of residual tumor. Measurement of blood levels of the β subunit of HCG admirably fulfills this requirement for patients with choriocarcinoma and embryonal carcinoma; therapeutic decisions can be made even in the absence of clinically detectable disease.[2,12] For the majority of human tumors, however, tumor markers such as CEA are not useful to detect occult or residual disease. When such markers are found and can reliably be used to judge which patients are in need of adjuvant therapy, it will be a major step forward.

Finally, the increasing number of drugs available with activity against human tumors gives promise that effective and selective drug combinations may be found, thus eliminating some of the hazards associated with adjuvant chemotherapy.

Summary

The use of chemotherapy as an adjuvant to surgery and/or radiotherapy is well founded in experimental tumor systems and appears to be effective in patients in some circumstances. It is clear from both clinical and experimental studies that (1) the dose is important, (2) the earlier chemotherapy is started after primary therapy the better, and (3) combination chemotherapy may be more effective than single-agent treatment. The better the estimation of risk of recurrence, the better the assessment of the risk–benefit ratio with adjuvant therapy. Salvage therapy as well as relative risk of recurrence are considerations in the choice of patients to be treated. Finally, some evidence is presented to indicate that alkylating agents may not be necessary in combination regimens for adjuvant therapy if effective antimetabolite combinations are available.

REFERENCES

1. Adegra, J., Simon, R., and Lippman, M.: The association between steroid hormone receptor status and the disease-free interval in breast cancer. In *Adjuvant Therapy of Cancer*, S.E. Jones and S.E. Salmon, eds. New York: Grune and Stratton, 1979, pp. 47–59.
2. Anderson, T., Walldmann, T.A., Javadpour, M., and Glatstein, E.: Testicular germ cell neoplasms: Recent advances in diagnosis and therapy. *Ann Intern Med* **90**:373–385, 1979.
3. Bertino, J.R., and Hryniuk, N.M.: Disorders of cell growth. In *Clinical Pharmacology, Basic Principles in Therapeutics*, K.L. Melmon and H.F. Morelli, eds. New York: Macmillan, 1978, pp. 802–841.
4. Bertino, J.R., Sawicki, W.L., Lingquist, C.A., and Gupta, V.S.: Schedule-dependent antitumor effects of methotrexate and 5-fluorouracil. *Cancer Res* **37**:327–328, 1977.
5. Bonnadonna, G., Valagussa, P., Rossi, A., Zucali, R., Tancini, G., Bajetta, E., Brambilla, C., DeLena, M., DiFronzo, G., Banfi, A., Rilke, F., and Veronesi, U.: Are surgical adjuvant trials altering the course of breast cancer? *Semin Oncol* **5**:450–464, 1978.
6. Cadman, E., Heimer, R., and Davis, L.: Enhanced 5-fluorouracil formation after methotrexate administration: Explanation for drug synergism. *Science* **205**:1135–1137, 1979.
7. Carter, S.K.: Integration of chemotherapy into combined modality treatment of solid tumors. 1. The overall strategy. *Cancer Treat Rev* **1**:1–13, 1974.
8. Fernandes, D.J., and Bertino, J.R.: 5-fluorouracil-methotrexate synergy. Enhancement of 5-fluorodeoxyuridylate binding to thymidylate synthetase by dihydrofolate polyglutamates. *Proc Natl Acad Sci USA* **77**:5663–5667, 1980.
9. Gewirtz, A.M., and Cadman, E.: Preliminary report on the efficacy of sequential methotrexate and fluorouracil in advanced breast cancer. *Cancer*, in press.
10. Glucksberg, H., Rivkin, S.E., and Rasmussen, S.: Adjuvant chemotherapy for stage II breast cancer:

A comparison of CMFVP versus L-PAM (Southwest Oncology Group Study), In *Adjuvant Therapy of Cancer* S.E. Jones and S.E. Salmon, eds. New York: Grune and Stratton, 1979, pp. 261–268.
11. Hryniuk, W., Fischer, G.A., and Bertino, J.R.: S-phase cells of rapidly growing and resting populations. Differences in response to methotrexate. *Mol Pharmacol* **S**:558–564, 1969.
12. Javadpour, N.: The National Cancer Institute experience with testicular cancer. *J Urol* **120**:651–659, 1978.
13. McArdle, C.S., Cooper, A.F., Moran, C., Russell, A.R., and Smith, D.C.: The emotional and social implications of adjuvant chemotherapy in breast cancer. In *Adjuvant Therapy of Cancer* S.E. Jones and S.E. Salmon, eds. New York: Grune and Stratton, 1979, pp. 319–328.
14. Mieler, T.P., Jones, S.E.: Chemotherapy of localized histiocytic lymphoma. *Lancet* **I**:358–360, 1979.
15. Nissen-Meyer, R., Kjellgren, K., Malmio, K., et al.: Surgical adjuvant chemotherapy. Results with one short course with cyclophosphamide after mastectomy for breast cancer. *Cancer* **41**:2088–2098, 1978.
16. Norton, L., Simon, R.: Tumor size, sensitivity to therapy, and design of treatment schedules. *Cancer Treat Rep* **61**:1307–1317, 1977.
17. Pinkel, D.: Treatment of acute leukmeia. *Pediatr Clin North Am* **23**:117–129, 1976.
18. Pitman, S.W., Kowal, C.D., Papac, R.J., and Bertino, J.R.: Sequential methotrexate-5-fluorouracil: A highly active drug combination in advanced squamous cell carcinoma of the head and neck. *Proc Am Assoc Cancer Res* **21**:473, 1980.
19. Portlock, C.S., Rosenberg, S.A., Glatstein, E., and Kaplan, H.S.: Impact of salvage treatment on initial relapses in patients with Hodgkin's disease, stage I–III. *Blood* **51**:825–933, 1978.
20. Prosnitz, L.R., Farber, L.R., Fischer, J.J., Bertino, J.R., and Fischer, D.B.: Long-term remissions with combined modality therapy for advanced Hodgkin's disease. *Cancer* **37**:2826–2833, 1976.
21. Rosenberg, S.A., Kaplan, H.S., Brown, B.W.: The role of adjuvant MOPP in the therapy of Hodgkin's disease: An analysis after ten years. In *Adjuvant Therapy of Cancer*, S.E. Jones and S.E. Salmon, eds. New York: Grune and Stratton, 1979, pp. 109–117.
22. Rossi, A., Bonnadonna, G., Valagussa, P., Banfi, A., and Veronesi, U.: CMF adjuvant program for breast cancer: Five-year results. *Proc Am Assoc Cancer Res* **21**:204, 1980.
23. Salmon, S.E., Hamberger, A.W., Srehlen, B., Durie, B.G.M., Alberts, D., and Moon, T.E.: Quantitation of differential sensitivity of human tumor stem cells to anticancer drugs. *N Engl J Med* **298**:1321–1327, 1978.
24. Schabel, F.M.: Rationale for adjuvant chemotherapy. *Cancer* **39**:2875–28882, 1967.
25. Schabel, F.M.: Surgical adjuvant chemotherapy of metastic murine tumors. *Cancer* **40**:558–568, 1977.
26. Schackney, S.E., McCormack, G.W., and Cuchural, G.J., Jr.: Growth rate patterns of solid tumors and their relation to responsiveness to therapy. An analytical review. *Ann Intern Med* **89**:107–121, 1978.
27. Swenerton, K.D., Legha, S.S., Smith, T., Hortobage, G.N., Gehan, E.A., Yap, H.Y.: Gutterman, J.U., and Blumenschein, F.R.: Prognostic factors in metastatic breast cncer with combination chemotherapy. *Cancer Res* **39**:1552–1562, 1979.
28. Ultmann, J.E., and Konosfky, J.R.: Adjuvant therapy: Principles and state of the art. In *Adjuvant Therapy of Cancer* New York: Grune and Stratton, 1979, pp. 637–659.

CHAPTER 46

Clonogenic Assays for Predicting the Response of Solid Tumors to Therapy

John M. Yuhas, Ph.D.[a]

Our present understanding of the response of solid tumors assigns a major role to the number of clonogenic tumor stem cells which survive treatment. A number of other variables, either intrinsic or extrinsic to the stem cell, can contribute to overall end results, but with the development of methods for quantitating the fractional survival of tumor colony-forming units or TCFU following therapy,[1] the role these factors might be playing has received less and less attention.

In using TCFU survival to evaluate the effectiveness of therapy, two assumptions are being made. First is that the number of tumor stem cells which survive treatment is the single most important determinant of end results. The second, and perhaps more tenuous assumption, is that the TCFU which are assayed *in vitro* are both quantitative and qualitative reflections of the tumor stem cells which would have survived and determined end results had the tumor been left intact. Unless the second assumption is valid, one cannot comment on the first. If one could show that the analysis of TCFU survival is predictive of end results, one would have strong indirect evidence in support of both assumptions, but, unfortunately, TCFU analysis is often performed with no consideration of its relationship to end results.

Over the years, however, a number of investigators have addressed this problem and in many instances TCFU analysis has failed to predict end results. Instead of listing each of the reported exceptions to the desired correlation, we list below examples of each type.

Divergence Based on Treatment Intensity

If we assume that the number of surviving TCFU is the sole determinant of end results and that these cells divide exponentially at a constant rate independent of treatment, then growth delay should be a linear function of the log of the surviving TCFU fraction. The expected linear relationship is not observed, however, especially when a broad range of response is studied. Stephens and Steel[6] compared TCFU survival to growth delay in the Lewis lung carcinoma system of mice. While the physiologic state of the tumor (ambient, Ro-07-0582 treated or clamped tumors) did not alter the relationship, all three sets of data were characterized by a curvilinear relationship between log TCFU survival and growth delay (see Fig. 1). In other words, in the high-dose, low-TCFU survival range, TCFU analysis underestimated the effectiveness of therapy as estimated by growth delay.

Divergence Based on Physiologic Status

In the studies of Stephens and Steel[6] the relationship between TCFU survival and growth delay was the same whether the animals breathed air, received Ro-07-0582, or

[a]Department of Radiation Therapy,
University of Pennsylvania and
Children's Hospital of Philadelphia, Pa.

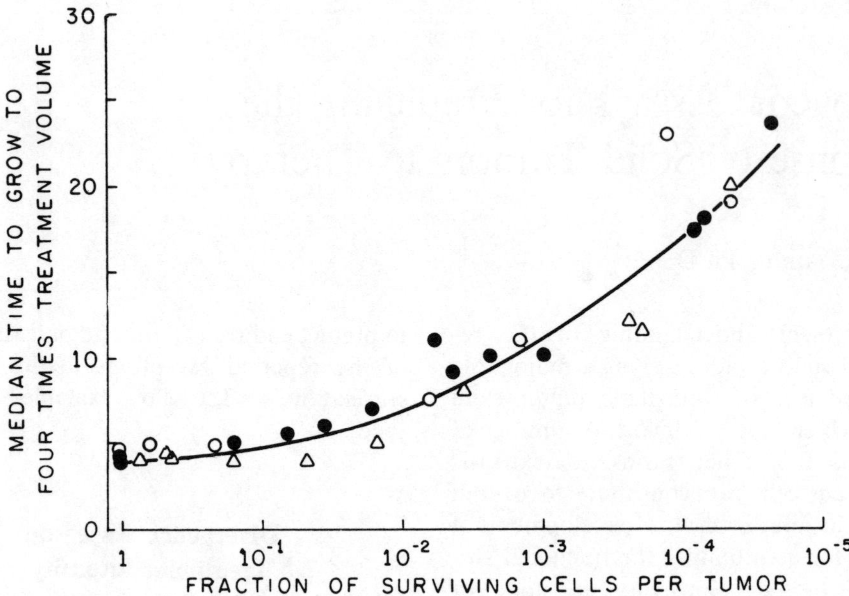

Figure 1. Relationship between fraction of surviving cells per tumor (TCFU) and growth delay observed in mice bearing the Lewis lung carcinoma who were exposed to ^{60}Co gamma rays. ● = air-breathing mice; Δ = mice whose tumors were clamped; and o = mice given 1 mg/kg of Ro-07-0582. (Data from Stephens and Steel, 1980[6].)

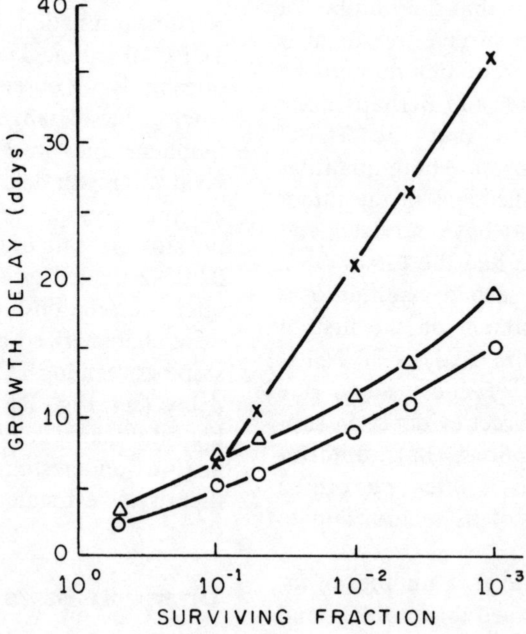

Figure 2. Growth delay induced by x-rays in the RIB_5C tumor system as a function of the surviving fraction of TCFU. x = animals breathing air; Δ = animals breathing oxygen; and o = animals whose tumors were clamped. (Data from McNally, 1973[3].)

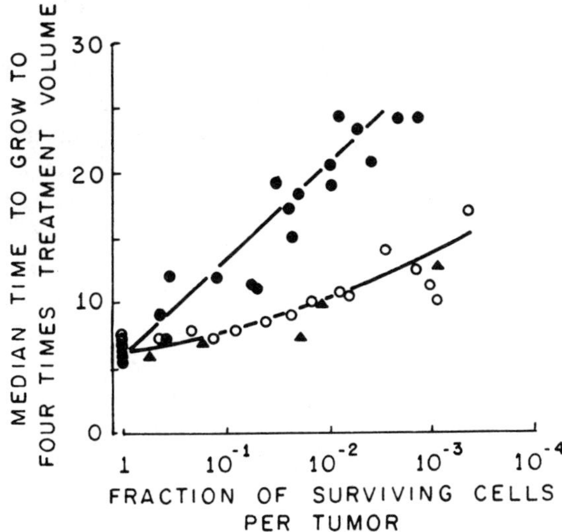

Figure 3. Growth delay as a function of fractional TCFU survival in the B16 melanoma system. ● = cyclophosphamide; o = CCNU; and Δ = L-phenylaline mustard. (Data from Peacock and Stevens, 1978[4].)

had their tumors clamped during exposure. Using a similar design as for the RIB_5C tumor, McNally[3] obtained quite a different pattern (see Fig. 2). The TCFU versus growth delay curve was far steeper in air-breathing mice than for the others. Further, the curve for animals breathing oxygen was displaced to the left of that for animals with clamped tumors, leading to an estimated oxygen enhancement ratio of 2.5 in the TCFU system, but 3.0 in the growth delay system.[3]

Divergence Based on Type of Treatment

The most severe dissociations of TCFU survival and growth delay appear when one compares a series of drugs. Stephens and Peacock[5] and Peacock and Stephens[4] have reported comparisons of TCFU survival versus growth delay in the B16 melanoma system which diverge widely depending on the particular drug being studied (see Fig. 3). The relationship is the same for drugs such as CCNU and L-phenylalanine mustard but far steeper for cyclophosphamide (Fig. 3). In this instance, the therapeutic potential of cyclophosphamide would have been grossly underestimated by simple TCFU analysis.

As a last example of dissociation of TCFU analysis and growth delay, we report our own data on growth delay and TCFU survival in MCa-11 multicellular tumor spheroids or MTS[10] exposed to peak negative pi mesons or x-rays. If the MTS are left intact after exposure, the sole difference between two types of radiations is that the threshold, which must be exceeded before growth delay becomes a linear function of dose, is smaller in the pion-exposed MTS than in their x-ray counterparts (see Fig. 4). However, if, immediately after exposure, the MTS are trypsinized and plated for TCFU survival, no difference between peak pions and x-rays is apparent (see Fig. 4[b]).

In summary, TCFU survival is not a rigid predictor of end results in cancer therapy, but can diverge depending on the particular tumor being studied, the physiologic status of the tumor, and the intensity and type of treatment being studied. The pessimistic view is that TCFU analysis may not be used to evaluate therapeutic effectiveness without first establishing that the two end points do not diverge and, therefore, the savings in

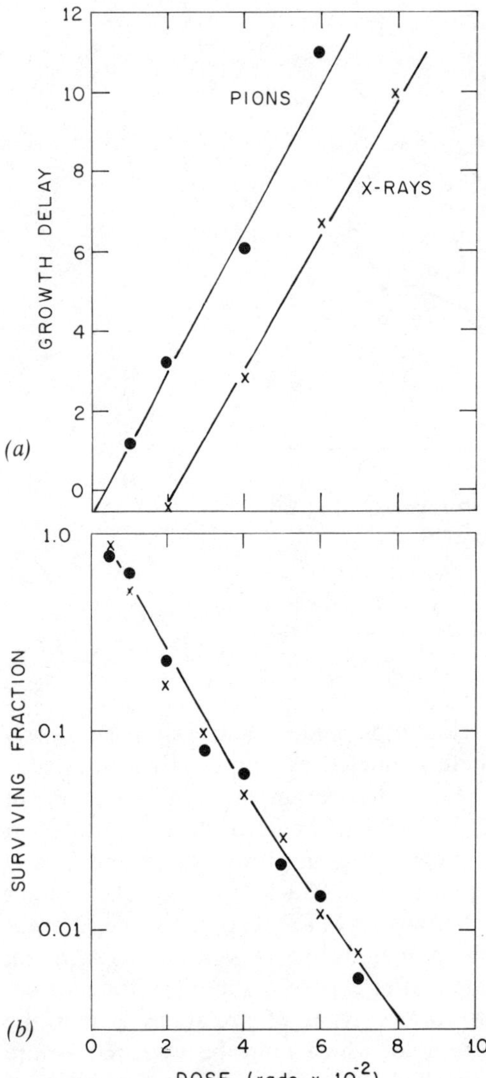

Figure 4. (*a*) Growth delay and (*b*) TCFU survival for MCa-11 multicellular tumor spheroids exposed to graded doses of peak negative pions or 300 kVp. ● = peak pions and x = x-rays.

time and effort promised by TCFU analysis is obviated. A more optimistic view of the foregoing would argue that the dissociations noted above may provide the most promising leads for identifying those factors, in addition to the number of TCFU which survive which contribute to end results. Toward this end, we will reexamine the divergences noted above in the hope of differentiating additional variables from artefacts.

Basis of Intensity Divergence

At the present, it is not possible to offer a definitive conclusion as to why TCFU analysis should underestimate growth delay in the high dose range relative to data obtained in the lower dose range (Fig. 1). As the radiation dose is increased the fraction of the surviving TCFU which were hypoxic at the time of exposure increases, thereby raising the possibility that the plating efficiency of the various subpopulations is responsible for this pattern. In order to account for the pattern in Figure 1, it would have to be argued that the well-oxygenated cells have a lower plating efficiency and/or retrieval than their hypoxic counterparts. As shown below, however, it would appear that the reverse is true.

An alternate proposal which might account for the divergence based on intensity was proposed by Stephens and Steel.[6] These investigators demonstrated that the rate at which the TCFU repopulated the tumor did not vary appreciably over the dose range of 1500 - 3500 rad in air-breathing mice, but that as the dose increased so did the lag period before this normal growth was resumed. It would be speculative at present to champion one or another possible basis for this dose-dependent lag period. Whether this effect resides within the TCFU themselves or in other host factors as discussed by Brown[2] remains to be determined, but elucidation of these factors, especially if they persist under conditions comparable to the clinic, is clearly an area of investigation worthy of attention.

Basis of Tumor Physiology Divergence

In the original study by McNally,[3] it was observed that the OER estimated by TCFU analysis was 2.5, while that estimated by growth delay was 3.0. McNally suggested that this discrepancy might have resulted from the failure of the TCFU method to accurately describe the number of hypoxic TCFU which survived the treatment. This

TABLE 1. Retrieval of ^{3}H-Leucine- and ^{125}IUdR-Labelled Cells from Three Types of MTS

MTS Line	^{3}H-Leucine Intact	Tryp.	% Loss	^{125}IUdR Intact	Tryp.	% Loss
Line 1	68,391 ± 1704	65,268 ± 803	4.6%	32,843 ± 564	30,898 ± 271	5.9%
MCa-11	59,472 ± 1203	37,266 ± 777	37.3%	21,874 ± 342	19,111 ± 299	12.6%
MDA-361	36,040 ± 281	19,741 ± 904	45.2%	16,181 ± 202	15,744 ± 808	2.7%

raises one of the major difficulties of TCFU analysis for solid tumors; in none of the assays presently in use can one quantitate the plating efficiency of hypoxic TCFU versus well-oxygenated ones. Sutherland et al.[7] have attempted to overcome this problem by sequential trypsinizations of multicellular tumor spheroids, and Kallman (personal communication) is developing methods whereby one can determine whether a given colony was produced by a cell which was or was not dividing at the time of treatment. Neither of these approaches addresses the critical question, however, of the yield of TCFU in these two compartments relative to those which exist in the intact state. Data presently accumulating in our laboratory suggest that the yield of viable tumor cells can vary widely in the two compartments of well-oxygenated and hypoxic cells (see Table 1). Following prolonged incubation of MTS in ^{3}H-leucine, virtually all cells are labelled, but a final 24-hour incubation in ^{125}IUdR only labels those cells which are actively in division.[9] By comparing the ^{3}H and ^{125}I incorporated into these MTS before and after trypsinization, one can estimate the loss of total cells (^{3}H) relative to the loss of cells which were actively dividing (^{125}I). In a preliminary survey of three MTS lines, it became apparent that ^{3}H-labelled and ^{125}I-labelled cells were lost in proportion following trypsinization in some lines, but that selective loss of ^{3}H-labelled cells occurred in others (Table 1). This would suggest that nondividing, presumably hypoxic, cells can be selectively destroyed by trypsinization in at least certain tumors. If TFCU follow similar patterns, the results presented by McNally[3] would not be unexpected. Until such time that differential plating of hypoxic and well-oxygenated TCFU can be resolved (as well as other physiologic variables such as hyperthermia), it is not likely that simple TCFU survival will be able to predict the consequences of physiologic alteration of the tumor.

Basis of Treatment-Type Divergence

This is perhaps the most serious of the problems with TCFU analysis since most of our effort is devoted to quantitation of effectiveness of a series of agents. At least three mechanisms have been reported which can generate treatment-dependent differences in the relationship of TCFU survival to growth delay.

In the B16 melanoma system, Stephens and Steel[6] reported that cyclophosphamide produced a far greater growth delay at a given level of TCFU survival than did either CCNU or L-phenylalanine mustard (Fig. 3). By following the rate of growth of the surviving TCFU in these animals, these investigators were able to demonstrate that the surviving TCFU proliferated at a far slower rate in cyclophosphamide-treated mice than in mice treated with the other two drugs. Again, one must invoke heritable changes in TCFU proliferation rate or, more likely, non-TCFU factors as discussed by Brown.[2]

Following the demonstration of gross overestimates of growth delay when bleomycin was studied in the TCFU system, Twentyman[8] was able to trace this diver-

TABLE 2. Plating Efficiency of EMT6 Tumor Cells Which Were Harvested and Plated Alone (Control) or Harvested and/or Plated with Cells from Treated Tumors[c]

Treatment	Control	Plated with Treated Cells	Suspended and Plated with Treated Cells
Bleomycin	30.7%[a]	34.7%	0.41%
	31.0	31.7	0.01
	42.0[b]	52.0	4.4
Radiation	36.3	49.3	33.3
Cyclophosphamide	55.3	59.0	61.3
BCNU	56.0[b]	67.3	85.3

[a]Unless otherwise noted, treatment given 30 minutes before trypsinization.

[b]Treatment given 2 hours before trypsinization.

[c]Data from Twentyman, 1977.

gence to the presence of bleomycin during the cell-suspension procedure (see Table 2). Control tumors manifested a high plating efficiency when they were suspended and plated separately or when suspended separately but plated in the presence of cells suspended from bleomycin-treated tumors. If, however, the two types of tumors were both suspended and plated together, the plating efficiency for control TCFU was reduced by a factor of 2 logs or more. This would suggest that artifacts can be introduced into TCFU analysis if the drug persists in the tumor at the time the cells are suspended, and this effect is not noted with all drugs (Table 2). Therefore, drug-dependent artifacts are to be expected in the TCFU system.

A last point concerns our own studies on MTS. As has been observed by many others, our own divergence of growth delay and TCFU survival has been traced to an interaction of the trypsinization procedure and potentially lethal damage. If the pion-treated MTS are left intact, the radiation dose required to cure 50% of them[10] is on the order of a kilorad, and it is only marginally reduced if the MTS are trypsinized immediately after or 24 hours after exposure but before being introduced into the cure assay system (see Table 3). The same does not hold true for x-ray-treated MTS since intact spheroids have a TCD_{50} of more than

TABLE 3. Peak Pion and X-Ray doses Required to Cure 50% of Exposed MTS When the MTS Were Left Intact, Trypsinized Immediately after Exposure, or 24 hours Later.

MTS Handling	ED_{50} (rad ± s.e.) Peak Pions	X-rays
Intact	1086 ± 56	1791 ± 47
Tryp. (t = 0)	974 ± 91	1174 ± 96
Tryp. (t = 24 hours)	1101 ± 117	1856 ± 27

1700 rad which drops to 1200 rad if the MTS are trypsinized 1 hour after treatment, but rises again to 1800 rad if trypsinization is delayed until 24 hours. Clearly, the interaction of potentially lethal damage is far more important in x-ray- than in pion-treated MTS.

Summary

It would be an overgeneralization to argue that TCFU analysis has no place in experimental cancer therapy because of the many problems cited above. Our somewhat negative approach has been taken intentionally in order to emphasize the fact that, although TCFU studies are simple to perform, they are difficult to analyze. Based on the discussion presented above, it proposed that any conclusions drawn from TCFU analysis must be tempered by the realization that end results may show totally different patterns.

Acknowledgments

Research for this chapter was supported by Grant N01-CB-74203 from the National Cancer Institute.

REFERENCES

1. Barendsen, G.W., and Broerse, J.J.: Experimental radiotherapy of a rat rhabdomyosarcoma with 15MeV neutrons and 300 Kv x-rays. 1. Effects of single exposures. *Eur J Cancer* **5**:373–391, 1969.
2. Brown, J.M.: Drug or radiation changes to the host which could effect the outcome of combined modality therapy. *Int J Radiat Oncol Biol Phys* **5**:1151–1163, 1979.
3. McNally, M.J.: A comparison of the effects of radiation on tumor growth delay and cell survival. The effect of oxygen. *Br J Radiol* **46**:450–455, 1973.
4. Peacock, J.H., and Stephens, T.C.: Influence of anesthetics on tumor-cell kill and repopulation in B16 melanoma treated with melpholan. *Br J Cancer* **38**:725–731, 1978.
5. Stephens, T.C., and Peacock, J.H.: Tumor volume response, initial cell kill and cellular repopulation in B16 melanoma treated with cyclophosphamide and 1-(2-chloroethyl)-3-cyclohehyl-1-nitrosourea. *Br J Cancer* **36**:313–321, 1977.
6. Stephens, T.C., and Steel, G.G.: Regeneration of tumors after cytotoxic treatment. In *Radiation Biology in Cancer Research* R.E. Meyn and H.R. Withers, eds. New York: Raven Press, 1980, pp. 385–395.
7. Sutherland, R., Eddy, H., Bareham, B., Reich, K., and Vanantwerp, D.: Resistance to adriamycin in multicellular tumor spheroids. *Int Radiat Oncol Biol Phys* **5**:1225–1230, 1979.
8. Twentyman, P.: An artifact in clonogenic assays of bleomycin cytotoxicity. *Br J Cancer* **36**:642–644, 1977.
9. Yuhas, J.M., and Li, A.P.: Growth fraction as the major determinant of multicellular tumor spheroid growth rates. *Cancer Res* **38**:1528–1532, 1978.
10. Yuhas, J.M., Tarleton, A.E., and Harman, J.G.: *In vitro* analysis of multicellular tumor spheroids exposed to chemotherapeutic agents *in vitro* or *in vivo*. *Cancer Res* **38**:3595–3598, 1978.

CHAPTER 47

Notes on Pharmacokinetic and Other Aspects of Drug Resistance in Cancer Chemotherapy

Maurizio D'Incalci, M.D.[a]

In general the therapeutic outcome of drug treatment depends on the concentration of the substance itself, or active metabolite(s), available at the receptor site, and on the sensitivity of the receptor. In the case of antitumoral drugs, the receptor is in the cancer cell and may differ for each drug (e.g., DNA or RNA or specific proteins). The factors determining the relation between the dose administered and the drug concentration at the receptor can be defined as pharmacokinetic; the factors determining the relation between the concentration at the target and the clinical response can be defined as pharmacodynamic (see Fig. 1).

In other areas of pharmacology, pharmacokinetic studies aimed at evaluating the absorption, metabolism, distribution, and elimination of drugs have provided valid information to increase the efficacy of the treatment.[34] In the field of anticancer agents, pharmacokinetic knowledge is still insufficient for many drugs and only recently have suitable analytical methods been developed to permit appropriate studies in cancer patients. One more reason why pharmacokinetic studies have such relevance is that cancer, particularly at an advanced stage, is a systemic disease involving so many alterations in the host that it is hardly surprising that the fate of a drug in the organism may also be influenced.

[a]Research Associate, Istituto di Ricerche Farmacologiche "Mario Negri." Milan, Italy

There are examples of very wide variability in absorption of antitumorals in cancer patients. Figure 2 shows plasma levels of hexamethylmelamine (HMM) in 11 ovarian cancer patients after oral administration of the drug. For the same doses the concentration × time ($C \times T$) varies up to 100 times in different patients,[11] so that low bioavailability of the drug might be responsible for the inefficacy of HMM treatment in some patients. Figure 3 shows VP16 levels after I.V. and oral (ampoules) administration to the same patient. Less than 5% of the oral VP16 was absorbed in this patient in spite of the fact that the majority of patients have good absorption, corresponding to about 50% of the dose. The lack of response in this particular patient after oral treatment may reasonably be due to the low absorption of the drug.

Figure 4 shows the levels of VP16 in plasma of a leukemic patient after I.V. doses of 100 mg/m^2 and 200 mg/m^2. This child received a first course of five consecutive daily doses of VP16 at 100 mg/m^2/day and a second course (after 15 days) of 5 consecutive daily injections of VP16 at 200 mg/m^2/day. After the first course with the low dose no response was observed, and there was a continued increase of peripheral blasts. After the second course with double the dose there was a dramatic improvement with the disappearance of blasts from peripheral blood; bone marrow examinations revealed a nearly complete response. This example shows that sometimes, even after

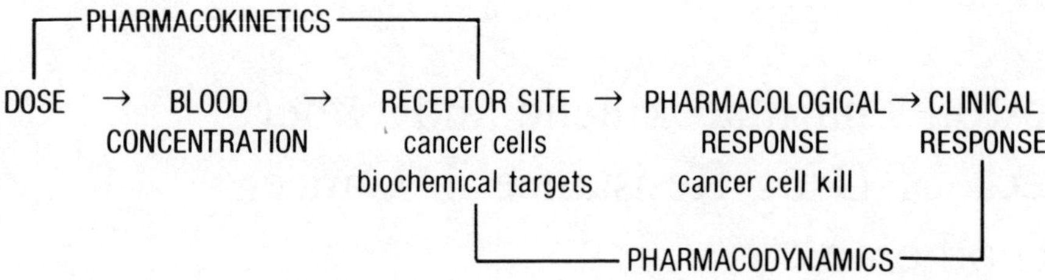

Figure 1. Schematic representation of principal factors and terms involved in drug dosage and response.

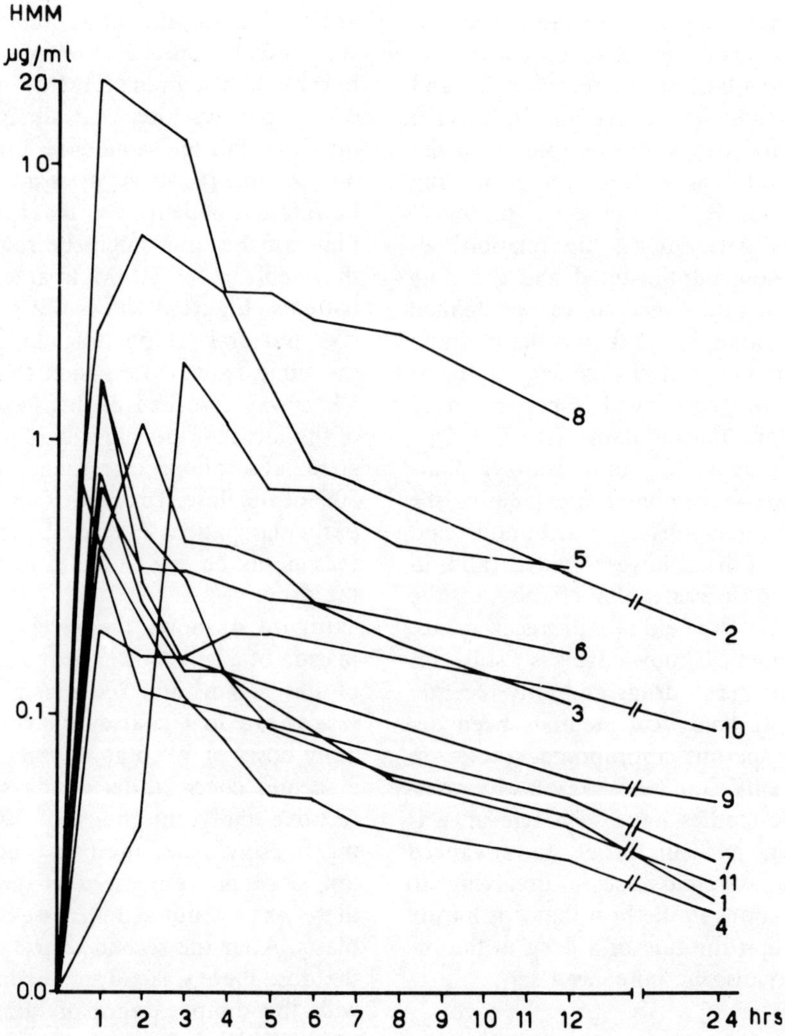

Figure 2. Hexamethylmelamine plasma levels after oral administration to ovarian cancer patients.

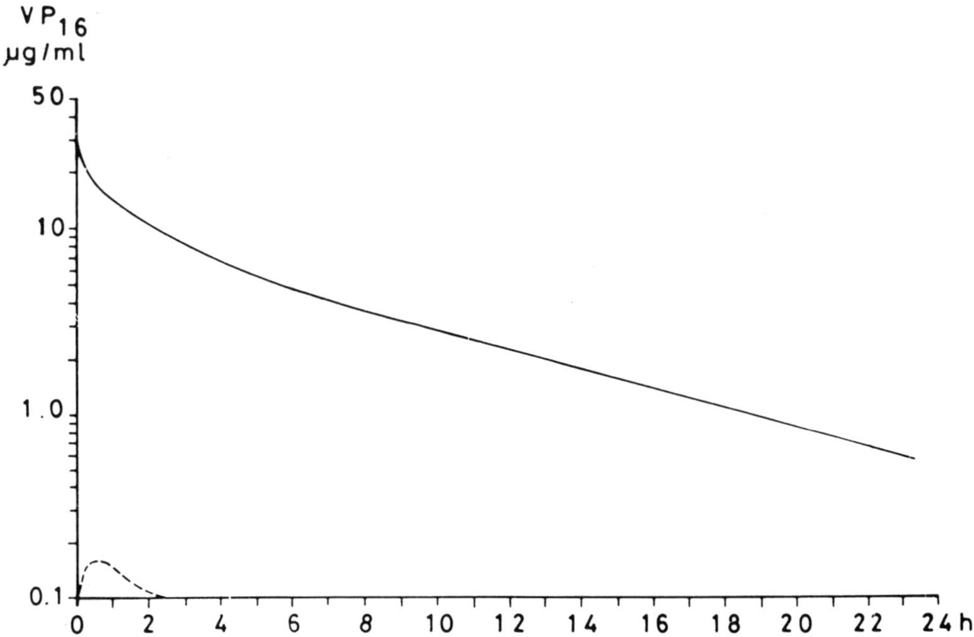

Figure 3. VP16 plasma levels after 100 mg/m² in a choriocarcinoma patient with impaired absorption function; continuous line = I.V.; dashed line = p.o.

parenteral administration, the elimination rate of a drug is such that effective concentrations are not achieved or not maintained long enough to exert a cytotoxic effect. In these cases resistance can often be countered by changing the doses or the duration of infusion.

Some drugs, such as cyclophosphamide (Cyc) for example, are not active per se, but act through the formation of active metabolites; thus, metabolism can be crucial in determining the effect. Figure 5 shows the plasma levels of Cyc after the first dose and after 6 months of continual treatment in two patients. There is a marked change in the elimination rate,[10] reflecting increased metabolism. It cannot be excluded that some cases of resistance to Cyc are due to these changes in metabolism with consequent changes in the concentrations of active metabolites.

The distribution of a drug may in some cases be the basis for therapeutic failure. There are compartments in which drugs penetrate only in minimal amounts, so that cancer cells localized in these so-called "sanctuaries" are not reached by the drug. The CNS is the most typical sanctuary (e.g., CNS metastases in ALL), and in fact most antitumorals currently used do not cross the blood-brain barrier. Nitrosoureas are virtually the only class of drugs which penetrate the CNS[19] (though perhaps podophyllotoxins do too, but these compounds have been found only in very small amounts in CSF,[8] possibly because of their high percentage of binding to plasma proteins). MTX at high doses[4] and Ara-C partially cross the blood-brain barrier.[7] None of the other drugs cross the barrier in significant amounts.

Other "sanctuaries" have not been so clearly identified in man because of the obvious difficulties in obtaining tissue samples from patients to measure drug concentrations. There are many experimental data, however, which indicate that drugs reach much lower concentrations in the less vascularized part of animal tumors. For example, as shown by Donelli et al.[13] in Lewis lung carcinoma, ADM concentrations in the external vegetating part are much

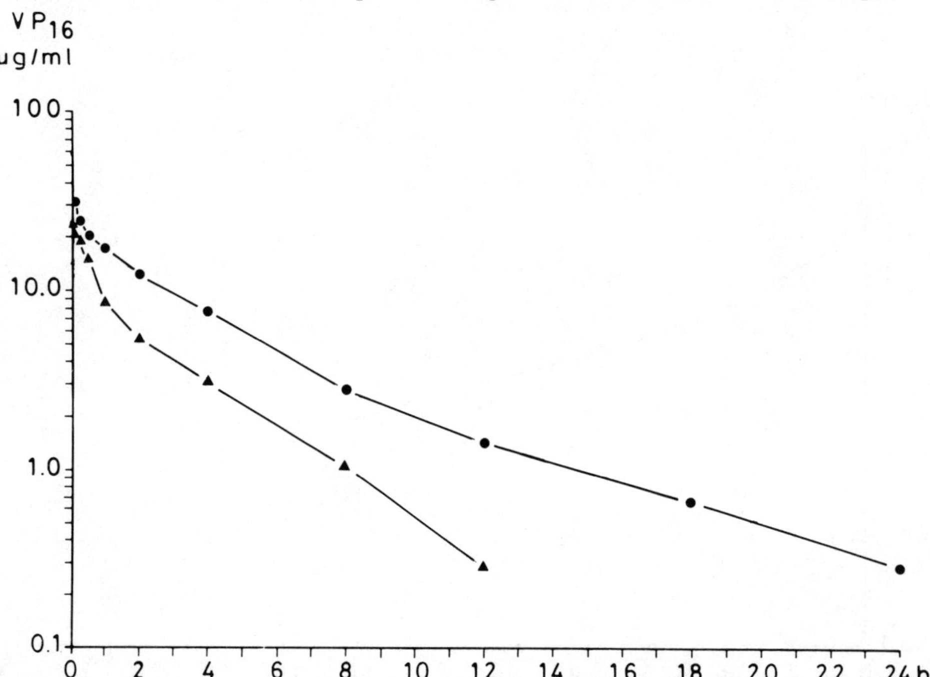

Figure 4. VP16 levels in a ALL child: ▲ levels after 100 mg/m² I.V.; ● levels after 200 mg/m² I.V.

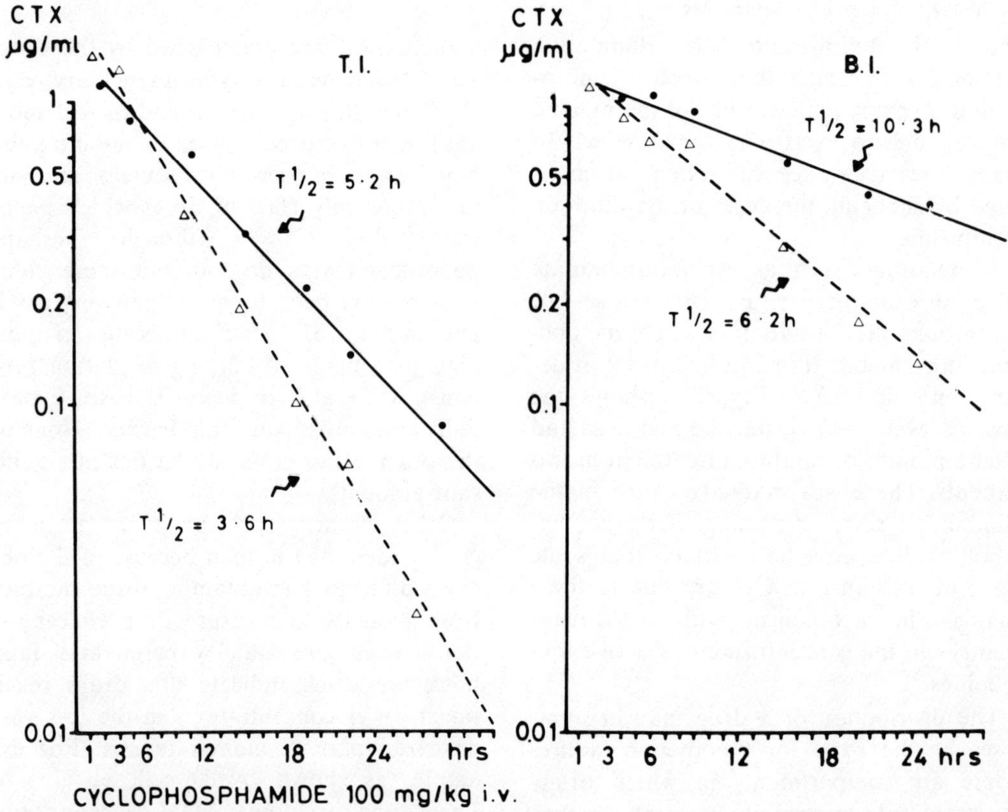

Figure 5. Cyclophosphamide plasma levels after the first dose (●) and after 6 months (Δ) of continual daily treatment in two patients (T.I. and B.I.).

TABLE 1. Distribution of Adriamycin in the Vegetating and Necrotic Parts of Lewis Lung Carcinoma[a]

Time after Treatment (minutes)	Vegetating Part (μg/g ± S.E.)	Necrotic Part (μg/g ± S.E.)
1	1.9 ± 0.1	<1
10	2.5 ± 0.4	<1
15	2.5 ± 0.7	<1
30	2.5 ± 0.2	<1
60	2.4 ± 0.3	<1
180	1.7 ± 0.5	<1
360	1.8 ± 0.1	<1
1440	2.1 ± 0.3	<1
AUC (μg/g X minutes)[b]		
60 minutes	143 ± 13	<1
24 hours	2745 ± 205	<1

[a] AM (15 mg/kg) was injected I.V. in C_{57}B1/6 mice with intramuscular 3LL 25 days old.

[b] AUC = area under the concentration vs. time curve.

TABLE 2. Distribution of Methotrexate in the Vegetating and Necrotic Parts of Lewis Lung Carcinoma[a]

Time after Treatment (minutes)	Vegetating Part (μg/g ± S.E.)	Necrotic Part (μg/g ± S.E.)
1	7.9 ± 1.0	1.7 ± 0.4
5	8.0 ± 1.1	3.4 ± 1.0
15	5.1 ± 0.8	<1
30	4.6 ± 0.2	<1
60	3.2 ± 0.4	<1
180	2.9 ± 0.7	<1
360	1.9 ± 0.3	<1
1440	2.1 ± 0.6	<1
AUC (μg/g X minutes)[b]		
60 minutes	233 ± 63	78
24 hours	3105 ± 321	78

[a] Methotrexate (15 mg/kg) was injected I.V. in C_{57} Bl/6 mice with intramuscular 3LL 25 days old.

[b] AUC = area under the concentration vs. time curve.

higher than in the central necrotic part (see Table 1). The same has been reported by this group for MTX (see Table 2) and for MeCCNU (see Table 3).[13]

Figure 6 shows the concentrations of HMM measured in some tissues of an ovarian cancer patient 9 hours after HMM administration. The drug concentrations are lower than in the other tissues, and in the necrotic part of the tumor no detectable levels were found.

Table 4 shows the mean ratios of HMM concentrations in tissue and plasma of 12 ovarian cancer patients who were operated at different intervals after HMM administration. The concentrations in the tumor were very low, and this partially explains the low efficacy of this drug.

The tumors of two patients were tested *in vitro* for sensitivity to HMM at the concentration found in the tumor after drug ingestion. Both had very similar drug concentrations, but one was sensitive, the other not at all (see Fig. 7). This is just one example, but it clearly shows that other factors, not connected with pharmacokinetics,

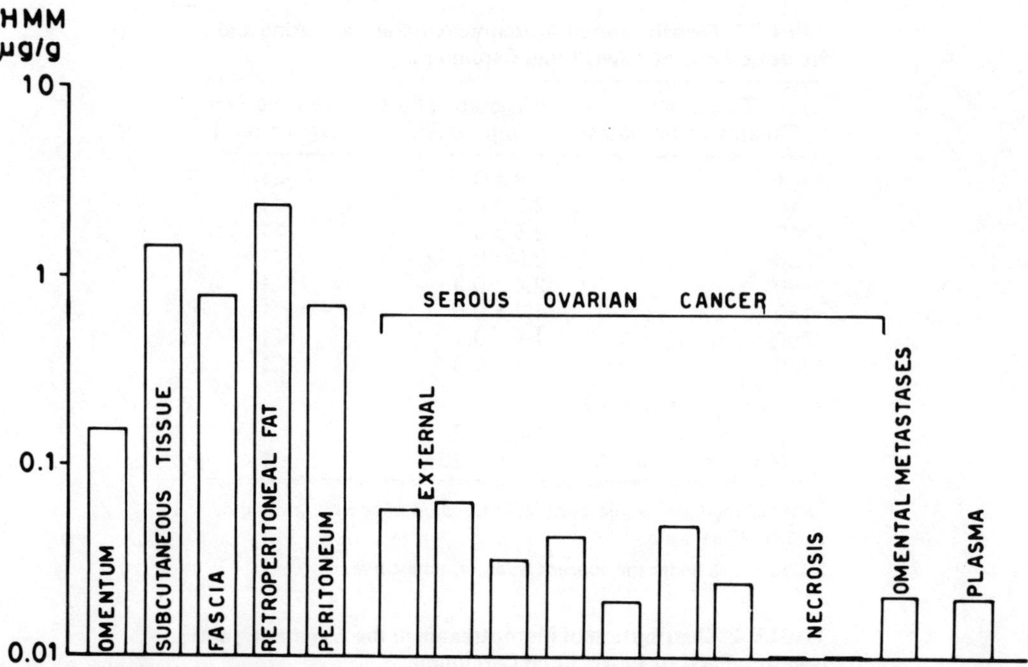

Figure 6. Hexamethylmelamine concentrations in some normal and neoplastic tissues 3 hours after the drug administration of 140 mg/m² P.O.

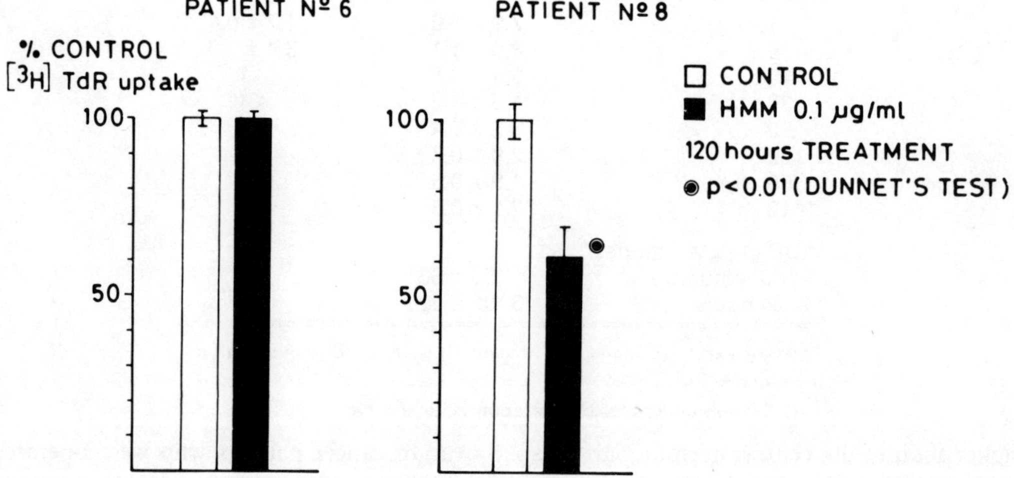

Figure 7. [³H] thymidine uptake of two human ovarian cancer primary cultures exposed to hexamethylmelamine.

are also responsible for the lack of sensitivity.[12]

These factors have been partially clarified for some drugs. Table 5 shows the mechanisms of resistance to some of the most widely used anticancer drugs. Most of the mechanisms have been established in cells from animal tumors, and only a few of them have been confirmed in human cancer cells.[2,18] The lack of such important information is basically due to the difficulties of obtaining viable human cancer cells in sufficient amounts, and particularly of obtaining repeated samples from the same patients without the use of invasive surgical procedures. The only clinical situations which, in

TABLE 3. Distribution of Methyl-Nitrosourea in the Vegetating and Necrotic Parts of Lewis Lung Carcinoma[a]

Time after Treatment (minutes)	Vegetating Part (μg/g ± S.E.)	Necrotic Part (μg/g ± S.E.)
1	2.8 ± 0.1	<1
5	8.4 ± 0.3	<1
15	6.6 ± 0.7	<1
30	3.8 ± 0.6	<1
60	2.3 ± 0.6	<1
180	1	<1
AUC (μg/g × minutes)[b]		
30 minutes	150 ± 18	<1
60 minutes	266 ± 12	<1

[a]Methyl-nitrosourea (20 mg/kg) was injected I.V. in C_{57}Bl/6 mice with intramuscular 3LL 25 days old.

[b]AUC = area under the concentration vs. time curve.

TABLE 4. HMM Tissue to Plasma Ratios in Pelvic Cancer Patients after Oral HMM (112–148 mg/m²)

Patient Number	Interval (hours)	Tumor	Subcutaneous Tissue	Omentum
1	2.00	1.88	10.90	31.01
2	3.00	1.66	16.55	16.36
3	3.16	0.92	29.75	68.90
4	3.50	1.02	8.58	—
5	4.25	1.77	35.77	1.44[a]
6	4.50	2.75	63.66	134.66
7	8.50	4.00	101.00	—
8	9.00	1.65	70.50	7.5[a]
9	12.00	1.33	17.00	—
10	16.00	1.43	23.33	—
11	18.00	1.7	7.00	5.3[a]
12	24.00	N.D.[b]	60	—
Range	(2–24)	(0.92–4)	(7.00–101.00)	(5.3–134.66)

[a]Metastatized omentum.

[b]N.D. = not detectable in plasma and tumor (<0.01 μg/ml or g).

fact, offer the chance for repeated study of malignant cells from the same patient are leukemia with large numbers of peripheral blasts, or pelvic or abdominal ascitic cancer with cancer cells floating in the effusion. A further problem is that cells taken by a small biopsy are not necessarily metabolically or kinetically representative of the different cell populations present in the tumor, and therefore the results of investigations may be meaningless.

Another approach to predict the sensitivity of human malignancies to chemotherapeutic agents involved tissue culture techniques. The idea that through studies on human tumor cells growing *in vitro* it might be possible to predict the clinical response to drugs has fascinated investigators for at least 20 years, particularly in view of the success of the conceptually similar approach used for guided antibiotic therapy.

Many conflicting results have been ob-

TABLE 5. Mechanisms Involved in Resistance to Clinically Widely Used Anticancer Agents

Drug	Mechanism	Reference
Methotrexate	impaired uptake[a]	Fischer, 1962; Hakala, 1965; Hoffbrand, et al., 1973; Sirotnak et al., 1968
	alteration of dihydrofolate reductase[a]	Jackson et al., 1976; Rosman et al., 1974
	increased synthesis of dydrofolate reductase	Bertino et al., 1977; Hryniuk and Bertino, 1969
5-Fluorouracil	reduced activities of uridine phospharilase	Reichard et al., 1959
	reduced activities of uridine kinase	Sköld et al., 1962
	reduced activities of uracil phosphoribosyl transferase	Brockman et al., 1960
6-Mercaptopurine	reduced activity of xantina-guanina phophoribosyl transferase	Davidson, 1960; Ellis and Le Page, 1963; Stutts and Brockman, 1963
Ara-C	increased deaminase activity[a]	Le Page, 1970; Steuart and Burke, 1971
Alkylating agents	impaired uptake (particularly for nitrogen mustard)	Kessel et al., 1969
	increased DNA repair capacity	Brockman, 1974

[a]Demonstrated in human malignancies too.

tained through a broad spectrum of methodologies to assess cell sensitivity.[17,35,36,38] The lack of reliability of these tests was such that they could not be applied in clinical practice.

Recently renewed interest has arisen in this approach because very promising results have been achieved with the clonogenic assay in agar proposed by Salmon et al.[29] This method appears to be much more accurate than the others previously reported and its validity has already been confirmed by independent groups.[26,37] In ovarian cancer the accuracy of this test in predicting resistance was reported to be 99% and the prediction response was 62%.[1] It is hardly necessary to emphasize the enormous perspectives offered by application of such a test which, if confirmed valid on larger populations of cancer patients and other types of tumor, could be clinically very relevant in the selection of effective therapies for each patient, avoiding useless toxic treatments.

Summary

The intricate phenomenon of resistance to cancer chemotherapy is analyzed here only from the pharmacological point of view. Examples of pharmacokinetics and pharmacodynamic reasons for drug resistance are given for some drugs to indicate what knowledge is available, the areas still not sufficiently explored, and to illustrate current research efforts to achieve a more rational means of counteracting resistance for human tumors.

Acknowledgments

The author wishes to thank G. Beggiolin, M. Broggini, T. Colombo, M.G. Donnelli, E. Erba, P. Farina, and C. Sessa for allowing to quote in detail their data, and J. Baggott, G. Scalvini, and A. Mancini for their assistance in the preparation of this manuscript.

REFERENCES

1. Alberts, D.S., Chen, H.S.G., Soehnlein, B., Salmon, S.E., Surwitt, E.A., Young, L., and Moon, T.E.: In vitro clonogenic assay for predicting response of ovarian cancer to chemotherapy. *Lancet* **2**:340–342, 1980.
2. Bertino, J.R.: Resistance of human tumors to cancer chemotherapeutic agents. An important research problem. *Med Pediat Oncol* **5**:105–114, 1978.
3. Bertino, J.R., Sawicki, W.L., Cashmore, A.R., Cadman, E.C., and Skeel, R.T.: Natural resistance to methotrexate in human acute nonlymphocytic leukemia. *Cancer Treat Rep* **61**:667–673, 1977.
4. Bleyer, W.A., and Poplack, D.G.: Clinical studies on the central nervous system pharmacology of methotrexate. In *Clinical Pharmacology of Anti-Neoplastic Drugs*, H.M. Pinedo, ed. Amsterdam: Elsevier North Holland Biomed Press, 1978, pp. 115–131.
5. Brockman, R.W.: Mechanism of resistance. In *Antineoplastic and Immunosuppressive Agents*, A.G. Sartorelli and D.G. Johns, eds. Berlin: Springer Verlag, 1974, pp. 352–409.
6. Brockman, R.W., Davis, J.M., and Stutts, P.: Metabolism of uracil and 5-fluorouracil by drug-sensitive and by drug-resistant bacteria. *Biochem Biophys Acta* **40**:22–32, 1960.
7. Carter, S.K., and Mathé, G.: Malignant diseases. In *Drug Treatment Principles and Practice of Clinical Pharmacology and Therapeutics* 2nd ed, G.S. Avery, ed. Sydney: ADIS Press, 1980, pp. 953–1009.
8. Creaven, P.J., and Allen, L.M.: EPEG, a new antineoplastic epipadophyllotoxin. *Clin Pharmacol Ther* **18**:221–226, 1975.
9. Davidson, J.D.: Studies on the mechanism of action of 6-mercaptopurine in sensitive and resistant L1210 leukemia *in vitro. Cancer Res* **20**:225–232, 1960.
10. D'Incalci, M., Bolis, G., Facchinetti, T., Mangioni, C., Morasca, L., Morazzoni, P., and Salmona, M.: Decreased half life of cyclophosphamide in patients under continual treatment. *Eur J Cancer* **15**:7–10, 1979.
11. D'Incalci, M., Bolis, G., Mangioni, C., Morasca, L., and Garattini, S.: Variable oral absorption of hexamethylmelamine in man. *Cancer Treat Rep* **62**:2117–2119, 1978.
12. D'Incalci, M., Farina, P., Sessa, C., Erba, E., Madonna, R., and Mangioni, C.: Hexamethylmelamine tissue concentrations in pelvic cancer patients. In *Frontiers in Therapeutic Drug Monitoring*, G. Tognoni, R. Latini, and W.J. Jusko, eds. New York: Raven Press, 1980, pp. 173–174.
13. Donelli, M.G., Broggini, M., Colombo, T., and Garattini, S.: Importance of the presence of necrosis in studying drug distribution within tumor tissue.

Eur J Drug Metab Pharmacokin **2**:63–67, 1977.
14. Ellis, D.B., and Le Page, G.A.: Biochemical studies of resistance to 6-thioguanine. *Cancer Res* **23**:436–443, 1963.
15. Fischer, G.A.: Defective transport of amethopterin (methotrexate) as a mechanism of resistance to the antimetabolite in L5178Y leukemic cells. *Biochem Pharmacol* **11**:1233–1234, 1962.
16. Hakala, M.T.: On the role of drug penetration in amethopterin resistance of sarcoma-180 cells in vitro. *Biochem Biophys Acta* **102**:198–209, 1965.
17. Hall, T.C.: Predictive tests in cancer. *Br J Cancer* **30**:191–198, 1974.
18. Hall, T.C.: Prediction of responses to therapy and mechanisms of resistance. *Semin Oncol* **4**:193–202, 1977.
19. Heal, J.M., Franza, B.R., and Schein, P.S.: Pharmacology of nitrosourea antitumor agents. In *Clinical Pharmacology of Anti-Neoplastic Drugs*, H.M. Pinedo, ed. Amsterdam: Elsevier/North Holland Biomed Press, 1978, pp. 263–275.
20. Hoffbrand, A.V., Tripp, E., Catovsky, D., and Das, K.C.: Transport of methotrexate into normal haemopoietic cells and into leukemic cells and its effects on DNA synthesis. *Br J Hematol* **25**:497–511, 1973.
21. Hryniuk, W.M., and Bertino, J.R.: Treatment of leukemia with large doses of methotrexate and folinic acid: Clinical-biochemical correlates. *J Clin Invest* **48**:2140–2155, 1969.
22. Jackson, R.C., Hart, L.I., and Harrap, K.R.: Intrinsic resistance to methotrexate of cultured mammalian cells in relation to the inhibition kinetic of their dihydrofolate reductase. *Cancer Res* **36**: 1991–1997, 1976.
23. Kessel, D., Hall, T.C., and Roberts, D.: Modes of uptake of methotrexate by normal and leukemic human leucocytes *in vitro* and their relation to drug response. *Cancer Res* **28**:564–570, 1968.
24. Kessel, D., Myers, M., and Wodinsky, I.: Accumulation of two alkylating agents, nitrogen mustard and busulfan, by murine leukemic cells *in vitro*. *Biochem Pharmacol* **18**:1229–1234, 1969.
25. Le Page, G.A.: Alterations in enzyme activity in tumors and the implications for chemotherapy. *Adv Enzyme Regul* **8**:323–332, 1970.
26. Marsh, J.C., and Kirkwood, J.M.: *In vivo* drug sensitivity of clonogenic human melanoma (M) cells. *Proc Am Assoc Cancer Res* **21**:279, 1980.
27. Reichard, P., Skold, O., and Klein, G.: Possible enzymic mechanisms for the development of resistance against fluorouracil in ascites tumours. *Nature* **183**:939–941, 1959.
28. Rosman, M., Lee, M.H., Creasey, W.A., and Sartorelli, A.C.: Mechanisms of resistance to 6-thiopurines in human leukemia. *Cancer Res* **34**:1952–1956, 1974.
29. Salmon, S.E., Hamburger, A.W., Soehlen, B., Durie, B.G.M., Alberts, D.S., and Moon, T.E.: Quantitation of differential sensitivity of human-tumor stem cells to anticancer drugs. *N Engl J Med* **298**:1321–1327, 1978.
30. Sirotnak, F.M., Kurita, S., and Hutchison, D.J.: On the nature of a transport alteration determining resistance to amethopterin in the L1210 leukemia. *Cancer Res* **28**:75–80, 1968.
31. Sköld, O., Magnusson, P.H., and Révész, L.: Studies on resistance against 5-fluorouracil. III. *Cancer Res* **22**:1226–1229, 1962.
32. Steuart, C.D., and Burke, P.J.: Cytidine deaminase and the development of resistance to arabinosyl cytosine. *Nature New Biol* **233**:109–110, 1971.
33. Stutts, P., and Brockman, R.W.: A biochemical basis for resistance of L1210 mouse leukemia to 6-thioguanine. *Biochem Pharmacol* **12**:97–104, 1963.
34. Tognoni, G., Bellantuono, C., Bonati, M., D'Incalci, M., Gerna, M., Latini, R., Mandelli, M., Porro, M.G., and Riva, E.: Clinical relevance of pharmacokinetics. *Clin Pharmacokinet* **5**:105–136, 1980.
35. Volm, M., Kaufmann, M., Mattern, J., and Wayss, K.: Sensitivity tests of tumors to cytostatics agents. I. Comparative investigations on transplanted tumors *in vivo* and *in vitro*. *Z Krebsforsch* **83**:85–96, 1975.
36. Volm, M., Mattern, J., Kaufmann, M., Hinderer, H., and Wayss, K.: Sensitivity tests of tumors to cytostatic agents. II. Investigation on human tumors. *Z Krebsforsch* **83**:97–104, 1975.
37. Willson, J.K.V., Ozols, R.F., Grotzinger, K.R., and Young, R.C.: New sources of clonogenic human ovarian cancer cells for drug sensitivity studies. *Proc Am Assoc Cancer Res* **21**:175, 1980.
38. Wright, J.C., Cobb, J.P., Gumport, S.L., Golomb, F.M., and Safadi, D.: Investigation of the relation between clinical and tissue-culture response to chemotherapeutic agents on human cancer. *N Engl J Med* **257**:1207–1211, 1957.

CHAPTER 48

Keynote Address: Problems and Alternatives to Classical Randomized Trials

Marvin Zelen, Ph.D.[a]

A clinical trial is an experiment on humans for the purpose of evaluating one or more potentially beneficial therapies where the investigator has control of some features of the trial. Usually the investigator can control the assignment of therapy to many of the patients. In this paper the discussion will be restricted to comparing two treatments. However, the generalizations also pertain to clinical trials with more than two treatments.

The fundamental scientific principle underlying the comparison of two groups of patients is that the groups must be alike in all important aspects and differ only with regard to the treatment each group receives. Otherwise differences between the groups may not be due to the treatments under study but may be attributed to the particular characteristics of the group.

In clinical experimentation the experimental units are patients who vary widely in their ability to respond to therapy. The one feature about clinical experimentation of which everyone is in agreement is that any group of patients is heterogeneous. Furthermore, the therapies cannot be exactly reproduced from occasion to occasion. This is in contrast to experiments in the physical sciences where experimental units are homogeneous and hence treatment groups are homogeneous. Furthermore, the treatments applied to the experimental units are exactly reproducible. Variability in clinical experimentation arises from the heterogeneity of the patient populations and lack of exact reproducibility of the treatment, whereas in the physical science variability is often a secondary factor and arises from slight changes in ambient conditions and the variability of the measuring instrument.

In order to generate comparable groups in clinical experimentation, we often resort to the method of *randomization*. Randomization refers to allocating the treatment to the patient using a chance mechanism—equivalent to tossing a coin in many instances. Classical randomized experiments require that neither the physician nor the patient know in advance the treatment to be given to a patient prior to entering a study. The device of randomization makes the treatment group "alike on the average" with respect to all factors likely to affect the principal end points used to compare the treatments. Using randomization, each patient has the same opportunity of receiving any of the treatments under study.

The use of randomization to form treatment groups makes treatment groups comparable and tends to eliminate the possible effects of biases when making treatment comparisons. These biases may be both known and unknown. This is the principal reason why results from randomized studies are regarded with credibility by the scientific community.

[a]Professor of Statistical Science, Harvard School of Public Health, Sidney Farber Cancer Institute, Boston, Mass.

Retrospective and Nonrandomized Studies

Randomized studies are not popular with many physicians. Some feel uncomfortable choosing a treatment by chance. Also, patients, when informed of randomization, may decline to participate in the study and even could lose confidence in their physician. It is for these reasons that many clinical investigators have resorted to nonrandomized studies for making conclusions about the value of treatment.

Generally, data are generated prospectively for a new treatment and compared with a group of patients who form a historical control group. Of course, if the value of treatment is overwhelmingly beneficial no retrospective comparisons will even be necessary. For example, if patients with documented primary liver cancer are living long periods of time without evidence of disease, no formal comparison is necessary. We know the prognosis of this disease is uniformly dismal. In some surgical procedures, the outcome is immediately known and the principle about why a procedure works may be very well understood. Two such examples are the setting of bones and suturing of wounds.

Unfortunately, in treating nearly all cancer sites, there are few treatments which result in substantial therapeutic benefit (curing high proportions of patients) or where the disease is very well understood. Such is the class of problems discussed in this chapter.

The use of historical controls for evaluating the benefits of a new therapy is fraught with many difficulties. There are ample opportunities for serious biases to completely distort the conclusions. Even when known biases are addressed, one never knows about the existence of unknown or unconscious biases.

Below is a list of the biases an investigator should discuss in making a comparison with a historical control group. Very few investigators address these problems.

1. *Physician selection bias*: Selection of patients for new treatment by physicians may be biased.
2. *Patient bias*: Patients self-select themselves for new treatment; there is no self-selection in the make-up of the historical group.
3. *Diagnosis and staging*: Methods of diagnosis and staging must be the same for treatment and historical group; if the methods have improved during recent years this may not be reflected in the historical group.
4. *Patient management and supportive care*: This must be the same for both groups.
5. *Evaluation methods*: This reflects on the quality of the data; if the methods of evaluation are different, comparisons may be difficult.
6. *Prognostic factors*: The key prognostic factors affecting outcome must be the same for both groups; statistical adjustments can often be used to make the groups comparable when the prognostic factors are known.

Using consecutive patients for generating data for the new treatment and the use of "matched" controls are two widely used methods for investigating new treatments without resorting to randomization. We shall comment on each.

Using consecutive patients for a study eliminates the opportunity for physician bias associated with the selection of patients. However, where patient consent is necessary, patient selection bias will still be present. If the patient mix has not changed over time, the prognostic variables associated with each group may be comparable. However, for issues such as patient bias, diagnosis and staging, patient management, and supportive care, different methods of evaluation must still be considered. The consecutive patient experimental design is targeted mainly at eliminating the bias arising from physician selection of patients.

Matched controls is another method often used to assess a new treatment with a historical control. This involves forming a group of one or more control patients for each patient receiving the new treatment. Patients are selected from the historical group so that they are comparable to the new treatment group on a patient-by-patient basis for known prognostic variables. This method is limited in that only a few key variables can be matched on any practical basis. For example, in matching one would aim to have comparable patients with respect to anatomic staging, pathology, performance status, and other extra-disease characteristics, such as demographic factors, prior treatment history, etc.

Statistical modeling is a generalization of matching which enables one to adjust for large numbers of factors. However, this also has limitations as the statistical adjustment for bias introduces additional variability in the analysis due to the "uncertainty" of the adjustment. Such adjustments can only be made for known prognostic factors. Patient and physician self-selection cannot be factored into the adjustments, neither can questions about different criteria for diagnosis and staging, different methods of patient support and management, and different evaluation methods.

In summary the nonrandomized methods for evaluation of new therapies are useful for exploratory studies and trying out new leads. They are not to be trusted for generating credible conclusions, unless the issues of potential biases are carefully discussed. This author has yet to see any such examples.

New Randomized Designs

This section discusses several new methods for carrying out randomized studies. They will be discussed in the context of multi-institutional cooperative studies where several institutions are pooling patients into a common study. We shall not discuss issues of stratification as this will detract from the main points of this section.

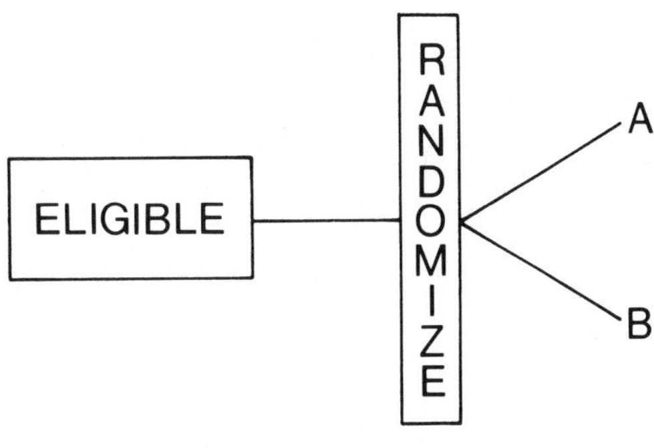

Figure 1a

The two treatments will be designated by A and B respectively. Figure 1(*a*) shows the experimental design for a conventional randomized study. Figure 1(*b*) shows the modification if patient consent is required. Even though physician and patient selection biases are present, the randomization equally distributes these biases.

Recently Zelen[1] has introduced a new class of designs for randomized clinical trials. This class of designs is called "randomized consent or prerandomized designs." Figure 2 shows the schema for this type of experimental design. This is called a "single consent randomized design."

After the patient's eligibility is established, the patient is randomized into one of two groups. One group (G_1) is called a "do not seek consent" group. Patients randomized for this group are not approached for consent to enter the clinical trial–they receive the best standard therapy (A). Patients assigned to the second group (G_2) are asked for their informed consent. These patients are asked if they wish to participate in the clinical trial and are willing to receive the experimental therapy B. All potential risks, benefits, and treatment options are explained. If the patient agrees, the experimental treatment (B) will be given; if the patient declines to receive the experimental treatment, the patient will (presumably) receive the best standard treatment (A).

The proposed new design has the desirable feature that the physician need only approach the patient to discuss a single

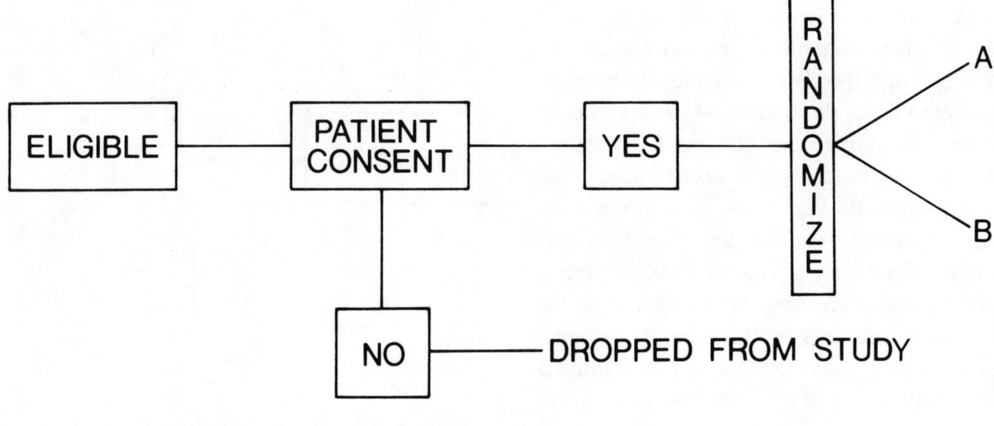

Figure 1b

ELIGIBLE
RANDOMIZE
DO NOT SEEK CONSENT
A (CONTROL)
SEEK CONSENT
YES
B (EXPERIMENTAL TREATMENT)
NO
A

A. CONTROL TREATMENT: BEST STANDARD TREATMENT

B. EXPERIMENTAL TREATMENT

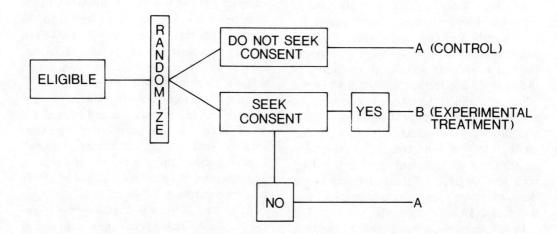

Figure 2

therapy. The physician need not appear, in the eyes of the patient, to be unaware of what he is doing as if he were "tossing a coin" to decide the treatment. Thus, the patient–physician relation is not compromised. On the patient's side, there is also an important advantage: before providing consent the patient knows which treatment will be given. Many patients agree to participate in a randomized study but have reservations about continuing after the treatment is known to them. At this point, some decline treatment and are considered "cancelled patients." However, others may continue the treatment, despite their reservations, because of the built-up momentum to do so and their reluctance to renege on their consent. My design requires a decision by the patient only on the experimental treatment. Hence, the patient's decision-making processes should be more straightforward. This new design cannot be used when there are important reasons for conducting a "double-blind" experiment–i.e., a trial in which nei-

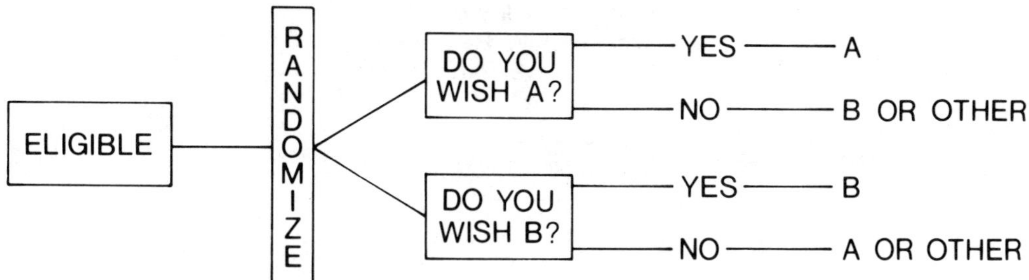

Figure 3

TABLE 1. Efficiencies of Single and Double Consent Randomized Designs

	Single Consent		Double Consent	
Probability of Acceptance	Efficiency	Break-Even Accrual Factor	Efficiency	Break-Even Accrual Factor
0.50	25%	4	0	–
0.60	36%	2.8	4%	25
0.70	49%	2.0	16%	6.2
0.80	64%	1.6	36%	2.8
0.90	81%	1.2	64%	1.6
0.95	90%	1.1	81%	1.2

ther the physician nor the patient knows the identity of the treatment during the course of treatment or its evaluation.

The analysis of this new design requires that Group G_1 (receiving only treatment A) is compared with Group G_2 (receiving treatment A or B). In other words, the comparison must be made with all patients in Group G_2, regardless of which treatment each received. It is clear that including all patients dilutes the measurable effect of treatment B. Nevertheless, all patients must be included if the analysis is to provide a valid comparison with treatment A. If only a small proportion of patients are willing to take treatment B, this experimental plan may be useless in evaluation of this treatment. However, the refusal of a large proportion of patients to agree to accept B may

mature to introduce the experimental therapy into a clinical trial.

Figure 3 describes another kind of randomized consent design. We call this a "double consent randomized design." It is suitable for comparing two treatments in which there is no control or best standard treatment. Patients are randomized to each of the two treatments and then are asked if they wish to accept the randomized treatment. If they decline, they are given the alternate treatment or perhaps another treatment not under investigation in this study. Comparison of the two treatments is made by comparing groups G_1 and G_2 regardless of the treatment actually received.

Table 1 summarizes the efficiencies of the single and double consent randomized design. These efficiencies depend on the probability of acceptance of the designated treatment by the patient. For example, consider a single consent randomized design in which only 50% accept the experimental treatment. The efficiency of the design is 25%. This means that four times as many patients in this design are required to obtain

θ = Prior Probability of Success
α = False Positive Rate: P(+/-)
β = True Positive Rate: P(+/+)

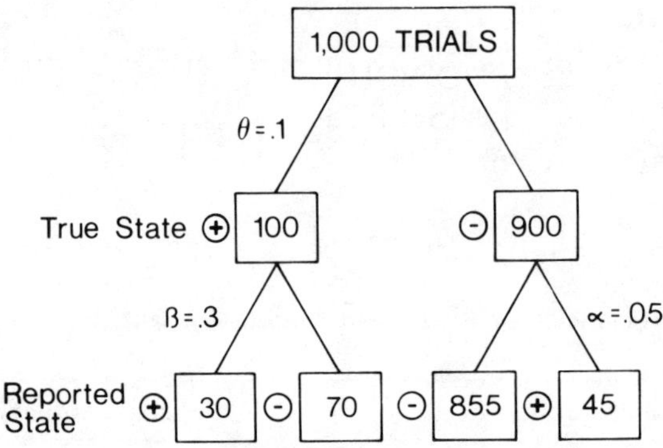

No. Reported + = 30 + 45

P(+) = Probability {Reported + Treatment is Effective} = $\frac{30}{75}$ = .40

Figure 4

the same sensitivity as a conventional randomized design. Thus, unless there is increased accrual by at least a factor of 4, this design may not be useful. This factor of 4 is called the "break-even accrual factor" in Table 1.

Strategy and the Clinical Trials Process

We next discuss the strategy of clinical experimentation. Failure to appreciate strategic considerations may lead to reporting large numbers of false positive treatments.

The three parameters which govern strategy are:

θ = prior probability of success
α = probability of a false-positive result
β = probability of a true-positive result

To illustrate the role of these parameters, consider the clinical situation in which these parameters have the following values:

$\theta = 0.10$
$\alpha = 0.05$
$\beta = 0.30$

Figure 4 illustrates this process if we have 1000 trials. Note that with these parameters 75 trials will be reported as being positive. However, there are only 30 true positives among these 75 trials. Thus, the proportion of true positives among the reported 75 positive trials is 30/75 = 0.40. If we denote the probability by $P\,(+)$, then we can write:

$$P\,(+) = \theta\beta/[\theta\beta+(1-\theta)\alpha]$$

Table 2 is a summary of $P\,(+)$ for a variety of different θ and β with $\alpha = 0.05$. As the sample size gets very large, we have the sensitivity (β) approaching unity. However, $P\,(+)$ does not approach 1. On the other hand, as θ goes to unity, $P\,(+)$ will approach 1.

The parameter θ represents the prior probability of success. It depends on the level of clinical innovation and basic science. If θ is high, there is a good chance for success. If it is low, the chances for success are small. The prior probability (θ) is subjective and cannot be measured objectively.

TABLE 2. Probability of Prior Success and True Positive[a]

θ	β		
	0.3	0.6	0.9
0.1	0.40	0.57	0.67
0.2	0.60	0.75	0.82
0.4	0.80	0.89	0.92
0.6	0.90	0.95	0.96
0.8	0.96	0.98	0.99

[a] θ:prior probability of success; β: sensitivity, power, true-positive probability; α = 0.05: false-positive probability.

However, it increases with knowledge of successful pilot or exploratory studies. Initiating large Phase III studies should only be done on the basis of successful exploratory studies. Failure to do so means that there will be a huge number of false-positive treatments in the clinic. At the present time there are at least approximately 4000 clinical studies of all kinds being conducted throughout the world. If one adopts a 5% false-positive rate, we would expect a minimum of approximately 200 of these studies to be reported as positive when in truth there is no positive effect. Thus, by starting definitive Phase III studies with low prior probabilities of success, the number of false-positive results is further increased.

Summary

Randomized clinical trials are regarded as the most credible way of generating scientific data comparing the benefits of different therapies. However, randomized studies present difficulties in their execution. Often physicians are unwilling to participate in such studies because they do not wish to inform the patient that the treatment program will be chosen by a chance mechanism. They feel such a discussion may compromise the physician–patient relationship. In this chapter alternatives to classical randomized trials are discussed, both the advantages and the pitfalls. Also discussed are some aspects of the strategy of clinical experimentation. It is pointed out that the initiation of definitive Phase III trials made on the basis of little prior expectation of success ("trying something out") tends to generate falsc-positive results.

Acknowledgments

Research for this chapter was supported in part by Public Health Grant CA23415 and CA06516 from the National Cancer Institute.

REFERENCES

1. Zelen, M.: A new design for randomized clinical. trials *N Engl J Med* **300**:1242–1245, 1979.

CHAPTER 49

Quality Control of Radiation Therapy in Clinical Trials

Simon Kramer, M.D.[a]
Robert Lustig, M.D.[b]
Graham Grundy, R.T.T.[c]

Large scale multicenter clinical trials in radiation therapy did not start in the United States until the 1960s. At that time studies in head and neck tumors, Hodgkin's disease, and prostate cancer began. While any one institution could accomplish internal quality control for in-house protocols, there was a need for a mechanism of interinstitution quality control of data collected from cooperative clinical trials. Variables, such as the treatment volume radiated, the point at which the dose was to be calculated, and verification of the dose delivered to the target volume, had to be addressed.

In 1968, the Radiologic Physics Center (RPC) was established at the M.D. Anderson Hospital. The two main functions were to evaluate the accuracy of the delivered dose from any one piece of equipment through calibration and phantom measurement and to review charts to verify dosimetry calculations.

The RPC performed initial evaluations for the institutions involved in the early cooperative trials. To date, there are 608 institutions participating in radiation therapy protocols that have been visited by RPC. Thus, there has been widespread acceptance by the radiation therapy community of such outside reviews.

In 1970, the Radiation Therapy Oncology Group (RTOG) was formed to undertake clinical trials in which radiation therapy was the principal mode of therapy in cancer management. But from its inception, the RTOG developed multimodality studies, including chemotherapy and/or surgery.

RTOG has now increased to 25 full members, 10 provisional members, 22 affiliates, and 31 affiliate members through the cancer control program of the full members. The scope of the RTOG has now expanded and is involved with the use of radiosensitizers and radioprotectors as well as high LET radiation.

A retrospective evaluation of the radiation therapy compliance was made in 1977, and it was discovered that there were still problems of variation from the protocol description. These were defined as "minor" or "major" as determined by the reviewing radiation therapist. "Minor deviations" are those which would be unlikely to adversely affect patient survival, primary tumor control, or complication incidence, although the details of the protocol had not been strictly followed. "Major deviations," on the other hand, are considered those which can seriously jeopardize the evaluability of a case for local and/or regional control or other areas of analysis. Failure to cover or adequately treat a specified region, either pri-

[a]Professor and Chairman, Department of Radiation Therapy and Nuclear Medicine, Thomas Jefferson University Hospital, Philadelphia, Penn.
[b]Department of Radiation Therapy, Cooper Medical Center, Camden, N.J.
Assistant Professor, Department of Radiation Therapy & Nuclear Medicine, Thomas Jefferson University Hospital, Philadelphia, Penn.
[c]Data Coordinator, Radiation Oncology Study Center, Philadelphia, Penn.

TABLE 1. Radiation Therapy Oncology Group Quality Control Definitions[a]

Dose, Fractions, and Time		Volume Encompassed
Per protocol	Within 5%	Each study chairman writes review guidelines; failure to adequately treat primary disease always "major."
Minor deviation	Variation 6–15%	
Major deviation—acceptable	Variation 16–20%	
Major deviation—unacceptable	Greater than 20%	

[a] As recommended by the Intergroup Radiation Therapy Committee Chairmen.

mary or nodal disease, is the main cause of major deviations.

These definitions have since been further refined by an intergroup committee of radiation therapists and are presented in Table 1.

In regard to dose, fractions, and time, numerical values of variation are used. If rest periods or breaks in therapy are permitted in the study, then these are taken into account. Volume is evaluated on the basis of an anatomical description prescribed in each study. In addition the study chairman is asked to describe his own review parameters and follow them for each case evaluated. This allows the study chairman to place emphasis on sites or regions of particular importance and similarly deemphasize other regions.

In early 1978 the RTOG instituted an early review mechanism in order to correct protocol deviations early in the treatment course. In addition, workshops and case presentations have been scheduled at each semiannual meeting. The results of these sessions have been documented in a Treatment Planning Handbook. This book is continuously under review, and revised recommendations for radiation therapy of lung cancer resulting from the June 1980 meeting will be incorporated shortly.

The initial review mechanism has been in place for 2 years, and 2204 cases have been reviewed. Within 2 weeks of patient entry into an RTOG study, information pertaining to the delivery of radiation therapy for that patient must be sent to RTOG Headquarters. This information includes a copy of a representative localization film, the initial dose calculations, and the radiation therapist's treatment prescription which should include the planned dose to the primary tumor, regional nodes, and critical structures. Each case on which information is due is monitored by computer-generated forms and reminders. The submitted information is reviewed by a radiation therapist and a dosimetrist. Problems related to protocol compliance are handled by the radiation therapist who, when necessary, calls the treating radiation therapist and requests that modifications be made in the treatment prescription to comply with the protocol.

The dosimetrist uses the physics information provided by the facility to review the dose calculations. This review has been initiated with the dose calculations. Machine calibration information is provided by the Radiologic Physics Center (RPC) and stored in the computer at RTOG Headquarters. Dose calculation programs are available at RTOG Headquarters. (Verification of these programs has been carried out with the assistance of a consulting physicist from the RTOG Medical Physics Committee.) If a problem is detected in the physics portion of the initial review, consultation is first made with the treating radiation therapist, and with his concurrence, the responsible physicist is contacted to review the problem.

Contacts are made by telephone during the early review phase to allow a rapid turnaround and to insure that corrections are made early in the treatment course. RTOG Headquarters does require that proof of corrections be submitted. For example, if a treatment field is not in compliance with the protocol, a new film must be submitted showing that the appropriate changes have been made.

TABLE 2. Radiation Therapy Oncology Group Summary of Quality Control Experience—December 1977 to August 1980

	Number of Cases Reviewed	Cases Not in Compliance	Major Deviations[a]
December 1977 (preinitiation of program)	198	68 (34%)	57 (19%)
March 1978	73	14 (19%)	6 (8%)
March 1979	108	8 (7%)	6 (6%)
June 1979	194	13 (7%)	7 (4%)
September 1979	180	11 (6%)	7 (4%)
December 1979	164	12 (7%)	6 (4%)
March 1980	170	4 (3%)	4 (3%)
June 1980	291	4 (2%)	4 (2%)
August 1980	137	7 (5%)	5 (4%)

[a]Major Deviations still subject to study chairman review.

A summary of the initial quality control early review program from December 1977 thourgh August 1980 is shown in Table 2.

There has been a steady decrease in the number of cases not in compliance, as well as in the number of major deviations. This is an important finding since more than 20 new protocols have been opened for case accession during 1978 and 1979.

The second part of the Radiation Therapy Quality Control Program is concerned with final data review. The purpose of the final radiation therapy review is to confirm the treatment delivered and protocol compliance for the statistician and study chairman so that a final overall evaluation of protocol radiation therapy treatment compliance can be made. This information can be used by the statistician in his analysis of the study. In order to complete the final review, additional information is required from the treating facility including films of any additional treatment areas or boost fields, any additional calculations performed, an isodose distribution at the level of the tumor, and a copy of the daily radiation therapy flow sheet. Upon receipt of this information, the dosimetrist at RTOG Headquarters completes a dose summary form. This form provides a summary of radiation therapy information to the study chairman so that by reviewing it in conjunction with the portal films a protocol compliance form can be completed.

The dose summary form and radiation therapy evaluation form have been developed at RTOG Headquarters and have been standardized for all external-beam treatment. Doses to the primary tumor, regional nodes, and appropriate critical structures are recorded for each case. Since the form has been standardized with descriptions appropriate to each primary tumor site, a review of radiation therapy data from several different studies of the same treatment site can be easily accomplished.

Any problems found in the final dosimetry review are referred to the Headquarters's consulting physicist. He is responsible for assisting the dosimetrist with difficult cases or with cases with a discrepancy between the stated initial treatment plan and the final review. More than 900 cases have had final physics review. Of these, over 700 have also been reviewed by the study chairman. A comparison is underway to determine the impact of the initial review on the number of major deviations found in final review; preliminary information shows a 93% agreement between initial and final reviews.

The third aspect of the RTOG Radiation Therapy Quality Control Program is feedback to the RTOG membership. The results of the early treatment planning review are reported to the membership on an individual basis at the time the review is made. A computer-generated form, completed by the reviewing radiation therapist, is mailed to the principal investigator. Similarly the final review by the study chairman is sent to the member and to the study statistician. A summary of the number of cases reviewed, the timeliness of data submission, and the results of the review are sent to each member. In addition, summary report of the RTOG Radiation Therapy Quality Control Program is presented to the membership at each semiannual meeting. The data summary is also sorted by study and sent to the study chairman and site chairman.

Medical Oncology Quality Control was initiated in 1978. A process of early review and correction is in operation similar to the radiation therapy system.

A Medical Oncology Treatment Planning Form must be submitted within a week of registration. This form documents the treatment regimen that is planned, including the calculated dosage and interval of administration. Upon receipt, the information is thoroughly reviewed. Surface area and drug dose calculations are checked as well as verification of the study regimen. This documentation verifies the intended compliance with the protocol. When errors or deviations from the protocol specifications are noted, the medical oncologist is notified by telephone. Documentation of modification is then required.

Medical Oncology data is periodically reviewed by the Medical Oncology Study Co-chairman and by the RTOG Medical Oncology Quality Control consultant. A comprehensive review of each new study is scheduled after approximately 50 cases have been entered. The purpose of this early review is to identify problem areas and to provide solutions. Special attention is directed toward uncovering difficulties in protocol interpretation, noncompliance in treatment delivery, and toxicity modifications which may warrant revisions in the protocol or a memorandum of explanation. A special work sheet is completed by a Headquarters's Data Manager prior to this review.

Patients who have completed the chemotherapy regimen or have had treatment terminated are reviewed for overall compliance to the treatment regimen. Results of this review are incorporated into the patient data file for use in study analyses.

RTOG is conducting a surgical quality control program under the auspices of the Head & Neck Subcommittee.

The site and staging (T and N category) for each patient, along with the operative report and the pathology report on the operative specimen, are provided to each reviewer in a coded fashion so that the identity of the surgical team, institution, and patient is not known. The operation on each patient is evaluated for the objective of the operation, achievement of the objective, rationale for the technical approach, and adequacy of neoplasm clearance. Each of these criteria is judged on a five-point scale: 0 = not evaluable; 1 = poor; 2 = marginal; 3 = good; and 4 = excellent.

The evaluation of the objective of the operation, the achievement of the objective, and the rationale for the technical approach are based on the operative report. The adequacy of neoplasm clearance is based on the operative report and the pathology report of the operative specimen.

Each operation is given a numerical rating. Ratings of 7 or less are considered poor, 8 - 11 are considered marginal, 12 -15 are considered good, and 16 is considered excellent.

Review of pathologic material as part of a quality control process has been instituted during the past 18 months. Studies of malignant glioma, prostate, head and neck, and soft tissue sarcomas are in process. Three hundred and fifty cases reviewed in the RTOG glioma study 7401 showed only a 2% rejection rate because of incomplete or inaccurate diagnosis. Slides and pathology reports are collected by RTOG Headquarters. They are subsequently sent to the reviewer. The completed review form is computer entered as part of the patient file for use with later analysis.

The use of a quality control system, as instituted by the RTOG, can be shown to be cost effective. The cost per randomized case for RTOG is \$1,500 per case. The cost per 100 randomized cases is 100 × \$1,500 = \$150,000. Using the 1977 figure of 19% major deviations, there were 81 evaluable cases per 100 randomized cases. The cost per evaluable case is \$150,000 ÷ 81 = \$1,852.

The cost per case for the RTOG per initial and final review is \$80. The cost per 100 randomized cases with quality control is 100 × \$1,580 = \$158,000. Using the 1980 figure of 3% major deviation, there are 97 evaluable cases per 100 randomized cases. The cost per evaluable case is \$158,000 ÷ 97 = \$1,629. This is a cost savings of \$223 per case using quality control.

In summary, the RTOG has responded to the need for quality control in inter-institution randomized protocols by developing a system of initial and final reviews. This has encompassed the areas of radiation therapy, surgery, medical oncology, and pathology review. Methods have been developed which have been shown to significantly increase compliance to protocol criteria per treatment and increase the percentage of evaluable cases. This has been accomplished in a fashion which has been shown to be cost effective.

Summary

The RTOG is a group of participating institutions which has a major interest in furthering clinical radiation oncology. They have formulated protocols for clinical investigation in which radiation therapy is the major modality of treatment. In addition, other modalities, such as chemotherapy, radiation sensitizers, and hyperthermia, are used in combined approach to cancer. Quality control in all aspects of patient management is necessary to insure quality data. These areas include evaluation of pathology, phsycis, and dosimetry, and clinical patient data. Quality control is both time consuming and expensive. However, by dividing these tasks into various levels and time frames, by using computerized data-control mechanisms, and by employing appropriate levels of ancillary personnel expertise, quality control can improve compliance and decrease the cost of investigational trials.

Acknowledgments

Research for this chapter was supported in part by Grant CA21661 from the Division of Cancer Treatment of the National Cancer Institute, National Institutes of Health.

CHAPTER 50

Costs of Cancer Care

W. E. Powers, M.D.[a]

The direct cost of care of cancer patients in the United States has been variously underestimated in the past to be in the range of 5–$7 billion per year.

The direct cost of all health care in the United States in 1979 was estimated to be $209.2 billion or 9.0% of the Gross National Product of $2,313 billion.

It is estimated that 20.4% of all deaths in the United States in 1977 were due to cancer. While it is clear we cannot attribute 20.4% of all health care costs to cancer care, reasonable estimates lead to the expectation that cancer care costs represent between 10 and 15% of health care costs or between $21 to $31 billion per year in the United States. This approximates a total integrated cost of from $30,000 to $40,000 per patient who gets invasive cancer.

We have identified that the treatment cost of care of a patient who fails to have control of cancer is approximately three times that of the patient who is cured. In 1976 dollars this represented approximately $12,000 per cured patient and $36,000 per failed patient for treatment costs.

Radiation therapy, which is responsible for a significant contribution to the treatment of more than 50% of all newly diagnosed invasive cancer patients each year in the United States, is estimated to cost between $0.9 and $1.0 billion per year or about 5% of all cancer care costs, and is thus a very inexpensive and effective modality of treatment.

[a]Professor and Chairman, Department of Radiation Oncology, Wayne State University, Detroit, Michigan

CHAPTER 51

Final Comments

Gilbert H. Fletcher, M.D.[a]

I have chosen to limit my comments to the variations of the time factor in irradiation schemes because, since the beginning of radiotherapy, of all the parameters in the design of schemes to render irradiation more effective, it has been the most investigated. I will start with the history of the time factor since 1900 in order to provide a perspective for understanding the present status. The single massive dose technique was the first scheme used, based on the principle of the therapia magna sterilisans–at that time the prevailing concept in antibacterial chemotherapy. The dose given was 1100 roentgens, i.e., 10% above the dose that produces a brisk erythema of the skin. The concept was that a dose slightly higher than the dose needed to kill the epithelium would sterilize all tumors originating from that epithelium. This single dose controlled some skin cancers, but no cures were achieved in deep-seated tumors. Because this treatment was not effective, it was felt[16] that the total dose should be given not in one but in several exposures in order to irradiate the cells in a state of greatest radiosensitivity–mitosis being considered the most sensitive phase of the cell cycle.

In 1918, the first skin experiment[11] showing that a certain physical dose of irradiation has a diminished effectiveness if given in multiple fractions instead of one exposure gave rise to the concept of recovery between fractions. During the 1920s and 1930s many skin experiments were designed to study the recovery factors in skin reactions. The best known studies include one on brisk erythema[15] and another on pigmentation of the skin[12] from which recovery exponents were determined to calculate the doses needed with increasing fractionation to produce the same degree of skin reaction.

Coutard, at the Curie Foundation, began in 1919 to use fractionated irradiation for tumors of the larynx and oropharynx and obtained a significant tumor control rate.[6] He also correlated moist desquamation of the skin and confluent mucositis with tumor control. In 1927 Regaud and Ferroux reported that sterilization of the testicles could be achieved with less skin damage if fractionation was used. These clinical and experimental data formed the basis of the concept of therapeutic ratio, i.e., the ratio of damage between normal tissue and tumor. Because of the effectiveness seen for intracavitary radium therapy in cancer of the uterine cervix and interstitial radium therapy in cancers of the oral cavity, a low dosage rate was thought to improve the therapeutic ratio.

In the latter part of the 1930s and early 1940s, Baclesse designed a technique which, by limiting the weekly dose, avoided both moist desquamation of the skin and confluent mucositis of the oral cavity and oropharynx mucosa. High doses could be given over protracted periods of time. Every field was treated every day, 6 days a week, and some patients received twice-a-day treatment. It was thought that the total dose should be divided into as many fractions as possible to further the sparing of normal tissues. Although acute reactions can be avoided by this method, late complications may develop.[17]

[a]Professor, Division of Radiotherapy,
The University of Texas. M.D. Anderson Hospital and Tumor Institute, Houston, Texas

In 1944, Strandqvist on a scatter diagram of failures and necroses using time and dose as coordinates, produced an isoeffect curve by drawing an exclusion curve above the failures and another one below the necroses. The curve drawn in between indicates isoeffect doses for various treatment times both for control of the cancer and for complications. On log-log coordinates the slope of the line is 0.22. The recovery exponents of Reisner and MacComb and Quimby can be fitted on that slope. Isoeffect lines for erythema, moist desquamation, and necroses parallel the line for tumor control; therefore, there was no advantage from the standpoint of the therapeutic ratio in fractionating treatment.

In the latter part of the 1950s and the early 1960s, Andrews[1] explored the extremes of dose and time. No differences in survival rates were shown between a series of patients treated with 9000–10,000 roentgens in treatment times up to 100 days and series of patients treated more or less conventionally. Seemingly the high tumor doses merely kept up with repopulation. In another series 20 patients with squamous cell carcinoma of the oral cavity, oropharynx, and larynx were treated with one single exposure of 2500 to 2750 roentgens, most of them with 2500 roentgens. Only 4 of the 20 patients had control of the disease at 1 year, and the complications were horrendous. In 1952 Cohen[5] stated that the recovery exponent both for adenocarcinoma of breast and the skin was 0.34. Therefore, there was no advantage to fractionation in the treatment of breast cancer. In two series, massive breast tumors were treated palliatively with a total dose of 2500 roentgens in two exposures with 22 MeV x-rays. The area irradiated included also the axilla and the supraclavicular area. The single-dose equivalent calculated from the Strandqvist formula is 2000 roentgens when treatment was given in 2 consecutive days[2] and 1500 roentgens when given within a week.[7] These doses are far below 3000 roentgens, the single-dose equivalent for necroses.[18] Since all patients treated with high dose fractions who lived long enough developed horrible complications, the advantage of fractionation is clearly indicated.

In 1966,[8] a formula was produced that took into consideration not only the overall treatment time and the total dose but also the number of fractions. This formula and its derivatives, the TDF and the CRE, have been widely used to design isoeffect schemes, principally to save patients' visits.

A popular fractionation scheme has been the split course which, with a rest interval, results in a total treatment time of 9 – 10 weeks instead of 6 – 7 weeks. In some series, a diminished control of T3 and T4 tumors but not of the T1 and T2 tumors has been seen.[13] The rest interval between treatment courses was to allow for further tumor shrinkage and potentially better reoxygenation before the second half of the treatment was given. Seemingly, however, repopulation outweighs the benefit of reoxygenation. Another scheme has been to treat 3 days instead of 5 days a week. In one series of patients with T3 and T4 tumors of the oropharynx, it has been found that 330 rad 3 times a week is less effective than 5 × 200 rad despite the NSD levels being the same.[4]

A more significant reason to manipulate the time factor would be to design irradiation schemes that would improve the therapeutic ratio. The potential advantages of multiple daily fractionation (MDF) are:

1. Small doses per fraction are characterized by preferential sparing of late effects relative to acute effects (including tumor control)[19]; reduced OER (compared with higher doses).
2. When short interfraction intervals (e.g., 3 hours) are used, repair of sublethal injury in hypoxic cells is less complete than in well-oxygenated cells.
3. With hyperfractionation, the frequency of redistribution of radioresistant surviving cells into more radiosensitive phases of the cell cycle is increased.

4. With rapid treatment, rapidly growing tumors are less likely to "escape" control.

Different schemes can be adapted to specific situations. For inflammatory carcinoma of the breast, which is a very fast-growing tumor, better control rates were obtained by using 5100 rad in 4 weeks in 40 fractions (i.e., a weekly dose of 1275 rad), than by using the Baclesse technique, delivering 6000 rad in 8 weeks (i.e., 750 rad per week).[3] The cell kill of 750 rad per week does not outweigh repopulation. For large and rapidly growing neck node(s) and node(s) growing under treatment with 900 to 1000 rad per week, a second treatment of 150 rad given on 2 consecutive days per week, 3 hours after the first treatment, is very effective.[9] Treatment of advanced head and neck tumors with three-times-a-day fractions is being tried by the European Organization for Research on Treatment of Cancer Trial. From the report of Arcangeli in Chapter 31 on the material of the Istituto di Ricerca Scientifica and from a recent personal communication from Horiot (1980) on the results of the cooperative study, the early results seem very promising.

It is of great conceptual importance that the rationale of the multiple daily fractions is based on basic radiobiological parameters and on cell kinetics, showing a close interaction between basic scientific principles and clinical radiotherapy.

REFERENCES

1. Andrews, J.R.: Dose-time relationships in cancer radiotherapy, a clinical radiobiology study of extremes of dose and time. *AJR* **93**:56–74, 1965.
2. Atkins, H.L.: Massive dose technique in radiation therapy in inoperable carcinoma of the breast. *AJR* **91**:80–89, 1964.
3. Barker, J.L., Nelson, A.J., and Montague, E.D.: Inflammatory carcinoma of the breast. *Radiology* **121**:173–176, 1976.
4. Byhardt, R.W., Greenberg, M., and Cox, J.D.: Local control of squamous carcinoma of oral cavity and oropharynx with 3 versus 5 treatment fractions per week. *Int J Radiat Oncol Biol Phys* **2**:415–425, 1977.
5. Cohen, L.: Radiotherapy in breast cancer. I. The dose-time relationship: Theoretical considerations. *Br J Radiol* **25**:636–646, 1952.
6. Coutard, H.: Roentgentherapy of epitheliomas of the tonsillar region, hypopharynx, and larynx from 1920 to 1926. *AJR* **28**:313–331, 1932.
7. Edelman, A.H., Holtz, S., and Powers, W.E.: Rapid radiotherapy for inoperable carcinoma of the breast. Benefits and complications. *AJR* **93**:585–599, 1965.
8. Ellis, F.: The relationship of biological effect on dose-time fractionation factors in radiotherapy. In *Current Topics in Radiation Research* vol. 4, Ebert and Howard, eds. Amsterdam: North-Holland Publishing Co., 1968, pp. 357–397.
9. Fletcher, G.H.: *Textbook of Radiotherapy*, 3rd ed. Philadelphia: Lea & Febiger, 1980, pp. 180–219.
10. Horiot, J.C.: Personal communication, 1980.
11. Krönig, S., and Friedrich, W.: Physikalische und biologische Grundlagen der Strahlentherapie. *Sonderband der Strahlentherapie*, 1918.
12. MacComb, W.S., and Quimby, E.H.: The rate of recovery of human skin from the effects of hard or soft roentgen rays or gamma rays. *Radiology* **27**:196–204, 1936.
13. Parsons, J.T., Bova, F.J., and Million, R.R.: A reevaluation of split course technique for squamous cell carcinoma of the head and neck. *Int J Radiat Oncol Biol Phys* **6**:1645–1652, 1980.
14. Regaud, C., and Ferroux, R.: Discordance des effets de rayons X, d'une part dans la peau, d'autre part dans le testicle, par le fractionment de la dose. *C R Soc Biol* **97**:431–434, 1927.
15. Reisner, A.: Hauterythem und Rontgenstrahlung. *Ergeb Med Strahlenforsch* **6**:1–60, 1933.
16. Schwarz, G.: Heilung teifliegender Karzinome durch Rötgenbestrahlung von der Korperoberflache. *Munch Med Wochenschr* **61**:1733, 1914.
17. Spanos, W.J., Montague, E.D., and Fletcher, G.H.: Late complications of radiation only for advanced breast cancer. *Int J Radiat Oncol Biol Phys* **6**:1473–1476, 1980.
18. Strandqvist, M.: Studien über die kumulative Wirkung der Röntgenstrahlen bei Fraktionierung. *Acta Radiol [Suppl]* **55**:1–300, 1944.
19. Withers, H.R., and Peters, L.J.: Biologic aspects of radiation therapy. In *Textbook of Radiotherapy* 3rd ed. G.H. Fletcher, ed. Philadelphia: Lea & Febiger, 1980, pp. 103–180.

CHAPTER 52

Symposium Summary

Jack F. Fowler, D.Sc., Ph.D., M.Sc., F. Inst. P.[a]

It is clear that clinical trials take 10 years or more to produce a definite answer. Therefore, there are a number of new approaches with a laboratory basis that have simply not been adequately tried yet. There are, in fact, quite a lot of new methods in the pipeline. Briefly, the conclusions to date are:

1. *Hyperbaric oxygen*—a modest gain, except in bladder
2. *Fast neutrons*—a modest gain, except in brain tumors
3. *Radiosensitizers of hypoxic cells*—too early to tell, but with some promising early reports
4. *Multiple doses per day*—too early to tell (split-course therapy has shown no advantage)
5. *Hyperthermia*—too early to tell.

How big an improvement in survival or local control can be counted as a major gain in cancer treatment? In clinical trials of advanced cancer where metastases are already widespread, local control or delay in regrowth of the primary is the best measure of success. An improvement in treatment shows up first in those parameters. Even a 10% gain would be worthwhile, but it would take such a large clinical trial to prove it that more than 10 years would be required.

The "modest" gain for hyperbaric oxygen therapy was an increase of about 20% in local control for the two British trials, Ca cervix and head and neck carcinomas (both signficant) and also for the American RTOG trial, although the latter was not a statistically significant difference (see Chapter 8). A fourth trial, that of Ca cervix at Houston, had shown no difference or even a slightly worse result for HBO, but with 24% (HBO) and 12% (air) lethal complications. There seems to be, on balance, evidence that hypoxic cells do matter in radiotherapy, but the results from radiosensitizers of hypoxic cells should clarify just how important they are.

The neutron results (see Chapter 42) showed a similar increase, from 42 to 61% in local control, and an improvement in survival (from 25 to 41%) with complications similar on both sides (8 and 9%). With only 73 patients (38 + 35) the differences were not significant. The pi meson results (see Chapter 43) do not allow us at this time to say more than that the method is feasible without prohibitive normal-tissue injury. The same was shown for hyperthermia (see Chapter 41) and for nonstandardized fractionation (see Chapters 29 and 31), and a large number of centers are using these methods.

One of the newer laboratory-based modalities is the use of a radioprotective drug, such as WR-2721, which concentrates more in normal tissues than in tumors (see Chapter 39). This drug is only just completing its Phase I (toxicity) clinical trial in the United States.

The impressive results of standard radiotherapy, superbly carried out at Houston, were presented in Chapters 35 and 36. The influence of increasing radiation dose in im-

[a]Gray Laboratory of the Cancer Research Campaign, Mount Vernon Hospital, Northwood, Middlesex, England

proving the elimination of tumors or of regional metastatic nodes was clearly demonstrated. The importance of good physical distributions of dose and a knowledge of where the tumor had spread to was emphasized (see Chapter 9).

The question of how much gain would be achieved if hypoxic, radioresistant cells could be eliminated altogether was dealt with in Chapter 14 which showed that, if reoxygenation is modest, a large gain factor of 1.8 or more in equivalent dose would be achieved. If reoxygenation is large, then 1.0 – 1.3 could be expected for multiple small fractions. It is therefore, important that the presence or absence of hypoxic cells in human tumors should be detected and that ways of measuring the rates of reoxygenation in human tumors should be devised. Dr. Chapman's very recent work provides promise of achieving these aims. He has found that radioactively labelled misonidazole is bound into hypoxic cells by metabolic action at a critical concentration.

It is clear that ways of measuring some parameters in tumors in individual patients, before and during treatment, so that a suitable modality might be chosen or adjusted, are important priorities that are not provided by biopsies and histology (see Chapter 14), although average indications for a group (as in clinical trials) might be obtained. Two important parameters are identified in this volume.

The first is the proportion of hypoxic cells in the tumor—the new method of measurement reported by Dr. Chapman (see Chapter 10) which was received with much interest. The other parameter is the proportion of proliferating P cells (triggered into proliferation from quiescent Q cells in the tumor); there is, as yet, no obvious way of measuring it in patients, except possibly by biopsy and FMF (see Chapters 5 and 9). Another source of radiation resistance was identified as repair of potentially lethal damage. This occurs more in Q cells than in P cells.

In discussion it was pointed out that although every radiation oncology department has medical physics support to provide good radiation dosimetry and beam localization in the tumor volume, our knowledge of the concentration of chemotherapeutic drugs in tumors or in normal tissues is abysmal. No trained scientist would consider that it is adequate for use on patients at this time! No medical oncology groups have employed pharmacologists or biologists to assay these concentrations routinely, as has been done by physicists for radiotherapy.

Some chemotherapeutic drugs can be potentiated by electron-affinic radiosensitizers (see Chapters 11 and 40), and the side-effects of chemotherapy, as well as of radiotherapy, can be diminished by thiol-containing drugs (see Chapter 39). These interactions bring the clinical disciplines of radiation oncology and medical oncology closer together, as they ought to be.

Index